Atlas of Palpation

Springer Nature More Media App

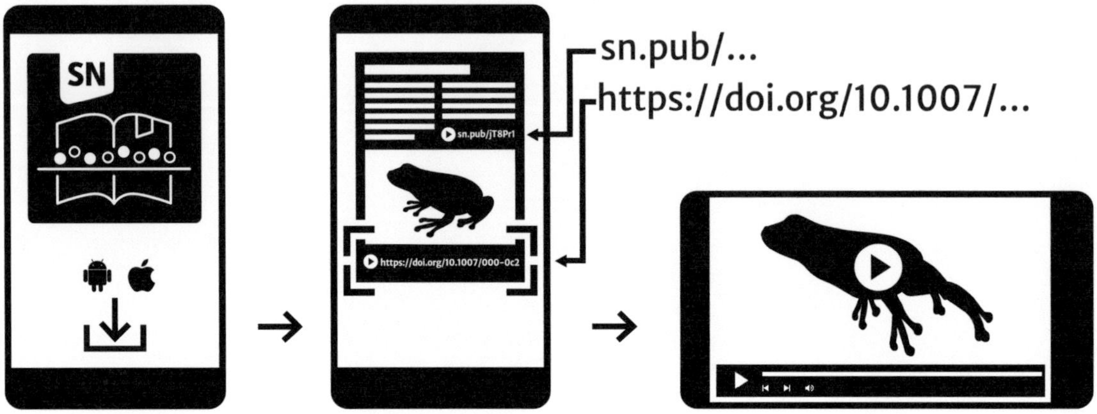

1.
Download

2.
Scan Link

3.
Enjoy Video

Support: customerservice@springernature.com

Robin Bauer • Sandro Wolfram

Atlas of Palpation

Springer

Robin Bauer
BWS-Education GmbH
Thalheim, Germany

Sandro Wolfram
BWS Education GmbH
Bad Elster, Germany

ISBN 978-3-662-69185-4 ISBN 978-3-662-69186-1 (eBook)
https://doi.org/10.1007/978-3-662-69186-1

Translation from the German language edition: "Palpationsatlas" by Robin Bauer and Sandro Wolfram, © Der/die Herausgeber bzw. der/die Autor(en), exklusiv lizenziert an Springer-Verlag GmbH, DE, ein Teil von Springer Nature 2022. Published by Springer Berlin Heidelberg. All Rights Reserved.

This Springer imprint is published by the registered company Springer-Verlag GmbH, DE, part of Springer Nature.
The registered company address is: Heidelberger Platz 3, 14197 Berlin, Germany

Preface

Dear readers,

Probably the most fascinating thing about the therapeutic sector is its multifaceted nature. Palpation is one of the most diverse examination and therapy approaches.

One of the aims of this book is to bring this technique to the fore and to shed light on it in as much detail as possible, without elevating it above the status of other approaches.

As physiotherapists with a scientific mindset, we are passionate about advancing and pioneering digitalisation in the field of therapy. As you are reading these lines at this moment, we are very happy to take you on this exciting journey.

At first glance, this book will seem like an ordinary reference book. On closer inspection, however, you will realise that this book has an interactive and multimedia structure. In addition to contemporary technical texts and pictorial representations, you can expect around 270 videos demonstrating the practical implementation of the palpation techniques. With the corresponding app, you can access these by scanning codes. Ultimately, palpation is carried out more often on people in practice than with reading glasses in the living room armchair.

Another aim is to put you in a position where you can practically apply the knowledge presented. On this path, the book can show you the appropriate approaches and procedures. At least as important, however, is your motivation to want to develop further. Palpation is not a skill that is learned quickly and then remains available. It has to be learned theoretically and constantly refined in practice. The process of training is comparable to a pyramid. The broad basis is your anatomical knowledge. The practice of practical palpation techniques builds on this basis and allows you to mature into an expert over the years and arrive at your individual pyramid peak.

If this kind of knowledge transfer inspires you, we cordially invite you to the Medplattform® (www.medplattform.com) we founded. Via knowledge boxes, a wide variety of medical-therapeutic content is prepared in an evidence-based manner and presented in multimedia form. Due to daily growth, we are getting closer every day to our vision of merging the medical-therapeutic sector with the most innovative technologies of our time.

Now we wish you much joy and the greatest possible success with the book.

Stay curious.

Thalheim, Germany — Robin Bauer
Bad Elster, Germany — Sandro Wolfram

Contents

About the Authors

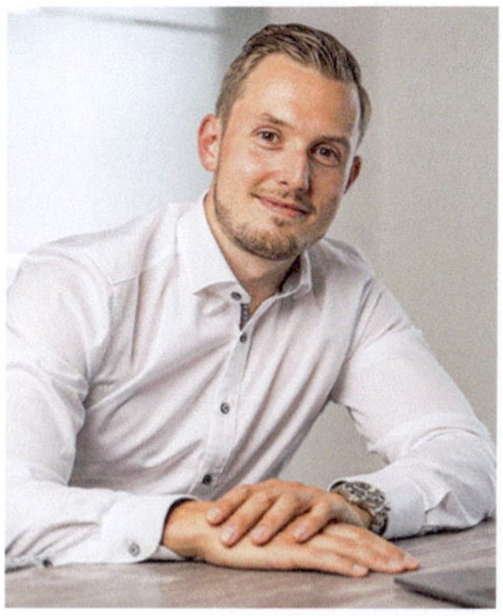

Robin Bauer

- Physiotherapist, B.Sc.
- Manual therapist
- Sports physiotherapist, German Olympic Sports Confederation
- Sectoral alternative practitioner in physiotherapy
- Teacher for medical-therapeutic staff
- Examiner for exams for medical-therapeutic personnel
- Course instructor
- Lecturer for further education
- Shareholder, BWS-Education GmbH
- CEO, BWS-Education GmbH
- Founder and inventor of www.medplattform.com
- Owner of "Sport & Bookshop", Thalheim

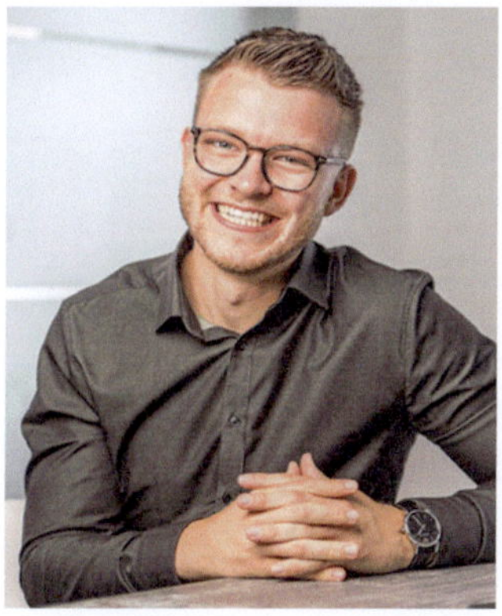

Sandro Wolfram

- Physiotherapist
- Manual therapist
- M.Sc., musculoskeletal physiotherapy
- Sports physiotherapist, German Olympic Sports Confederation
- Teacher for medical-therapeutic staff
- Examiner for exams for medical-therapeutic personnel
- Course instructor
- Lecturer for further education
- Shareholder, BWS-Education GmbH
- CEO, BWS-Education GmbH
- Founder and inventor of www.medplattform.com

Abbreviations

a.	Arterie/artery
art.	Articulatio/joint
C1	Cervical segment 1
dt.	Deutsch/German
engl.	Englisch
L1	Lumbar segment 1
lig.	Ligamentum
m.	Musculus/muscle
MCP	Metacarpophalangeal joint
n./nn.	Nervus/nerve
proc/c.	Processus/processi
rr.	Rami
S.I.A.S.	Spina iliaca anterior superior
S.I.A.I.	Spina iliaca anterior inferior
S.I.P.I.	Spina iliaca posterior inferior
S.I.P.S.	Spina iliaca posterior superior
SIJ	Sacroiliac joint
Th1	Thoracic segment 1
v.	Vene/vein

1 Basics of Palpation

Contents

1.1 Introduction

What cannot be seen with one's own eyes is felt with one's hands. This principle applies to everyone who works on people in the medical-therapeutic sector. No technical device is even close to being able to perform high-quality palpation. This fact shows the elementary importance of the human hand as an indispensable instrument for the adequate diagnosis of the client to be examined. Numerous and very differentiated receptors [1] in the area of the hands make it possible to feel information in a precisely graduated manner and to interpret the findings. Blind people read Braille with their fingers. Similarly, body structures must be read with the hands. An important factor in the interpretation of palpation results is the comparison with empirical values. The clinician's palpation skills are therefore able to improve or become more refined at any given time through the services of neuroplasticity. So here too, as so often, "practice makes perfect".

The absolute basic prerequisite for safe palpation of structures on the human body is a detailed knowledge of anatomy. When we approach the examiner, we should see a precise map in front of our inner eye that includes all structures from the surface to the depth of the tissues. The word "palpation" originally comes from the Latin word "palpare". This term stands for touch or feel with the hands. While performing palpation, the focus should be exclusively on feeling the texture of the respective structures. Try to create an atmosphere during the process in which it is possible to concentrate on the essentials.

Good palpation is comparable to securing evidence at a crime scene after a crime has taken place. The aim is to secure as much evidence as possible in order to be able to put these pieces of the mosaic together to form an overall picture. It is similar in palpation. Here, too, there is a lot of "evidence" just waiting to be discovered and interpreted. Here, too, we speak of the so-called clinical reasoning. It would be suboptimal if clues were lost during our palpation. It is therefore very important to start palpating structures on the surface and then slowly work our way into deeper tissue

Supplementary Information The online version contains supplementary material available at https://doi.org/10.1007/978-3-662-69186-1_1. The videos can be accessed individually by clicking the DOI link in the accompanying figure caption or by scanning this link with the SN More Media App.

R. Bauer, S. Wolfram, *Atlas of Palpation*, https://doi.org/10.1007/978-3-662-69186-1_1

layers. In addition to the careful approach, it is also very important to always test the structures found in a side-by-side comparison. In this way, no traces are blurred. At this point, it is important for us to emphasise that although palpation is an important tool in the diagnostic process, it is only one part of it. Even if we concentrate strongly on one topic in this book, we should never lose sight of holism.

This work serves to enable them to palpate selected structures of the human body in a targeted manner. If palpation is possible, the next step will be the recording and interpretation of information. This will enable you to confirm or reject hypotheses you have made in relation to the clinical picture of the client. Through this continuous thinking process, you will learn the skills to derive an adequate therapy based on precise findings. You can evaluate this through subjective or objective retests and are thus in a position to constantly improve your therapeutic action through recurring self-reflection. Let us now delve deeper into the exciting world of palpation together.

1.2 Palpation of the Skin

As the largest organ of the human body, the skin and its appendages have a number of important functions. In addition to immunological tasks, the enormous variety of information sent by the skin to the central nervous system should be brought to the fore at this point. Thus, this organ with differentiated receptors, which are found in the three layers (epidermis, dermis, subcutis), enables us to absorb a multitude of stimuli from the environment. By absorbing stimuli in the areas of pressure, touch, vibration and temperature, a functioning surface sensitivity is ensured. All layers are interconnected in this process. They are not only connected to each other, but also enter into a close connection with the surrounding tissue via fascial structures.

During palpation, the skin is the tissue with which the examiner is in direct contact. Various information is recorded with the fingertips of the long fingers. It is important to note that each palpation of structures begins on the surface and is then continued in deeper tissue layers. Thus, by lightly brushing the skin with the back of the hand, information about the temperature and perspiration in the area to be examined should first be evaluated. Afterwards, the mobility of the individual skin layers within themselves and in relation to each other is examined. The turgor (state of tension) of the skin plays a central role here. When palpating the cutis, a soft and elastic palpation sensation is expected. Of great relevance for the palpator is the sensation of the client's surface sensitivity. Attention should be paid to hyper- or hyposensitivity symptoms. Furthermore, dermatome areas should be distinguished from areas of the area nervina.

In addition to the classic skin, scars that are initially only visible on the skin can also be palpated deep down. This connective tissue is palpated with the fingertips of the index and/or middle finger. The replacement tissue should be easily movable, smooth and not too firm. Due to the fact that scars are not only superficial, but extend deep into the tissue and are connected there with other structures fascially, they are often felt as a firm structure and can cause restrictions in mobility.

The dimple test enables the clinician to detect protein-rich oedema. A dent is pressed into the tissue with a fingertip in the area to be examined. If this dent remains visible even after the application of pressure has ended, this indicates a protein-rich oedematous process. In addition to the described dent test, the so-called standing skin fold can also be tested. In this way, the skin is pressed together with the thumb and index finger to form a raised fold. If the fold continues to exist even after the compression has ended, i.e. if it does not elastically return to its original state, this indicates that the person being examined is dehydrated. If the mobility between the individual skin layers is restricted, this manifests itself during the skin mobility test in the form of pain and a discordant palpation sensation (Fig. 1.1).

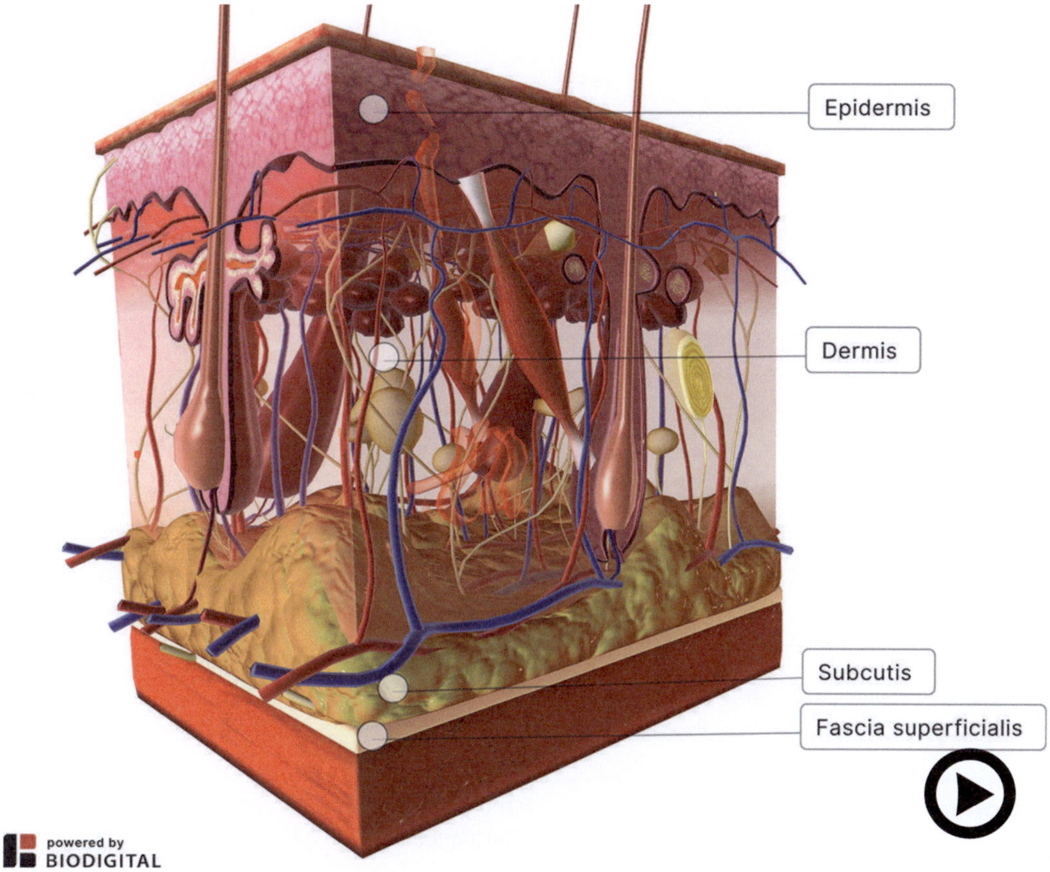

Fig. 1.1 Anatomy and palpation of the skin (▶ https://doi.org/10.1007/000-cp9)

1.3 Palpation of the Bones

In the past, osseous material was often dismissed as merely passive supporting tissue. In the meantime, the enormous relevance of the quite mobile viscoelastic material as a component of the tensegrity model [2], according to which our organism is constructed, has become clear. In addition to protecting organs and participating in movement, this type of tissue can participate in numerous additional functions. These include haemopoiesis [3] or the storage function for calcium and phosphorus [4]. From the outside, the periosteum, as a protective layer [5], envelops the bone tissue. In osseous palpation, the areas of interest are mainly those where a muscle joins the bone via its tendon of origin or attachment in a periosteal-diaphyseal or chondral-apophyseal transition zone. Due to the correspondence with the myofascial system, irritation [6] can often occur in the respective transition zone. These are usually characterised by pain symptoms. Thus, all reference points are of great importance in bony palpation.

Bony tissue feels hard and inelastic on palpation compared to other structures. As mentioned above, pain may occur during palpation, the cause of which is usually irritation of the tendon of origin or attachment or of the periosteum itself. In addition to pressure points, attention is also paid to the condition of the bone. This can be smooth or rough on the surface, as well as showing elevations or depressions. As you go deeper into the tissue, you should pay attention to these conditions. Depending on the region of the body, bones are palpated on the surface as well as in depth using the flatly placed or steeply placed long-fingered fingertips. Some areas, especially those of the small bones, are often palpated in tweezers or even forceps grip.

If a fracture is suspected, this hypothesis can be confirmed or weakened with the so-called percussion test [7]. The clinician taps the area where a possible fracture is suspected. If, after percussion, there is a slowly increasing painful sensation that is described as bright and intense and persists for a period of 20–30 s, the likelihood of a fracture or fissure is very high. However, similar symptoms can also be observed in tumorous processes. Depending on the fracture line, this may be palpated in combination with crepitation. In the presence of these examination findings, closer medical clarification in terms of imaging procedures is strongly recommended (Fig. 1.2).

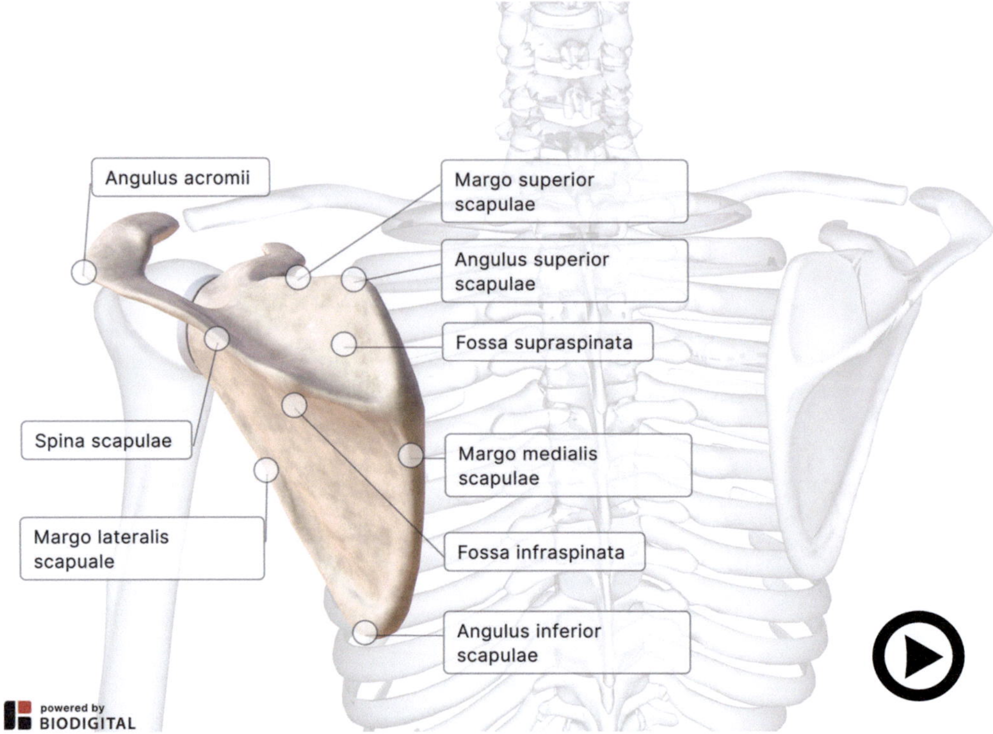

Fig. 1.2 Anatomy and palpation of the bones (▶ https://doi.org/10.1007/000-cp7)

1.4 Palpation of the Joints

Joints are formed whenever two bones meet and articulate with each other. The construction of the joint partners differs depending on the type of joint. Movements should be harmonious and painless so that they can be used for activities of daily living. When examining the clients, the joints must also be palpated. The joint space as well as the joint capsule and the ligaments are palpated.

1.4.1 Palpation of the Joint Space

The exploration begins with the palpation of the joint space. This can best be found with simultaneous movement of the joint partners. While the joint space is palpated with simultaneous mobilisation of the corresponding joint, the clinker concentrates on any conspicuous features that deviate from a harmonious movement of the joint partners in relation to each other. Small joints, such as those in the carpus or tarsus, are grasped with tweezers by holding one joint partner in place with the index and middle fingers. For larger joints, a suitable grip technique must be used in order to be able to perform palpation. Joints that are mobilised by the influence of the myofascial system enable our organism to move. Therefore, all periarticular structures should be included in the palpation findings. These include myofascial, ligamentous, capsular and, of course, osseous structures that have an influence (Fig. 1.3).

1.4.2 Palpation of the Joint Capsule

With three-dimensional fibrous tracts [8], joint capsules surround almost every joint in the human body. They consist of an outer membrana (stratum) fibrosa and an inner membrana (stratum) synoviale. While the membrana fibrosa, due to its more stable structure, tends to fulfil a movement-limiting requirement, the membrana synovialis, with its synovial villi, participates in the joint metabolism in a friction-reducing and nourishing way through the production of thixotropic synovia (synovial fluid) [9]. Mechanoceptors, which are located together with nociceptors in the joint capsule, form the relation to the proprioceptive system [10].

Depending on the position of the joint, palpation of the capsular structure is more or less possible. Due to the deep position of the joint-enveloping capsule, it is difficult to describe a specific palpation sensation. In terms of palpation, a possible pressure dolence in depth is the most important diagnostic criterion. Joint capsules are most likely to be palpable when they are irritated or inflamed, as they carry more fluid at this stage [11] and can thus be felt in depth as a kind of taut balloon with the flat fingertips. High attention should be paid to the structures that are fused with the joint capsule.

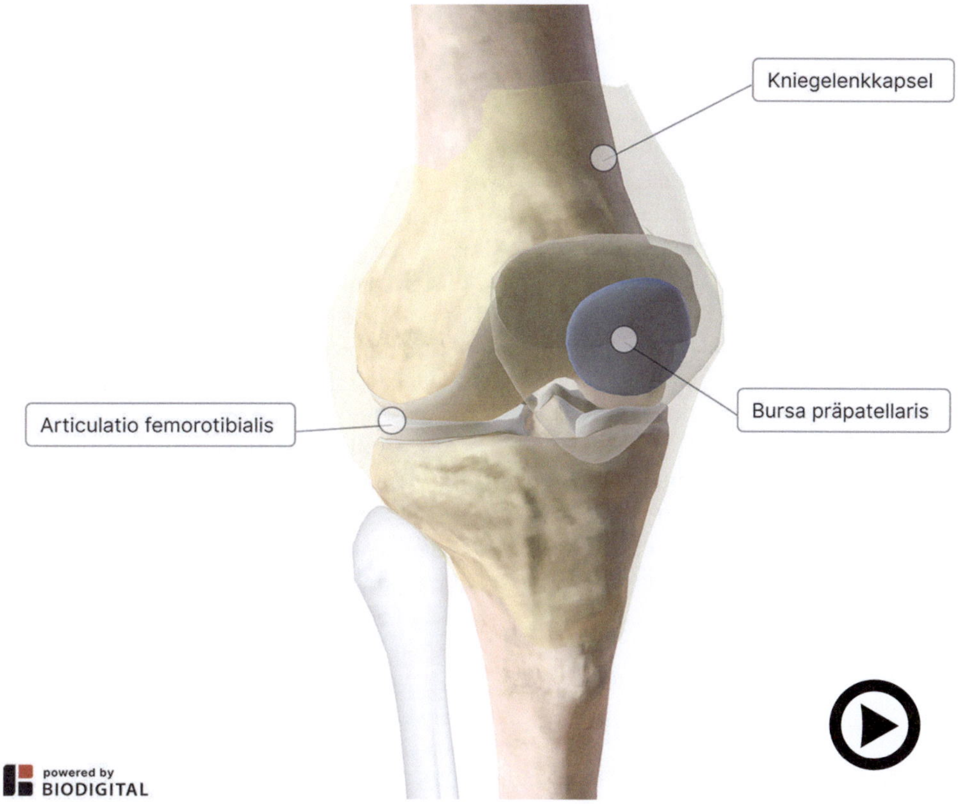

Fig. 1.3 Anatomy and palpation of the joints (▶ https://doi.org/10.1007/000-cp8)

Thus, in addition to muscular influences that are able to adapt the tension of the capsule to the current requirements, there are also ligaments that are anchored in the layers of the structure surrounding the joint.

In the course of certain diseases, structural changes of the capsule can occur. The three-dimensional tissue shrinks and increasingly restricts the mobility of the joint in certain directions [12]. The development of movement restrictions in a specific sequence strengthens the hypothesis of capsular symptoms (Fig. 1.3).

1.4.3 Palpation of the Bursae

Bursae form natural sliding bearings that minimise friction between different structures [13]. They are thus considered to have an economising and harmonising function during movement. In the structure of bursae, the outer membrana fibrosa can be distinguished from the inner membrana synovialis. While the outer layer with its firmer attachment provides sufficient stability, the inner layer is responsible for the production of synovial fluid. The synovial fluid in the tissue sac enables the bursa to adapt to the forces acting on it in a buffering and finely graduated manner.

Due to the similar structure and the usually deep location, bursae are comparable to joint capsules. The palpation of bursae is therefore rather difficult. A classic palpation sensation can therefore not be given, which makes the identification of a possible pressure dolence in the area of a bursa all the more important. If a bursa is overstimulated, inflammatory changes often occur. Palpable bursae then usually appear doughy, and the palpation sensation during palpation is comparable to the kneading of a snowball (Fig. 1.3).

1.5 Palpation of the Ligaments

The main task of our ligamentary system is to limit movements together with the joint capsule. In order to fulfil this function, they consist of tight collagenous connective tissue [14]. Through a mechanoceptive and also nociceptive receptor supply [15], ligaments can communicate with the central nervous system via targeted afferents. This enables our body to process the proprioceptive messages and to close the so-called sensorimotor circuit via the reaction of the motor system. The places where a ligament corresponds with bone tissue, capsule or muscle tissue are of great anatomical importance [16]. The ligamentary tension can also be changed by these external influences.

The sensation during palpation of ligamenta is reminiscent of that of tendons. The clinician therefore tends to look for firm as well as sharply defined tissues. Again, anatomical knowledge of the location of the individual ligaments is essential to differentiate them from surrounding structures. Superficial ligaments can be grasped with tweezers or forceps. Direct palpation via the fingertips involves palpating the structure across the fibres. Deep ligaments are best felt with the index or middle finger. In addition, the joint can be moved during palpation to tighten the ligaments and make them more palpable.

If ligaments are palpable, the tonus situation and also any existing pressure dolences can be evaluated in a lateral comparison. If a nociceptive impulse, triggered by pressure on ligamentous structures, is cortically conscious, it is usually felt as local pain.

When the capsuloligamentous system is injured, our body often tries to compensate for the deficit by over-programming structures that are not affected [17]. On palpation, these abnormalities can be observed in addition to directly locally developed negative changes (Fig. 1.4).

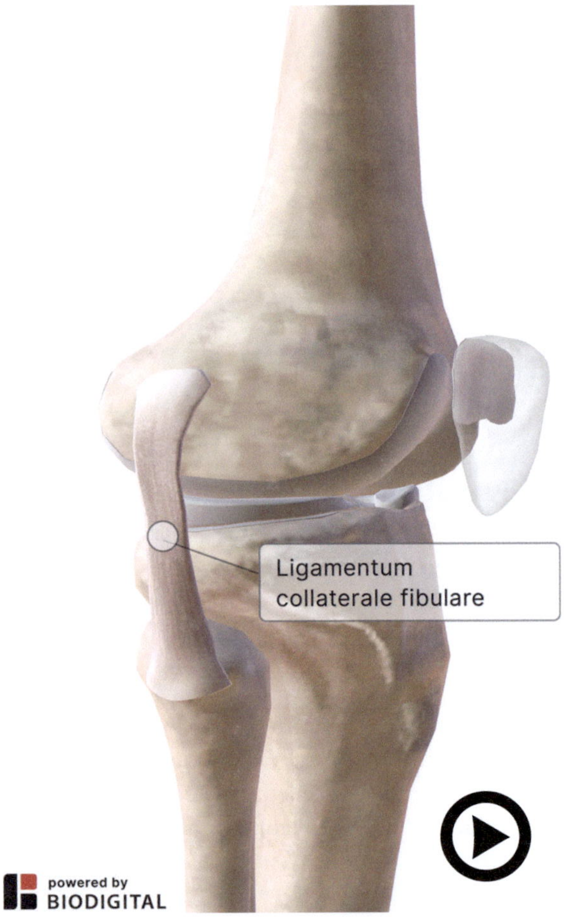

Fig. 1.4 Anatomy and palpation of the ligaments (▶ https://doi.org/10.1007/000-cp6)

1.6 Palpation of the Musculature

The tendons of origin and attachment, together with the muscle belly, are the contractile elements and thus the motors of our musculoskeletal system. Depending on the point of view, the origin is defined as the proximal part or the punctum fixum. The distal part or the punctum mobile is accordingly regarded as the base. This is also referred to as the myofascial system. This describes the direct connection between muscle and connective tissue. The collagenous connective tissue embeds all structures that are relevant for the supply and disposal of the corresponding muscle. Vascular, lymphatic and also nervous structures run mainly in the fascial tissue [18]. Both types of tissue are therefore inextricably intertwined and mutually dependent. In addition, the connective tissue has a supply of nociceptors [19]. The receptors of the musculature are represented by the muscle spindles and the tendon spindles. Here, the muscle spindle takes on the task of a length control system, whereas the tendon spindle is responsible for measuring the current tension situation [20, 21]. Muscle tone is formed from this constant discrepancy between the two systems and the resulting competitive situation. As already described, almost every muscle corresponds with the skeletal system via its tendon of origin or attachment.

Due to the high fluid content in the muscular tissue [22], it presents a soft and elastic resistance to palpation. When palpating, it is advisable to first palpate the muscle in an approximate starting position. The easiest way to feel this tissue is to palpate it across its course and to tense it into its function during palpation. Superficial muscles are palpated with the palm of the hand but also with the long finger berries. In the case of deep-lying contractile structures, the overlying muscles must first be pushed to the side before palpation into the depths is carried out with the long fingers or thumb placed rather steeply. Narrow muscles can best be grasped with the tweezer grip. A tendon appears firmer than muscle tissue but softer than bone tissue when palpated. Superficial tendons can be grasped very well with the pollex (thumb) and index finger, while deep tendons are best felt with the radial side of the index (index finger).

The clinician focuses on factors such as muscle tone and the possible presence of pressure dolence. Pain symptoms arising from the myofascial system can be either local or referred pain. The examiner should be able to correctly interpret the knowledge of sufficiently observed and known areas of radiation of pain or other referred symptoms on palpation of muscles. There are various explanatory models and theories about the mechanisms of origin and the differences between transmitted and local pain [23]. At this point, however, it is not the pathophysiology that leads to the development of a myofascial dysfunction that is decisive, but rather the clinical picture that is displayed.

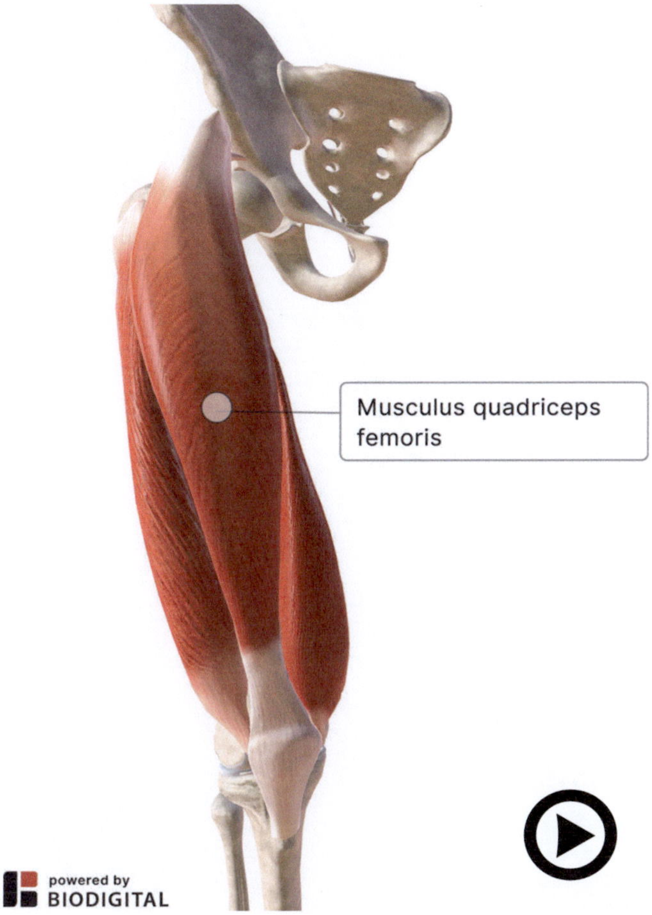

Fig. 1.5 Anatomy and palpation of the musculature (▶ https://doi.org/10.1007/000-cpa)

If post-traumatic haemorrhage is suspected as a result of an injury to the vascular system, this can often be recognised in the palpation findings with the so-called "mushy sign". The examiner feels a non-physiological fluid cushion under his fingers in the symptomatic area. This is due to the haematoma that has developed. After muscle fibre or muscle bundle ruptures, a dent can often be felt in the muscle belly. In the case of tendon ruptures, the muscle belly is also displaced distally, e.g. in the case of a rupture of the original tendon of the biceps brachii muscle. These points show the enormous tension that the uninjured muscle tissue is under (Fig. 1.5).

1.7 Palpation of the Nerves

The peripheral nervous system plays a fundamental role in the exchange of information between the central nervous system and the structures of our body. Every afferent or efferent is received and then transmitted via sensory, motor or vegetative nerve fibres [24]. Without this transmission of electrical impulses, no processes would take place in the human body. Enveloped in fatty and connective tissue, data is specifically transported in the nerve fibres from the site of origin of the stimulus to the target site via the flow of axoplasm [25]. If axoplasm flows optimally in a nerve, a physiological conduction velocity is achieved [26]. It is thus highly relevant that a peripheral nerve has sufficient mobility to its surrounding tissue.

Due to their course, some peripheral nerves can be palpated at certain positions. The sensation of palpation is comparable to the bite of spaghetti or the side of a guitar. Depending on their position, palpable nerves are first differentiated from the surrounding tissue with the long-fingered berries transversely to their course. Palpation with the index or middle finger is recommended for this. The special regions where nerves are easily palpable require precise anatomical knowledge and are described in detail in the chapter on nerve palpation. When palpating, proceed gently at first, as nerves can also react symptomatically with paraesthesia, numbness or pain due to the pressure [27]. The reason for this is the reduction in axoplasmic flow when this structure is compressed.

Compared to muscles, nerves are more solidly constructed. In the region of the nerve, however, the structures that have a close positional relationship to the neural structure under examination should also be included in the palpation. Precise anatomical knowledge of natural entrapments in the course of the nerve therefore contributes enormously to a sufficient examination procedure. During the side-by-side assessment, the clinician should look for differences in the irritability or sensitivity of the neural structure. Among other things, it is important to register symptoms in the area of hypersensitivity and hyposensitivity. Disorders that manifest themselves in the area of hypersensitivity initially indicate a mild irritation, whereas hyposensitivities indicate a more severe symptomatology that is due to a lack of axon plasma flow. Pain symptoms can be expressed locally but also projected along the course of the nerve. In terms of the innervation areas of the skin, the dermatome area should be distinguished from the area nervina. Here, the dermatome area represents the sensitive catchment area of a spinal nerve into the skin, whereas the area nervina characterises the sensitive catchment area of a peripheral nerve into the skin [28]. This distinction allows conclusions to be drawn about the symptom-triggering structure (Fig. 1.6).

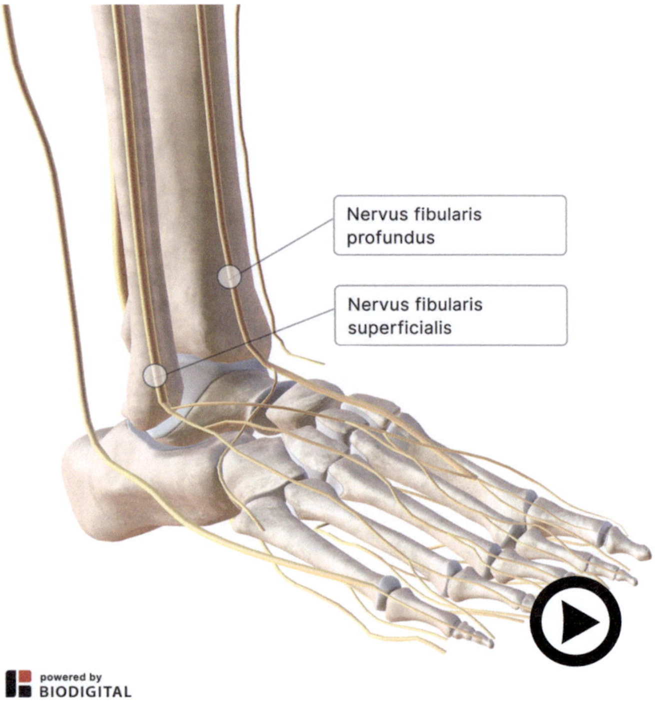

Fig. 1.6 Anatomy and palpation of the nerves (▶ https://doi.org/10.1007/000-cpb)

1.8 Palpation of the Vessels

To ensure a functioning metabolism, the fluids circulating in our vascular system are indispensable. The arterial system plays a decisive role in supplying the corresponding target cells. The resulting disposal is realised by the venous as well as additionally by the lymphatic system. Larger and multilayered vessels take on a transport function, while the areas of actual material exchange are found in the smaller capillary structures [29]. The flow of blood and lymph must therefore necessarily be possible for unrestricted function.

Arteries carry blood, oxygen-rich in the systemic circulation and oxygen-poor in the pulmonary circulation, away from the heart. They have three walls, and the innermost layer, which is in direct contact with the blood, is called the tunica intima. This smooth squamous epithelium is followed by the tunica media as the middle muscular layer. The outermost layer is called the tunica externa or adventitia, which consists of tight connective tissue. There are arteries that have a thin muscular layer; these tend to be located close to the heart. In the periphery, these vessels have a thicker muscular layer to ensure optimal blood flow. In some areas of the human body, we are able to palpate components of our vascular systems. When palpating larger arterial vessels, it is possible to feel a rhythmically pulsating pressure wave. The structure of the arteries is rounded and firmer than that of venous structures due to a more pronounced muscular layer. Blood vessels generally evoke a softer palpation sensation than, for example, nervous structures. Arteries can be displaced towards the surrounding tissue. For palpation, the index or middle finger is chosen to first feel the pulse wave superficially. Slow and attentive palpation can then be done in depth if no pulse is felt. The vascular roads of the body have to pass through many constrictions in their course, similar to nerves. The clinker should therefore be aware of the structures that have a direct influence on the vascular system.

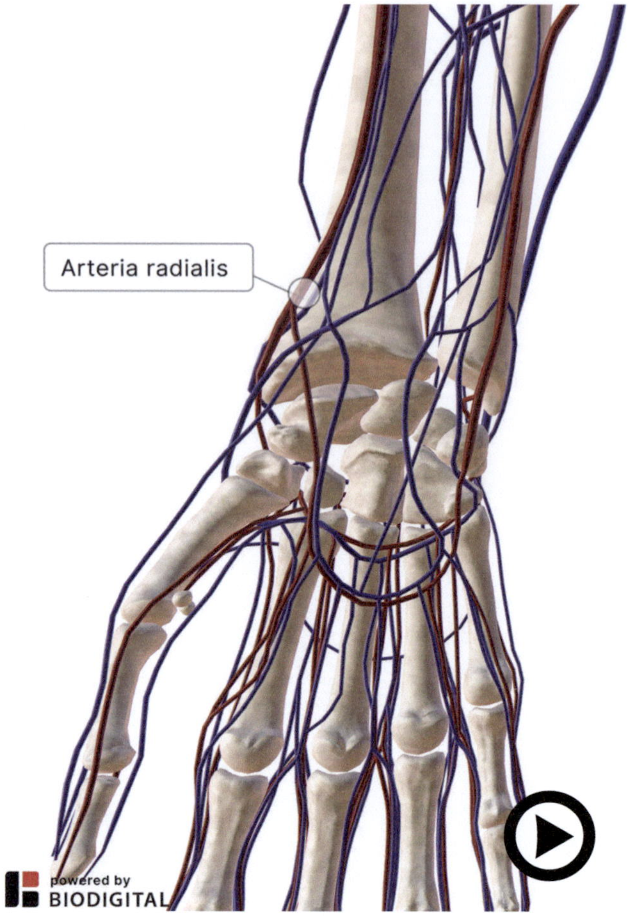

Fig. 1.7 Anatomy and palpation of the vessels (▶ https://doi.org/10.1007/000-cpc)

Veins transport blood, oxygen-poor blood in the systemic circulation and oxygen-rich blood in the pulmonary circulation, to the heart. They have a three-walled structure just like the arteries, with the difference that the muscle layer is not as pronounced. Veins have valves in them that prevent the blood from flowing back. When these vessels are palpated, superficial veins can often be perceived through the eyes as bluish, roundish and elongated structures. The respective vessel is then palpated directly with the index or middle fingertip. This reveals a roundish shape that is soft and elastic. The softer palpation sensation is due to the thinner muscle layer. No pulse can be felt, but venous vessels can be easily displaced to the surrounding tissue. Superficial compression of this network of veins results in congestion of blood, which may be partially reflected in a livid colouration of this region (Fig. 1.7).

References

1. Johnson, K. (2001, August). The roles and functions of cutaneous mechanoreceptors. *Current Opinion in Neurobiology, 11*(4), 455–461. https://doi.org/10.1016/s0959-4388(00)00234-8
2. Wendling, S., Canadas, P., Oddou, C., & Meunier, A. (2002, February). Interrelations between elastic energy and strain in a tensegrity model: Contribution to the analysis of the mechanical response in living cells. *Computer Methods in Biomechanics and Biomedical Engineering, 5*(1), 1–6. https://doi.org/10.1080/10255840290032162
3. Groarke, E., & Young, N. (2019, August). Aging and hematopoiesis. *Clinics in Geriatric Medicine, 35*(3), 285–293. https://doi.org/10.1016/j.cger.2019.03.001
4. Nordin, B. (1997, July–August). Calcium and osteoporosis. *Nutrition, 13*(7–8), 664–686. https://doi.org/10.1016/s0899-9007(97)83011-0
5. Bisseret, D., Kaci, R., Lafage-Proust, M.-H., Alison, M., Parlier-Cuau, C., Laredo, J.-D., & Bousson, V. (2015, March). Periosteum: Characteristic imaging findings with emphasis on radiologic-pathologic comparisons. *Skeletal Radiology, 44*(3), 321–338. https://doi.org/10.1007/s00256-014-1976-5
6. Moen, M., Tol, J., Weir, A., Steunebrink, M., & De Winter, T. (2009). Medial tibial stress syndrome: A critical review. *Sports Medicine, 39*(7), 523–546. https://doi.org/10.2165/00007256-200939070-00002
7. Roberts, P. (1979, June). The axial percussion test for fracture. *Canadian Family Physician, 25*, 749–751.
8. Iwanaga, T., Shikichi, M., Kitamura, H., Yanase, H., & Nozawa-Inoue, K. (2000, March). Morphology and functional roles of synoviocytes in the joint. *Archives of Histology and Cytology, 63*(1), 17–31. https://doi.org/10.1679/aohc.63.17
9. Hlavácek, M. (2001). The thixotropic effect of the synovial fluid in squeeze-film lubrication of the human hip joint. *Biorheology, 38*(4), 319–334.
10. Witherspoon, J., Smirnova, I., & McIff, T. (2014, September). Neuroanatomical distribution of mechanoreceptors in the human cadaveric shoulder capsule and labrum. *Journal of Anatomy, 225*(3), 337–345. https://doi.org/10.1111/joa.12215
11. Awerbuch, M. (2008, January 7). The clinical utility of ultrasonography for rotator cuff disease, shoulder impingement syndrome and subacromial bursitis. *The Medical Journal of Australia, 188*(1), 50–53. https://doi.org/10.5694/j.1326-5377.2008.tb01507.x
12. Gagey, O., & Boisrenoult, P. (2004, February). Shoulder capsule shrinkage and consequences on shoulder movements. *Clinical Orthopaedics and Related Research, 419*, 218–222. https://doi.org/10.1097/00003086-200402000-00036
13. Ruangchaijatuporn, T., Gaetke-Udager, K., Jacobson, J., Yablon, C., & Morag, Y. (2017, April). Ultrasound evaluation of bursae: Anatomy and pathological appearances. *Skeletal Radiology, 46*(4), 445–462. https://doi.org/10.1007/s00256-017-2577-x
14. Mienaltowski, M., & Birk, D. (2014). Structure, physiology, and biochemistry of collagens. *Advances in Experimental Medicine and Biology, 802*, 5–29. https://doi.org/10.1007/978-94-007-7893-1_2
15. Ikeuchi, M., Wang, Q., Izumi, M., & Tani, T. (2012, June). Nociceptive sensory innervation of the posterior cruciate ligament in osteoarthritic knees. *Archives of Orthopaedic and Trauma Surgery, 132*(6), 891–895. https://doi.org/10.1007/s00402-012-1478-7
16. Jadhav, S., More, S., Riascos, R., Lemos, D., & Swischuk, L. (2014, March–April). Comprehensive review of the anatomy, function, and imaging of the popliteus and associated pathologic conditions. *Radiographics, 34*(2), 496–513. https://doi.org/10.1148/rg.342125082
17. Shanbehzadeh, S., Bandpei, M., & Ehsani, F. (2017, May). Knee muscle activity during gait in patients with anterior cruciate ligament injury: A systematic review of electromyographic studies. *Knee Surgery, Sports Traumatology, Arthroscopy, 25*(5), 1432–1442. https://doi.org/10.1007/s00167-015-3925-9
18. Stecco, A., Stern, R., Fantoni, I., De Caro, R., & Stecco, C. (2016, February). Fascial disorders: Implications for treatment. *PM & R, 8*(2), 161–168. https://doi.org/10.1016/j.pmrj.2015.06.006
19. Tesarz, J., Hoheisel, U., Wiedenhöfer, B., & Mense, S. (2011, October 27). Sensory innervation of the thoracolumbar fascia in rats and humans. Neuroscience, 194, 302–308.
20. Kistemaker, D., Knoek Van Soest, A., Wong, J., Kurtzer, I., & Gribble, P. (2013, February). Control of position and movement is simplified by combined muscle spindle and Golgi tendon organ feedback. *Journal of Neurophysiology, 109*(4), 1126–1139. https://doi.org/10.1152/jn.00751.2012
21. Macefield, V., & Knellwolf, T. (2018, August 1). Functional properties of human muscle spindles. *Journal of Neurophysiology, 120*(2), 452–467. https://doi.org/10.1152/jn.00071.2018
22. Lorenzo, I., Serra-Prat, M., & Yébenes, J. (2019, August 9). The role of water homeostasis in muscle function and frailty: A review. *Nutrients, 11*(8), 1857. https://doi.org/10.3390/nu11081857
23. Masuda, M., Lida, T., Exposto, F., Baad-Hansen, L., Kawara, M., Komiyama, O., & Svensson, P. (2018, March 21). Referred pain and sensations evoked by standardized palpation of the masseter muscle in healthy participants. *Journal of Oral & Facial Pain and Headache, 32*(2), 159–166. https://doi.org/10.11607/ofph.2019
24. Garcia, M., & Stippich, C. (2013, July). Functional neuroanatomy: Sensorimotor system. *Der Radiologe, 53*(7), 584–591. https://doi.org/10.1007/s00117-013-2483-8
25. Moro, F., Alberghina, M., & Amantia, L. (1983, January). Axoplasmatic transport. The optic nerve and the retina. *Klinische Monatsblätter für Augenheilkunde, 182*(1), 2–6. https://doi.org/10.1055/s-2008-1054696
26. Podnar, S., Omejec, G., & Bodor, M. (2017, December). Nerve conduction velocity and cross-sectional area in ulnar neuropathy at the elbow. *Muscle & Nerve, 56*(6), E65–E72. https://doi.org/10.1002/mus.25655
27. Spies, C., Müller, L., Oppermann, J., Neiss, W., Hahn, P., & Unglaub, F. (2016, April). Surgical decompression of the superficial radial nerve: Wartenberg syndrome. *Operative Orthopädie und Traumatologie, 28*(2), 145–152. https://doi.org/10.1007/s00064-015-0431-7
28. Kachlik, D., Musil, V., & Baca, V. (2017, April). Contribution to the anatomical nomenclature concerning upper limb anatomy. *Surgical and Radiologic Anatomy, 39*(4), 405–417. https://doi.org/10.1007/s00276-016-1749-z
29. Haber, S., Clark, A., & Tawhai, M. (2013, October 1). Blood flow in capillaries of the human lung. *Journal of Biomechanical Engineering, 135*(10), 101006–101011. https://doi.org/10.1115/1.4025092

Palpation of Bony Reference Points

2

Contents

Supplementary Information The online version contains supplementary material available at https://doi.org/10.1007/978-3-662-69186-1_2. The videos can be accessed individually by clicking the DOI link in the accompanying figure caption or by scanning this link with the SN More Media App.

R. Bauer, S. Wolfram, *Atlas of Palpation*, https://doi.org/10.1007/978-3-662-69186-1_2

2.1 Basics of Bony Palpation

The passive supporting apparatus gives people support and stability. Furthermore, bones provide sufficient surface for muscle attachments as well as origins and thus form the basis of our active movement system. In palpation of the bones, the tweezer grip with the index and middle finger is used for smaller bones. Larger bones and special bone points are palpated with the fingertips of the long fingers two and three. Here, palpation is done slowly from the surface into the depth, and a hard structure is expected that cannot be moved in itself. Before the bone can be felt, contact must first be made with the skin. To be able to feel osseous material afterwards, it is often necessary to palpate through other tissues, such as musculature or connective tissue. It is important to proceed carefully to recognise the different types of tissue. Once on the bone, there is direct contact with the periosteum, the periosteum that covers almost the entire bone. This so-called magic tissue is full of receptors and can therefore react symptomatically with nociceptive action potentials. Recorded information should be carefully analysed and interpreted by the clinician.

In the following chapters, various bones are presented with their palpable reference points. We will start with the pelvis and then carry out bony palpation on the lower extremity, thorax, upper extremity and head.

2.2 Palpation of Bony Reference Points on the Pelvis

The pelvis forms a bony structure which is biomechanically constructed in such a way that two decisive forces meet exactly here. The weight of the upper body meets the ground reaction force, which is directed cranially via the legs [1]. Thus, the pelvis is the fulcrum of the balance of forces. It is therefore used by numerous ligaments and muscles as the point of origin or attachment. The most important bony reference points are developed by palpation in the following text and presented as instructions in the accompanying instructional video. All reference points are palpated with the fingertips. A comfortable starting position in the supine or prone position is chosen for the palpation journey.

The palpation journey on the pelvis starts at the crista iliaca, which is felt via the fingertips on the contralateral side. A direct bony ridge is felt on the side of the abdomen, approximately at the level of the navel. If the finger berries move medially, they fall into the iliac fossa. This fossa is palpable over almost the entire course of the crista iliaca. If the finger berries move ventrally from the crista iliaca, they meet the spina iliaca anterior superior (SIAS) directly. Below the SIAS is the spina iliaca anterior inferior (SIAI). If the palpation continues in the direction of the middle of the body along the pecten ossis pubis, the ramus superior ossis pubis is connected, which ends at the symphysis via a small hump, the tuberculum pubicum. This cartilage forms the mobile connection between the two ossa coxae and is thus also an important point in the balance of forces between the right and left sides of the pelvis. Distally, the ramus inferior ossis pubis follows the symphysis and ends dorsally in the tuber ischiadicum. This structure can be palpated very well in depth on the buttocks. The ischial tuberosity is an important site for the origo of the ischiocrural muscles. Cranial to the tuber ischiadicum, there is a small bony point in depth, the spina ischiadica, which can best be palpated over the ligamentum sacrospinale. The next palpation point is the spina iliaca posterior inferior (SIPI), which can be palpated via the fingertips rather superficially cranial to the spina ischiadica. Directly above the SIPI is the spina iliaca posterior superior (SIPS), which is also easily palpable superficially. Medial to these tips is the os sacrum, which is connected to the os ilium via the sacroiliac joint (SIJ). This "sacred bone" is palpated in more detail in the chapter on spinal column. The SIPS passes directly into the iliac crest. Lateral to the crista iliaca is the ala ossis ilii with the facies glutea. This is palpated with the long finger berries.

Implementation Note

The following points may be more symptomatic during palpation. Therefore, proceed with particular caution.

- SIAS/SIAI
  - Muscle origin: m. sartorius (SIAS), m. rectus femoris (SIAI)
- Ramus superior/inferior ossis pubis/tuberculum pubicum
  - Muscle origin: Mm. adductores
- Spina ischiadica
  - Anatomical proximity to the piriformis muscle and the sciatic nerve (Figs. 2.1 and 2.2)

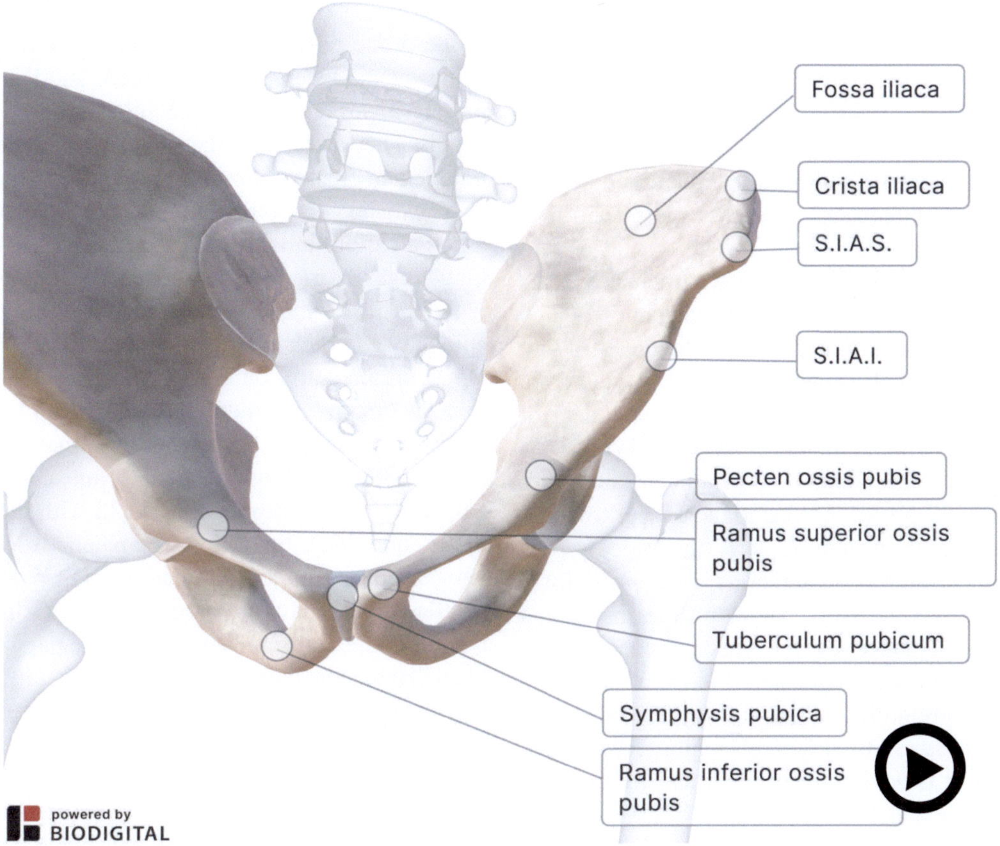

Fig. 2.1 Anatomy and palpation of the pelvis (▶ https://doi.org/10.1007/000-cqj)

Fig. 2.2 Anatomy and palpation of the pelvis

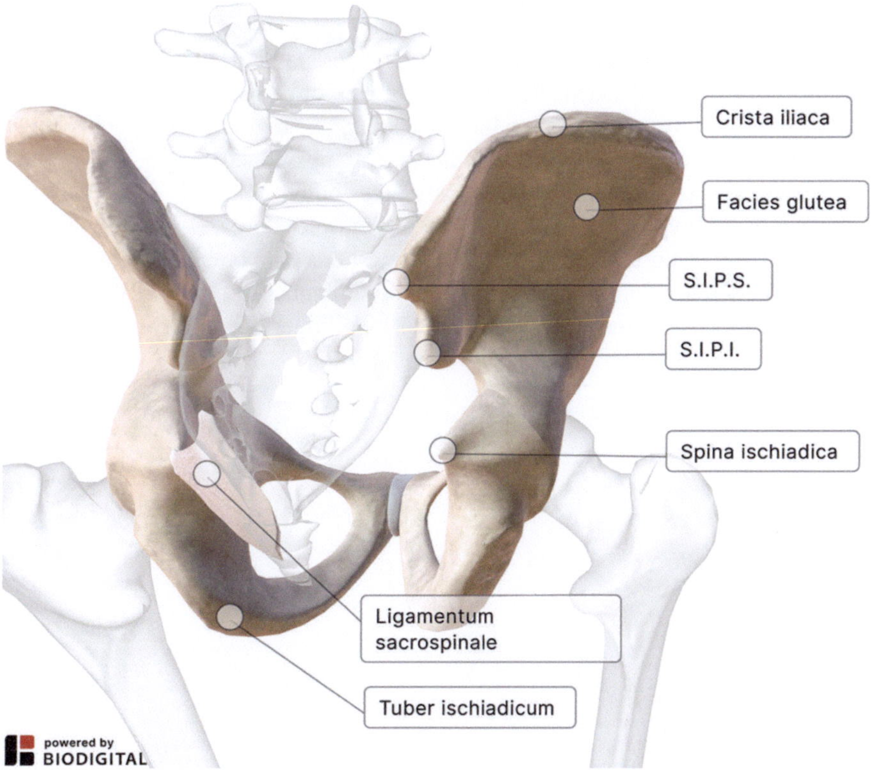

2.3 Palpation of Bony Reference Points on the Femur

The longest tubular bone of the human body ensures that the ground reaction forces can be transferred well into the pelvis [1]. The following reference points can be identified on this bone by palpation. For palpation, the client is placed in a supine or prone position.

Proximolateral to the thigh is the greater trochanter. This prominent protrusion is the starting point for palpation, which is first performed from the supine position. The fingertips are located on the outside of the thigh at about the level of the symphysis. In combination with a rotational component of the hip joint, the large rolling mound is palpated. With internal rotation, this point becomes more prominent, and with external rotation, it disappears. Medial to the greater trochanter, at the transition to the collum femoris, the finger berries travel over the linea intertrochanterica as well as the fossa trochanterica. Opposite the large bump, on the inside and slightly distal, is its counterpart, the lesser trochanter. The best way to palpate the lesser trochanter is from the lateral position. In this position, the patient lies on the side to be palpated. As numerous soft tissues in this region make palpation very difficult, it is advisable for the client to tense the lower leg in abduction and flexion. By means of the tension in abduction, a reciprocal inhibition of the adductors of the hip joint is achieved, which leads to a reduction in tension. The flexion component causes an increase in tension in the psoas major muscle, which leads to the trochanter minor in the insertion area. Here, the steeply positioned finger berries follow the muscle up to the insertion and, after relaxation, move deeper onto the bony prominence. The posterior crista intertrochanterica, which connects the two humps, cannot be palpated directly. Only a stimulus can be produced in this region from the lateral or supine position via the steeply positioned long finger berries. Proximally, hardly any other bony reference points can be palpated because numerous muscles cover the bone. Posterior to the shaft, the linea aspera can be detected in depth via the corpus femoris, longitudinally as a rough elevation, with the steeply positioned long finger berries by means of stimulation. For this purpose, the patient is in the prone position, and the fingertips move between the bellies of the biceps femoris muscle and the semitendinosus muscle approximately in the middle of the thigh into the depths. They directly hit the caput breve of the biceps femoris muscle and create a stimulus on the linea aspera.

The distal part of the femur is palpated in the supine position. Palpation starts from the lateral side via the flatly placed long finger berries. An elevation can be perceived in this region. This prominent reference point is the lateral femoral epicondyle, which is located on the lateral femoral condyle. Opposite, medially on the femur, the epicondylus medialis femoris or condylus medialis femoris can be palpated using the same technique. Somewhat proximal to the medial epicondyle, the tuberculum adductorium can be accessed by palpating a small elevation in depth with the steeply placed index and middle fingertips. The patella is located anteriorly between the femoral condyles. During palpation, the apex patellae distally and the base patellae proximally, as well as the margo medialis and lateralis of the patella, can be developed. Here, the palpation technique using the long finger berries of the index and middle finger is used again.

Implementation Note

The following points can be more symptomatic during palpation. Therefore, proceed with particular caution here.

- Greater trochanter
  - Insertion site: m. gluteus medius and minimus and m. piriformis
  - Anatomical proximity to the trochanteric bursa
- Lesser trochanter
  - Insertion site: m. psoas major and m. iliacus
  - Anatomical proximity to the adductor muscles, especially the adductor magnus and minimus muscles
- Apex patellae
  - Anatomical proximity to the attachment tendon of the quadriceps femoris muscle
- Tuberculum adductorium
  - Anatomical proximity to the adductor canal (Figs. 2.3 and 2.4)

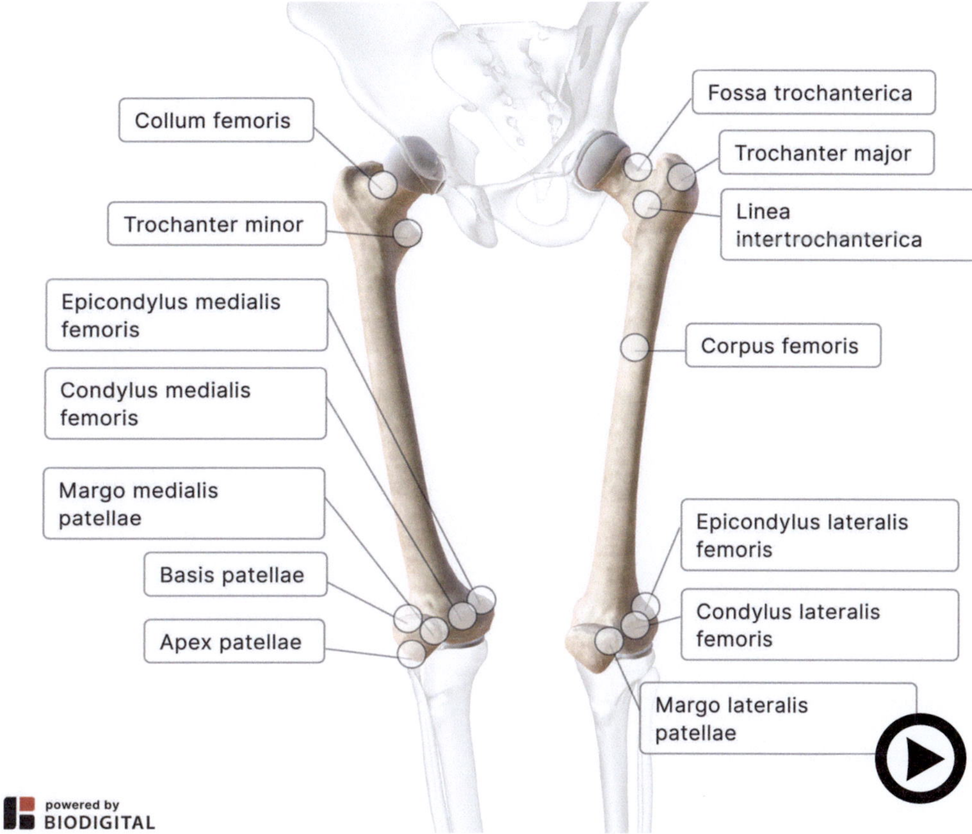

Fig. 2.3 Anatomy and palpation of the femur (▶ https://doi.org/10.1007/000-cpe)

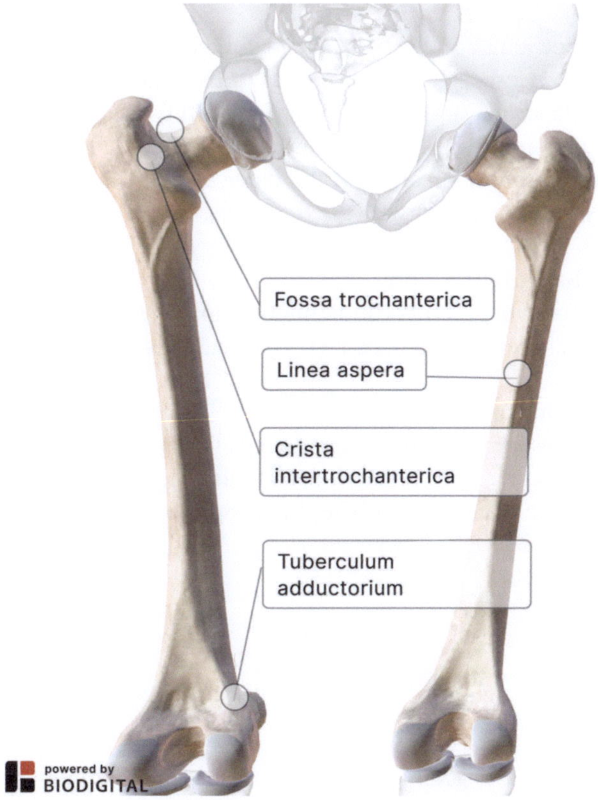

Fig. 2.4 Anatomy and palpation of the femur

2.4 Palpation of Bony Reference Points on the Lower Leg

The lower leg, like the forearm, consists of two bones that are connected by the membrana interossea cruris and ligaments. This compound between the tibia and fibula serves to transfer forces between the foot and thigh and also forms numerous joints that are of great importance for activities such as walking. Starting proximally, the following reference points can be palpated on the crus. The starting position in the supine position should be chosen for this.

2.4.1 Palpation of the Tibia

If the patella ligament is followed by the long finger berries, it ends distally in the tibial tuberosity. Starting from this roughness, a protrusion can be felt laterally, which is called the condyle lateralis tibiae. It is important not to pass over the first protrusion as the caput fibulae are located quite laterally. Halfway to this condyle, the Gerdy's tuberculum can be stimulated with flatly applied fingertips, which can be felt as roughness. Medially at the level of the tibial tuberosity, the medial tibial condyle is palpable as a rounded raised structure via the flatly applied fingertips. Distal to the tibial apophysis, there is a

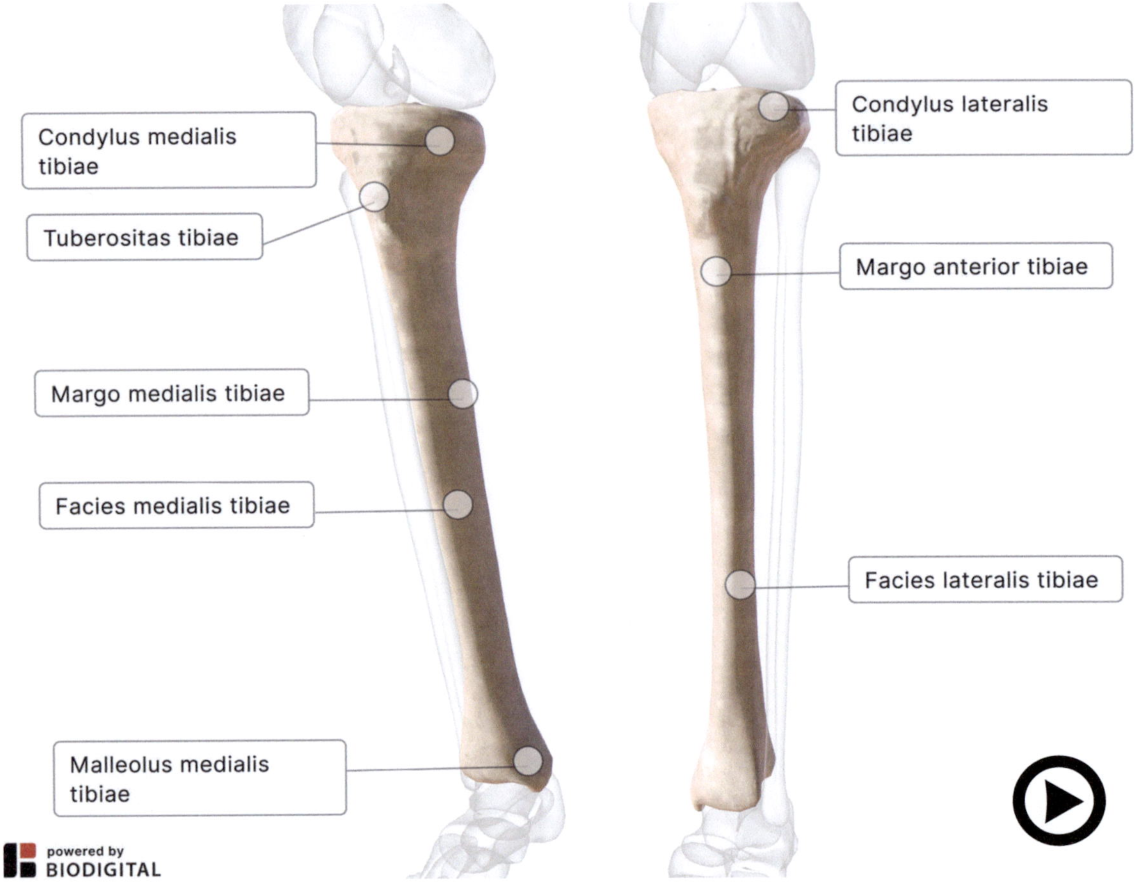

Fig. 2.5 Anatomy and palpation of the tibia (▶ https://doi.org/10.1007/000-cpf)

sharply defined longitudinal edge. The described margo anterior tibiae are palpable over almost the entire course of the tibia. Medial and lateral to this prominent edge are the facies medialis and lateralis of the tibia, which can be felt in depth with the index and middle fingers raised. The medial facies is followed inwards by another clearly palpable, longitudinal edge, the medial tibial marrow. Distally, the tibia extends into the medial malleolus. The inner ankle of the foot can be clearly perceived as a rounded structure via the fingertips.

Implementation Note
In the symptomatology of shin splints, the region around the margo anterior may react in a pressure-dolent manner (Figs. 2.5 and 2.6).

2.4.2 Palpation of the Fibula

The fibula is palpable proximolaterally on the lower leg via a distinct elevation. The caput fibulae are located laterally on the knee joint and can be palpated directly with the fingertips or with a forceps grip. The corpus of the fibula is difficult to palpate as it is surrounded by various soft tissues such as the fibularis longus and brevis muscle. Distally, the fibula ends in the lateral malleolus. As the outer ankle of the foot, it is very easy to palpate with the fingertips.

Implementation Note
The following points can be more symptomatic during palpation. Therefore, proceed with particular caution here.

- Tibial tuberosity
  - Insertion site of the quadriceps femoris muscle
- Margo medialis tibiae, especially in the proximal third
  - Facies posterior tibiae, insertion area of the popliteus muscle (Fig. 2.6)

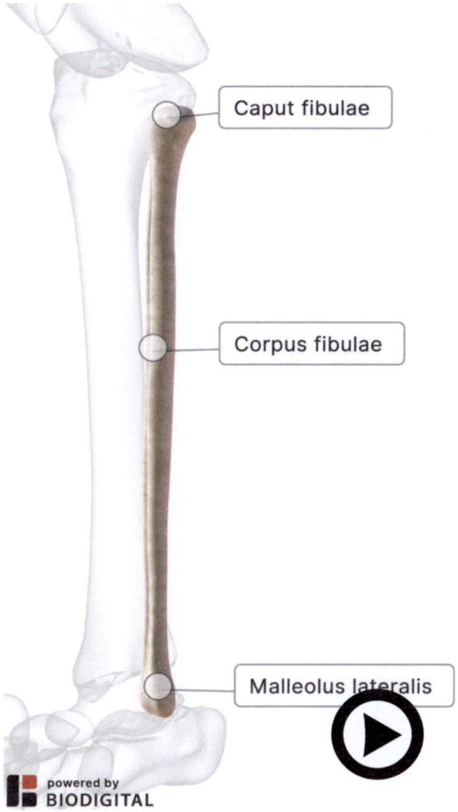

Fig. 2.6 Anatomy and palpation of the fibula (▶ https://doi.org/10.1007/000-cpg)

2.5 Palpation of Bony Reference Points on the Pes

The foot carries a person through life. Every day, numerous kilometres must be covered in order to cope with everyday life. In addition to adapting to a wide variety of surfaces, it is forced into different types of footwear for the purpose of optimising the gait pattern or aesthetics. Humans are designed for a daily walking distance of at least 10 km [2], so it is therefore clear that in today's sedentary society, there are many deformities and malpositions of the foot. The bent and fallen foot, to name just one typical diagnosis, has gradually become a "widespread disease" [3]. If a malformed foot carries a person through life, it is therefore understandable why there are so many ongoing orthopaedic problems that can be traced back to the pes [4]. To be able to examine and treat the foot well therapeutically, it is of the highest priority to know and palpate all 28 bones. A relaxed starting position with the client in the supine position is ideal for this.

The palpation journey on the foot begins with the bone, which occupies a kind of relay station on the foot and is also a bone on the human body where no muscles attach or originate.

2.5.1 Palpation of the Talus

The talus, which forms the "summit" of the foot, can best be felt by palpating the medial malleolus with the long finger berries a little way distally until a small depression is perceptible. With active supination of the lower ankle in combination with plantar flexion of the upper ankle, the posterior tibialis tendon should be clearly felt under the fingers immediately distal to the medial malleolus. Immediately anterior and posterior to this tendon section is the talus. An additional palpation site exists anteriorly between the tendon of the anterior tibialis muscle and the extensor hallucis longus muscle. Starting from the foot lifter tendon, which is clearly visible during dorsal extension and supination, the steeply positioned index finger is placed lateral to this tendon at the level of the upper ankle joint. Lateral to the finger, the tendon of the extensor hallucis longus is also palpable. The talus is palpated in depth in this region, in the direction of the heel. Viewed as a whole, the talus is surrounded by many soft tissue structures. This makes it difficult to perform an all-encompassing, free bony palpation (Fig. 2.7).

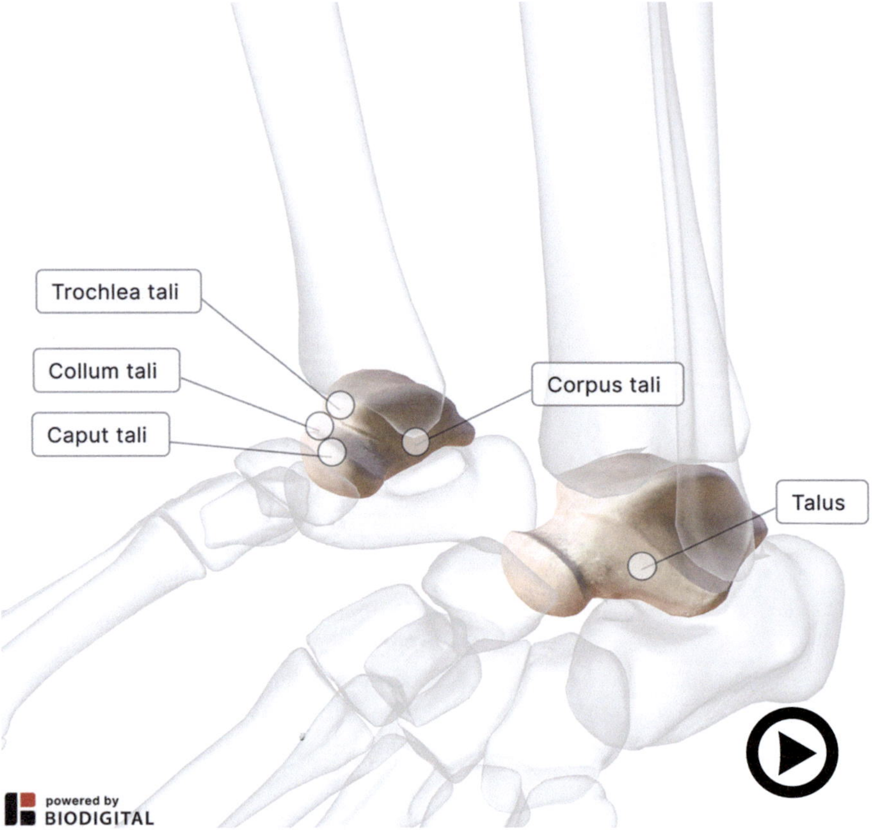

Fig. 2.7 Anatomy and palpation of the talus (▶ https://doi.org/10.1007/000-cph)

2.5.2 Palpation of the Os Naviculare

If palpation is continued distally on the medial side of the talus, a joint space and a subsequent distinct elevation can be perceived. This elevation is the tuberositas ossis navicularis, which is part of the os naviculare. At this point, the bone can be palpated very well in a pincer grip from the plantar and dorsal sides between the thumb and index finger. Another method is to approach the metatarsal I from the medial side. If the fingertip follows the first metatarsal proximally, the first joint to the os cuneiforme medial and then proximally also the tuberositas ossis navicularis can be clearly felt. The bone margins of the os naviculare can be clearly demarcated by movement in relation to neighbouring bones. The movable lateral edge forms the border to the os cuboideum, which is shown next (Fig. 2.8).

2.5.3 Palpation of the Os Cuboideum

For palpation of the cuboid bone, the fingertips make contact centrally on the outside of the foot and move proximally on this fifth metatarsal. A distinct prominence, the tuberositas ossis metatarsalis V, is noted. Proximal to this prominence is the os cuboideum, which can then be grasped directly via the fingertips or in a direct pincer grip. By fixating the os naviculare, the bone margin can be grasped even more clearly by moving it. Furthermore, the examiner can move his toes II to V in extension. This causes a contraction of the extensor digitorum brevis muscle, whose muscle belly lies directly above the os cuboideum (Fig. 2.9).

2.5.4 Palpation of the Cuneiform Ossa

Starting from the distal edge of the os naviculare, three small bones, the ossa cuneiformia, can be palpated. A distinction is made between the os cuneiforme mediale, the os cuneiforme intermediale and the os cuneiforme laterale. During palpation, the tuberositas ossis navicularis is felt as the starting point, the os naviculare is fixed and then palpated further distally at the medial edge of the foot until the edge of the bone and then a joint space appear. From the medial edge, these three cuneiforms can be fixed with the pincer grip, via the thumb from plantar and the index finger from dorsal and moved against the already fixed os naviculare. This is the

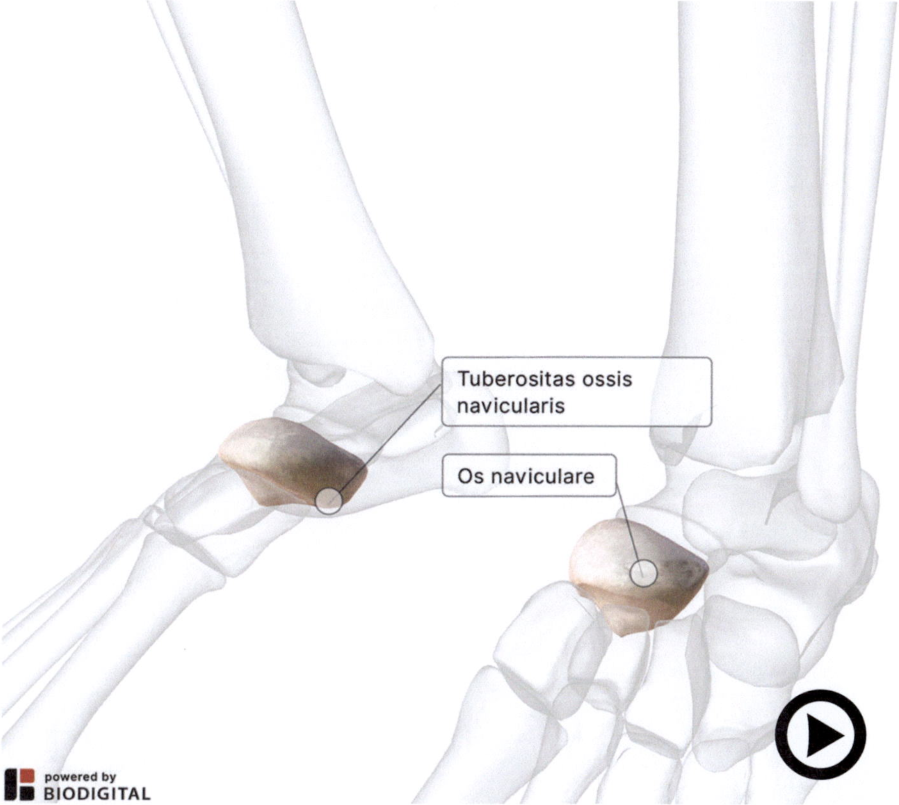

Fig. 2.8 Anatomy and palpation of the os naviculare (▶ https://doi.org/10.1007/000-cpj)

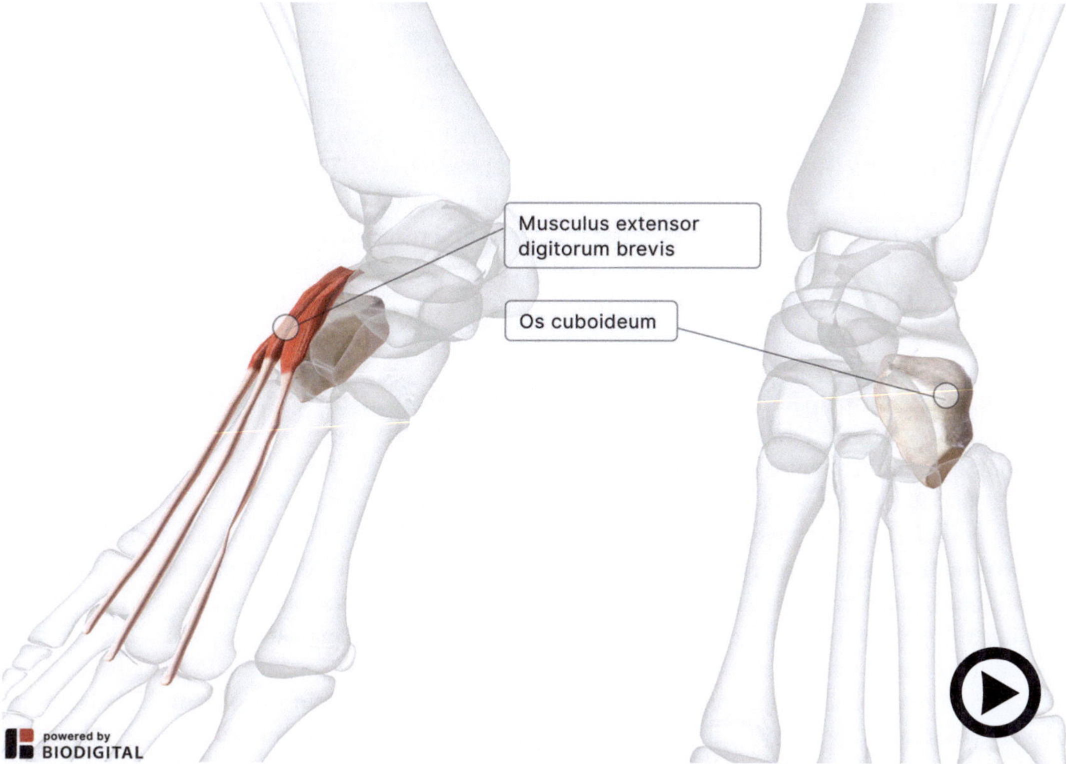

Fig. 2.9 Anatomy and palpation of the os cuboideum (▶ https://doi.org/10.1007/000-cpk)

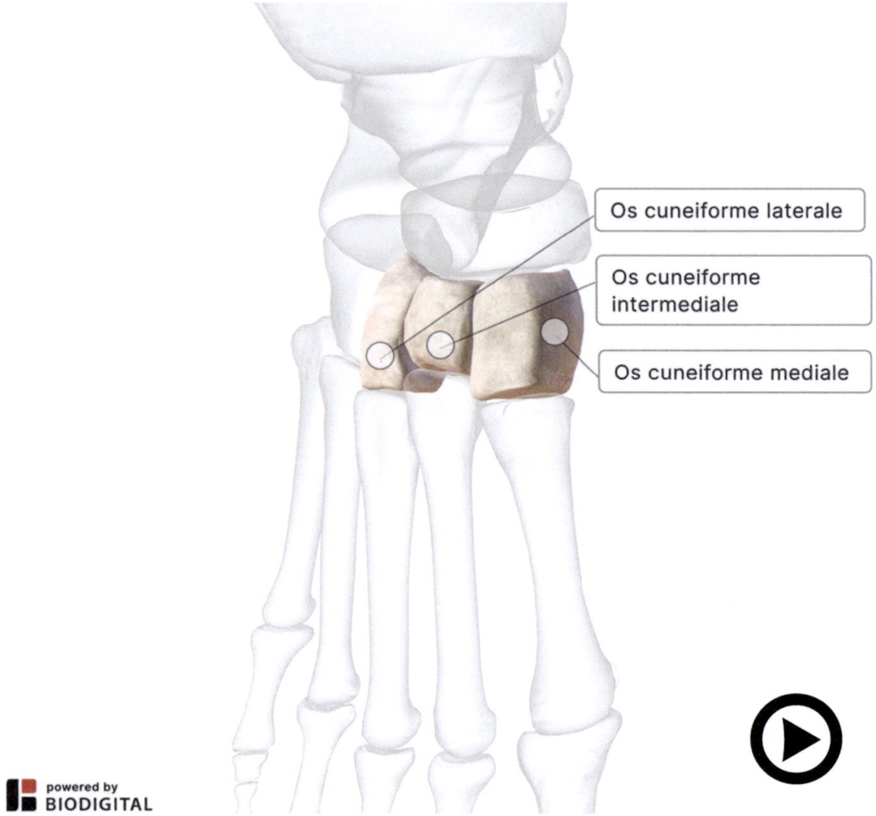

Fig. 2.10 Anatomy and palpation of the ossa cuneiformia (▶ https://doi.org/10.1007/000-cpm)

best way to feel the bone edges of the ossa cuneiformia. The os cuneiforme mediale is most pronounced in this group (Fig. 2.10).

2.5.5 Palpation of the Ossa Metatarsalia

Starting from the medial cuneiform bone, the adjacent base of the metatarsal bone can be palpated distally along the medial edge of the foot. For this purpose, the os cuneiforme I is grasped distally in a pincer grip in order to palpate the adjoining base of the os metatarsale I. The long finger berries are then used to palpate the base. With the long finger berries, this elongated tubular bone is now accessible to palpation from the plantar side, but even better from the medial and dorsal sides. A special feature of the metatarsal I is located distally plantar to this bone. Here, there are two small sesamoid ossicles, which can be perceived as small, hard, pea-sized structures by deep palpation with the index finger. Metatarsal I can generally be palpated in its entire course with the pincer grasp and medially with two-dimensional palpation. A similar approach can be taken for the other metatarsals. Metatarsals II and III join the os cuneiforme intermediale and laterale, respectively, while metatarsals IV and V follow the os cuboideum distally. The metatarsals of the second, third and fourth rays can only be palpated from the plantar and dorsal sides in a pincer grip. The fifth metatarsal can also be felt from the lateral side. To do this, palpate distally with the long finger berries, starting from the os cuboideum, and then feel an extremely prominent elevation after a small depression. This elevation is the tuberositas ossis metatarsalis V. This clearly palpable reference point is partly visible from the outside of the foot. All metatarsals end in a respective caput at the metatarsophalangeal joint. This region can be palpated very well with the long finger berries or also in a pincer grip (Fig. 2.11).

2.5.6 Palpation of the Ossa Phalangeales Pedis

Distal to the metatarsal heads, the art. metatarsophalangeales is formed by means of the base of the proximal phalanx. These two bony reference points, the caput of the metatarsal and the base of the phalanx, can be fixed by the pincer grip and then moved against each other. The corpus and the caput of the phalanx are connected to this base. A further phalanx is attached to each of the proximal phalanges, which can be palpated first with the pincer grip and then with the long finger berries. It should be noted that there are only two phalanges on the big toe, whereas toes two to five each have three phalanges, which are connected by interphalangeal joints (Fig. 2.12).

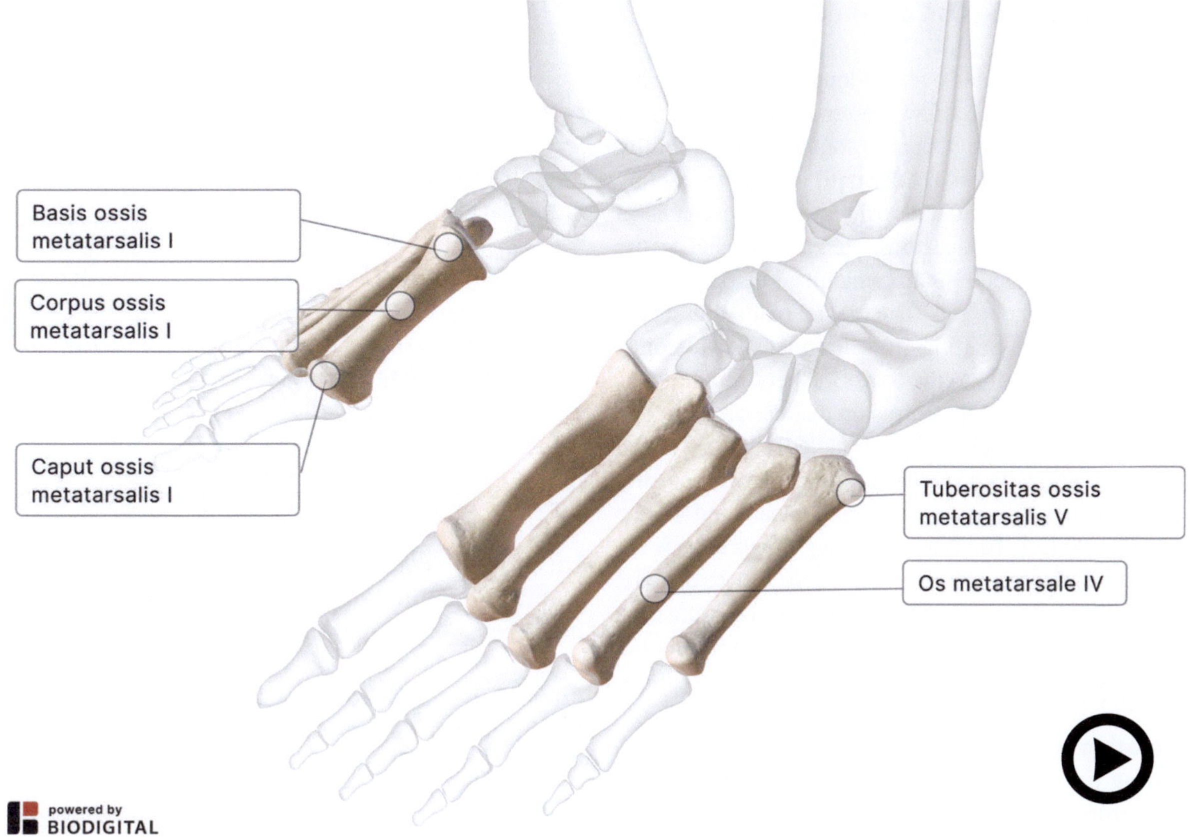

Fig. 2.11 Anatomy and palpation of the Ossa metatarsalia (▶ https://doi.org/10.1007/000-cpn)

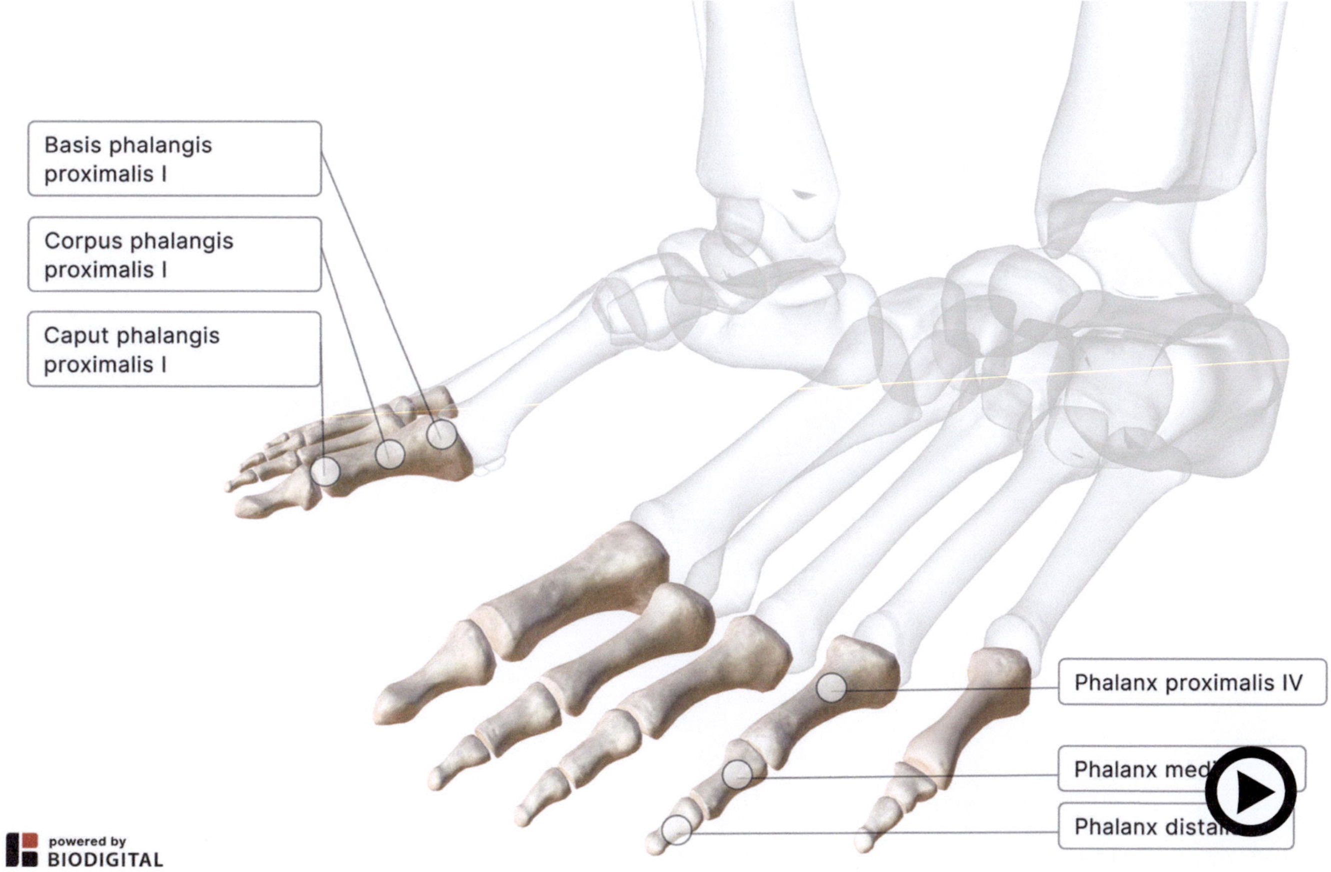

Fig. 2.12 Anatomy and palpation of the ossa phalangeales (▶ https://doi.org/10.1007/000-cpp)

2.5.7 Palpation of the Os Calcaneus

The calcaneus can be palpated over the long finger bones. This bone can be palpated using a few reference points. The first point, the calcaneal tuberosity, can be found by palpation by following the Achilles tendon distally until it becomes a bony structure. This is the calcaneal tuberosity, which is palpable as an elevation lateral and medial to the tendon. Medial to the calcaneus is the sustentaculum tali, which can be palpated in depth via the long finger berries. The medial malleolus serves as an orientation point. Starting from the medial malleolus, palpation continues distally to the transition between the talus and calcaneus. There, a small protrusion can be felt, which is the sustentaculum tali. Below this so-called balcony is the medial plantar artery, which is clearly palpable by a recurring pulse wave. Another reference point can be palpated on the facies lateralis calcanei. To do this, the long finger berries are first placed flat on the lateral malleolus. Then palpate distally. The fingers first fall into a depression that forms the transition to the calcaneus. About one transverse finger width further on, the trochlea fibularis exists as a perceptible elevation.

Implementation Note

The following points can be more symptomatic during palpation. Therefore, proceed with particular caution here.

- Talus
  - Insertion of the fibulo- and tiobiotalaris anterius and posterius ligaments
- Tuberositas ossis metatarsalis V
  - Insertion of the fibularis brevis muscle
  - Danger of bony avulsion
- Calcaneus
  - Insertion sites Ligg. fibulo- or tibiocalcaneare
- Os cuneiforme I as well as base os metatarsale I of plantar
  - Insertion site of the anterior and posterior tibialis and fibularis longus muscles (Fig. 2.13)

2.5.8 Palpation of the Sesamoid Pedis Ossa

Distal to the caput of the os metatarsale I, there are two plantar sesamoid bones. The fingertip of the index finger is the best way to identify the directly adjacent sesamoid bones. To do this, the flat index fingertip is placed directly at the level of the metatarsophalangeal joint of the big toe from the plantar side and palpated in depth (Fig. 2.14).

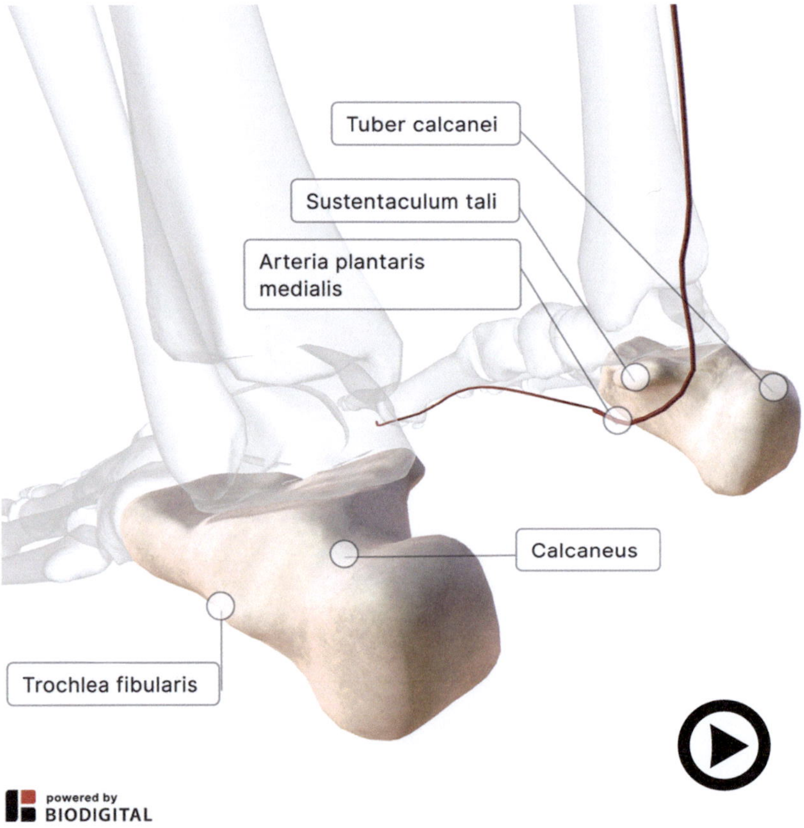

Fig. 2.13 Anatomy and palpation of the calcaneus (▶ https://doi.org/10.1007/000-cpq)

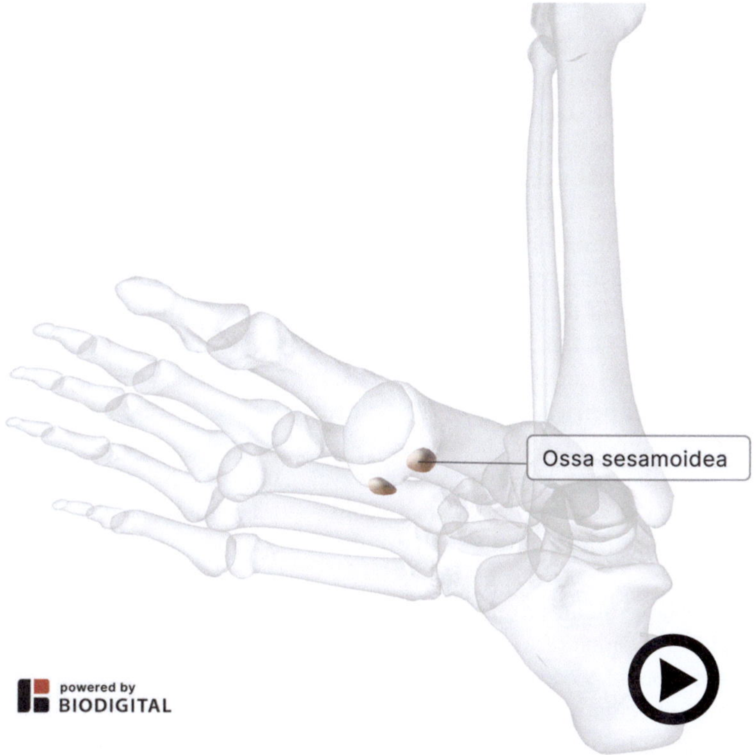

Fig. 2.14 Anatomy and palpation of the ossa sesamoidea (▶ https://doi.org/10.1007/000-cpr)

2.6 Palpation of Bony Reference Points on the Columna Vertebralis

The spinal column not only forms the stable backbone of the human being, but it also protects the highly sensitive spinal cord located in it and also ensures sufficient mobility. Consisting of 24 vertebral bodies and 23 intervertebral discs, the column curved as a "double S" is located dorsally on the trunk. The cervical spine with seven vertebrae, the thoracic spine with 12 vertebrae and the lumbar spine with 5 vertebrae are joined by the os sacrum with 5 and the os coccygis with 3–5 fused vertebrae [5, 6]. The os sacrum forms the connection to the pelvis and is therefore, from a biomechanical point of view, an important force transmitter [7]. The os coccygis, which is directly connected to the os sacrum, forms the caudal end of the columna vertebralis. In its entirety, the spinal column is a highly complex structure, both from an orthopaedic and a neurological point of view. It is fundamentally important to be familiar with the palpation of this region to be able to derive specific therapeutic approaches. The following shows the bony palpation of the spine from the starting prone position.

The palpation journey, with the client in the prone position, begins at the os sacrum. The caudal hand is placed on this bone with the fingertips pointing cranially, extending the anal fold. While the patient breathes in and out deeply, small movements should be noticeable. These provide a rough guide to the position of the sacrum. Directly in the centre of the os sacrum is the crista sacralis mediana. Posteriorly, this forms prominent projections which, as fused spinous processes of the sacrum, can best be palpated as hard elevations via the long finger berries. Laterally, at the caudal end of the sacrum, there is the lateral inferior angulus of the sacrum, which can also be palpated in depth with the long finger berries. Between the two anguli laterales inferiores is the tip of the os sacrum, the so-called apex ossis sacri. This tip is followed caudally by the os coccygis, which can be palpated globally with the heel of the hand and locally with the fingertips of the index or middle finger. Cranially of the os sacrum, the processi spinosi are palpable as a small elevation in the centre of the spine. For rough orientation, all spinous processes are first palpated cranially. The last processus spinosus that can be palpated is that of the second cervical vertebra. Starting from the cervical spine, the palpation of the processes spinosi caudally is described below. The first palpable process spinosus from the cranial side is that of the axis. To do this, palpate cranially, in the middle of the cervical spine, with the long finger berries in a caudal direction until the first prominent elevation can be felt. Palpating further caudally, the interspinal space can be felt as a depression between the bony elevations of the spinal processes. The seventh cervical vertebra is often called the vertebra prominens because of its long and clearly protruding processus spinosus. The spinous process of the sixth cervical vertebra is only slightly shorter than that of C7. The clinician can differentiate between the two processes of the sixth and seventh cervical vertebrae through an extensor movement of the cervical spine. If the processus spinosus of C6 is palpated, it disappears during extension due to an anterior displacement. The spinous process of C7, on the other hand, remains clearly perceptible to the examiner even during extension [8]. In addition, the superior inferior articular process and the inferior articular process articulating with it can be palpated directly lateral to the spinous processes of the cervical spine using the steeply placed index or middle fingers. In addition to the procc. articulares, the transverse process of the atlas can be felt on the cervical spine. Immediately in front of the sternocleidomastoid muscle, the transverse process of C1 can be palpated in depth on both sides at the level of the caput mandibulae using the steeply positioned long finger berries.

In the thoracic spine, the spinous processes can be found more quickly using orientation lines than counting them individually. The spine of the second thoracic vertebra is located at the level of the jugular fossa. In an imaginary connecting line between the two spinae scapulae, the processus spinosus of Th3 is located in the middle. The same applies to the anguli inferiores of the scapula and Th7. The spine of Th9 is found topographically at the level of the xiphoid process. If the 12th rib is followed in the direction of the columna vertebralis, it ends at the level of the thorn of Th12. It should be noted that the interspinous space between Th11 and Th12 appears much larger than that between Th12 and L1. It is important to note that the processi spinosi of the thoracic spine overhang each other like roof tiles. From this, it can be concluded that the respective spinous process always lies caudal to the associated processi transversi. To be able to palpate the associated processi transversi starting from the spinous process, one transverse finger is palpated between Th1 and Th3, two transverse fingers from Th4–6, three transverse fingers from Th7–9, two transverse fingers from Th10–Th11 and one transverse finger from Th12 cranially and two transverse fingers laterally.

In the lumbar spine, the massive spinous processes run in an anteroposterior direction. They can be easily palpated as prominent elevations. An imaginary connecting line of the bilateral highest points of the cristae iliacae leads the clinker centrally to the spinous process of L3 or L4. This variability can be attributed to a steeply or shallowly developed pelvis. While the steeply set up male pelvis tends to lead to L3, in the more flatly developed female pelvis, the reference line is located at the level of L4 [9]. The midpoint of a horizontal connecting line between the two SIPS leads the clinker to the spinous process of S2.

Implementation Note

The following points can be more symptomatic during palpation. Therefore, proceed with particular caution here.

- Processi spinosi
  - Muscle origins and attachments
- Generally in the area of the cervical spine
  - Increased occurrence of neurovascular structures (Fig. 2.15)

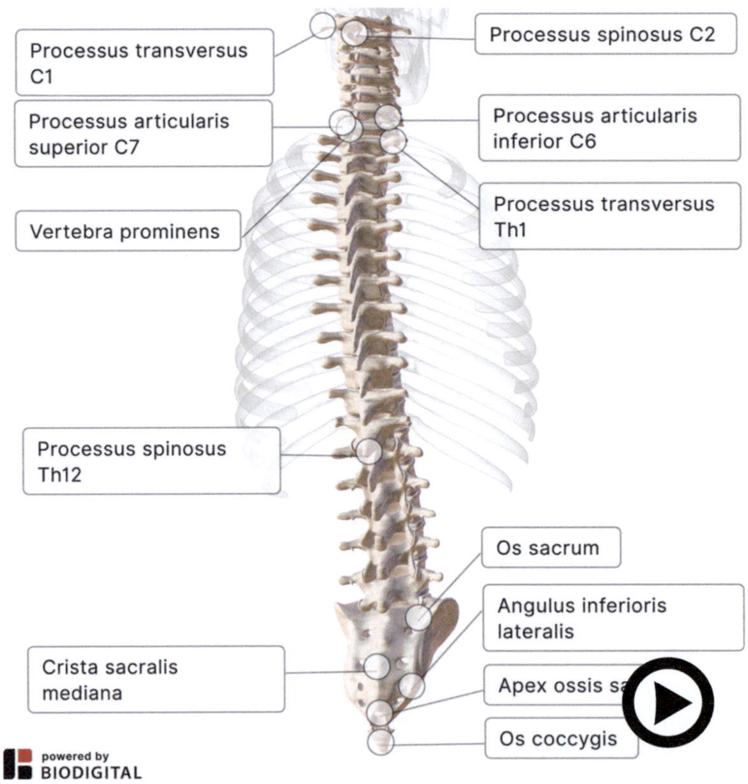

Fig. 2.15 Anatomy and palpation of the columna vertebralis (▶ https://doi.org/10.1007/000-cps)

2.7 Palpation of Bony Reference Points on the Thorax

Internal organs in the human body are predominantly protected by bony structures. This important protective function is provided in the trunk area by the thorax. In addition, the thorax, which consists of 24 costae and the sternum, also forms the direct connection point to the upper extremity. In addition to the protective function, which requires a certain stability, the thorax must also ensure the necessary mobility to be able to adapt optimally to movements of the thoracic spine as well as to the demands of breathing. This combination of stability and mobility increases the risk of negative local changes in the thorax, but also in the structures corresponding to it. For this reason, it is important to palpate bony reference points to subsequently create a targeted diagnosis or therapy. The most important palpatory reference points on the sternum and costae are described below. Here, work is mainly done with the long finger berries. Depending on the region, the client is in a supine or lateral position.

Palpation begins at the sternum, which can be classified from cranial to caudal into manubrium sterni, corpus sterni and the inconstant processus xiphoideus. At the most cranial point of the manubrium is the incisura jugularis; this depression can be palpated very well with steeply placed fingertips. To the right and left of this depression, the manubrium forms an articular surface to the clavicle via the incisura clavicularis. This indentation can be felt with the flat fingertips at the transition to the clavicle. In the middle of the manubrium, at the lower edge, is the angulus sterni, which can be felt as a small elevation in the course. The manubrium then merges smoothly into the corpus sterni. On this middle section of the sternum, small, ring-shaped elevations can be felt on the lateral edges. These prominent points are the thickenings of the incisurae costales of the second to seventh ribs. Here, the ribs insert over the cartilago costae on the sternum. At the caudal end of the corpus, the inconstant processus xiphoideus joins. This xiphoid process can be palpated as a single- or double-pinnate tip.

The ribs form the most mobile part of the ribcage. The 12 pairs of ribs extend from the sternum to the spine and must move with each breath. This movement extends from the sternum to the spine. Based on their anatomy, the ribs can be divided into costae verae 1–7 (real), costae affixae 8–10 (fake) and costae fluctuantes 11–12 (free ribs). In some cases, the ability to palpate the ribs can be severely limited, as numerous muscles extend both ventrally and dorsally over large parts of the ribs. Start by palpating the first rib. The costa prima can be palpated lateral to the incisura costalis I at the transition to the manubrium. It is also possible to palpate the most cranial rib in the depth between the trapezius pars descendens and the clavicle, in the clavicular fossa. With all this, the corpus costae become partially palpable. The second to seventh ribs can be palpated ventrally over the cartilaginous costae at the junction with the corpus sterni, in each case lateral to it. This cartilaginous part is palpable as a flexible structure which is slightly movable dorsally when pressure is applied in depth. The corpus costae adjoin the cartilago costae, again dorsally. These bodies of the ribs can be palpated very well via the flat fingertips or the radial edge of the index finger in the course, on the convex facies externa. Here, it is clear that the ribs take on a curved shape. The ribs are bordered cranially and caudally by the superior and inferior costal margo. These edges can be felt with the steeply placed fingertips. The corpus costae are followed dorsally by the respective angulus costae. This can be palpated in the same way as the corpus costae. The cartilaginous extensions of ribs 8–10 extend ventrally into the cartilago costae of the seventh rib and thus have no direct contact with the sternum. Through their course, they form the arcus costalis, which can be easily delineated on palpation. The further course can be palpated as usual over the corpus and angulus costae. The 11th and 12th ribs belong to the free ribs and can only be palpated on the corpus and the angulus costae.

Implementation Note

The following points can have an increased symptomatic reaction during palpation. Therefore, proceed with particular caution here.

- Incisura jugularis
  - Direct proximity to the brachial plexus
- Proc. xiphoideus
  - Direct proximity to the solar plexus
  - May be dislocated after chest compressions
- Angulus costae
  - Malpositions occur more frequently in the area of the articulationes costotransversales (Fig. 2.16)

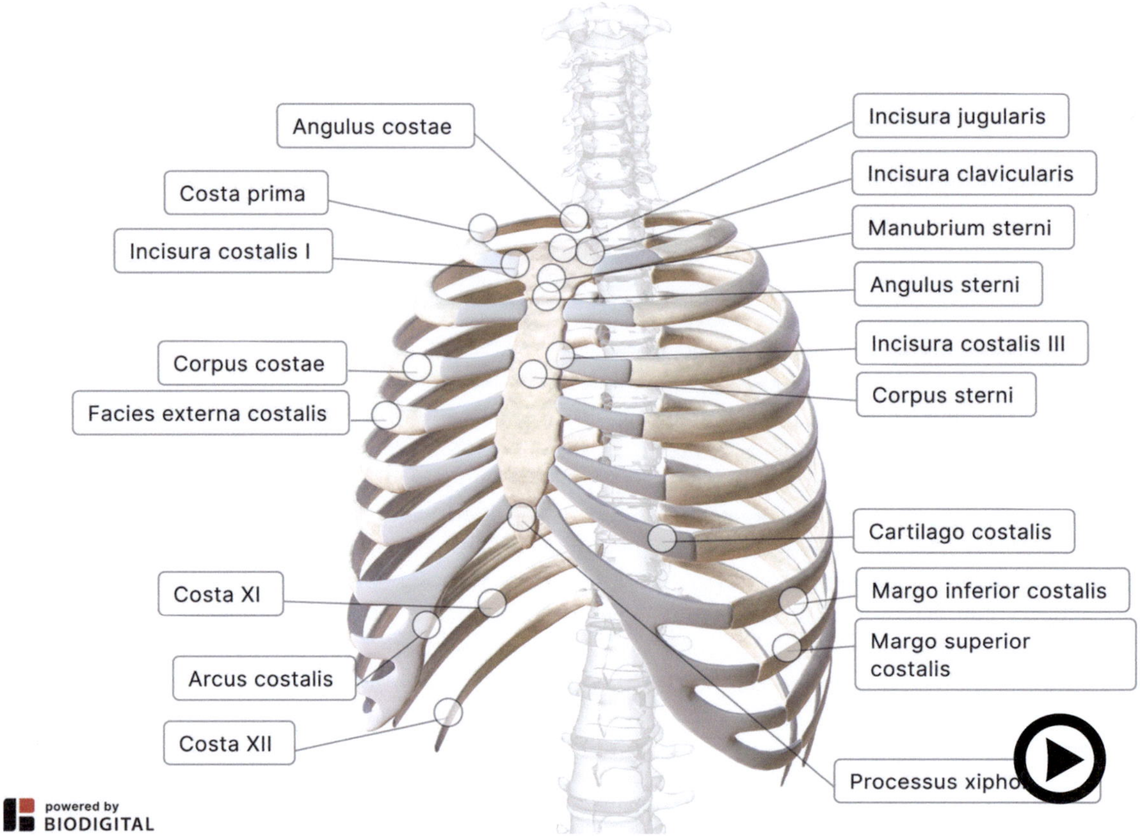

Fig. 2.16 Anatomy and palpation of the thorax (▶ https://doi.org/10.1007/000-cpt)

2.8 Palpation of Bony Reference Points on the Shoulder Girdle

The shoulder girdle forms a highly complex, functional unit that is interdependent in its entirety. By means of the articulatio sternoclavicularis, it not only connects the torso with the upper extremity, but also ensures that the person can properly perform the everyday functions that require the arms. This functional unit is formed by the clavicle and the scapula. For the diagnosis and therapy of the shoulder girdle, it is indispensable to be able to orientate oneself palpatory via bony reference points, as numerous muscles originate or attach to the bony points, among other things. For palpation, it is advisable to place the patient in a sitting position. Alternatively, ventral palpation of the clavicle can also be performed with the patient in the supine position and dorsal palpation of the scapula in the prone position.

2.8.1 Palpation of the Clavicle

In this description, the osseous palpation circle of the shoulder girdle begins with the clavicle. Medially on the clavicle, the transition from the manubrium to the extremitas sternalis of the clavicle can be palpated over a small elevation by means of the long finger berries placed flat. Often, this transition is already visually perceptible, as this reference point is prominently oriented ventrally on both sides. In the intermediate third, the clavicle narrows laterally as it progresses. This can be felt by the clinician by means of the fingertips but also in the pincer grip from ventral, dorsal and cranial. The S-shape of this bone becomes very clear. The anterior margo is located ventrally, with the anterior facies, and the superior margo is located cranially. Further laterally, the clavicle ends over a broad surface in the extremitas acromialis. At the transition of the corpus claviculae to the extremitas acromialis, a small elevation, the so-called tuberculum conoideum, is palpable from the dorsal side. This can be optimally felt from the cranial and dorsal sides by placing the long fingers flat against it.

Implementation Note

The following points can be more symptomatic during palpation. Therefore, proceed with particular caution here.

- Extremitas sternalis claviculae
  - Origin of the sternocleidomastoid muscle
- Corpus claviculae
  - Anatomical proximity to the lateral cervical region and thus to numerous nerves and vessels (Fig. 2.17)

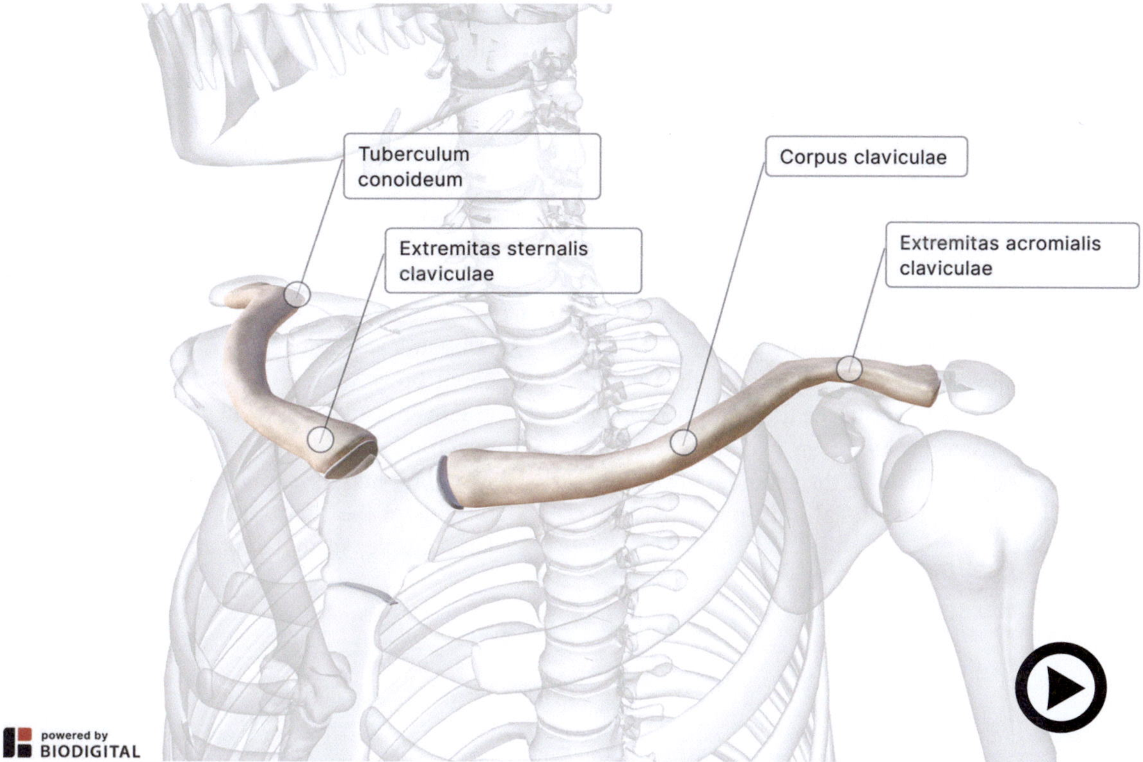

Fig. 2.17 Anatomy and palpation of the clavicula (▶ https://doi.org/10.1007/000-cpv)

2.8.2 Palpation of the Scapula

The scapula, which is so thin in the middle that light shines through it, has many more osseous palpation points compared to the clavicle [10]. Due to its triangular basic structure, the scapula can be divided into three corner points and three edges, which are described in detail below. The starting point is the inferior angulus. This can be easily felt in the lowest area of the scapula. During the palpation, the examiner feels a hard structure under his fingers that can be clearly distinguished from the surroundings and is pointed caudally. Starting from the lower tip of the scapula, the medial margo, which rises cranially, is found medially. The inner edge is clearly palpable in its course via steeply positioned long finger berries. If the fingers move under this edge onto the ventral surface of the scapula, the subscapular fossa can be felt directly in this area. The superior angulus is the upper end of the medial margo. This can only be palpated to a limited extent due to the anatomical proximity of the trapezius pars descendens muscle. The superior margo cannot be palpated, whereas the lateral scapular margo can be clearly palpated. The oblique caudomedial border, which ends in the inferior angulus, can be palpated in depth via the erect long finger berries. In addition to this border, there are other palpable osseous reference points on the scapula. Viewed from the dorsal side, the spina scapulae is located in the upper third. This can be easily palpated as an elongated bony ridge, starting from the upper third of the margo medialis and running slightly obliquely craniolaterally. The scapula ridge ends laterally in the acromion. In many clients, the shoulder height is already clearly perceptible in the visual findings. The acromion is palpated with the fingertips. The angulus acromii on the outer edge of the acromion is clearly perceptible. Immediately above the spina scapulae is the supraspinous fossa and below the infraspinous fossa. Both are palpable in depth but are covered by the supra- and infraspinatus muscles, respectively. Another important reference point on the clavicle is the coracoid process. The coracoid process is palpated in depth using the steeply positioned long finger berries or alternatively with the thumb. Initially, the extremitas acromialis of the clavicle serves as orientation. Starting from this reference point, the palpation finger is moved caudally. Caudal to the acromial limb, there is a depression filled with soft tissue. A clearly rounded, bony structure with the fingertips is perceptible breechward of this depression. This structure is the coracoid process. Lastly, the subscapular fossa should be mentioned on the scapula, which is the anterior surface of the scapula that contacts the thorax. Depending on the starting position, different parts of the subscapular fossa become palpable. If the examiner is lying prone, the clinker can achieve a separation between the scapula and the thorax by means of a passive retraction movement in the shoulder girdle. This makes it possible to contact the medial parts of the subscapular fossa in the region of the inferior angulus or the medial margo with the long finger berries placed flat. The same procedure can also be implemented in the lateral position. Passive retraction of the shoulder girdle is recommended beforehand to approach soft tissue structures. If the client is in the supine position, the clincer should first perform a slight abduction in the shoulder joint, the side to be examined. Now the examiner contacts the margo lateralis, immediately caudal to the axilla, with the extended long fingers. Once this has been identified, the space between the thorax and the scapula can be palpated in a dorsal direction. If the clinker exerts slight pressure in the direction of the scapula, stimuli can be applied to the lateral parts of the subscapular fossa. Try to see the described bony reference points as mosaic pieces of an overall picture in your examination. As components of the shoulder girdle, the scapula and clavicle form a functional unit in the sense of holism.

Implementation Note

The following points can be more symptomatic during palpation. Therefore, proceed with particular caution here.

- Angulus inferior scapulae
  - Origin of the teres major muscle
- Margo lateralis
  - Areas of origin of the teres major and teres minor muscles
- Coracoid process
  - Anatomical influence of the pectoralis minor muscle, caput breve of the biceps brachii muscle, coracobrachialis muscle, coracoclavicular ligament and coracoacromial ligament
- Fossa supra- and infraspinata and subscapularis
  - Origins of the supra- and infraspinatus and subscapularis muscles from the rotator cuff (Figs. 2.18 and 2.19)

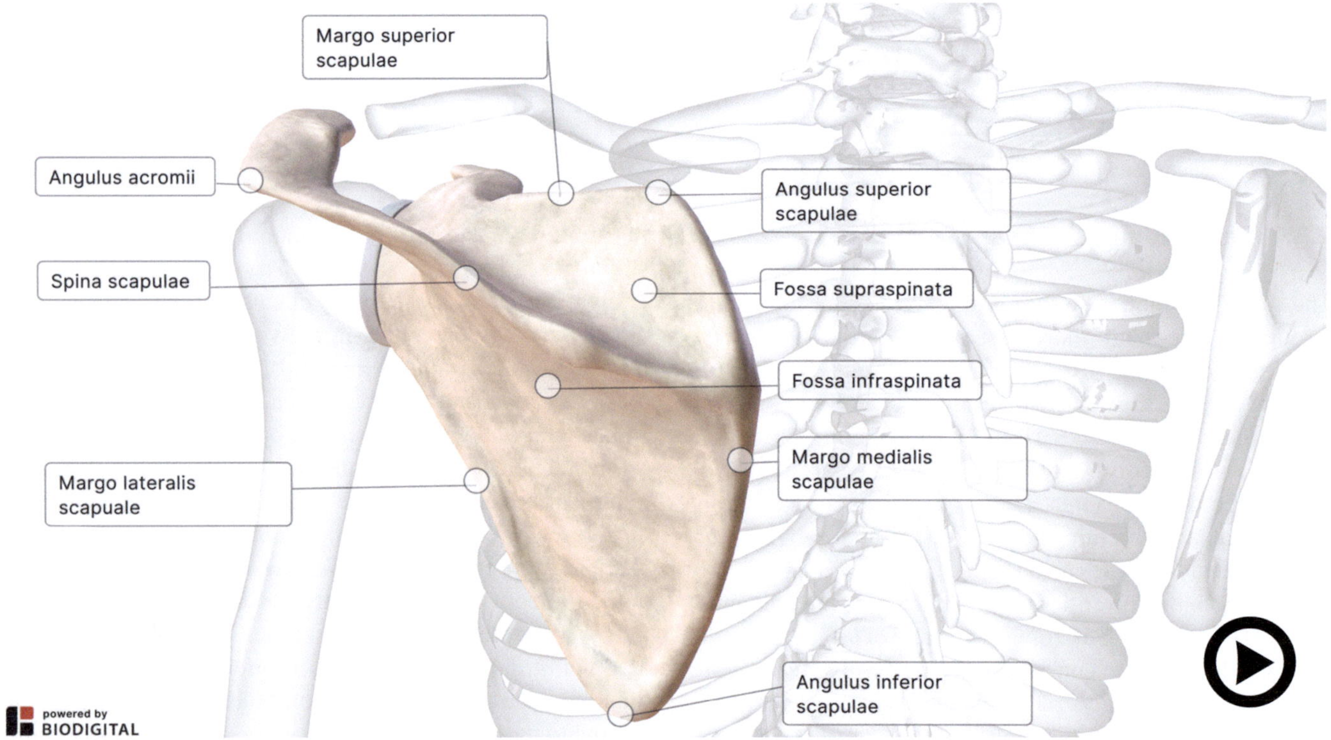

Fig. 2.18 Anatomy and palpation of the scapula (▶ https://doi.org/10.1007/000-cpw)

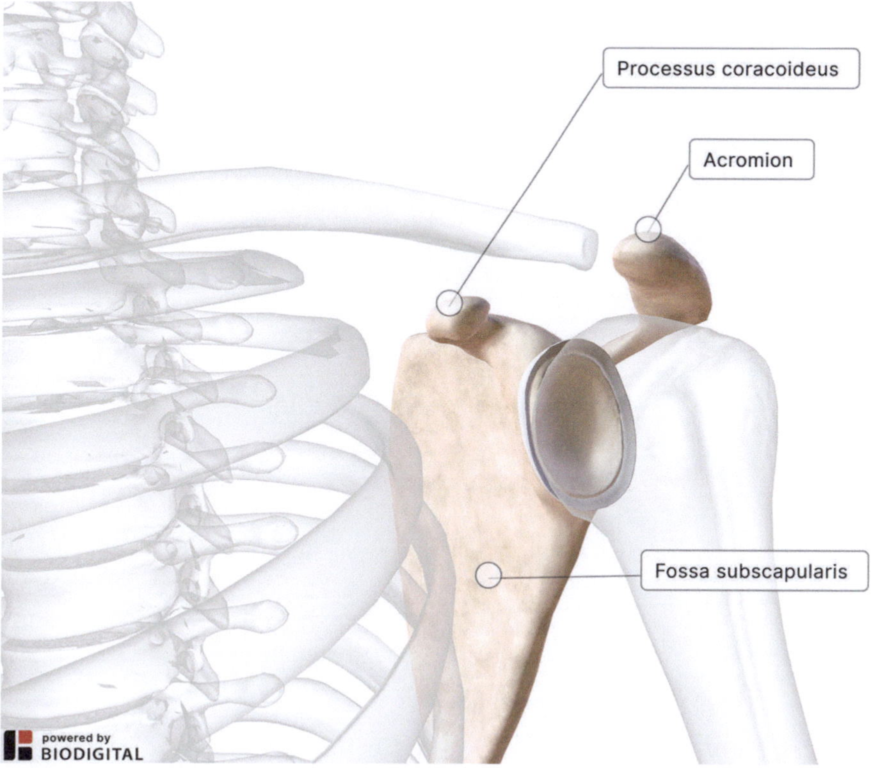

Fig. 2.19 Anatomy and palpation of the scapula

2.9 Palpation of the Humerus

As the longest bone of the upper extremity, the humerus has numerous reference points that need to be explored by palpation. Early fractures of the humerus occur abundantly, which shows that this bone is definitely exposed to high stresses in everyday life [11]. In addition to fractures, epicondylopathia lateralis and medialis humeri are also frequent diagnoses that prompt clients to see a doctor or therapist [12]. The various clinical forms of this structure bring the importance of high-quality palpation to the fore. For palpation, the client is in the sitting or alternatively supine position.

Palpation begins proximally with the two bumps on the humerus, the tuberculum majus and minus. The former is distal to the acromion and thus lateroproximal to the humerus and is best palpated with the long finger berries of the index and middle fingers placed flat. External and internal rotation in the humeroscapularis articularis can be used to register movement of the greater cusp. Starting from the greater tuberosity, palpation is performed horizontally in a medial direction. First, the long tendon of the biceps brachii muscle is palpated, which extends transversely to the course of palpation in the intertubercular sulcus. Further medially, the tuberculum minus ventroproximal on the humerus is palpable. Lateral to the humerus, the deltoid tuberosity is located in the centre. This bony landmark is palpated by first placing the long finger berries on the lateral distal end of the humerus and slowly palpating proximally with the humerus actively abducted at approximately 30°. Halfway along the path, a small depression can be felt in the tissue, which is joined further proximally by the muscle belly of the deltoid muscle. The deltoid tuberosity can be found at the point described in the depression. Then palpate laterally again distally until a bony prominence is felt near the elbow. This small prominence is called the lateral humeral epicondyle. It is best accessed via the fingertips when the client's elbow joint is flexed at about 90°. From this point, the anterior surface of the humerus is oriented medially. The capitulum humeri can be palpated distally in depth laterally as a convex curve, and then the trochlea humeri can be palpated medially. In this area, the quality of palpation is limited by the overlying soft tissue structures. Further medially, the epicondylus medialis humeri are palpable as a distinct elevation in a 90° flexed position. In this initial position, the posterior surface of the distal humerus is palpated. When the posterior distal surface of the humerus is palpated, a clearly perceptible depression is heard in the centre. If the clinician feels this with his palpation finger, he has arrived at the olecranon fossa.

Implementation Note

The following points can be more symptomatic during palpation. Therefore, proceed with particular caution here.

- Tuberculum majus
  - Insertions of the supraspinatus, infraspinatus and teres minor muscles
- Tuberosity minus
  - Insertion site of the subscapularis muscle

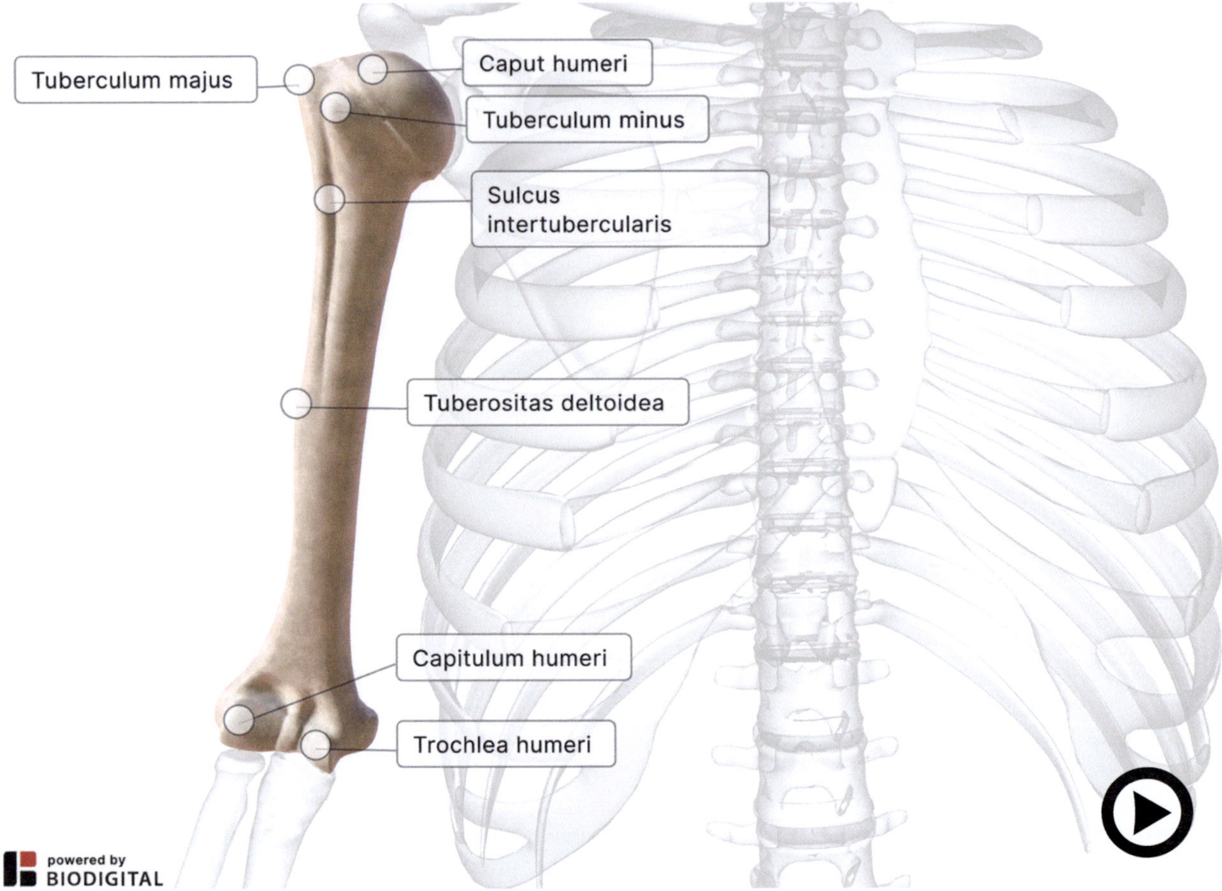

Fig. 2.20 Anatomy and palpation of the humerus (▶ https://doi.org/10.1007/000-cpx)

- Sulcus intertubercularis
  - Houses the tendon of the biceps brachii caput longum muscle
- Deltoid tuberosity
  - Insertion site of the deltoid muscle
- Epicondylus lateralis humeri
  - Insertion site of the wrist extensors, caution with epicondylopathia lateralis
- Epicondylus medialis humeri
  - Insertion-site wrist flexors, caution in case of epicondylopathia medialis (Figs. 2.20 and 2.21)

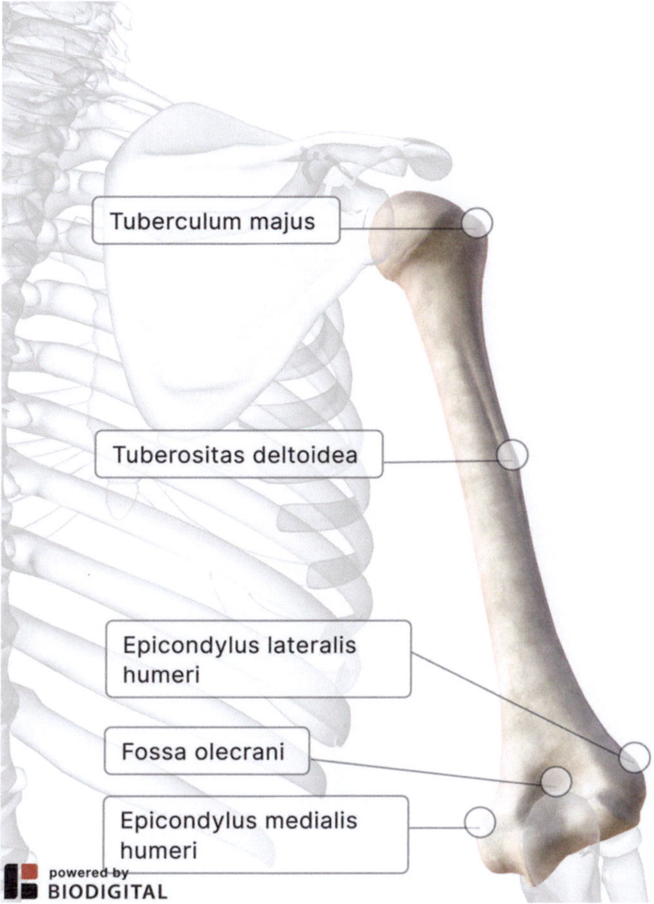

Fig. 2.21 Anatomy and palpation of the humerus

2.10 Palpation of Bony Reference Points on the Antebrachium

The forearm, like the lower leg, consists of two bones. The ulna and radius form a mutually dependent functional unit. Both bones are structurally connected to each other articularly and via the membrana interossea antebrachii. In addition, this region is particularly susceptible to injury. The distal radius fracture is the most frequently diagnosed bone fracture [13]. This clearly illustrates the great stresses on the forearm bones in a person's everyday life. It is therefore even more important to palpate the region of the forearm in order to be able to derive a suitable therapy afterwards. The recommended starting position for the client is supine or, alternatively, sitting.

2.10.1 Palpation of the Ulna

The palpation of the bony reference point at the antebrachium is described below, starting with the ulna. The ulna can be divided into an extremity proximalis, a corpus ulnae and an extremity distalis. The olecranon is found as a prominent palpation point dorsoproximally on the ulna. This part of the ulna is clearly perceptible with all palpation techniques. It is recommended that contact be made with the flat-placed fingertips to get a good feel of the structure itself. The margo posterior serves as a posterior, osseous orientation line. This edge is in extension of the olecranon and can be clearly felt through the fingertips. Anteriorly in the proximal part of the ulna is the coronoid process and slightly more distally the ulnar tuberosity. These elevations can be felt directly in the crook of the elbow, on the ulnar side as a hard elevation, via the steeply positioned index and middle finger berries. The ulna ends remote from the body via the caput ulnae in the ulnar styloid process. This protrusion is usually already clearly visible to the naked eye and can therefore be easily palpated. The discus articularis and the os triquetrum follow distally.

The following points can be more symptomatic during palpation. Therefore, proceed with particular caution here.

- Ulnar tuberosity
  - Insertion-site brachial artery (Figs. 2.22 and 2.23)

2.10.2 Palpation of Bony Reference Points on the Radius

Palpation of the radius begins proximally and laterally at the epicondylus lateralis humeri. This reference point is used to palpate the articular transition to the circumferentia radii during movement in flexion and extension in the elbow joint. The next point of reference is the radial tuberosity. To locate it, it is useful to follow the tendon of the biceps brachii muscle distally. This tightens during active flexion and supination in the elbow joint and inserts at the sought osseous site. Once at the insertion site, the patient is asked to perform an alternating pro- and supination movement in the elbow joints. As the radius rotates around the ulna during these movements, the roughness disappears during pronation, whereas the radial tuberosity can be felt as a hard elevation in depth during supination. On the thumb side, the radius can then be palpated along the margo anteriorly or posteriorly to the distal end. For this purpose, it is advisable to palpate the radius over the surface of the fingertips or in a pincer grip. The radial styloid process is located at the distal end and can be felt as a reinforcement. The dorsal tuberosity is also located centrally on the dorsodistal radius. This can be felt as a small elevation.

Implementation Note

The following points can be more symptomatic during palpation. Therefore, proceed with particular caution here.

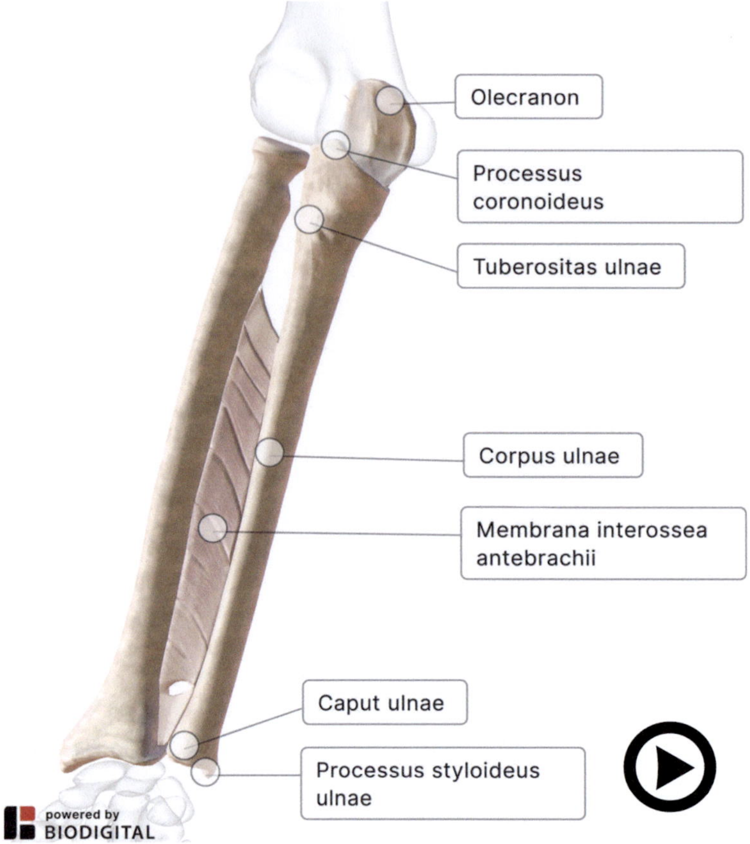

Fig. 2.22 Anatomy and palpation of the Ulna (▶ https://doi.org/10.1007/000-cpy)

Fig. 2.23 Anatomy and palpation of the ulna

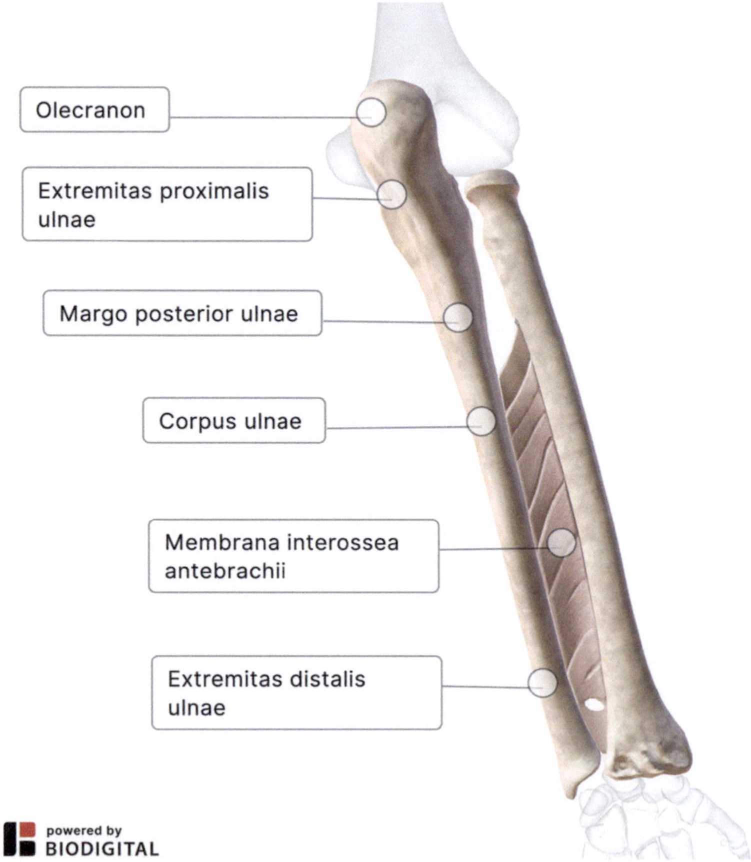

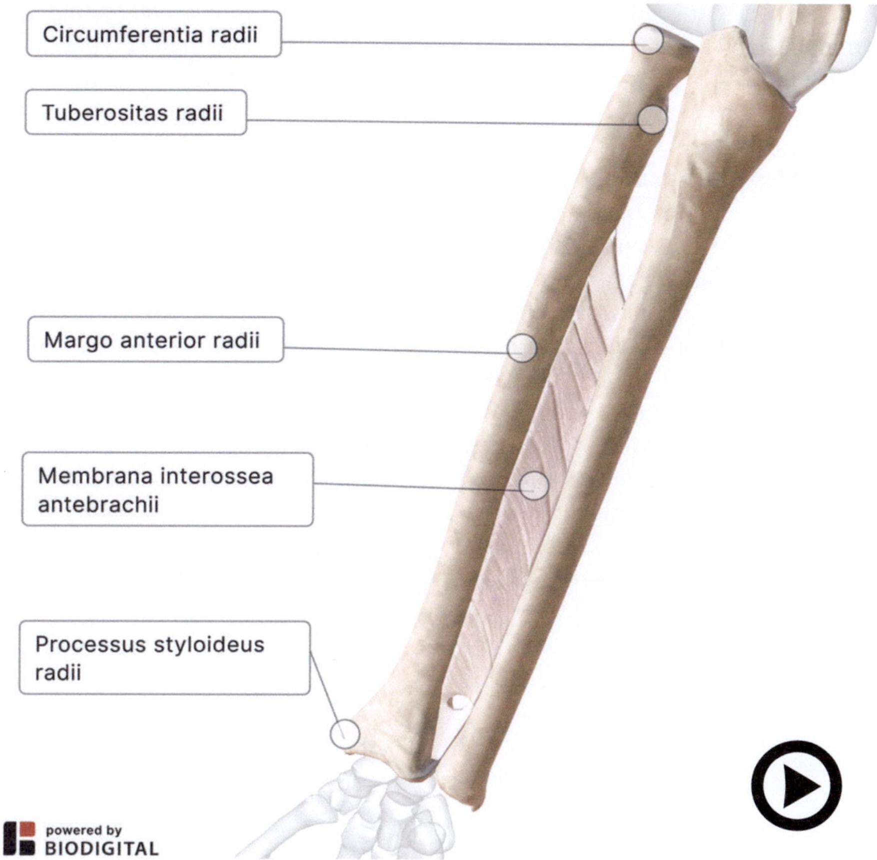

Fig. 2.24 Anatomy and palpation of the radius (▶ https://doi.org/10.1007/000-cpz)

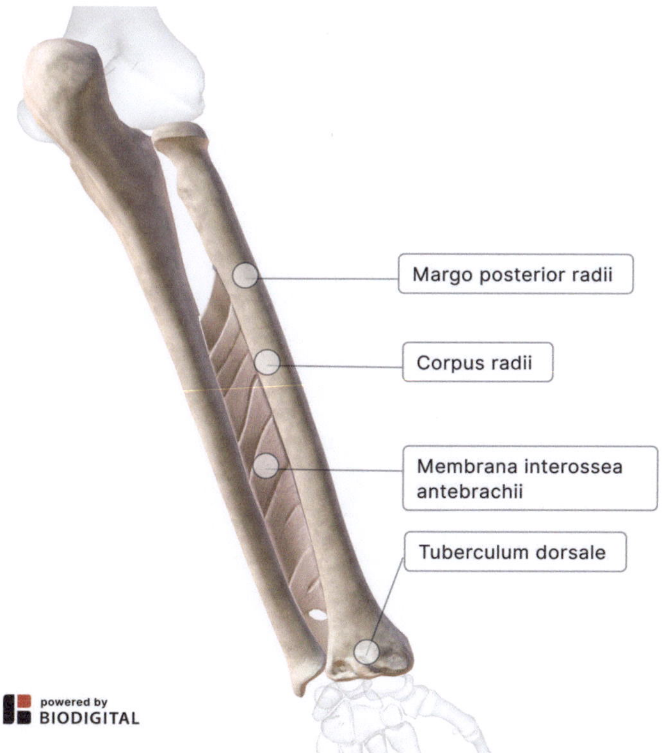

Fig. 2.25 Anatomy and palpation of the radius

- Radial tuberosity
  - Insertion site m. biceps brachii (Fig. 2.24 and 2.25)

2.11 Bony Reference Points on the Manus

The filigree as well as highly precise working hand gives the human organism a fascinating unique selling point in nature. Whether eating, drinking, using tools, driving, working on the PC, opening doors or other numerous everyday activities, the hand is always needed. As a gripping organ, it enables the precise grasping of objects through the corresponding fine motor skills. The basic osseous structure of the hand consists of 29 bones. These include the eight carpal bones (carpus), five metacarpal bones (metacarpus), five proximal phalanges, four medial phalanges, five distal phalanges (digiti I–V) and two sesamoid bones. This multitude of bones forms the basic framework for highly complex movements. Palpation of various osseous points enables topographical orientation of the hand. For this purpose, it is advantageous to position the client in a supine or sitting position. The bones are then palpated with a pincer grip or flat palpation to delineate them from the surrounding structures. Especially in the area of the carpus, palpation should only be done with the fingertips due to the manageable size of the bones. It is advisable to work through the chapters chronologically, as the individual contents usually build on each other.

2.11.1 Palpation of the Ossa Metacarpalia

Palpation of the hand begins at the metacarpus. This procedure simplifies the exploration of all other bones of the manus. The caput of the respective metacarpals I–V is located proximally at the base joints of the fingers. This is noticeable as a rounded thickening. In their course, the elongated tubular bones can be felt from their heads, proximally over the respective corpus, to their base in a pincer grip. The osseous palpation sensation is more pronounced from the dorsal in contrast to the palmar contact surface. Slight dorsopalmar translatory mobilisation impulses that cause movement between the individual metacarpals can be helpful in accurately delineating the respective osseous structure. The carpometacarpal joint space adjoins the respective base of the ossa metacarpalia. This forms the junction between the metacarpus and the carpus. On metacarpal I, two sesamoid bones exist as a special feature palmar distal to the caput. They can best be felt by direct palpation with the flat index finger (see Sect. 2.11.11) (Fig. 2.26).

2.11.2 Palpation of the Os Capitatum

Palpation of the eight carpal bones begins via the metacarpal III. This is followed from distal to proximal until the carpometacarpal joint space is felt. The os capitatum joins as the proximal joint partner. The highly vascularised capitate is the largest bone in the carpus [14]. If the metacarpal tertium is palpated from proximal to distal on the dorsal side, a clearly

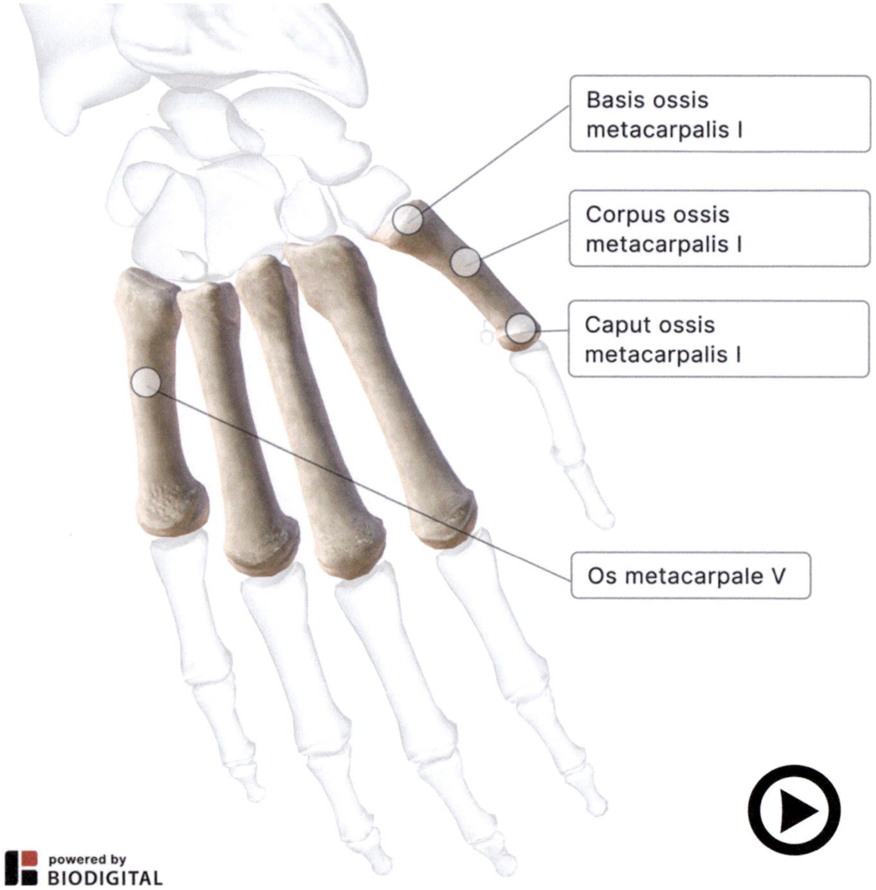

Fig. 2.26 Anatomy and palpation of the ossa metacarpalia (▶ https://doi.org/10.1007/000-cq0)

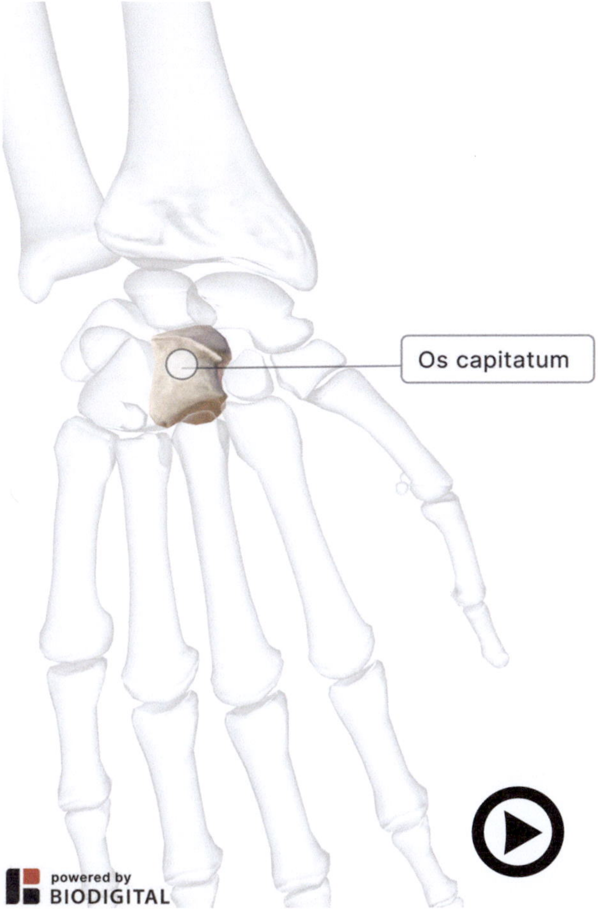

Fig. 2.27 Anatomy and palpation of the os capitatum (▶ https://doi.org/10.1007/000-cq1)

perceptible depression follows the transition to the os capitatum. This indentation marks the successful location of the os capitatum. This bone serves as an orientation point and is initially held in a pincer grip (Fig. 2.27).

2.11.3 Palpation of the Os Trapezoideum

With the os capitatum held in a pincer grip, the radially located os trapezoideum, also known as the small polygonal bone, is then palpated with the free hand in a pincer grip. Small dorsal and palmar movements are the best way to distinguish it from surrounding structures (Fig. 2.28).

2.11.4 Palpation of the Os Trapezium

The os trapezoideum is radially adjacent to the os trapezium in the proximal carpal row. The large polygonal bone is also the proximal joint partner of the thumb saddle joint. The joint space of art. carpometacarpalis I is easily palpable from the radial side as a depression and leads the examiner proximally directly to the os trapezium via the fovea radialis, which is also known as the tabatière. It is also advisable to palpate the edges of this bone of the distal carpal series using small movement impulses. Furthermore, the tuberculum ossis trapezii can be perceived palmar to the os trapezium as a small elevation above the fingertips (Fig. 2.29).

2.11.5 Palpation of the Os Scaphoideum

Starting from the fixed os trapezium, the proximally connected os scaphoideum is grasped with the pincer grip. On the palmar side of the scaphoid is the tuberculum ossis scaphoidei, which is palpable as a clear protrusion. The scaphoid tubercle can also be delimited proximally from the radius by gentle mobilisation impulses. Furthermore, it can be felt more prominently via radial abduction, whereas it tends to flatten out during ulnar abduction (Fig. 2.30).

2.11.6 Palpation of the Os Lunatum

The os lunatum is located ulnar to the os scaphoideum in the proximal carpal row. To separate the bone edges from each other, the scaphoid bone is fixed in a pincer grip and the lunate bone is moved slightly dorsally and palmar with the same grip technique. The bone wheels can be clearly felt (Fig. 2.31).

2.11.7 Palpation of the Os Pisiforme

From the palmar view of the hand, the os pisiforme is located in the proximal ulnar quadrant immediately distal to the ulna. Palpation of the pea bone can be done both flat and in a forceps grip. As a sesamoid bone, the os pisiforme is located directly palmar to the os triquetrum and is embedded in the

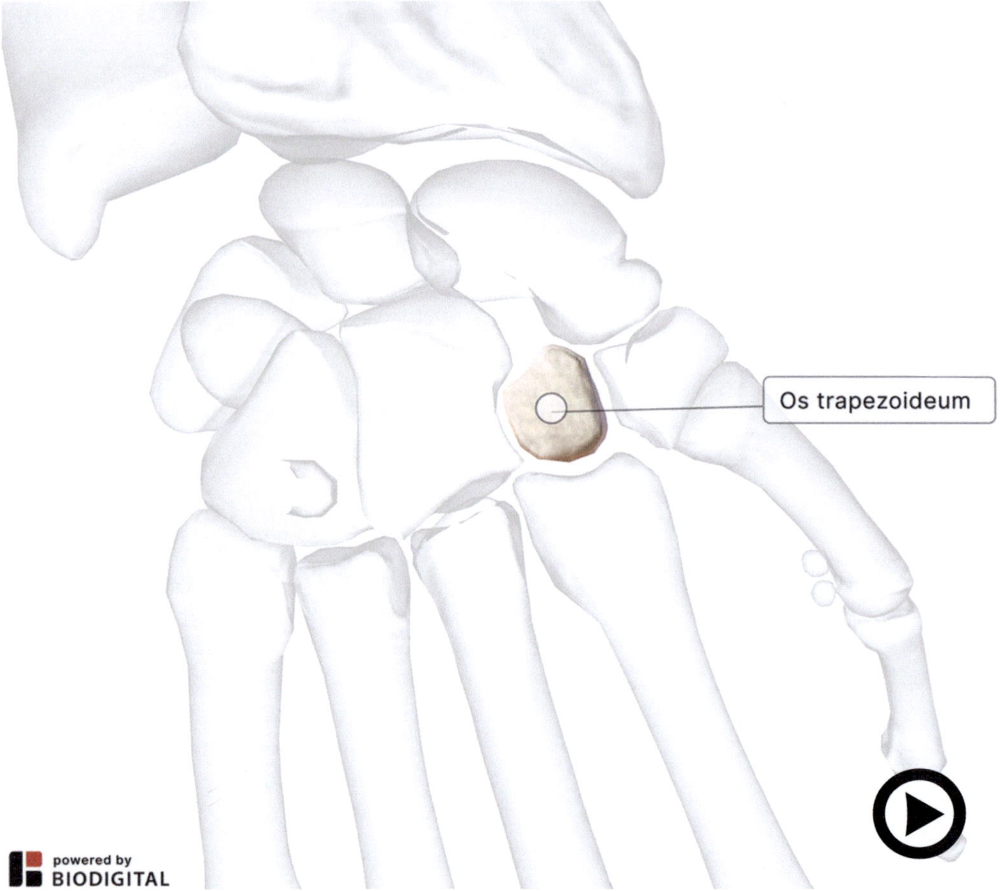

Fig. 2.28 Anatomy and palpation of the os trapezoideum (▶ https://doi.org/10.1007/000-cq2)

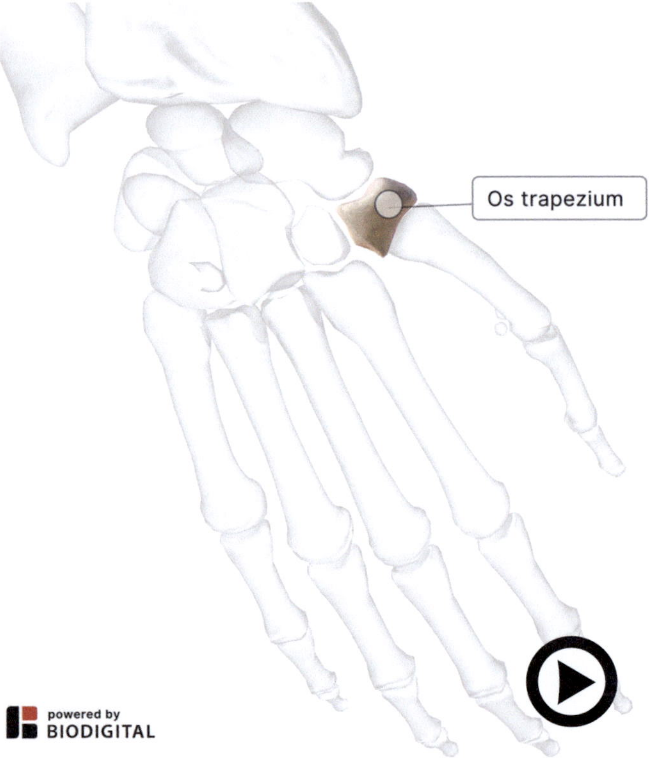

Fig. 2.29 Anatomy and palpation of the os trapezium (▶ https://doi.org/10.1007/000-cq3)

tendon of the m. flexor carpi ulnaris, which contracts during active ulnar abduction and leads directly to the pea bone (Fig. 2.32).

2.11.8 Palpation of the Os Triquetrum

The os triquetrum is attached distally to the discus articularis, which corresponds with the caput ulnae from the distal side. The pincer grip can be used to move the triquetrum proximally to the discus articularis or radially in relation to the os lunatum (Fig. 2.33).

2.11.9 Palpation of the Os Hamatum

The hamate bone joins the triquetral bone distally on the ulnar side. The os hamatum can be palpated opposite the os triquetrum or alternatively opposite the os capitatum. In both variants, the respective bone should be fixed with the forceps grip and moved against the hooked bone. This makes the bone edges clearly perceptible. The hamulus ossis hamati, which can be easily palpated as a protrusion, is located on the palmar os hamatum. This hook can best be felt through the steeply positioned long finger of the index finger (Fig. 2.34).

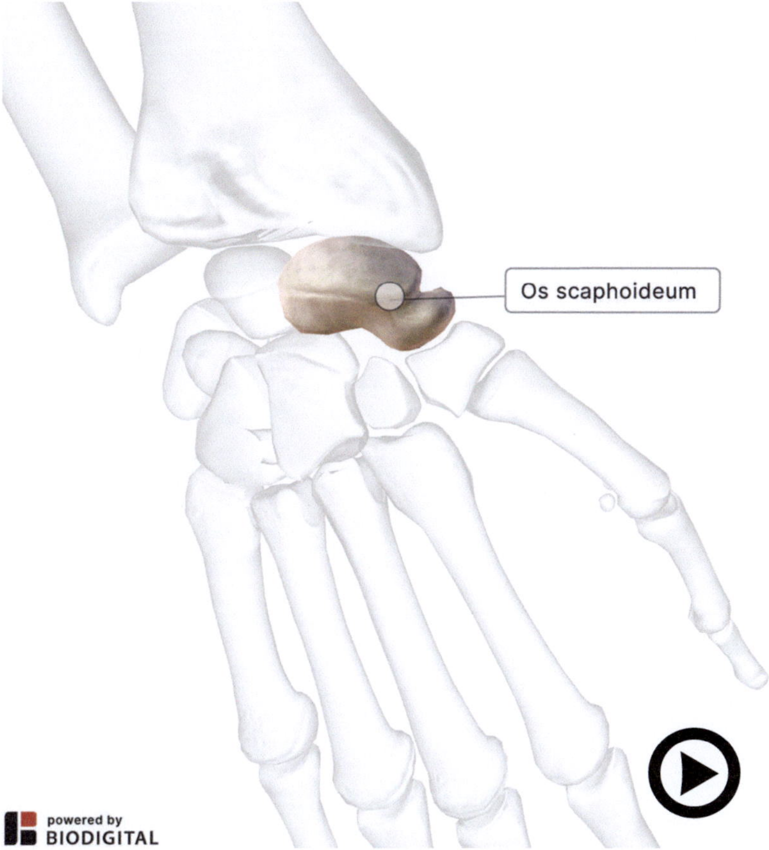

Fig. 2.30 Anatomy and palpation of the os scaphoideum (▶ https://doi.org/10.1007/000-cq4)

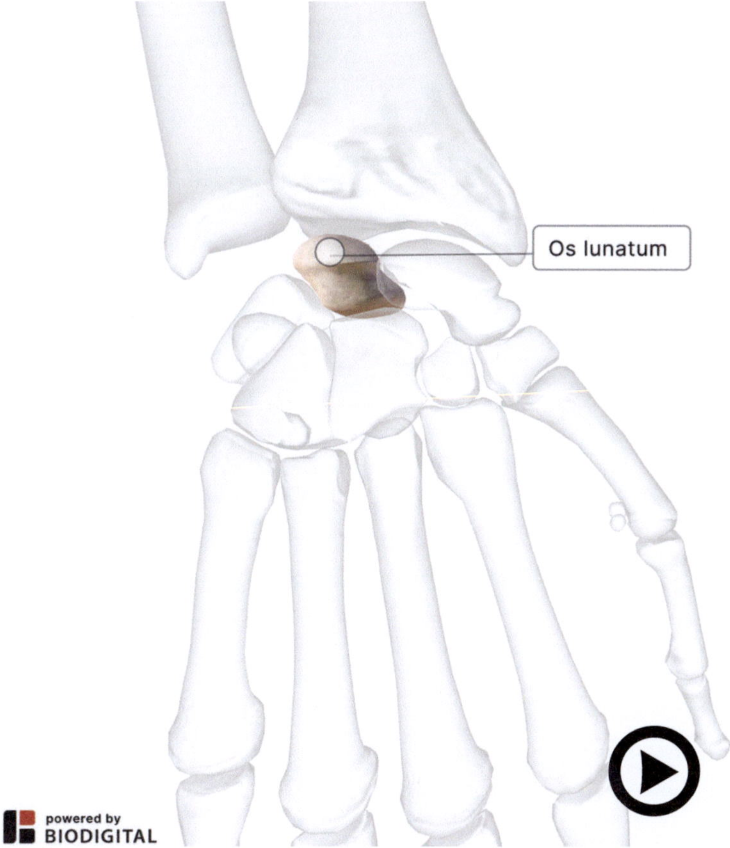

Fig. 2.31 Anatomy and palpation of the os lunatum (▶ https://doi.org/10.1007/000-cq5)

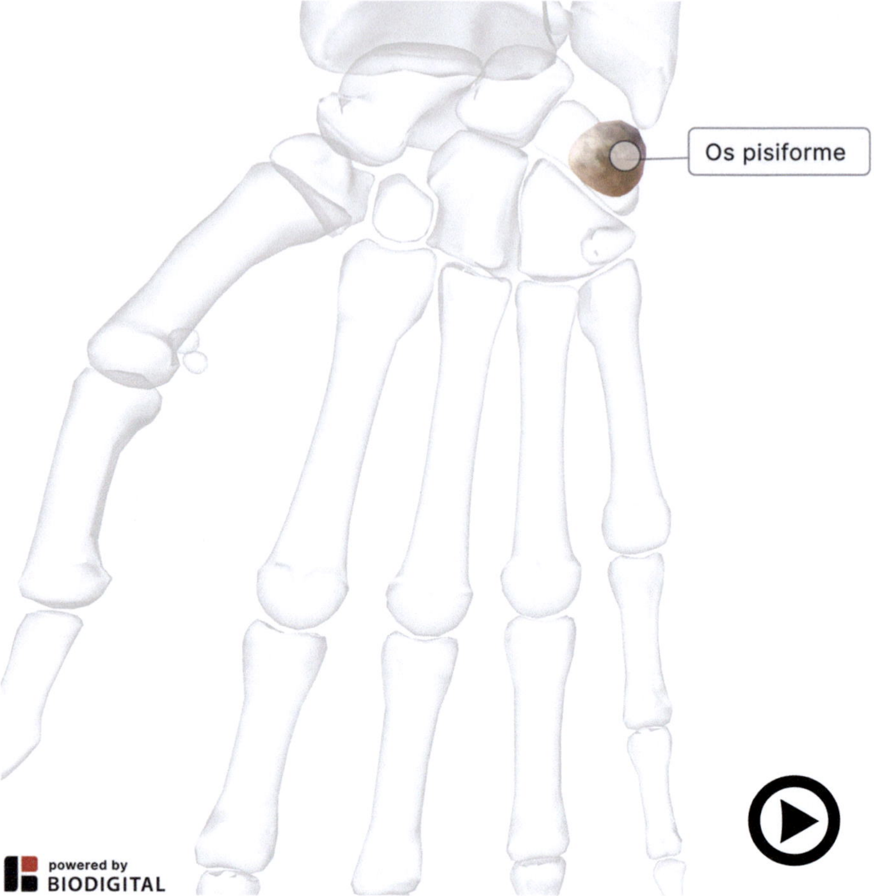

Fig. 2.32 Anatomy and palpation of the os pisiforme (▶ https://doi.org/10.1007/000-cq6)

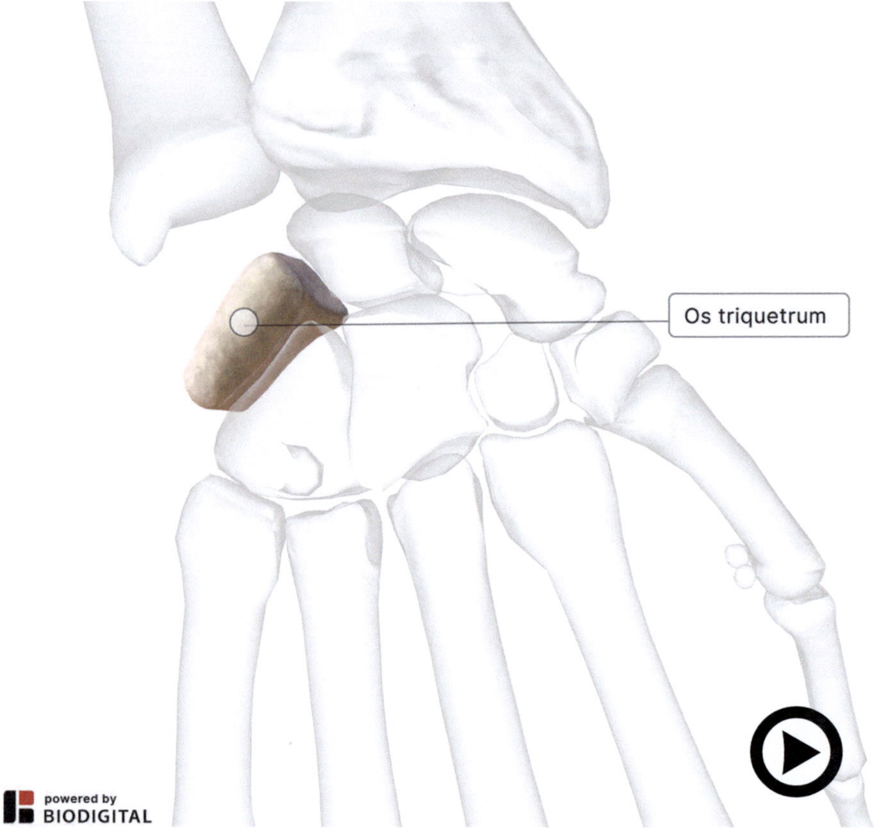

Fig. 2.33 Anatomy and palpation of the os triquetrum (▶ https://doi.org/10.1007/000-cq7)

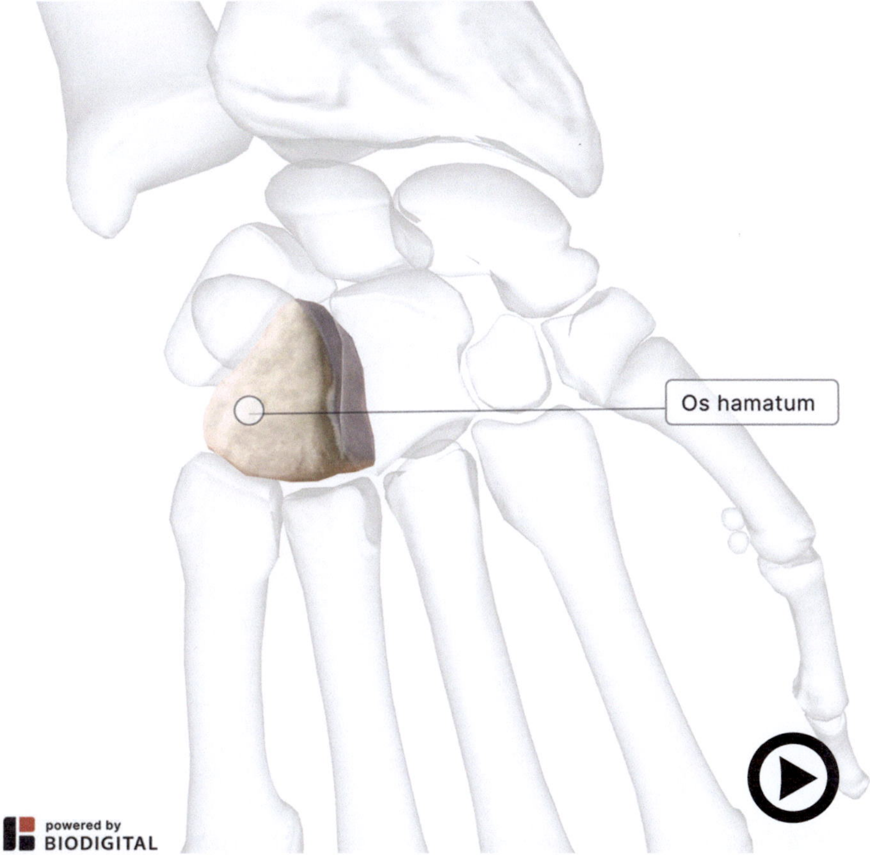

Fig. 2.34 Anatomy and palpation of the os hamatum (▶ https://doi.org/10.1007/000-cq8)

2.11.10 Palpation of the Ossa Phalangeales Manus

The ossa digitorum are each formed by two or three phalanges. The thumb has a proximal and a distal phalanx. The index finger, middle finger, ring finger and little finger each have a proximal, a medial and a distal phalanx. The phalanges are tubular bones and consist of a concave base, a corpus and a convex caput from proximal to distal [15]. Palpation starts from the metacarpophalangeal joints. In the case of an inflected metacarpophalangeal joint, the palpation finger is placed on the caput of the respective metacarpal and then palpated distally with gentle pressure until a small depression is felt. This depression marks the joint space and is in the immediate vicinity of the base of the proximal phalanx. From the base, which is again palpable as a small enhancement, the proximal phalanx is palpated via the interphalangeal joints to the distal phalanx in a forceps or forceps grip. The phalanges can also be palpated with small, translatory movement impulses to be able to delimit the bone edges from neighbouring structures (Fig. 2.35).

2.11.11 Palpation of the Sesamoid Manus Ossa

Distally on the caput of the os metacarpale I, there are palmar two sesamoid bones. The best way to identify the directly adjacent sesamoid bones is to use the fingertip of the index finger. To do this, the flat index fingertip is placed directly at the level of the metacarpophalangeal joint of the thumb from the palmar side and palpated in depth.

Implementation Note

The following points can be more symptomatic during palpation. Therefore, proceed with particular caution here.

- Bones of the proximal carpal row
  - Dorsal limit of the carpal tunnel
- Os trapezium
  - For rhizarthrosis (Fig. 2.36)

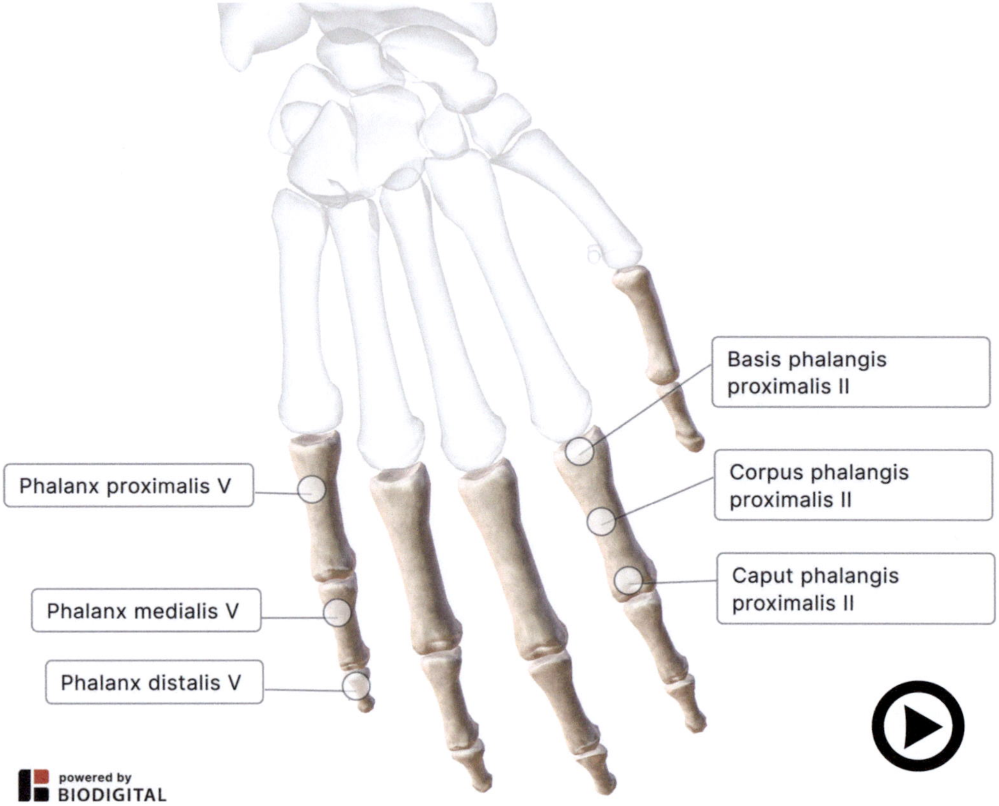

Fig. 2.35 Anatomy and palpation of the ossa phalangeales (▶ https://doi.org/10.1007/000-cq9)

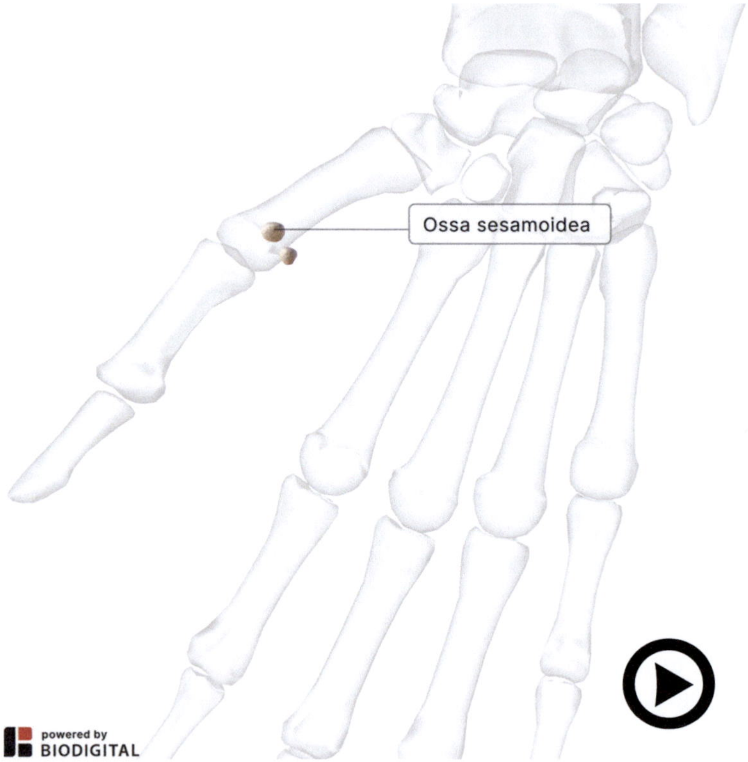

Fig. 2.36 Anatomy and palpation of the ossa sesamoidea (▶ https://doi.org/10.1007/000-cqa)

2.12 The Skull

Whether visual, auditory, olfactory or gustatory stimuli, all are received and processed in the cranial region [16]. In addition to the presence of various sensory systems, the cranium also houses the most important control centre of the human organism, the brain. To protect this and at the same time be optimally adapted to various requirements, a complex, bony construction is needed that makes it possible to meet these demands. In general, the osseous structure of the head is oval shaped. This structure is optimal for the transmission and distribution of acting forces. On closer inspection, it is noticeable that the skull is composed of several bones, most of which are connected to each other by suturae. The bony head can be divided into a neurocranium, which surrounds the brain, and a viscerocranium, which forms the facial features. Functionally, due to the anatomical correspondence, the os hyoideum ventral to the cervical spine can be counted as part of the bony skull. The cranial sutures, which connect the individual bones with each other in the neurocranium and viscerocranium, are necessary for the flexibility of the skull. This plays an important role at birth and during the growth process. To derive an adequate diagnosis or therapy, it is necessary to be able to palpate the bones as well as the accessible sutures of the cranium. These structures are palpated with moderate pressure using the fingertips. In addition, the palpable osseous reference points are indispensable for the general topographical orientation on the skull. The most important bony palpation points are presented below in the order neurocranium, viscerocranium and os hyoideum. It is advisable to position the patient in a supine position or alternatively in a sitting position.

2.12.1 Neurocranium

The neurocranium, which surrounds and protects the brain, consists of several bones. The os frontale, os parietale, os temporale and os occipitale belong to the bones accessible to palpation. Furthermore, the auditory ossicles and the sphenoidal bone define the neurocranium, but these are not palpable.

2.12.1.1 Palpation of the Os Frontale

The os frontale forms the forehead shape of the skull, which is individual from person to person. This bone, with its convex facies externa, is very easy to palpate with the flatly placed fingertips. Vertically ascending from the eyeball, there is a frontal tuberosity on both sides, which can be felt as a prominent elevation. In the caudal direction, the right and left arcus superciliaris are located. The respective eyebrow bulge is palpable as a distinct bony thickening cranial to the orbital rims. The eyebrows serve as a point of orientation for unerringly locating the respective arcus superciliaris. Starting from this point, the margo supraorbitalis is located immediately caudal. There are further palpable bone deformations at the upper edge of the orbit. Starting medially, the incisura frontalis appears as a small indentation on both sides of the supraorbital edge. One transverse finger laterally and half a transverse finger cranially to the incisura frontalis are the supraorbital foramen. At the lateral edge of the orbit, there is the palpable processus zygomaticus ossis frontalis. This corresponds via the sutura frontozygomatica with the processus frontalis ossis zygomaticus, which connects caudally.

The following points can be more symptomatic during palpation. Therefore, proceed with particular caution here.

- Supraorbital foramen
  - Exit of the supraorbital nerve (Fig. 2.37)

2.12.1.2 Palpation of the Parietal Bone

The os parietale is arranged in pairs and shapes the craniolateral surface of the skull. It is an almost rectangular bone that forms the cranial roof. The parietal bone can be optimally palpated by means of flatly placed long finger berries. At the border areas of the bone surface, cranial sutures can be identified which distinguish the os parietale from its surroundings. Directly in the middle of the skullcap, the sagittal suture with its posteroanterior course can be palpated as a prominent bony ridge. It forms the dividing or connecting line between the right and left parietal bone. Anteriorly, the os parietale is delimited from the os frontale on both sides by the sutura coronalis. The cranial suture separating the parietal bone from the occipital bone is the sutura lambdoidea. On the outer surface of the os parietale, the tuber parietale can also be identified on both sides as an elevation with the finger berries. Below this bump, two arcuate osseous lines can be palpated, the linea temporalis superior ossis parietalis and the linea temporalis inferior ossis parietalis (Fig. 2.38).

2.12.1.3 Palpation of the Temporal Bone

The temporal bone is located inferolaterally of the parietal bone. Via the sutura occiptotemporalis rising from the pars petrosa of the os temporale, this bone separates from the os occipitale, with which it forms the base of the skull. The very multifaceted temporal bone consists of four parts (pars squamosa, pars tympanica, pars mastoidea, pars petrosa), which form a variety of osseous contours. The following text contains those areas of the temporal bone which can be palpated. In the centre of the arcus zygomaticus, the sutura sphenosquamosa can be palpated with the fingertips as a vertically ascending cranial suture in a craniocaudal form. Starting from the sutura temporozygomatica, palpate cranially with

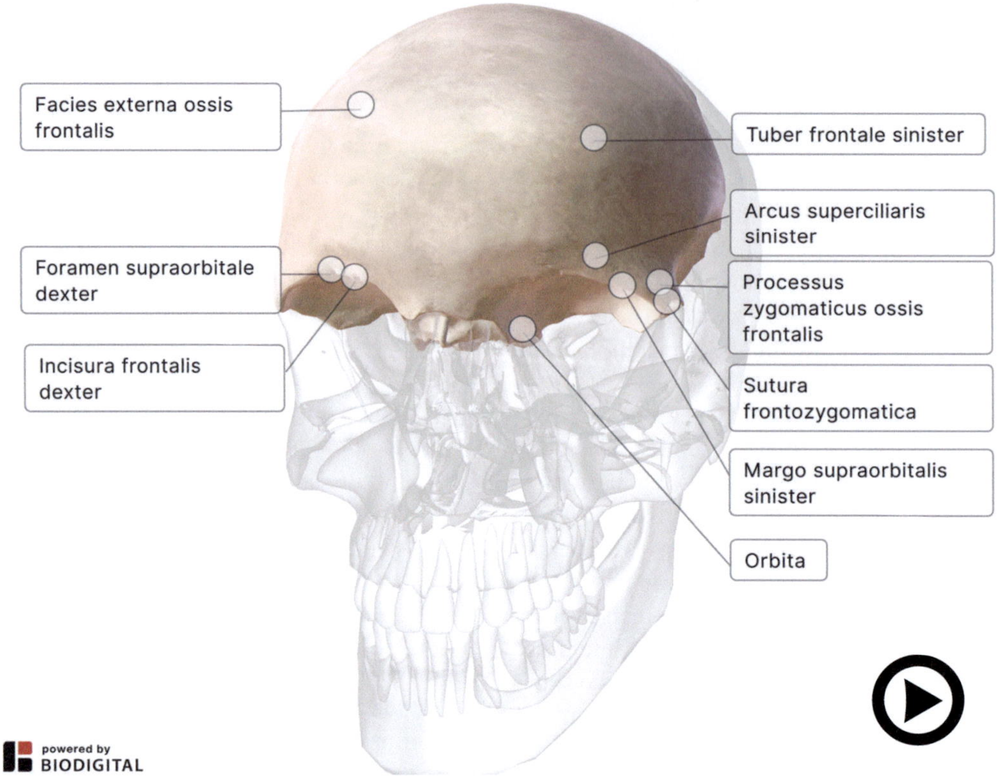

Fig. 2.37 Anatomy and palpation of the os frontale (▶ https://doi.org/10.1007/000-cqb)

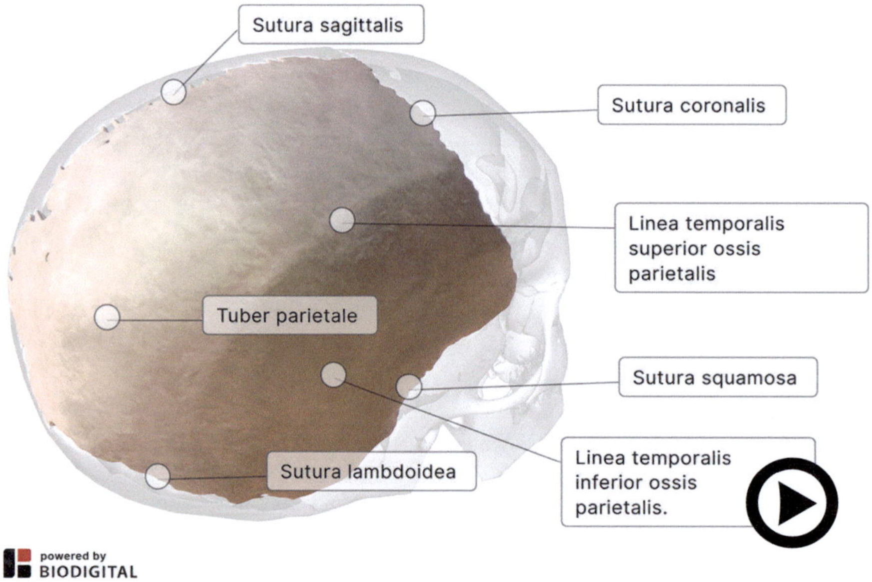

Fig. 2.38 Anatomy and palpation of the os parietale (▶ https://doi.org/10.1007/000-cqc)

the finger berries laid flat. After a small depression, the suture is palpable as an ascending dividing line. It forms the rostral border of the temporal bone.

The sutura squamosa, which forms the boundary to the os parietale, is located cranially in the front. In the occipital area, behind the ear, there is the sutura parietomastoidea, which continues caudally in the sutura occipitotemporalis. Along this cranial suture, at the most caudal end, the processus mastoideus can be felt in depth with the fingertips as a massive bony protrusion. If the os temporale is examined in detail, further palpation points can be found on the individual components. The pars squamosa is located cranially of the ear. The palpable point here is the facies temporalis. In the anterior area of this part, there is the palpable sulcus arteriae temporalis mediae, which leads the arteria temporalis media. This can be clearly felt via a rhythmically recurring pulse wave. In the anterior region, the pars squamosa forms a part via the processus zygomaticus ossis temporalis, the arcus zygomaticus, which is palpable as a protrusion. Caudal to the zygomaticus ossis temporalis process is the mandibular fossa.

The pars tympanica, which forms the meatus acusticus externus, can be palpated anterior to the tragus with steeply placed fingers in the posterior direction. Occipital to the ear is the pars mastoidea. In this part, the clearly palpable processus mastoideus is located as a massive bony prominence. This mastoid process is often more pronounced in men than in women. The pars petrosa is the hardest bone in humans [17]. It is located in the inner ear and is therefore not palpable.

The following points can be more symptomatic during palpation. Therefore, proceed with particular caution here.

- Sulcus arteriae temporalis mediae
  - The arteria temporalis media leads
- Os temporale
  - Origin of the temporalis muscle
- Mastoid process
  - Attachment of the sternocleidomastoid muscle (Fig. 2.39)

2.12.1.4 Palpation of the Os Occipitale

The best way to feel the os occipitale is when the client is in the prone position or alternatively in the sitting position. It forms the back of the head and mainly protects the cerebellum. The occipital bone can be divided into a pars squamosa, a pars basilaris and a pars lateralis. The pars squamosa is the only palpable part. First, the external occipital protuberance, which is located posteriorly in the centre of the occipital bone, can be palpated with the fingertips as a distinct elevation. The cranial parts of the crista occipitalis externa can be felt running vertically from this to the caudal. The sutura lambdoidea can be palpated as a boundary to the parietal bone. The sutura occipitotemporalis is the dividing line between the os occipitale and the os temporale. Above the protuberantia occipitalis externa, the linea nuchalis suprema is palpable as a slightly raised, almost horizontal structure. Below the external occipital protuberance, there are the nuchal lines, which are also almost horizontal. They are divided into a linea nuchae superior and inferior. These, as well as the linea nuchalis suprema, can be palpated transversely to their horizontal course with erect fingertips.

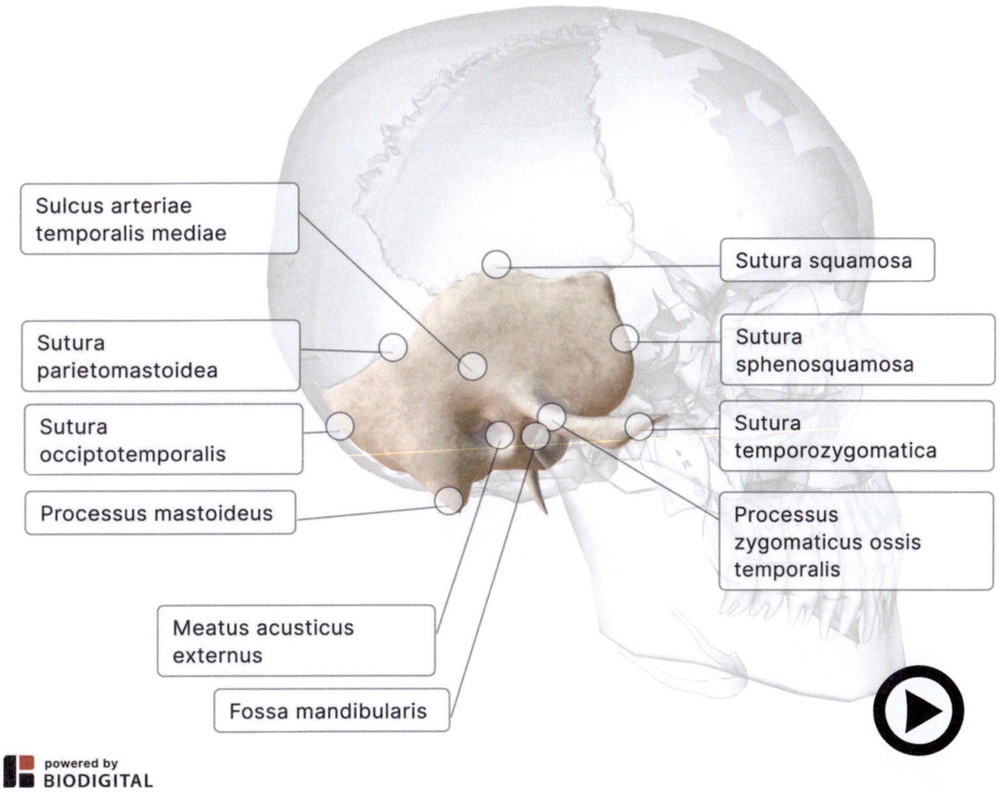

Fig. 2.39 Anatomy and palpation of the os temporale (▶ https://doi.org/10.1007/000-cqd)

Implementation Note

The following points can be more symptomatic during palpation. Therefore, proceed with particular caution here.

- Linea nuchae inferior
  - Insertion of the obliquus capitis superior, rectus capitis major and rectus capitis minor muscles (Fig. 2.40)

2.12.2 Viscerocranium

The numerous bones of the viscerocranium are essentially responsible for the features of the human face. The os zygomaticum, the os nasale as well as the maxilla and mandibula represent the bones of the facial skull that are accessible to palpation. Furthermore, the os lacrimale, the vomer, the concha nasales as well as the os palatinum and the os ethmoidale define themselves as belonging to the viscerocranium. However, these bones are not palpable.

Implementation Note

- All sutures are gently palpated first, as they may be pressure-dolent.
- All foramina are gently palpated as nerves and vessels emerge.
- All structures in the oral cavity are palpated with a glove.

2.12.2.1 Palpation of the Os Zygomaticum

The os zygomaticum is located laterally in the face and shapes the characteristic form of the cheeks. To palpate this bone, a raised bony ridge is palpated directly anterior to the external auditory canal over the long finger berries. This prominent region forms the processus zygomaticus ossis temporalis of the os temporale. Palpation is made anteriorly along this bony ridge via the erect long finger berries. The sutura temporozygomatica can be palpated as a cranial suture running almost perpendicular to the course of palpation. After this suture, which is located approximately after the posterior third of the arcus zygomaticus, the os zygomaticum is directly connected. The starting point is the processus temporalis ossis zygomaticus as a clear elevation. The further course of the cheekbone can be clearly differentiated from the surrounding soft tissues, as it lies superficially and the edges can be easily palpated. Starting narrowly, the arcus zygomaticus becomes increasingly broader anteriorly. Cranial to the temporalis ossis zygomaticus is the frontalis ossis zygomaticus. Anterocaudally to the arcus zygomaticus, the zygomatic bone continues with the help of the processus maxillaris ossis zygomaticus. The edges of the zygomaticus can be easily outlined by the fingertips of the long fingers using the described processes. Directly in the centre, the zygomaticofacial foramen can be palpated as a small depression over the erect tip of the index finger. The artery, vein and zygomatic nerve pass

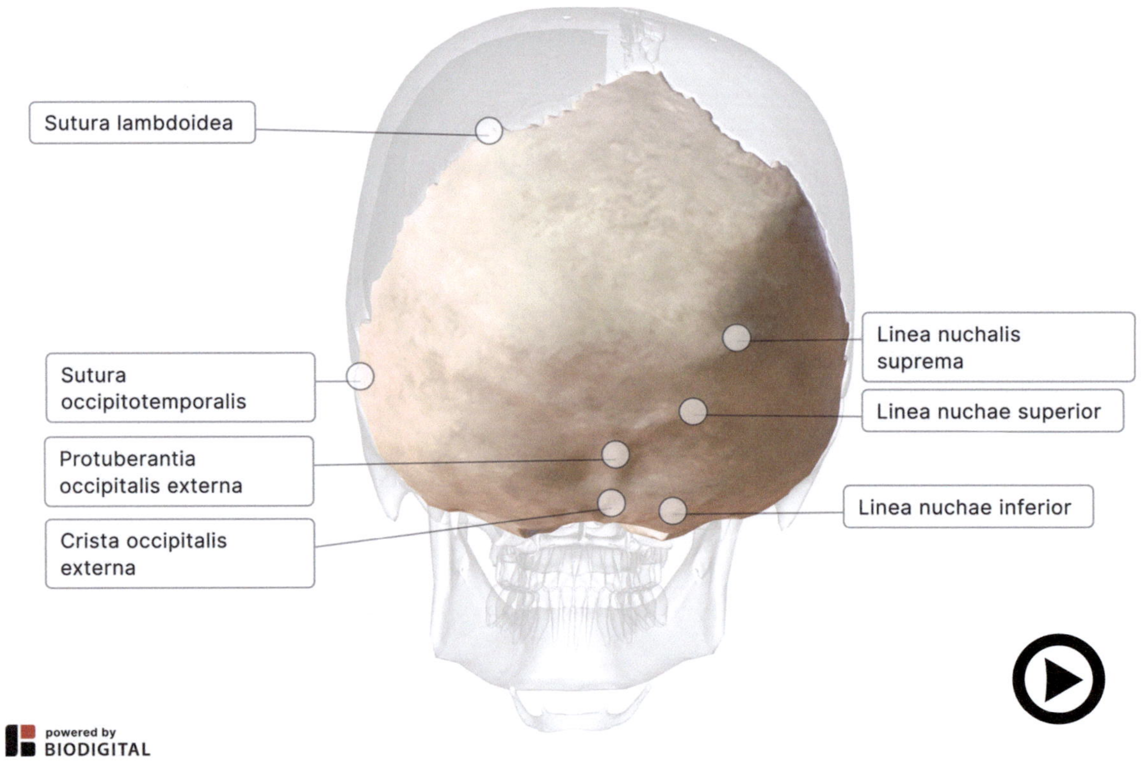

Fig. 2.40 Anatomy and palpation of the os occipitale (▶ https://doi.org/10.1007/000-cqe)

through this opening. Therefore, this structure can also be localised by a pulse wave. The upper area of this bone shapes the inferolateral part of the orbit and can therefore be felt as a distinct edge below the eye (Fig. 2.41).

2.12.2.2 Palpation of the Os Nasale

The os nasale is in pairs, is counted as part of the viscerocranium and forms the initial bony part of the nose. This small, elongated bone, located between the eye sockets, is very easy to palpate. Palpation of this bone begins directly in the osseous depression between the eyes. This is the site of the nasofrontal sutura, which separates the os frontale from the os nasale. Then palpate with the fingertips of the index finger over the bony bridge of the nose caudally to the transition into the nasal cartilage. The transition can be found by palpating the bridge of the nose from cranial to caudal using the forceps grip. During palpation, small mobilisation impulses to the right and left can be initiated by the examiner. If no movement is perceptible during these impulses, palpation still takes place on the os nasale; if movement to the right and left is perceptible, the palpating fingers are already on the cartilago nasi.

Implementation Note

The following points can be more symptomatic during palpation. Therefore, proceed with particular caution here.

- Foramen zygomaticofaciale: exit artery, vena and nervus zygomaticus (Fig. 2.42)

2.12.2.3 Palpation of the Os Maxillare

The multifaceted maxilla, located in the centre, forms the second largest bone of the viscerocranium and houses the teeth of the upper jaw. This paired bone has a decisive influence on the shape of the face. The outer structures of the

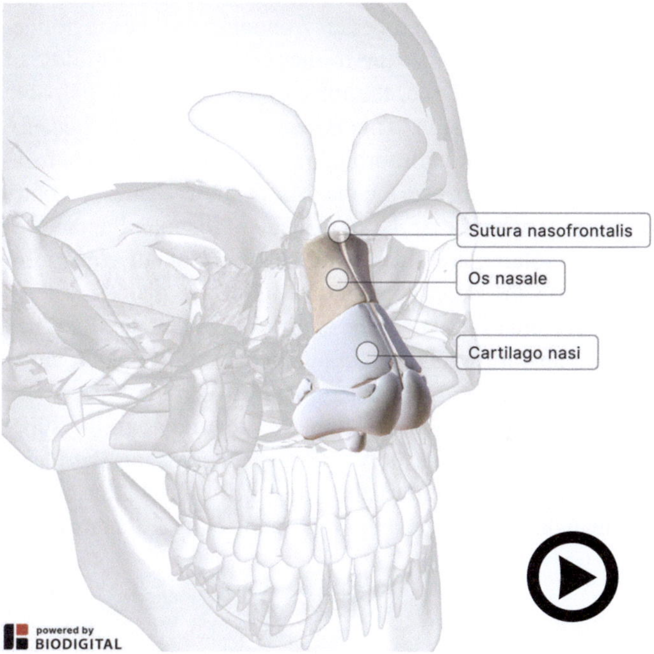

Fig. 2.42 Anatomy and palpation of the os nasale (▶ https://doi.org/10.1007/000-cqg)

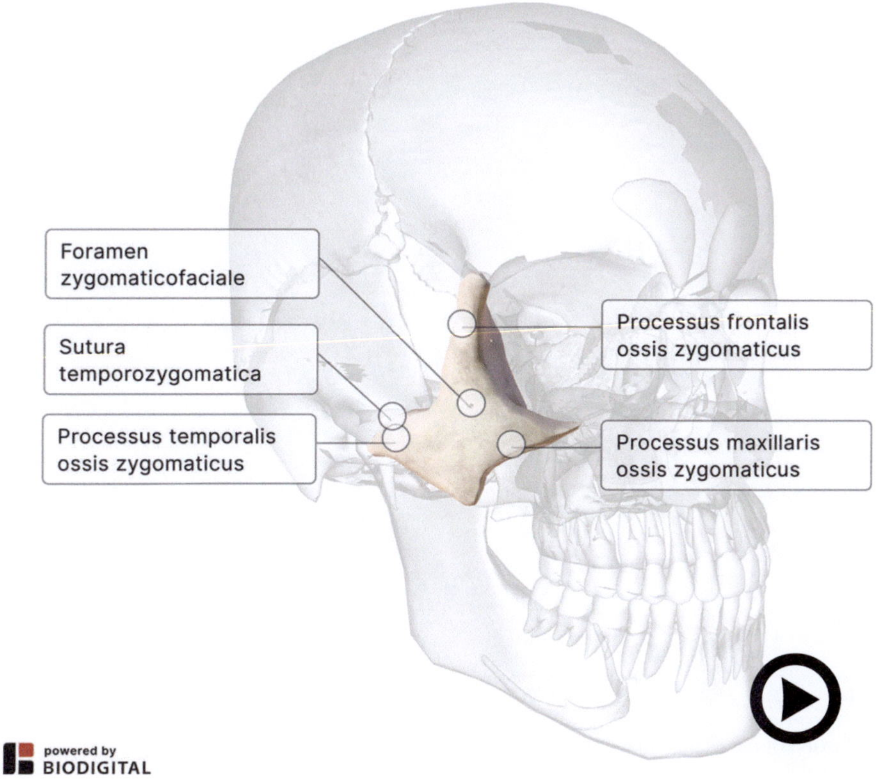

Fig. 2.41 Anatomy and palpation of the os zygomaticum (▶ https://doi.org/10.1007/000-cqf)

maxilla can be easily palpated with the long finger berries. It should be noted that soft tissue of the cheeks lies over this bone. Palpation is performed in the supine position and begins laterally at the os nasale, which is separated from the maxilla by the palpable sutura nasomaxillaris. Directly in this area of the facies anterior is the margo infraorbitalis, which forms part of the orbit and can be felt as a distinct edge. In this area, the processus frontalis maxillae are noticeable as an elevation. A little further caudally, in the middle of the inferior orbital rim, the infraorbital foramen is palpable as a small depression. This structure is significant because the artery, vein and infraorbital nerve pass through this foramen. Towards the nose, the maxilla closes as a ring-like bony apertura piriformis. At the caudal end of the maxilla, the processi alveolares are clearly noticeable as small elevations. They form the dental compartments of the maxillary teeth and therefore extend over the entire area of the maxilla. They are palpable through the skin but can also be palpated under the upper lip directly on the gums. Between these processes are the alveolar canals, which carry the artery and the superior posterior alveolar nerve. Further laterally on the facies infratemporalis maxillae, the crista infrazygomatica is palpable in depth just below the zygomatic bone as a bony ridge. In the posterior area of this surface, the maxillary tuberosity is clearly palpable as a hump. Cranially to this tuber, there is the processus zygomaticus, which delimits the maxilla from the os zygomaticus. This process is palpated in depth via the steeply positioned finger berries.

In addition to the reference points accessible from the outside, structures in the cavitas oris can be felt. It is important that the examiner wears gloves. Directly in the anterior region of the maxilla, behind the incisors, there is a foramen incisivum in the middle. This is palpable as a depression over the fingertips. Posterior to the foramen incisivum is the palpable sutura palatina mediana. To the right and left of this suture is the palatinus maxillae process, which can be felt as a bump.

Implementation Note

The following points can be more symptomatic during palpation. Therefore, proceed with particular caution here.

- Foramen infraorbitale: exit arteria, vena and nervus infraorbitalis
- Foramen incisivum: exit nasopalatine nerve and descending palatine artery (Figs. 2.43 and 2.44)

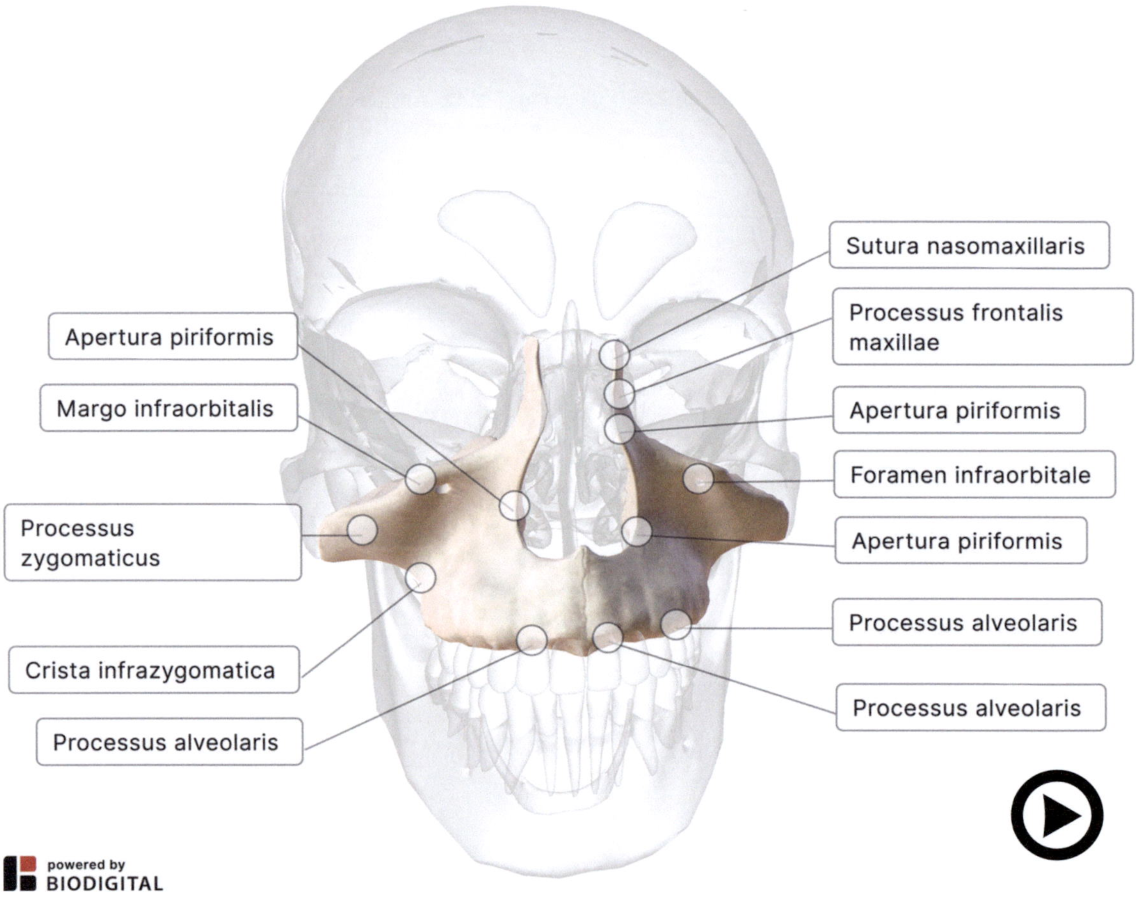

Fig. 2.43 Anatomy and palpation of the os maxillare (▶ https://doi.org/10.1007/000-cqh)

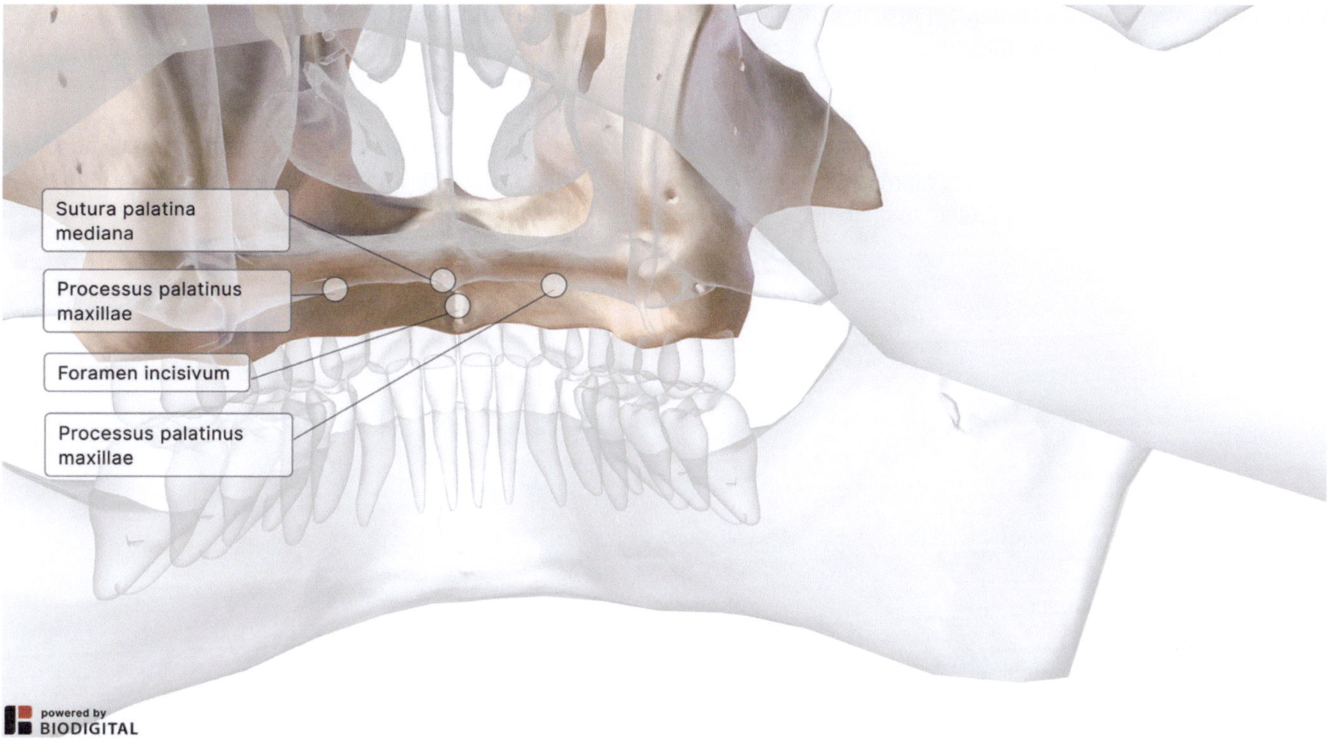

Fig. 2.44 Anatomy and palpation of the os maxillare

2.12.2.4 Palpation of the Os Mandibulare

Deriving from the Latin word "mandere" (meaning to chew), the mandible is the only movable bone of the viscerocranium. The mandible is horseshoe shaped and is divided into a corpus and an angulus and subsequent ramus mandibulae on the right and left sides. This multifaceted bone holds the lower 16 teeth and at the same time provides a surface for numerous muscles that originate or are attached here.

Palpation starts anteriorly at the corpus mandibulae with the protuberantia mentalis. This is where the two halves of the mandible meet and form the chin. This structure is clearly perceptible through the flatly placed fingertip. Directly to the right and left of the protuberantia, there is a mental tubercle. In the further course of the corpus posteriorly, the mental foramen can be palpated as a small depression. This opening, which is still in the anterior third of the corpus, carries the mental nerve. Starting from the mental foramen, the linea obliqua can be palpated obliquely posterocranially as a bony ridge. In the further course of the corpus, the alveolar processes are palpable as clearly prominent dental compartments with the flat fingertips. In the posterior region of the mandible is the angulus mandibulae, which as a turning point merges into the following ramus mandibulae. On the mandibular arch is the masseteric tuberosity, which is palpable as a rough surface. The course of the ramus mandibulae can be clearly felt at the posterior edge with the fingertips. It ends at the caput mandibulae via the condylar process. This forms the convex joint partner of the temporomandibular joint and can be palpated very well via the fingertips, which are placed anterior to the auditory canal. Subsequently, the osseous edge of the caput mandibulae can be palpated via the opening and closing of the mandible. Anterior to the caput mandibulae, the incisura mandibulae can be felt as an indentation which ends in the coronoid process. This process is located directly below the zygomatic bone and is therefore rather difficult to palpate. In addition, palpation in this region is complicated by masseter muscles. Therefore, the jaw muscles should be relaxed when feeling osseous structures.

Further osseous palpation areas on the mandible can be felt in the cavitas oris. Gloves are worn for hygienic reasons. Directly behind the anterior lower incisors is the fovea sublingualis, which extends over the right and left inner corpus. Below this fovea, the linea mylohyoidea runs obliquely posteriocranially and is palpable as an edge. Below this edge is another depression, the fovea submandibularis. Starting from the anterior lower incisors, the spinae mentales follow caudally, which are palpable as prominent tips, next to the digastric fossa. Further posteriorly, the corpus can be accessed via the forceps or forceps grip from the inside and outside. The shaft ends in the ramus mandibulae where the pterygoid tuberosity can be palpated. This roughness can also be felt from the outside. Behind the last molar, the retromolar fossa can be felt in the area of the trigonum retromolare mandibulare.

Implementation Note

The following points can be more symptomatic during palpation. Therefore, proceed with particular caution here.

- Foramen mentale: exit arteria, vena and nervus mentalis
  - Ramus mandibulae with tuberositas maseterica
- m. masseter approach (Fig. 2.45 and 2.46)

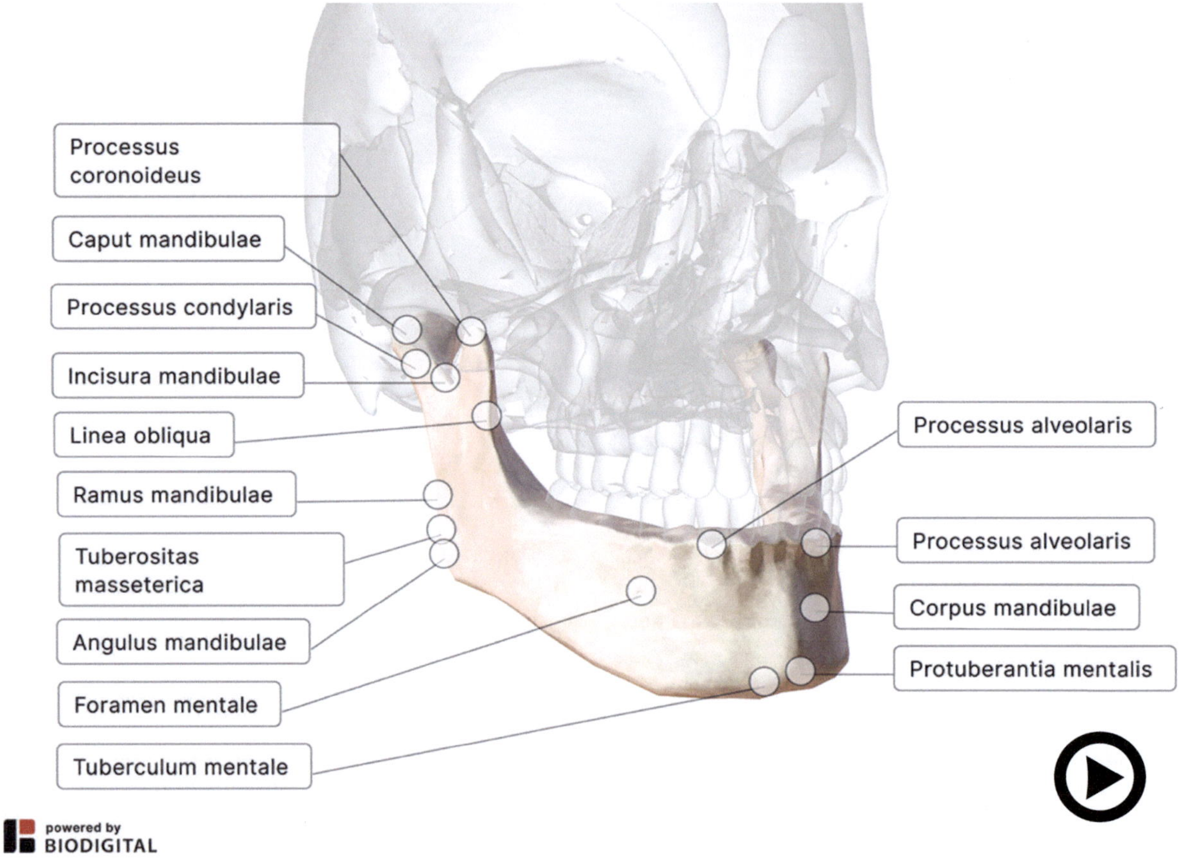

Fig. 2.45 Anatomy and palpation of the os mandibulare (▶ https://doi.org/10.1007/000-cpd)

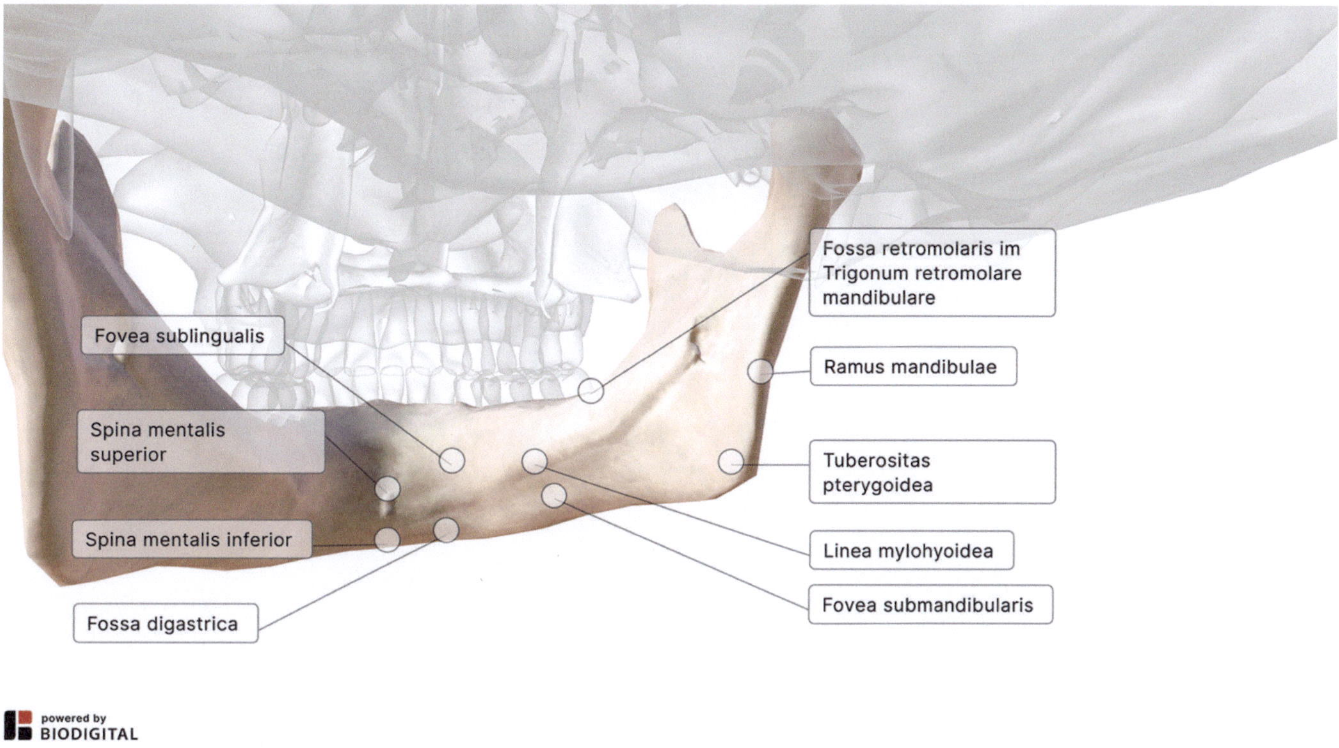

Fig. 2.46 Anatomy and palpation of the os mandibulare

2.13 Palpation of the Os Hyoideum

The hyoid bone is a small, horseshoe-shaped bone located anterior to the cervical spine at C3–4 and enclosing the trachea and oesophagus. Since the hyoid bone does not articulate bony with the cervical spine and is only connected to the head by muscles and ligaments, it is anatomically counted as part of the skull. Functionally, it is an important pivot and pivotal point and is important for the swallowing process, speaking, breathing and targeted chewing and tongue movements [18]. For these reasons, it is important to be able to palpate this bone. Cranially of the larynx and below the mandible, the hyoid can be easily grasped directly on the corpus ossis hyoidei using forceps. At the lateral edges, the cornu majus can also be felt. In the anterolateral region of the hyoid bone, a cornu minus is located in each case, which can be felt as a small tip in depth. For better differentiation, the hyoid bone can be moved to the right and left, as it is mobile. This mobility is particularly important for the functionality of the hyoid bone.

Implementation Note

- The movement of the hyoid has to be done carefully as it encloses sensitive structures, and this can be perceived as uncomfortable for the client (Fig. 2.47).

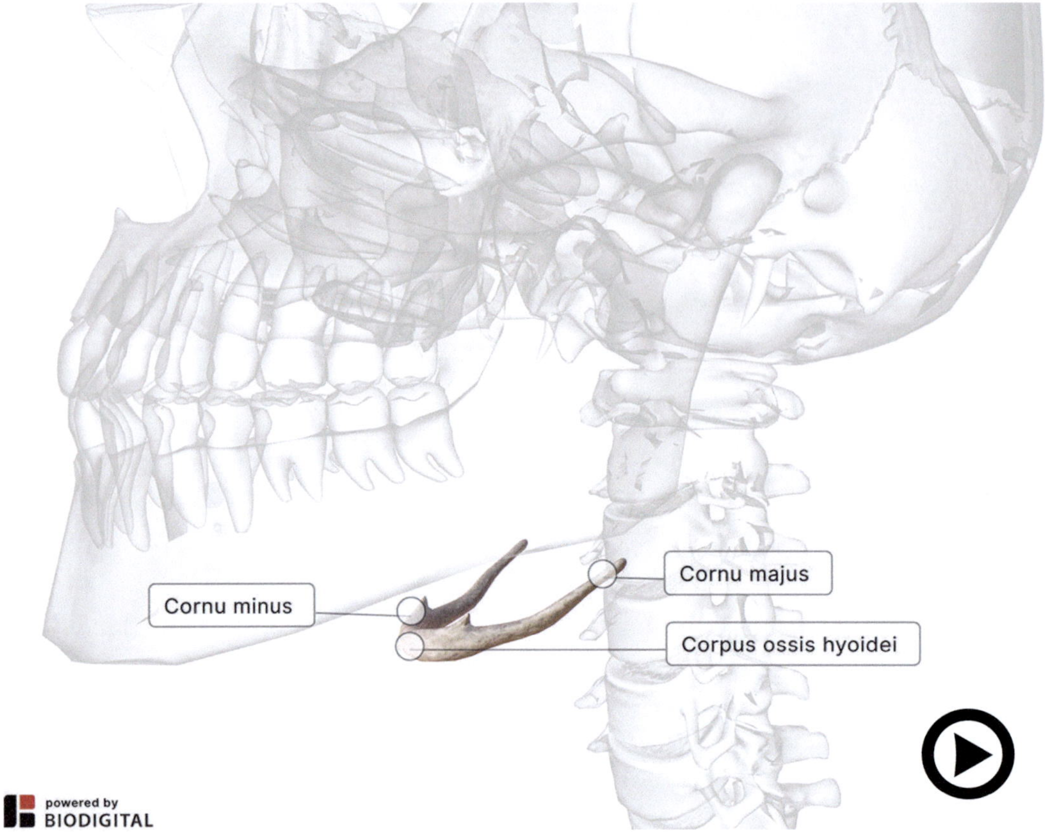

Fig. 2.47 Anatomy and palpation of the os hyoideum (▶ https://doi.org/10.1007/000-cqk)

References

1. Vleeming, A., & Schuenke, M. (2019). Form and force closure of the sacroiliac joints. *PM & R, 11*(Suppl 1), 24–31. https://doi.org/10.1002/pmrj.12205
2. Friedrichsen, H.-P. (2007). Industriekost trifft Steinzeitgenetik: Ist die moderne Zivilisationskost für den Menschen geeignet? *Zeitschrift für Orthomolekulare Medizin, 3*(3), 16–20. https://doi.org/10.1055/s-2007-965594
3. Maciałczyk-Paprocka, K., Stawińska-Witoszyńska, B., Kotwicki, T., Sowińska, A., Krzyżaniak, A., Walkowiak, J., & Krzywińska-Wiewiorowska, M. (2017). Prevalence of incorrect body posture in children and adolescents with overweight and obesity. *European Journal of Pediatrics, 176*(5), 563–572. https://doi.org/10.1007/s00431-017-2873-4
4. Iijima, H., Ohi, H., Isho, T., Aoyama, T., Fukutani, N., Kaneda, E., et al. (2017). Association of bilateral flat feet with knee pain and disability in patients with knee osteoarthritis: A cross-sectional study. *Journal of Orthopaedic Research, 35*(11), 2490–2498. https://doi.org/10.1002/jor.23565
5. Cheng, J., & Song, J. (2003). Anatomy of the sacrum. *Neurosurgical Focus, 15*(2), E3. https://doi.org/10.3171/foc.2003.15.2.3
6. Shams, A., Gamal, O., & Mesregah, M. (2023, February 11). Sacrococcygeal morphologic and morphometric risk factors for idiopathic Coccydynia: A magnetic resonance imaging study. *Global Spine Journal, 13*, 140. https://doi.org/10.1177/2192568221993791
7. Yoshihara, H. (2012, September). Sacroiliac joint pain after lumbar/lumbosacral fusion: Current knowledge. *European Spine Journal, 21*(9), 1788–1796. https://doi.org/10.1007/s00586-012-2350-8
8. Shin, S., Yoon, D.-M., & Bong Yoon, K. (2011, May). Identification of the correct cervical level by palpation of spinous processes. *Anesthesia and Analgesia, 112*(5), 1232–1235. https://doi.org/10.1213/ANE.0b013e3182110f9f
9. Pysyk, C., Persaud, D., Bryson, G., & Lui, A. (2010, January). Ultrasound assessment of the vertebral level of the palpated intercristal (Tuffier's) line. *Canadian Journal of Anaesthesia, 57*(1), 46–49. https://doi.org/10.1007/s12630-009-9208-5
10. Lehtinen, J., Tingart, M., Apreleva, M., & Warner, J. (2005, May). Quantitative morphology of the scapula: Normal variation of the superomedial scapular angle, and superior and inferior pole thickness. *Orthopedics, 28*(5), 481–486. https://doi.org/10.3928/0147-7447-20050501-15
11. Havránek, P., Pešl, T., Hendrych, J., & Kučerová, M. (2018). Supracondylar fracture of the humerus in childhood. *Rozhledy v Chirurgii, 97*(3), 122–127.
12. Duncan, J., Duncan, R., Bansal, S., Davenport, D., & Hacker, A. (2019, November 2). Lateral epicondylitis: The condition and current management strategies. *British Journal of Hospital Medicine (London, England), 80*(11), 647–651. https://doi.org/10.12968/hmed.2019.80.11.647
13. Mauck, B., & Swigler, C. (2018, April). Evidence-based review of distal radius fractures. *The Orthopedic Clinics of North America, 49*(2), 211–222. https://doi.org/10.1016/j.ocl.2017.12.001

14. Kadar, A., Morsy, M., Sur, Y.-J., Laungani, A., Akdag, O., & Moran, S. (2017, February). The vascular anatomy of the capitate: New discoveries using micro-computed tomography imaging. *The Journal of Hand Surgery, 42*(2), 78–86. https://doi.org/10.1016/j.jhsa.2016.12.002
15. Melamud, K., Drapé, J.-L., Hayashi, D., Roemer, F., Zentner, J., & Guermazi, A. (2014, November–December). Diagnostic imaging of benign and malignant osseous tumors of the fingers. *Radiographics, 34*(7), 1954–1967. https://doi.org/10.1148/rg.347130031
16. Adesnik, H., & Naka, A. (2018, December 5). Cracking the function of layers in the sensory cortex. *Neuron, 100*(5), 1028–1043. https://doi.org/10.1016/j.neuron.2018.10.032
17. Reisser, C., Schubert, O., & Hagen, W. (1995). Chirurgische dreidimensionale Felsenbeinanatomie aus Spiral-CT-Daten. *Otorhinolaryngologia Nova, 5*(1), 47–52. https://doi.org/10.1159/000313164
18. Auvenshine, R., & Pettit, N. (2020, January). The hyoid bone: An overview. *Cranio, 38*(1), 6–14. https://doi.org/10.1080/08869634.2018.1487501

Palpation of the Joints

3

Contents

Supplementary Information The online version contains supplementary material available at https://doi.org/10.1007/978-3-662-69186-1_3. The videos can be accessed individually by clicking the DOI link in the accompanying figure caption or by scanning this link with the SN More Media App.

R. Bauer, S. Wolfram, *Atlas of Palpation*, https://doi.org/10.1007/978-3-662-69186-1_3

3.1 Basics of Palpation of Joints

Joints enable a fundamental function of the human organism, mobility. Mobility arises from the harmonious articulation of joint partners, which, due to their respective anatomical construction, express different types of joints. For high-quality examination and therapy, it is crucial to know the individually different construction as well as the resulting biomechanics of the respective articulation. However, before a therapy can take place at the joint, the region must be palpated to secure all clues at the "crime scene". In general, this chapter describes the procedure that can be used to palpate joint spaces. It also focuses on the specific palpation sensation. Before these explanations, the most important facts about the respective joint are summarised. Articulations in which the joint space is not palpable are not discussed in this book. Both the topographical position and overlying body structures in the area of joints can prevent palpation of the respective joint space. Some articular joints have already been described in relation to their osseous reference points during bony palpation; therefore, this chapter only refers to the palpable joint spaces. In general, it is helpful during palpation if the corresponding joint is moved slightly so that the articulating partners can be better identified. The specific performance of each of these techniques is described in the text and practically presented in the instructional videos. The joint partners and the joint space are felt via the long finger berries.

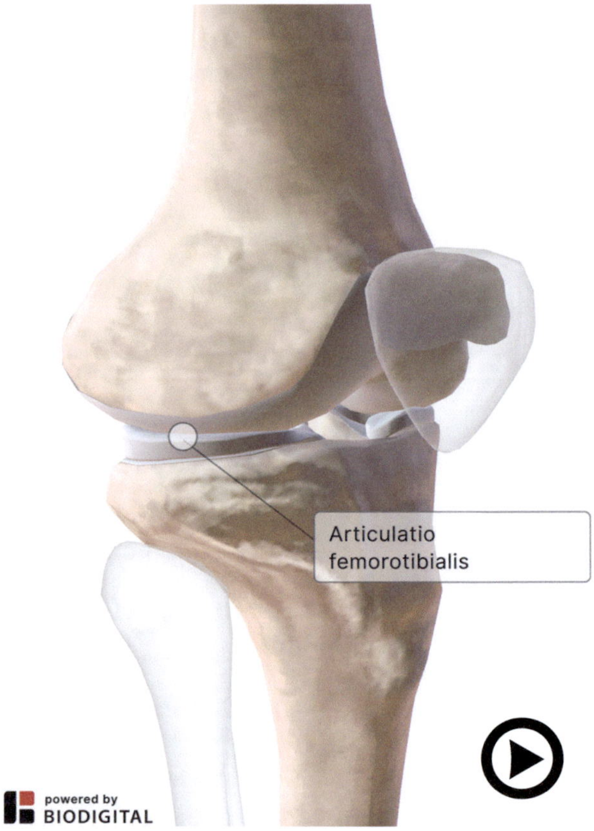

Fig. 3.1 Anatomy and palpation of the art. femorotibialis (▶ https://doi.org/10.1007/000-cr7)

3.2 Joints in the Area of the Knee

The knee joint forms a complex functional unit composed of several joints. The knee joint itself can first be divided into two joints (art. femorotibialis, art. femoropatellaris). Due to functionality, the art. tibiofibularis proximalis and distalis should also be considered here. From a biomechanical point of view, other sub-joints can be classified, but these play a subordinate role in palpation. In this palpation atlas, two articular joints in the area of the knee are highlighted. The recommended starting position is supine.

3.2.1 Palpation of the Femorotibial Joint

The transportable rotational hinge joint is a special joint because the possibility of movement in flexion, extension, and internal and external rotation, in combination with a high elastic deformability of the concave joint partner (the menisci), is unique [1].

The femoral condyles, which are convex in the sagittal plane, articulate with the superior concave menisci, which in turn should move on the tibial plateau. While the function of the medial meniscus can be influenced by its contact with the tibial collateral ligament, transverse genal ligament, semimembranosus muscle and medial meniscopatellar ligament, the lateral meniscus is associated with the popliteus muscle, lateral meniscopatellar ligament and transverse genal ligament. This knowledge is important for palpation of the developing joint space between femur and tibia with the patient in the supine position.

With the help of the lumbrical grip, contact is made medial and lateral to the knee below the apex patellae. Using a passive movement in flexion and extension, the femorotibial joint space can be located directly. Note that the collateral tibial and fibular ligaments are relaxed in slight flexion and thus palpation is best performed in this position. In addition, in the flexed position, a more precise differentiation can be made using a passively introduced external/internal rotation component. In extension, the collateral ligaments are tense and inhibit external rotation, whereas the non-palpable cruciate ligaments limit internal rotation in the flexed knee joint together with other structures (Fig. 3.1).

3.2.2 Palpation of the Femoropatellar Joint

Through its function as a hypomochlion, the patella enables an improvement in the leverage ratios, which in turn results in a higher force development [2]. Posterior to the patella is the facies articularis femoris patellae, which articulates with

Fig. 3.2 Anatomy and palpation of the art. femoropatellaris (▶ https://doi.org/10.1007/000-cqn)

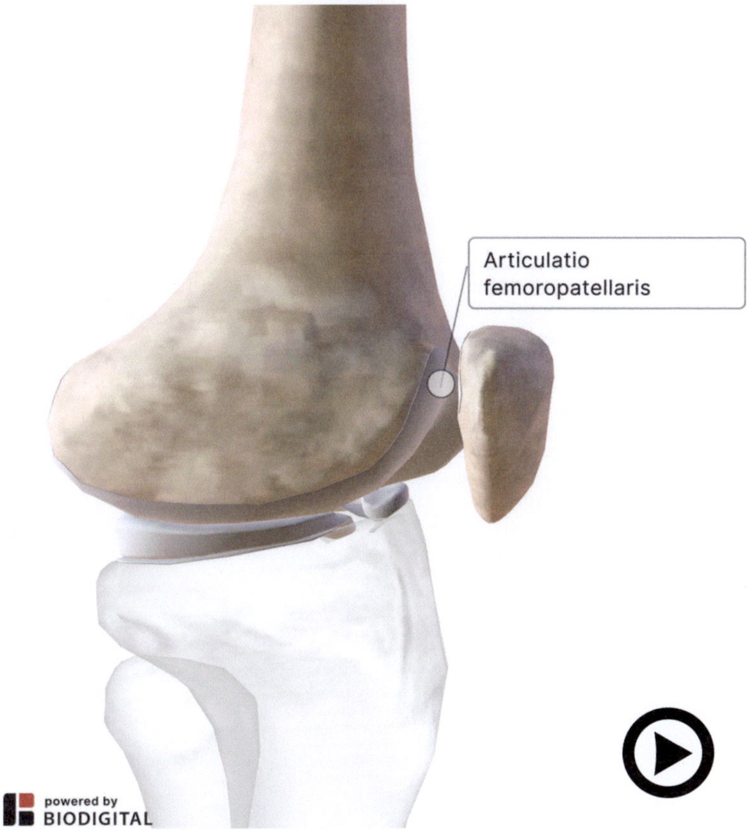

the facies articularis patellae femoris. Rotational movements of the art. femorotibialis are accompanied by combined translations in the art. femoropatellaris.

The patella can be felt anteriorly in the centre of the knee. Subsequently, the edges of the patella and thus medial and lateral parts of the retropatellar articulation surfaces can be palpated with the long finger berries or alternatively with the thumb. During palpation, it is advisable to move the sesamoid bone slightly medially and laterally to differentiate this joint even more precisely from the surrounding structures.

Implementation Note
The following criteria should be observed during palpation at the knee joint:

- The individual shape and alignment of the patella can vary greatly from person to person.
- Habitual dislocations in the retropatellar joint usually occur laterally, so care should be taken with slight movement impulses during palpation, especially laterally (Fig. 3.2).

3.3 Joints in the Area of the Foot

The foot is a highly complex system shaped by numerous joints that interact with each other. The talus, which forms the top of the foot, serves as a relay station and key force-transmitting point [3]. It forms the ankle joints, the majority of which cannot be palpated. Distal to the ankle joints, the bones of the tarsus, metatarsus and forefoot articulate under and with each other, thus completing the functional unit. Palpation, performed in the supine or sitting position, can be divided into the region of the tarsus, metatarsus and antetarsus. In general, palpation of the joint space in the foot is often challenging and requires a precise approach as there are numerous obscuring structures overlying the joints.

3.3.1 Palpation of the Intertarsal and Tarsometatarsal Joints

Low mobility results in the joints of the tarsus being called amphiarthroses. The joint spaces of these tight joints can best be palpated by fixing a bone via the pincer grip with thumb and index finger and simultaneously mobilising the articulating, osseous structure as best as possible. The joint space can then be located via the fingertips. This is the most elegant method of palpating the talonavicular, calcaneocuboid, cuneonavicular, cuneocuboid and tarsometatarsal artefacts.

Other joints such as the art. talocruralis, art. subtalaris as well as the artt. intercuneiformia are also located in the tarsus but cannot be palpated explicitly (Fig. 3.3).

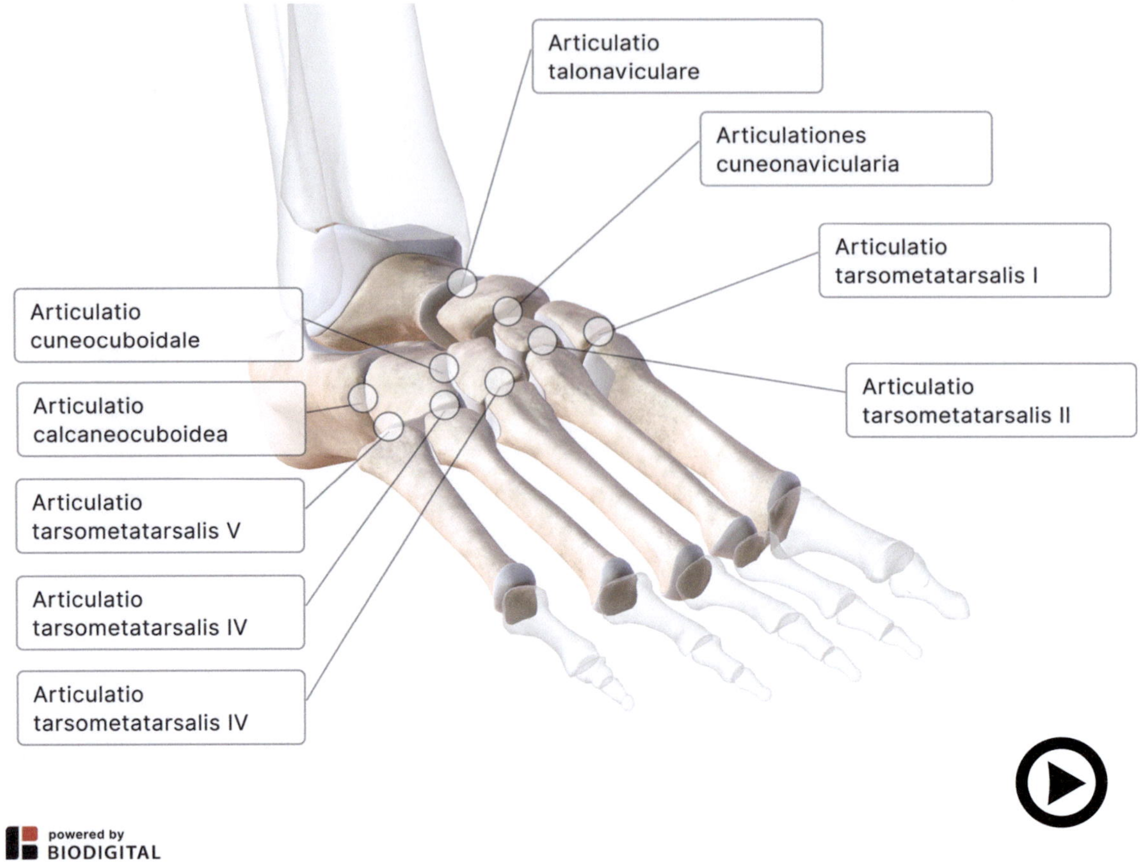

Fig. 3.3 Anatomy and palpation of the artt. intertarsales and tarsometatarsales (▶ https://doi.org/10.1007/000-cqp)

3.3.2 Palpation of the Intermetatarsal and Metatarsophalangeal Joints

The metatarsus consists of five elongated tubular bones, the metatarsals. These articulate proximally and distally with each other and as a middle piece with the tarsus and the forefoot. The concave base of each metatarsal is grasped via the pincer grip with the index finger and thumb and can then be moved with the respective articulating bone held via the same grip. This creates a mobilisation impulse directly at the joint space, which can then be palpated with the fingertips. The same approach can be performed distally with the convex caput of the metatarsal at the transition to the antetarsus. Here, the mobilising joint partner is the concave base of the respective proximal phalanx. Furthermore, the metatarsals also articulate with each other proximally and distally. This joint space is palpated in a similar way to those at the transition to the tarsus or forefoot by grasping and moving two adjacent metatarsals against each other in a pincer grip. The articulated connection to the tarsus via the os cuneiforme intermediale is offset slightly proximally to maintain stability as the anatomical longitudinal axis of the foot. For this reason, the range of motion of the second ray is physiologically the most immobile (Fig. 3.4).

3.3.3 Palpation of the Interphalangeal Pedis Joints

The forefoot is constructed of phalanges. Toes two to five each have a proximal, medial and distal phalanx. The first toe differs from the others by the absence of a medial phalanx. The phalanges of the second to fifth toes each form a proximal and distal interphalangeal joint. Only one interphalangeal joint exists at the hallux. The corresponding caput is convex to the adjacent concave base. Furthermore, the base of the proximal phalanx articulates with the head of the metatarsal at the transition to the metatarsus, thus creating the metatarsophalangeal joints. Palpation of the joint space is best achieved when the fingertips are placed directly on the joint in a pincer grip from the medial and lateral sides, and the distal joint partner is passively moved in flexion and extension. In this case, the movement of the joint partners leads directly to the joint space. A slight traction of the distal partner will increase the quality of the palpation.

Implementation Note
The numerous amphiarthroses of the foot are massively stabilised by ligaments. A very precise and concentrated approach during palpation is therefore indispensable (Fig. 3.5).

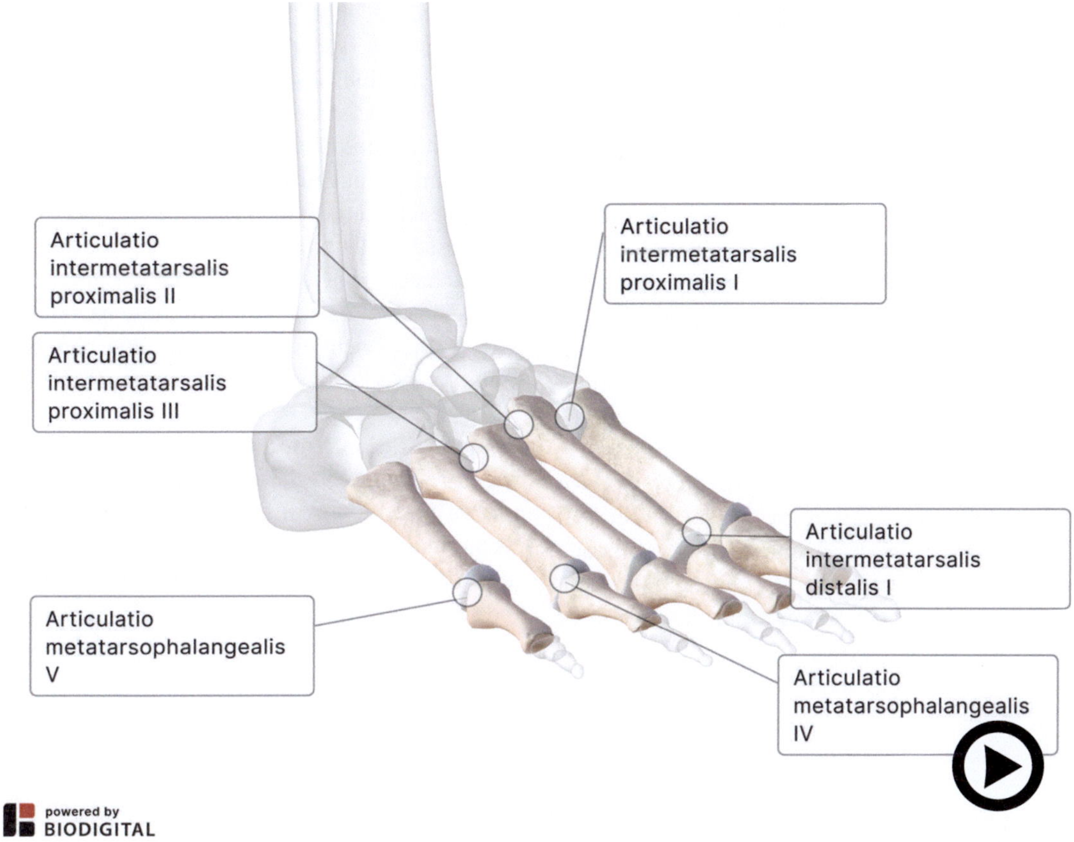

Fig. 3.4 Anatomy and palpation of the artt. intermetatarsales and metatarsophalangeales (▶ https://doi.org/10.1007/000-cqq)

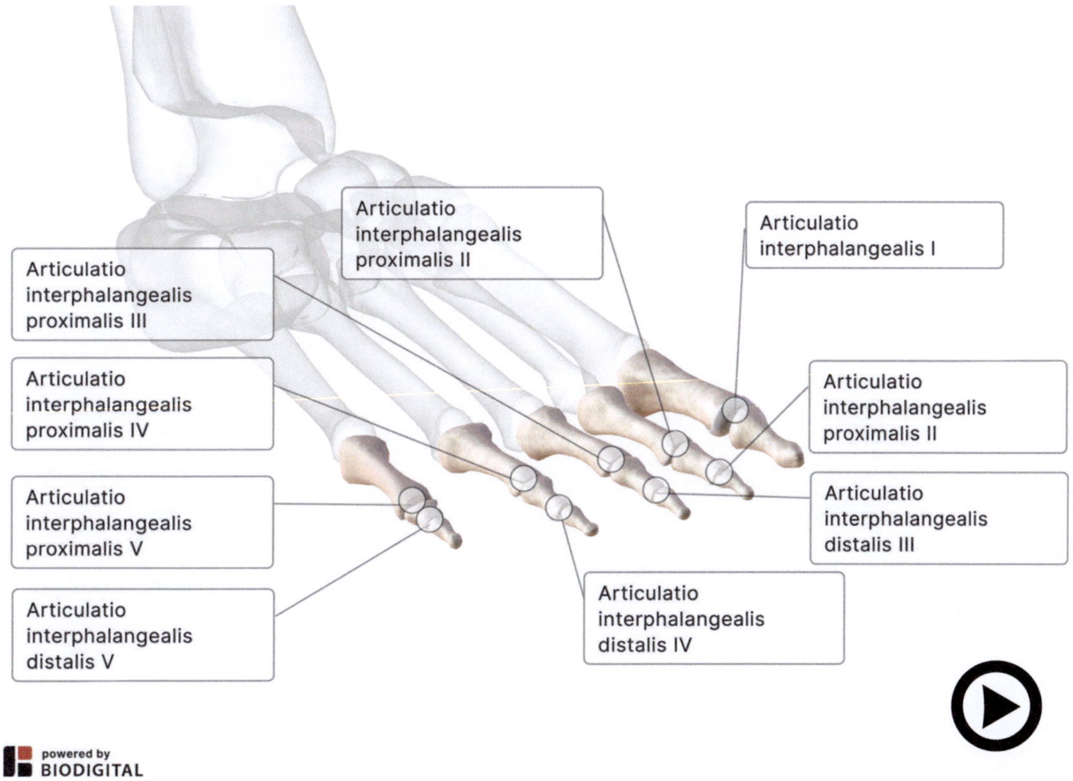

Fig. 3.5 Anatomy and palpation of the artt. interphalangeales (▶ https://doi.org/10.1007/000-cqr)

3.4 Palpation of the Zygapophysial Joints

For a long time, the columna vertebralis was regarded as a rigid, bony structure. Over time, this view changed. In the meantime, it has been proven that the spine, together with corresponding structures, is an integral part of the mobility of the trunk [4]. In addition to the typical bony palpation points, articular connections can also be palpated. These include the artt. zygapophysiales from C2 to C7. For optimal detection of these facet joints, it is advisable to place the patient in the prone position. In this starting position, the muscles around the joints experience maximum relaxation.

To find the zygapophysial joints, it is advisable to first use the respective procc. spinosus as a guide. The procc. spinosi can be palpated caudally from C2 onwards. When the cervical spine is flexed, the spinous processes move away from each other, whereas they move closer together during extension. The fingertip of the index finger moves from the respective proc. spinosus about one transverse finger laterally. During deep palpation, superficial soft tissue is moved laterally as much as possible. The hard, osseous structures, which can be felt through the steeply positioned long finger, represent the procc. articulares of the respective facet joint. Passive flexion leads to an opening (divergence) in the facet joint. Accordingly, an extension leads to a closure (convergence) of the art. zygapophysialis. During this closure, the procc. articulares approach each other, which can be felt through the fingertips. During an opening, a removal of these becomes apparent. The passive movement necessary for this can be realised, for example, by adjusting the head section of the therapy bench.

Implementation Note

The artt. zygapophysiales are in depth and therefore require a lot of palpation skill. All structures above them (muscles, fascia, ligaments, etc.) can react painfully to increased pressure. Palpation of the facet joints should therefore be slow and sensitive (Fig. 3.6).

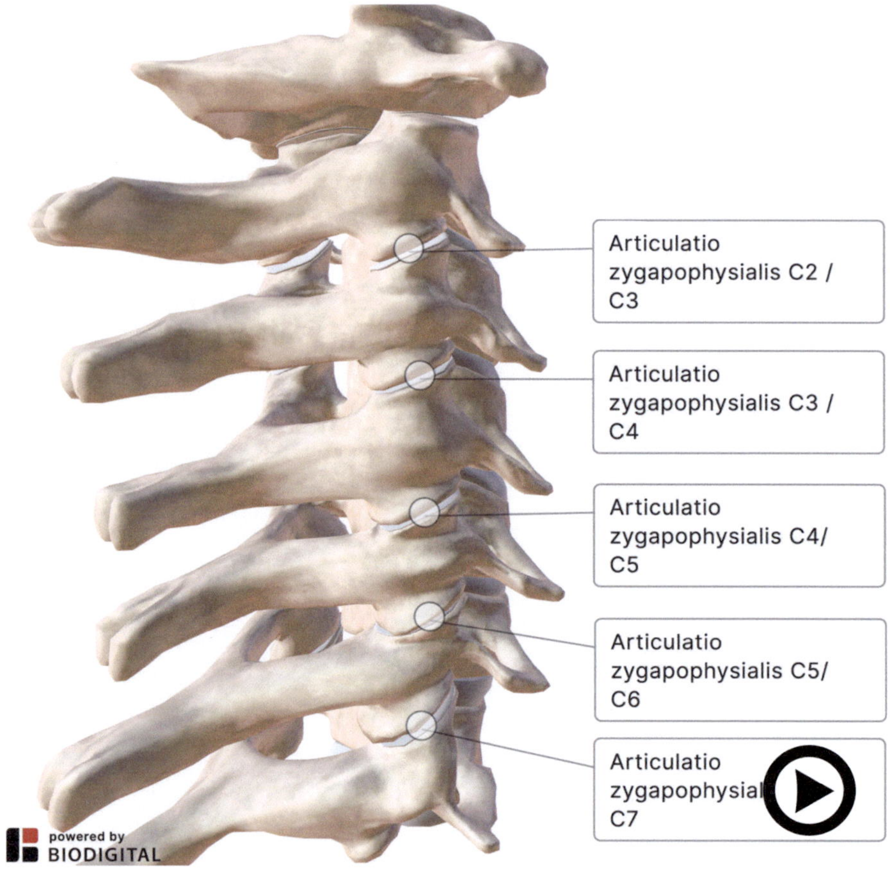

Fig. 3.6 Anatomy and palpation of the artt. zygapophysiales (▶ https://doi.org/10.1007/000-cqs)

3.5 Palpation of the Sternocostal Joints

The rib cage forms the bony armour protecting the internal organs. Twenty-four ribs, which are connected to each other via a myofascial tension-belt mechanism, form articulation surfaces to the sternum as well as to the spine [5]. In addition to their protective function and stabilising task, they must also be mobile, which is noticeable with every breath. While they rise during inhalation, they lower during exhalation. This biomechanical process is indispensable for the functionality of the chest. During inspiration and expiration, ribs one to five move in a cranial and caudal direction, respectively, thus changing the anterior-posterior dimension of the thorax. Ribs 6–12, on the other hand, move in a lateral and medial direction and thus change the width. This mobility is ensured by the artt. sternocostales and the artt. costovertebrales. Only the former can be palpated. The patient lies supine with the head underneath.

The long finger berries are first placed directly centrally on the sternum. If you now orientate laterally to the right or left side, small bony elevations become noticeable. These small bumps (edges of the incisurae costales) are reinforcing structures of the artt. sternocostales. During inhalation and exhalation, movement in these joints can be felt at the joint space located directly at the transition between the sternum and the cartilago costalis of ribs one to seven.

Implementation Note

If these joints are in dysfunction, direct palpation on the joint spaces can cause pain. Therefore, palpation should be flat and gentle, as the joint spaces are very superficial (Fig. 3.7).

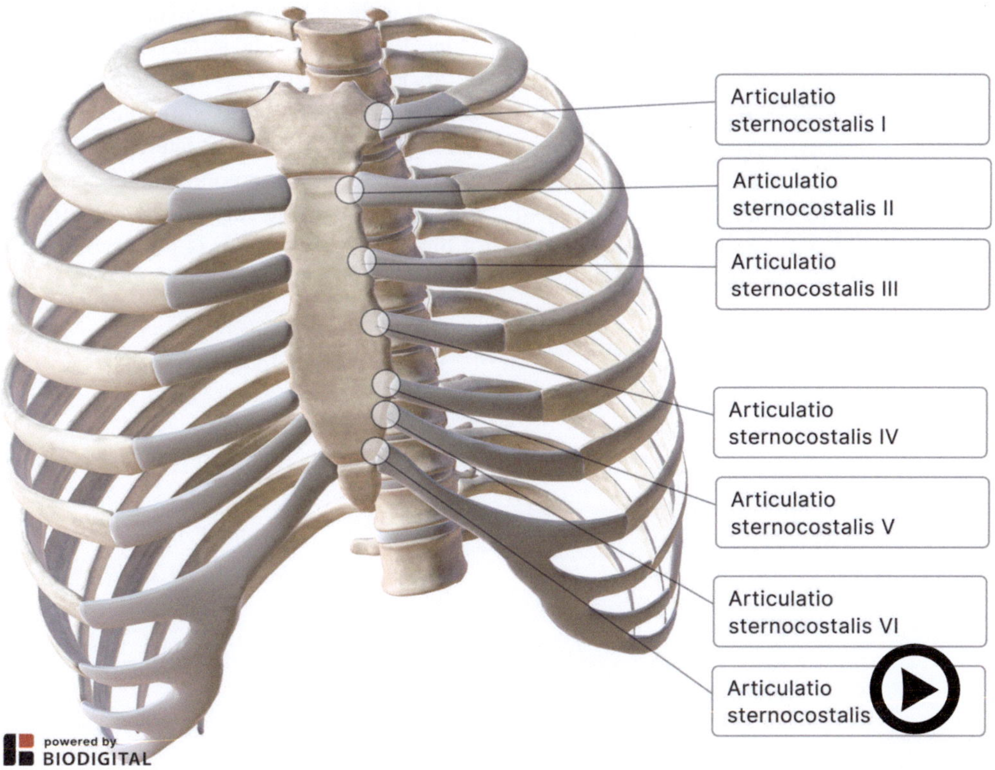

Fig. 3.7 Anatomy and palpation of the artt. sternocostales (▶ https://doi.org/10.1007/000-cqt)

3.6 Joints in the Shoulder Area

The harmonious interaction of five joints leads to the creation of an interlocking functional unit [6]. The articulated joints are always interdependent in everyday activities.

In addition, the shoulder girdle forms the articulated connection to the trunk via the articulatio sternoclavicularis and is therefore also in contact with it. The following five subchapters describe the palpation of the joints in the shoulder region. The starting position can be freely chosen.

3.6.1 Palpation of the Sternoclavicular Joint

The clavicle forms the only direct, bony connection to the trunk via a saddle joint [7]. The joint space can be palpated by first placing the fingertips flat and centrally on the manubrium sterni. The easily perceptible incisura jugularis serves as orientation for locating the manubrium sterni. Lateral to this depression, there is a raised area which represents the transition to the clavicle. Active rotation of the cervical spine to the contralateral side leads to a visible increase in tension of the muscle belly of the homolateral sternocleidomastoid muscle. Its tendon of origin is found both at the sternal manubrium and at the sternal extremity of the clavicle. This anatomical feature makes it possible to locate the sternoclavicularis articularis unerringly. Movements actively initiated by the patient in pro- and retraction as well as elevation and depression of the shoulder girdle lead to clearly perceptible movement deflections, which can be evaluated directly at the respective joint space of the art. sternoclavicularis. While pro- and retraction behave biomechanically in the same direction, the type of joint results in opposing arthro/osteokinematics during elevation and depression. The joint must also be free to move when the arm is moved. Thus, for example, during anteversion and retroversion, a posterior or anterior rotation of the clavicle can be felt at the joint space (Fig. 3.8).

3.6.2 Palpation of the Acromioclavicular Joint

The plane acromioclavicular joint, which connects the clavicle with the scapula, must perform the movements of the clavicle during the motion of the arm, just like the sternoclavicular joint. It is therefore in direct contact and shows the functional connection between the joints of the shoulder girdle. Palpation of this joint is performed in the lateral position. The long-fingered berries of the index/middle finger are placed on the spina scapulae and trace it laterally. The scapular bone opens laterally into the acromion, which is palpated from the posterior edge with the steeply placed fingertips. If the lateral edge of the shoulder elevation is followed anteriorly, the fingertip meets a small depression. At this region, the clavicle articu-

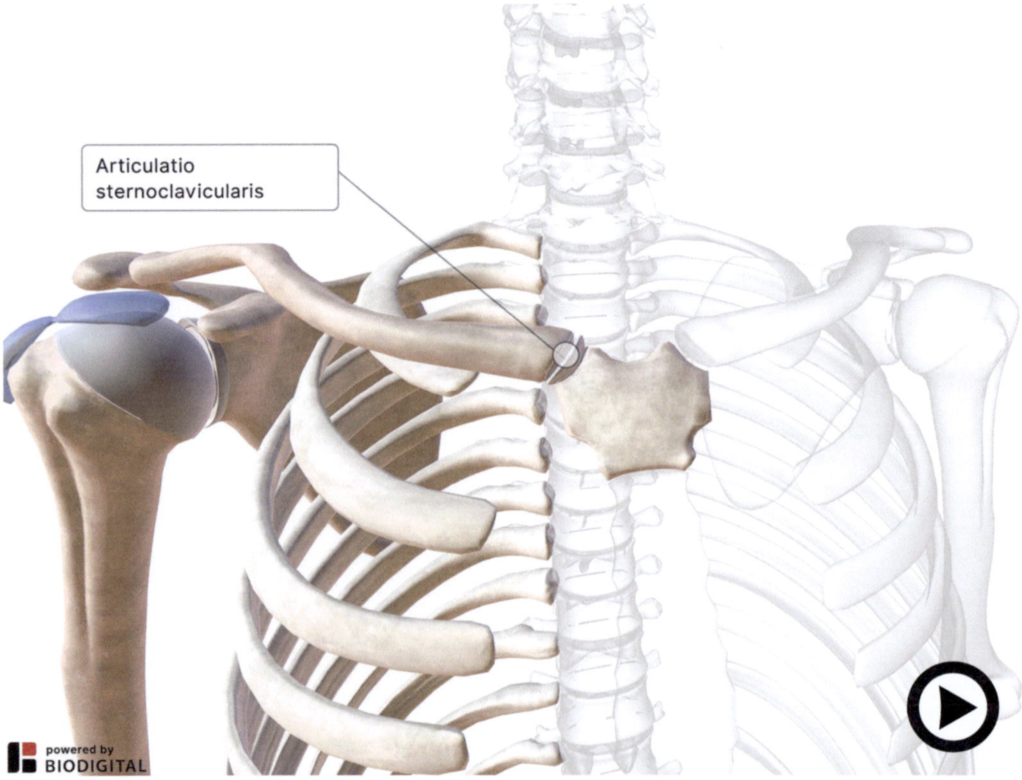

Fig. 3.8 Anatomy and palpation of the art. sternoclavicularis (▶ https://doi.org/10.1007/000-cqv)

lates with its extremitas acromialis directly at the shoulder level. The joint space is clearly felt at the junction of the two bones. Another approach is a palpatory orientation starting from the clavicle. The clavicle is felt on the superior surface with the fingertips and then palpated from medial to lateral. At the end of the extremitas acromialis, the joint space is felt first and the adjacent acromion further laterally (Fig. 3.9).

3.6.3 Palpation of the Subacromial Joint

The acromion forms the cranial limit of the subacromial accessory joint. This joint, which is formed by the subacromial bursa and the subdeltoid bursa, serves only to reduce the friction of influencing structures. The subacromial bursa serves to reduce friction between the shoulder joint capsule, the long tendon of the biceps brachii muscle and the tendon of the supraspinatus muscle on the one hand and the acromion on the other. The subdeltoid bursa is a friction-minimising device between the capsule of the shoulder joint and the deltoid muscle. Palpation is performed directly from the lateral side underneath the acromion using the steeply positioned fingertips of the long fingers to feel this joint. Alternatively, contact can also be made from anteriorly. In this case, the client is in a relaxed starting position. Due to the construction of the accessory joint, only a depression can be palpated, and no clearly delineated joint space can be heard. By gently tractioning the arm longitudinally to the humerus, the joint space will be enlarged and thus be easier to palpate.

Implementation Note

In case of distal shoulder dislocation or subluxation, the "joint space" is enlarged, and no additional traction should be performed (Fig. 3.10).

3.6.4 Palpation of the Humeroscapular Joint

The shoulder joint, which has a high degree of mobility, is elementary for coping with everyday life, as it plays a decisive initiating role in controlling the upper extremity. The ball and socket joint, which consists of the strongly convex caput humeri and the slightly concave cavitas glenoidale, has an incongruent size ratio of four to one [8]. For palpation of the joint, the patient lies relaxed in the supine position, while the steeply positioned long finger berries first grasp the tuberculum minus humeri from anterior. Slightly craniomedial to this small bump, the examiner can approach the joint space with the fingertips. The quality of palpation decreases as the client's muscular status increases.

Implementation Note

Increased palpation quality can be achieved by rotating the arm (Fig. 3.11).

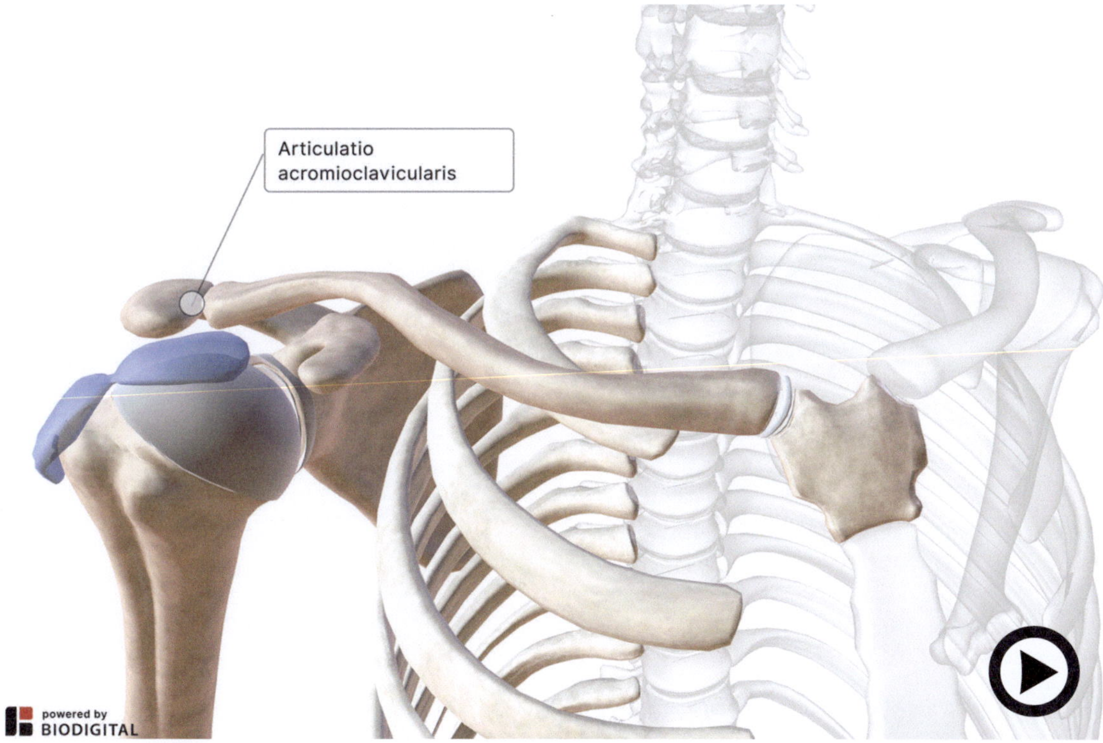

Fig. 3.9 Anatomy and palpation of the art. acromioclavicularis (▶ https://doi.org/10.1007/000-cqw)

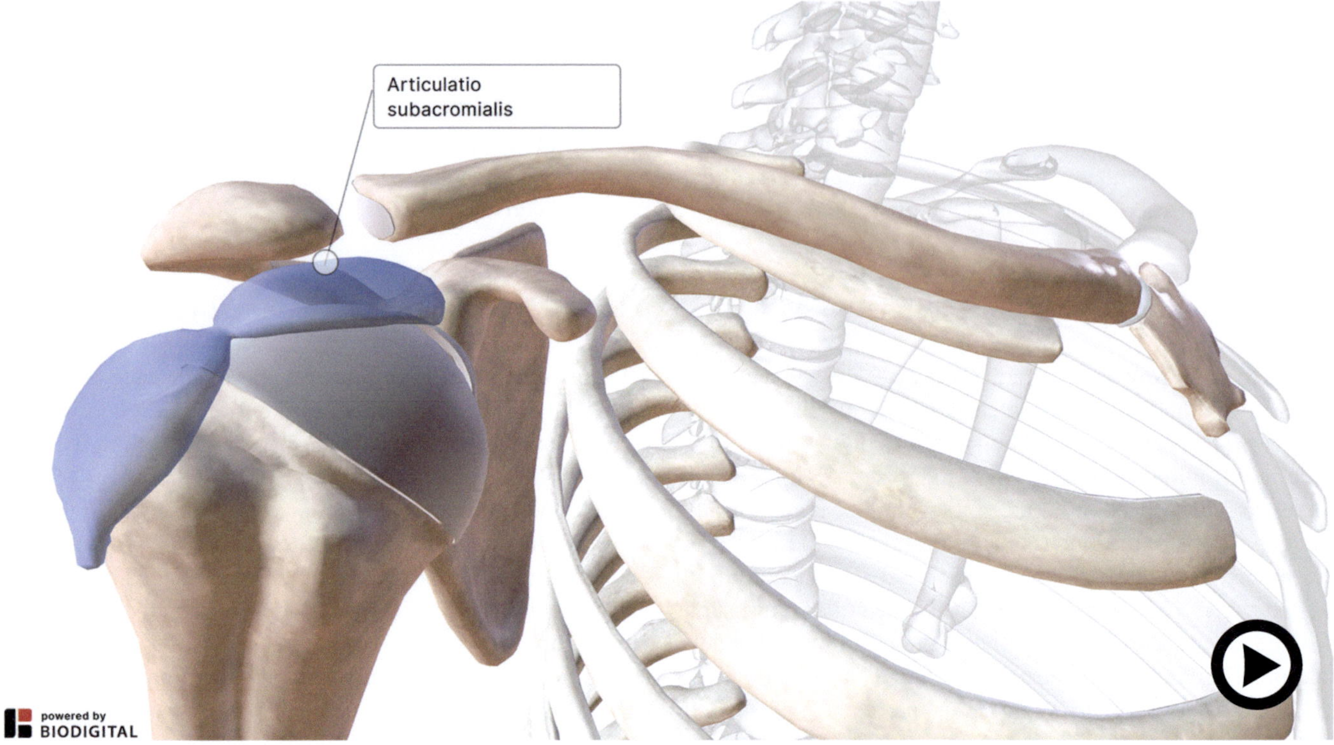

Fig. 3.10 Anatomy and palpation of the art. subacromialis (▶ https://doi.org/10.1007/000-cqx)

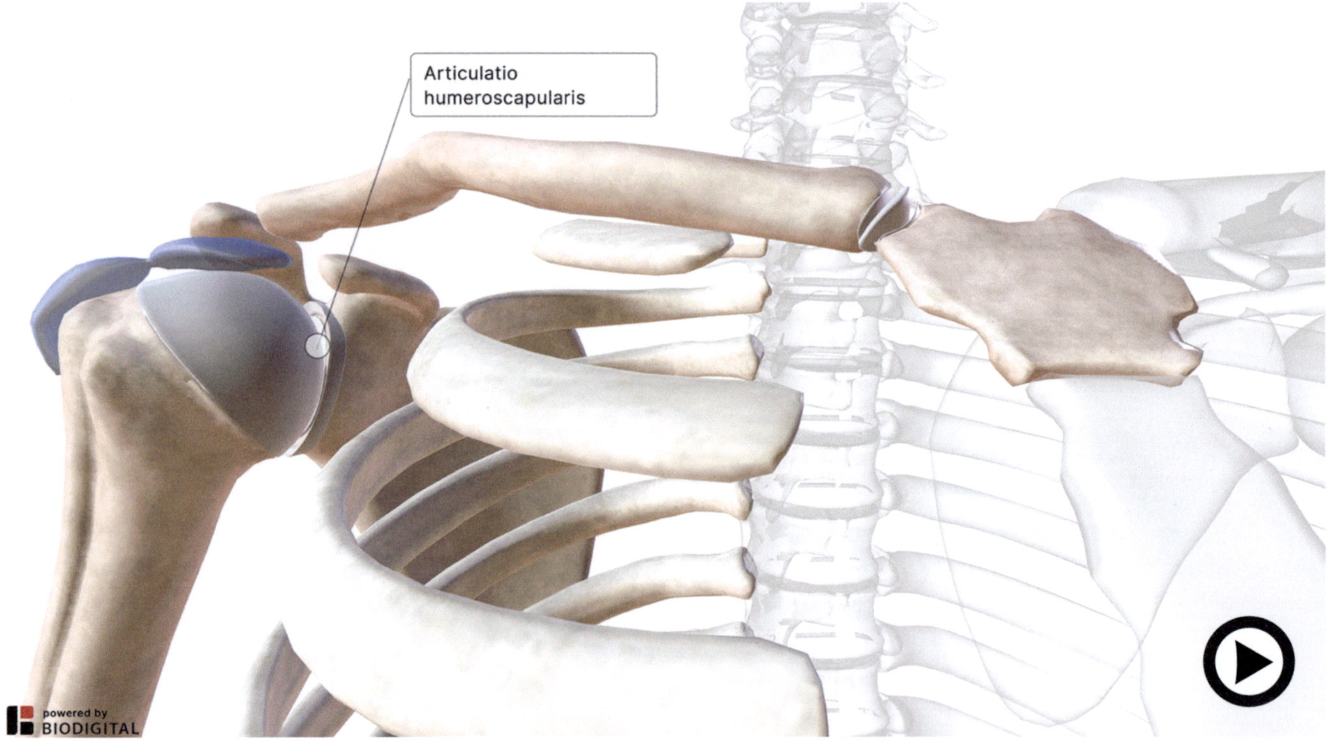

Fig. 3.11 Anatomy and palpation of the art. humeroscapularis (▶ https://doi.org/10.1007/000-cqy)

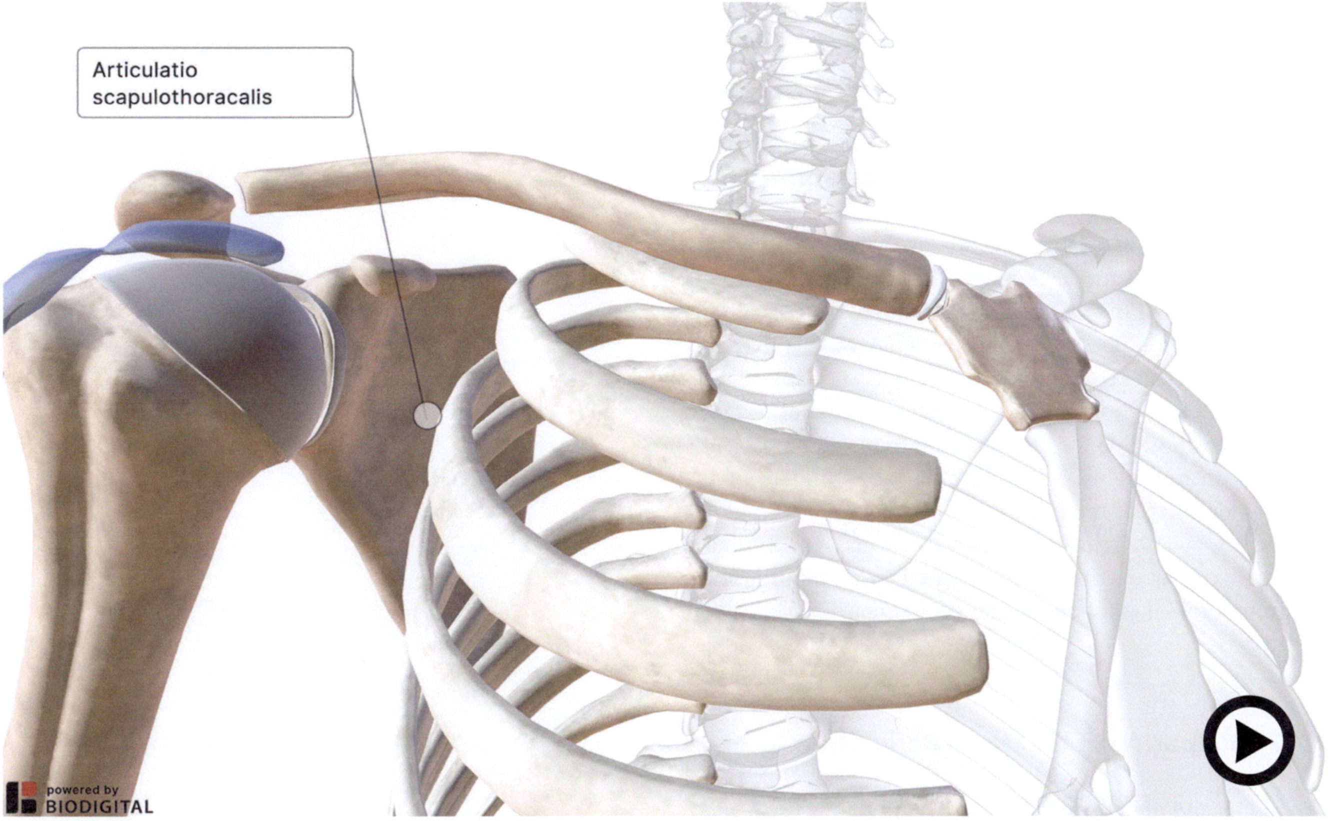

Fig. 3.12 Anatomy and palpation of the art. scapulothoracalis (▶ https://doi.org/10.1007/000-cqz)

3.6.5 Palpation of the Scapulothoracic Joint

The humeroscapular rhythm describes the interplay between the movement of the humerus and the inevitably coupled movement of the scapula, which is necessary, for example, to achieve a range of movement over approx. 40° in abduction or anteversion [9]. The sliding of the scapula on the thorax is significantly influenced by the thoracic gliding surface, which is formed by the subscapularis and serratus anterior muscles. In order to palpate the region under the scapula, a relaxed position in the prone or lateral position is recommended.

If the client is in prone position, the side to be palpated is underlaid with an underlay material under the shoulder from anterior, and the arm on the same side is passively positioned in the apron tie grip. This setting causes a slight separation between the scapula and the thorax. The examiner can reinforce this separation by a retraction movement in the shoulder girdle of the side to be palpated. Contact is then made with the margo medialis scapulae, and from there, palpation is made with the extended long finger berries in the space between the two joint partners.

When proceeding in the lateral position, the head is placed underneath and the upper arm is positioned lengthwise on the torso of the client. The examiner can now contact the upper shoulder from anteriorly via his upper body. Subsequently, a retraction movement is initiated by a slight push posteriorly. This again causes a separation between the scapula and the thorax, and the examiner is able to feel the space between the scapula and the thorax via the margo medialis scapulae with flexed fingers (II–V).

Implementation Note

The thoracic gliding surface is sometimes very difficult to reach in clients who do not have the necessary mobility of the scapula. During palpation, which simultaneously involves mobilisation of the thoracic gliding surface, pain may be triggered in the case of biomechanical dysfunctions. Palpation should therefore be initiated and performed with caution (Fig. 3.12).

3.7 Joints in the Area of the Elbow

The functional unit of the articular cubiti is formed by the union of several joints. The articulating surfaces of the humerus, radius and ulna form four joints. Comparable to clockwork, the “gears” of the elbow joint must also mesh harmoniously to enable everyday activities such as eating. Of these four joints (humeroulnaris, humeroradialis, radioulnaris proximalis and distalis), two can be palpated. This palpation is performed in a relaxed starting position. The supine or seated position with the elbow joint passively flexed through approx. 90° is the method of choice.

3.7.1 Palpation of the Humeroradial Joint

In a passive flexion position of 90° at the elbow, the long finger of the index finger is placed flat on the epicondylus lateralis humeri. If the palpation finger moves distally, it falls into a depression directly after the epicondylus lateralis humeri, which can be felt as a distinct elevation. This depression represents the joint space of the humeroradial joint. In addition, it is possible for the examiner to place the patient's forearms on top of his. Now both the index fingers of the practitioner can feel the respective joint space. The remaining fingers, which grip the client's forearms, can initiate a passive flexion or extension movement. During mobilisation, the humeroradial joint space can be delineated even better (Fig. 3.13).

3.7.2 Palpation of the Distal Radioulnar Joint

The radius and ulna form a functional unit that is connected, among other things, by the membrana interossea antebrachii. While the proximal articular radioulnaris is not palpable in depth as a pivot joint, the distal radius joint can be palpated well from the dorsal side. The same starting positions as in 3.6.1 are recommended for this. The long fingertip of the palpating index or middle finger is placed dorsodistally on the ulnar styloid process. When palpating radially, the finger falls into a small depression. This represents the joint space of the distal radioulnaris. During pro- and supination, this joint space can be felt even more clearly. During pronation, this gap flattens, whereas it deepens during final supination.

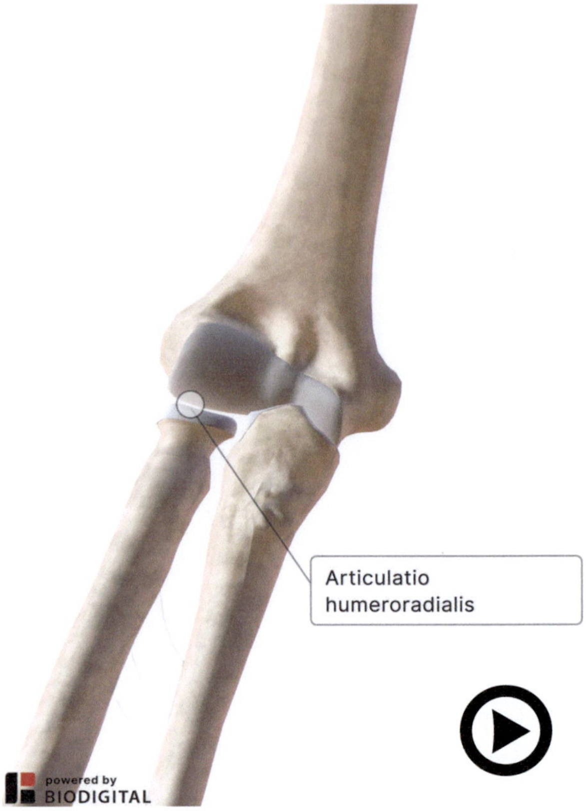

Fig. 3.13 Anatomy and palpation of the art. humeroradialis (▶ https://doi.org/10.1007/000-cr0)

These movements can be actively performed by the client in 90° elbow joint flexion.

Implementation Note
Palpation of the humeroradial joint may be painful if the client has lateral humeral epicondylopathy. The irritated tendons lie in the area of palpation and may therefore be symptomatic when pressure is applied (Fig. 3.14).

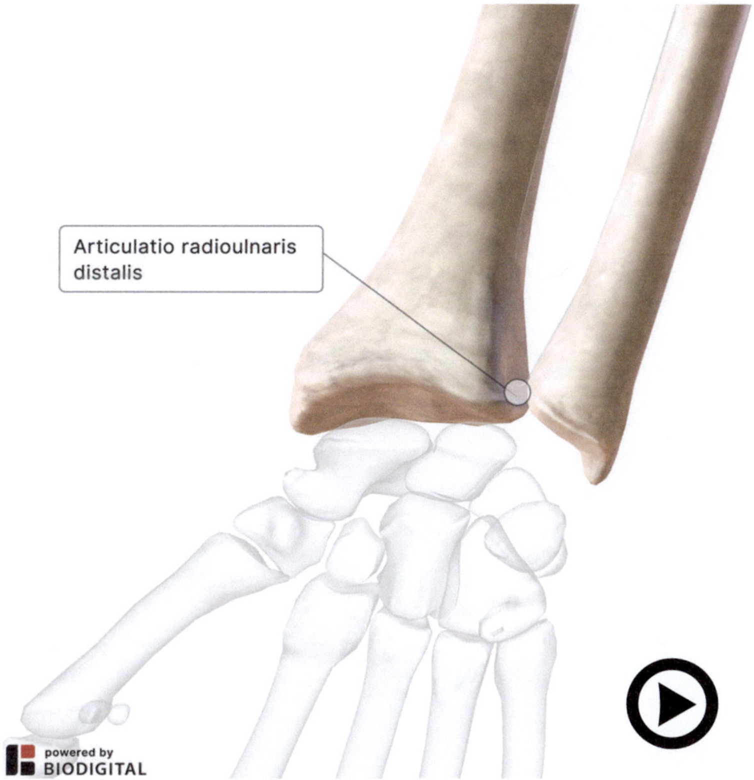

Fig. 3.14 Anatomy and palpation of the art. radioulnaris distalis (▶ https://doi.org/10.1007/000-cr1)

3.8 Joints in the Area of the Hand

The "instrument of instruments", as Aristotle already called the hand, is the finest motor tool of the human being [10]. It enables us to master everyday tasks such as eating, working, hygiene and non-verbal communication, to name but a few. Like a jigsaw puzzle, the hand is made up of many joints that can be palpated to form a meaningful overall construct. The procedure is the same as in Sect. 2.11 on osseous palpation. In this chapter too, it is shown that the carpal bones and the metacarpals and phalanges are frequently moved against each other to feel the edges of the bones. At the same time, if the anatomical components permit, the joint space can of course also be clearly palpated. For these reasons, the explanations on palpation in this chapter are kept short, and reference is made to Sect. 2.11 for more detailed information. For a good palpation result, it is recommended to place the client in a relaxed supine position or in a sitting position with the forearms resting on the back. The procedure for palpating the joints of the hand is described below.

3.8.1 Palpation of the Radiocarpal Joint

Of fundamental importance for the gross motor mobility of the hand is the proximal wrist, which extends as an egg yolk joint between the radius, discus articularis and proximal carpus. The sensation of the joint space begins at the ulnar styloid proc., which is found distally on the ulna as a distinct elevation. The long finger berries, laid flat, feel distally and "fall" directly into a depression in which the discus articularis is located. This articulates with the os triquetrum during ulnarduction. If the palpation fingers move radially, the joint space between the radius and the proximal carpus can be felt directly from the dorsal side as a longitudinal groove. This groove deepens in the radiocarpal joint during dorsal extension, whereas it flattens out during palmar flexion (Fig. 3.15).

3.8.2 Palpation of the Intercarpal Joints

The tight intercarpal joints that form between the carpal bones are amphiarthroses that allow little movement. However, the little movement that is allowed is crucial for functioning biomechanics. A strongly pronounced ligamentous fuse makes palpation of the articular connections within the carpus difficult. At this point, reference is made to Sect. 2.11, in which the bone edges, which simultaneously lead to the joint spaces, are described in detail in the palpatory finding (Fig. 3.16).

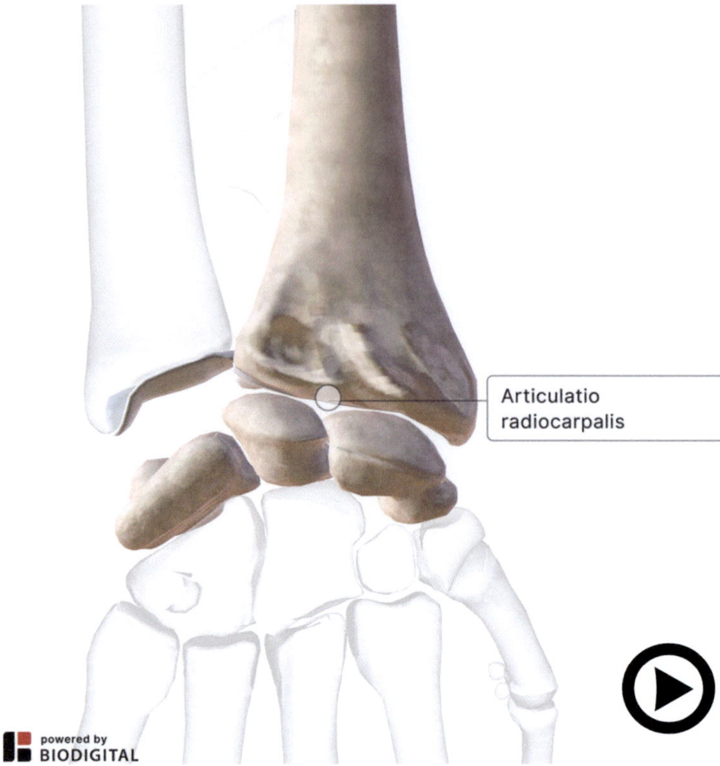

Fig. 3.15 Anatomy and palpation of the art. radiocarpalis (▶ https://doi.org/10.1007/000-cr2)

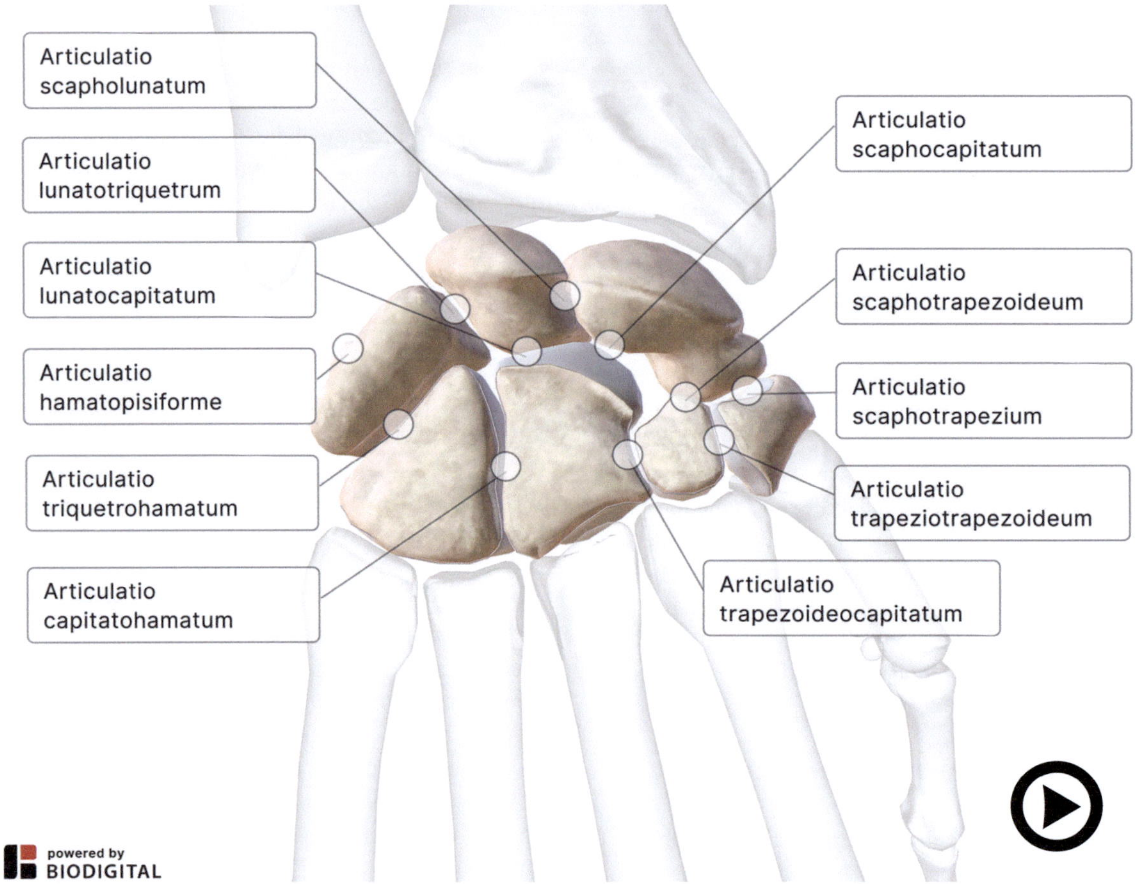

Fig. 3.16 Anatomy and palpation of the artt. intercarpales (▶ https://doi.org/10.1007/000-cr3)

3.8.3 Palpation of the Carpometacarpal Joints

The articular transitions between the carpus and the metacarpal are initially best felt on the third ray. From the dorsal side, the palpating tip of the index or middle finger is placed in the centre of the metacarpal III. It then palpates in a proximal direction until the finger sinks into a depression. This point is the transition to the os capitatum. The joint spaces of the other artt. carpometacarpales can be palpated in the same way. This requires trained palpation skills. Alternatively, palpation of the joint space can also be performed using the forceps grip.

Art. carpometacarpalis I, which is better known as the thumb saddle joint, has a special feature. Palpation of this joint is done directly via the tabatière from the dorsal side [11]. Using the forceps grip, the index finger is placed between the tendon of the extensor pollicis longus muscle and the tendon of the abductor pollicis brevis or extensor pollicis brevis muscles, which are clearly visible when the thumb is extended. Between these tendons, a depression is formed, the fovea radialis (tabatière) in which the thumb saddle joint is in depth. The joint space between the os trapezium and os metacarpale I can be clearly distinguished from the surrounding area. This particular saddle joint behaves in arthro/osteokinematics in abduction and adduction convexly around a radioulnar axis, whereas in flexion and extension, it behaves concavely around a dorsopalmar axis.

Implementation Note
Particularly when palpating the art. carpometacarpal I in the tabatière, pain can be caused by rhizarthrosis. Therefore, first go gently from the surface to the depth (Fig. 3.17).

3.8.4 Palpation of the Intermetacarpal Joints

For fist closure, it is important, among other things, that the metacarpals II–V move against each other. In doing so, they each form a proximal and a distal joint. These amphiarthroses are components of the functional unit of the entire hand. Palpation is limited to the distal joints, which are clearly perceptible between the heads of the metacarpals. The joint space of the distal artt. intermetacarpales is palpated using the pincer grip, with the index finger dorsal and the thumb palmar. A distinct depression between the adjacent and elevated caput metacarpales points the direct way to The joint space, which is located in depth. A translatory movement of the metacarpals towards each other dorsally and palmar reveals the gap even more clearly. Meanwhile, the fingers should be passively positioned in the zero position.

Implementation Note
The mobility of the artt. intermetacarpales distales increases physiologically significantly from radial to ulnar (Fig. 3.18).

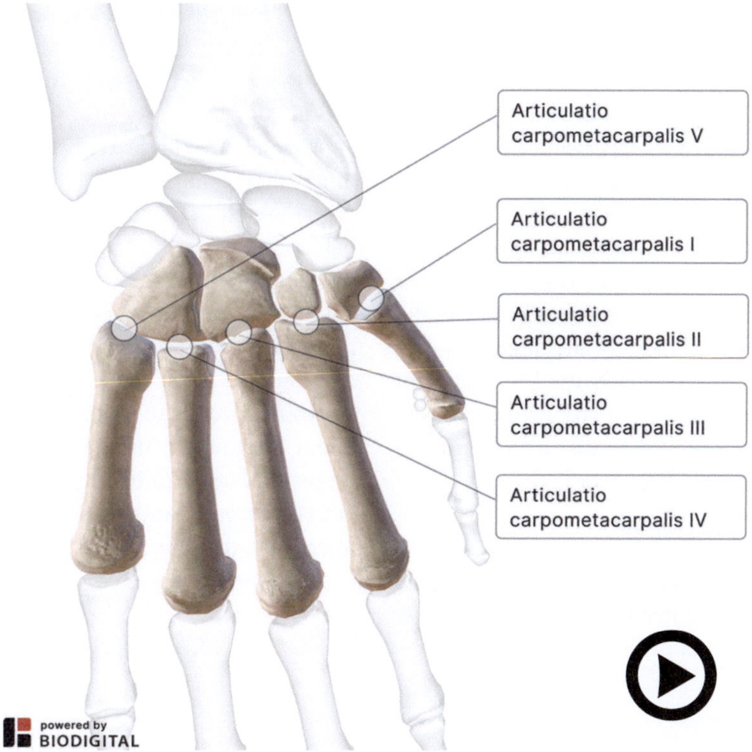

Fig. 3.17 Anatomy and palpation of the artt. carpometacarpales (▶ https://doi.org/10.1007/000-cr4)

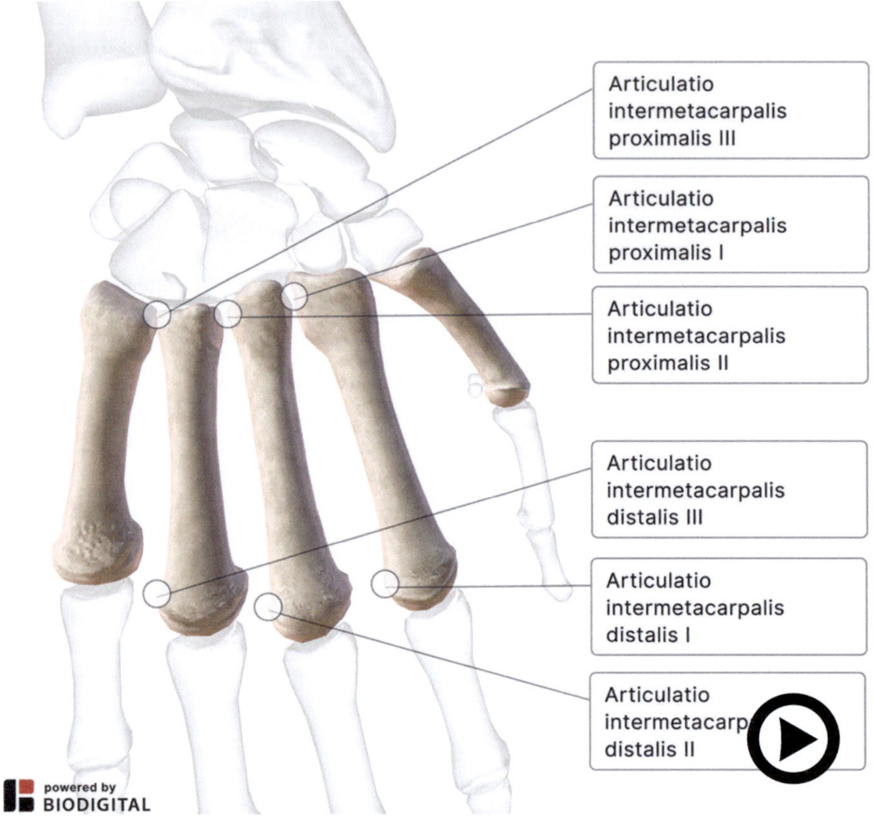

Fig. 3.18 Anatomy and palpation of the artt. intermetacarpales (▶ https://doi.org/10.1007/000-cr5)

3.8.5 Palpation of the Metacarpophalangeal Joints

The basic joints of the individual fingers are formed by the respective convex caput of the ossa metacarpalia and the concave base of the respective proximal phalanx. Thus, the ellipsoidal joints (MCP II–V) or the hinge joint (MCP I) behave concave to each other during movement in the open system. The already clearly visible joints are palpated with the pincer grip. The fingertips of the thumb and index finger contact the proximal phalanx by being applied radially and ulnarly or dorsally and palmar. Then palpate proximally until a clear joint space appears. If the respective art. metacarpophalangealis is in flexion, the joint gap increases even further. During movement, the gap can be differentiated even more precisely.

Implementation Note
In the preliminary stages, traction in this joint can lead to a visible depression that is created just above the joint space. This can be used for a first rough orientation (Fig. 3.19).

3.8.6 Palpation of the Interphalangeal Joints

The fingers are designed for gross and fine coordinative activities of everyday life. Consisting of two or three phalanges that articulate with each other via interphalangeal joints, they complete the human hand distally. The hinge joints, which consist of a distal convex caput and a proximal concave base, move arthro/osteokinematically in the same direction in the open system. The joint space is palpated in these joints via the pincer grip by the thumb and index finger. One of the practitioner's fingers is placed radially, and the other ulnar between two adjacent phalanges. The joint space is then palpated with moderate but still sufficient pressure in the artt. interphalangeales. Meanwhile, the respective joint can be moved in flexion and extension so that the gap can be felt even more clearly. It should be noted that the thumb has only one interphalangeal joint, whereas the fingers II–V each have a proximal and a distal joint (Fig. 3.20).

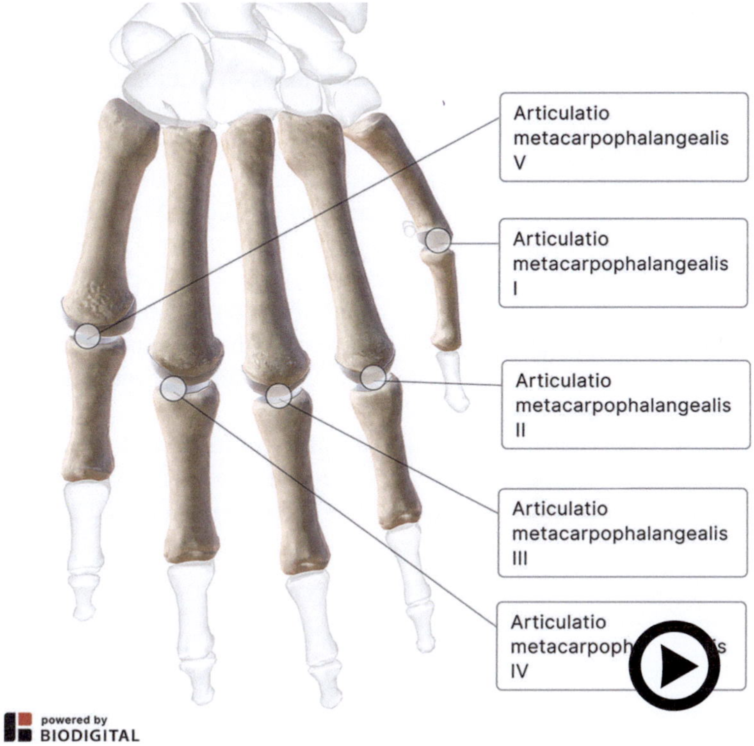

Fig. 3.19 Anatomy and palpation of the artt. metacarpophalangeales (▶ https://doi.org/10.1007/000-cr6)

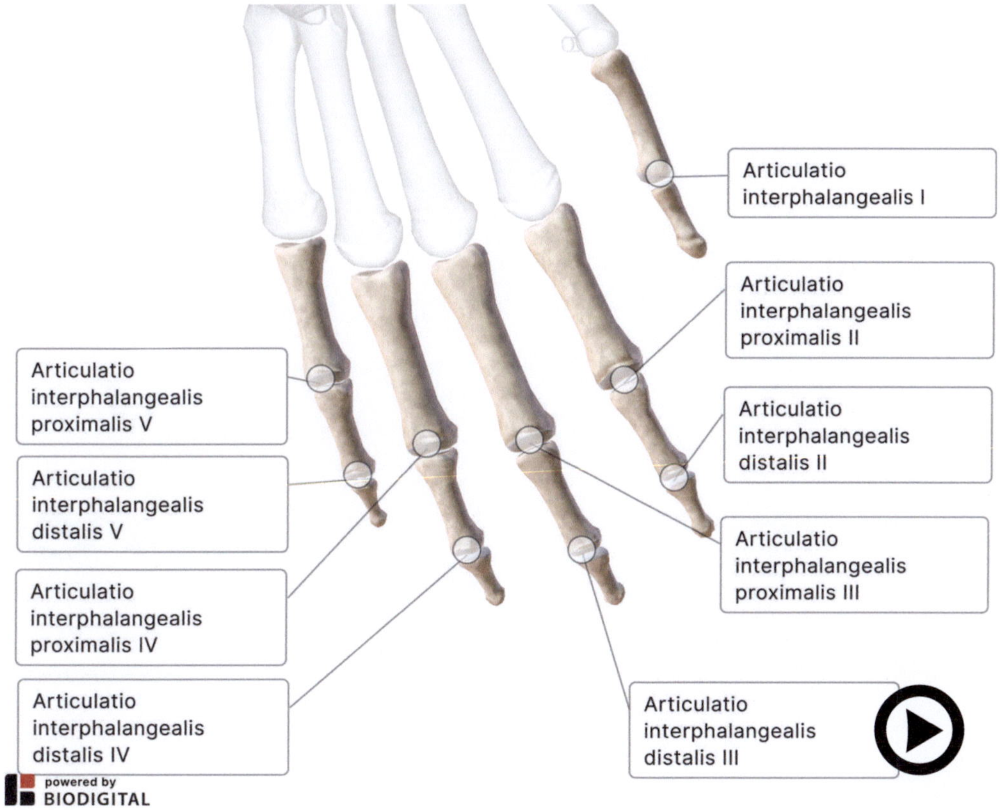

Fig. 3.20 Anatomy and palpation of the artt. interphalangeales (▶ https://doi.org/10.1007/000-cqm)

3.9 Palpation of the Temporomandibular Joint

The jaw joint is essential for eating, speaking and processing emotions. The nutrients that the human body needs for energy production are extracted from the food that is crushed by the teeth through the jaw. The resulting energy supply enables all physiological processes of the organism to run smoothly. The temporomandibular joint is formed by the biconvex caput mandibulae, which articulates with the concave fossa mandibularis. Between these two joint partners, there is an additional discus articularis, which is indispensable for functionality and divides the joint into a discotemporal and discomandibular compartment. Hinge movements such as opening and closing; carriage movements such as protrusion, retrusion, laterotrusion and mediotrusion; as well as grinding movements are necessary for the chewing process. These movements must always occur simultaneously in both joints so that the necessary mobility can be applied.

Palpation of the temporomandibular joint is done using the long finger berries of the index or middle finger placed flat. These are placed immediately anterior to the external meatus acusticus. While the client makes small movements in the direction of opening and closing, the joint gap is clearly felt. As the opening increases, the caput mandibulae performs a movement anterolaterally. This can be easily perceived by the examiner. With final opening, a depression is created behind the caput mandibulae.

Implementation Note

Use caution when palpating as craniomandibular dysfunction can lead to increased pain perception (Fig. 3.21).

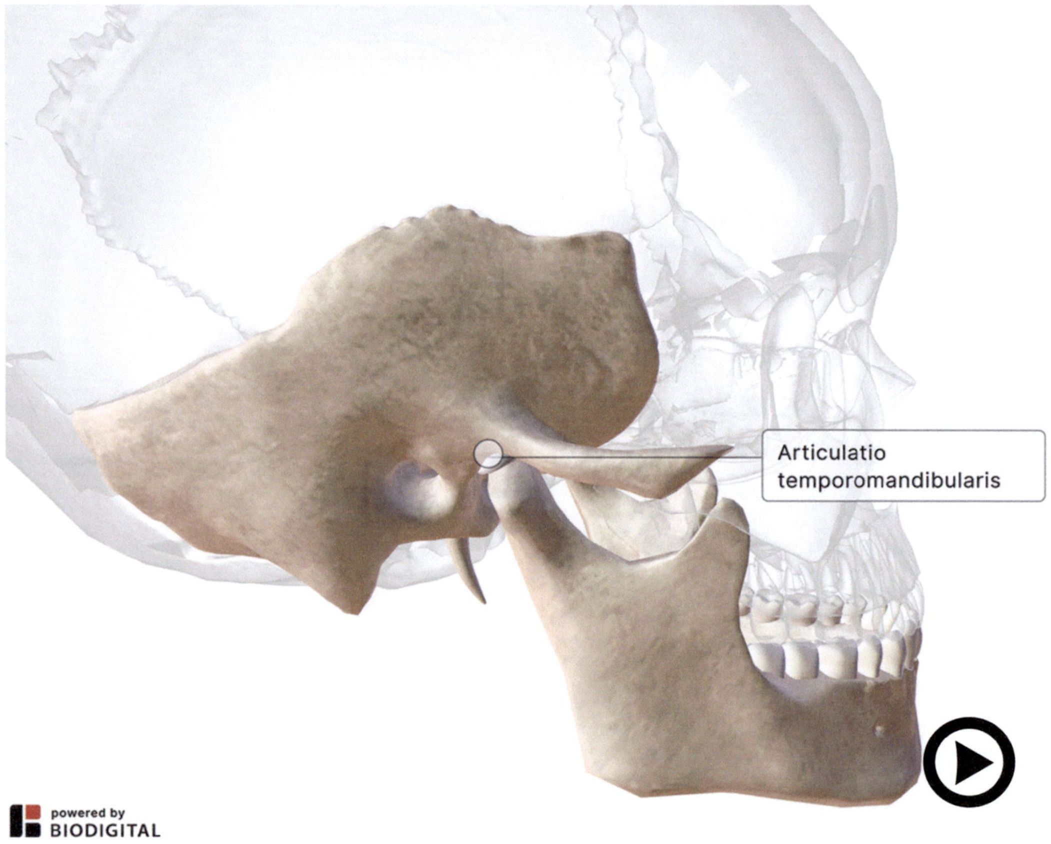

Fig. 3.21 Anatomy and palpation of the art. temporomandibularis (▶ https://doi.org/10.1007/000-cr8)

References

1. Schäfer, F., Order, B., Bolte, H., Heller, M., & Brossmann, J. (2002, October). Sport injuries of the extensor mechanism of the knee. *Der Radiologe, 42*(10), 799–810. https://doi.org/10.1007/s00117-002-0794-2
2. Sherman, S., Plackis, A., & Nuelle, C. (2014, July). Patellofemoral anatomy and biomechanics. *Clinics in Sports Medicine, 33*(3), 389–401. https://doi.org/10.1016/j.csm.2014.03.008
3. Mahato, N. (2011, December). Morphology of sustentaculum tali: Biomechanical importance and correlation with angular dimensions of the talus. *The Foot, 21*(4), 179–183. https://doi.org/10.1016/j.foot.2011.06.001
4. Preece, S., Mason, D., & Bramah, C. (2016, February). The coordinated movement of the spine and pelvis during running. *Human Movement Science, 45*, 110–118. https://doi.org/10.1016/j.humov.2015.11.014
5. Lee, D. (1993). Biomechanics of the thorax: A clinical mode of in vivo function. *Journal of Manual & Manipulative Therapy, 1*(1), 13–21. https://doi.org/10.1179/106698193791069771
6. Veeger, H., & van der Helm, F. (2007). Shoulder function: The perfect compromise between mobility and stability. *Journal of Biomechanics, 40*(10), 2119–2129. https://doi.org/10.1016/j.jbiomech.2006.10.016
7. Dhawan, R., Singh, R., Tins, B., & Hay, S. (2018, October). Sternoclavicular joint. *Shoulder Elbow, 10*(4), 296–305. https://doi.org/10.1177/1758573218756880
8. Halder, A., Itoi, E., & An, K. (2000, April). Anatomy and biomechanics of the shoulder. *The Orthopedic Clinics of North America, 31*(2), 159–176. https://doi.org/10.1016/s0030-5898(05)70138-3
9. Kozono, N., Takeuchi, N., Okada, T., Hamai, S., Higaki, H., Shimoto, T., et al. (2020, September–December). Dynamic scapulohumeral rhythm: Comparison between healthy shoulders and those with large or massive rotator cuff tear. *Journal of Orthopaedic Surgery (Hong Kong), 28*(3), 230949902098177. https://doi.org/10.1177/2309499020981779
10. Mustak-Blagusz, M., & Pertinatsch, C. (2015, March 6). Wunderwerk Hand. rheuma plus, *14*, 50–54. https://doi.org/10.1007/s12688-014-0020-0
11. Derian, A., Amundson, J., Abi-Aad, K., Vasquez-Duarte, R., & Johnson-Greene, D. (2018, November). Accuracy of ultrasound-guided versus palpation-based carpometacarpal joint injections: A randomized pilot study in cadavers. *Ultrasound, 26*(4), 245–250. https://doi.org/10.1177/1742271X18789711

Palpation of the Ligaments

4

Contents

4.1 Basics of Palpation of Ligaments

Humans are constructed according to the tensegrity model and are composed of bones that are stable in bending and muscles, tendons and ligaments that are stable in stretching. This tension-belt mechanism transforms unstable joint systems into mutually dependent, dimensionally stable bodies. The capsule-ligament apparatus makes a considerable contribution to this form stability. These fibre-rich strands of connective tissue are only moderately stretchable and usually stretch over a joint to stabilise it or limit movement. In addition to joints, ligaments also attach internal organs. This fixation ensures the necessary fixation with simultaneous mobility in the various body cavities. The main component of ligamentous structures is parallel fibres of collagen type I [1]. A smaller proportion of elastic fibres ensures a slight extensibility. For reasons of fibre placement and alignment, ligaments are often more stable in the longitudinal direction than osseous tissue. Therefore, severe overstretching of ligamentous structures can lead to bony avulsion [2]. In addition, ligaments are usually closely connected to the capsules, which surround the joint as enveloping tissue.

Of all the ligaments found in the human body, only a fraction are accessible to palpation. However, some important ligaments can be palpated and therefore constitute the main content of this chapter.

During palpation, it is important to ensure that the client is in a relaxed starting position. Furthermore, a well-trained sense of touch is required, as ligamentous structures are usually difficult to differentiate from the surrounding tissue. A technique frequently used in practice that aims to improve differentiation is the use of longitudinal stretching. Here, the joint is adjusted in such a way that a stretching of the structure to be palpated is achieved. If the ligament tightens longitudinally, differentiation from surrounding structures becomes

Supplementary Information The online version contains supplementary material available at https://doi.org/10.1007/978-3-662-69186-1_4. The videos can be accessed individually by clicking the DOI link in the accompanying figure caption or by scanning this link with the SN More Media App.

R. Bauer, S. Wolfram, *Atlas of Palpation*, https://doi.org/10.1007/978-3-662-69186-1_4

easier. Even though the ligament to be palpated cannot always be felt directly by the practitioner, it is still possible to force the ligamentous structures to respond to stimuli.

First palpate with the long fingertips of the index or middle finger across the course of the ligament. The result is a feeling of a firm-elastic structure that is slightly displaceable in relation to the surrounding tissue and is sharply delineated. Depending on the location, ligaments can be palpated by direct palpation in depth or by forceps grip.

For palpation, anatomical knowledge of the position of the ligaments is a basic prerequisite in order to hit the structure accurately. For this reason, the anatomy is illustrated in the individual chapters.

4.2 Palpation of the Lower Limb Ligaments

The ligaments of the lower limb have to resist the ground reaction force during standing, walking, running or during jumping. They perform this important task as part of the tension-belt system and thus provide stability during various everyday activities. Due to the sometimes high stress, especially in sports, the ligaments are often under very high strain, which they are sometimes unable to withstand. In order to recognise structural or functional changes, it is necessary to be able to feel the ligaments that may have changed negatively.

In the following chapters, the process of palpating the ligaments of the pelvis, hip joint, knee and foot is presented transparently. The special positioning is described in the individual chapters.

4.2.1 Palpation of the Pelvic Ligaments

Numerous ligaments are located in the area of the pelvis. Forces from the lower limb meet here with counterforces emanating from the torso. The ligaments play a fundamental role in distributing these forces optimally. For this reason, the pelvis is an important key point of the human body. The following chapters describe the procedure for palpating the ligamentous structures of the pelvis. Depending on the ligament, the person to be examined is positioned in the supine, prone or lateral position.

4.2.1.1 Palpation of the Iliolumbar Ligament

The iliolumbar ligament has two different fibre courses and serves to stabilise the lumbosacral transition. The parts run from the proc. costalis of the fourth and fifth lumbar vertebrae, respectively, to the crista iliaca. For precise stimulation, it is important to know that the iliopsoas muscle is located ventral to the ligament, the erector spinae muscle dorsal and the quadratus lumborum muscle exactly between the two parts. It is recommended that the patient be placed in the prone position. Starting from the procc. spinosi of the fourth and fifth lumbar vertebrae, the practitioner applies pressure ventrally with the index or middle finger placed steeply and slowly orientates laterocaudally towards the crista iliaca. A pronounced muscular status of the person being examined corresponds with a decreasing ability to apply a stimulus to the iliolumbar ligament.

Implementation Note

It is advisable to proceed gently during palpation of the iliolumbar ligaments. In the case of existing dysfunctions in the lumbosacral area, the iliolumbar ligaments often react with a clear irritation response in the sense of pressure dolence (Fig. 4.1).

4.2.1.2 Palpation of the Sacrospinous Ligament

The name of this ligament leads directly to the associated osseous suspension sites and conveys that the client is placed in the prone position for palpation. First, the lateral inferior angulus of the os sacrum is located and identified with the help of one finger. With the other hand, the spina ischiadica is also located and marked with the steeply placed index finger. A mental line between the two fingers represents the direct course of the sacrospinous ligament.

The entire course of the ligament can then be felt. A firm elastic structure is perceptible in depth. Palpation at right angles to the direction of the fibres makes it possible to differentiate the ligament from surrounding tissues. The sacrospinal ligament forms the lower limit of the foramen ischiadicum majus and is therefore in close proximity to the piriformis muscle. Active external rotation in the hip joint causes contraction of this muscle, making it possible to differentiate between the ligament and the muscle. The quality of palpation of this ligament is reduced with increasing muscular development.

Implementation Note

To avoid irritation of the piriformis muscle and the sciatic nerve, palpation should be performed slowly with increasing intensity in depth (Fig. 4.2).

4.2.1.3 Palpation of the Sacrotuberal Ligament

The lower edge of the foramen ischiadicum minus is formed by the sacrotuberal ligament, which runs from the caudal part of the sacrum and coccyx caudolaterally to the tuber ischiadicum.

As a triangular shaped ligament, it also has fibrous courses to the SIPI and thus serves to stabilise the sacroiliac joint. In addition to this function, it also serves as the point of origin for the biceps femoris muscle, which forms its origo via the caput commune in this region. Because of these important functions, it is relevant to be able to palpate this ligament. In this way, the state of tension can be determined and, if necessary, modulated. The steeply positioned fingers first seek out the tuber ischiadicum and, as a second reference point, the apex ossis sacri. An imaginary line between these two bony reference points shows the course of the sacrotuberal ligament. For better differentiation, the ligament can also be palpated transversely to the course of the fibres. The quality of palpation of this ligament decreases with increasing muscular development.

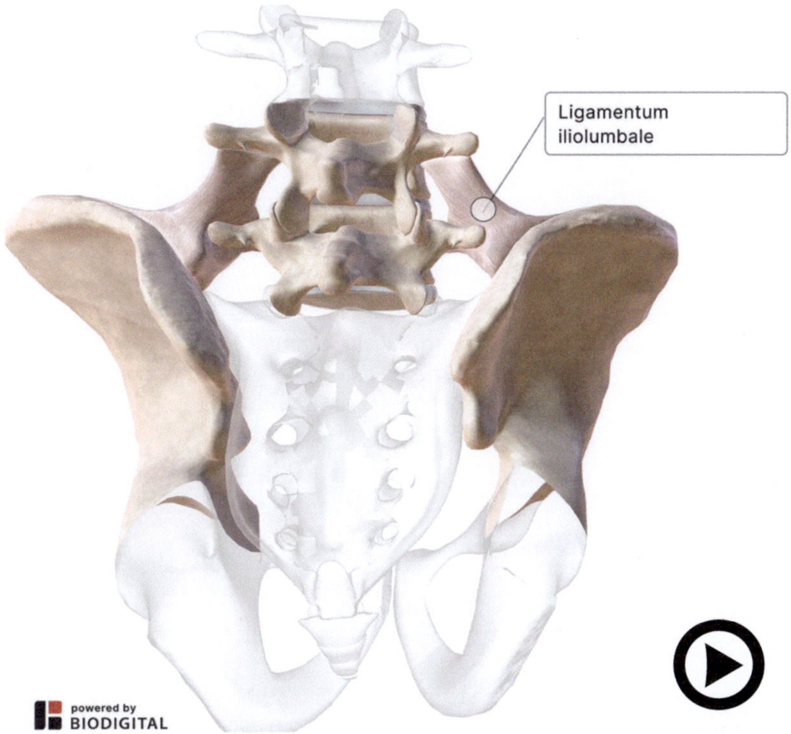

Fig. 4.1 Anatomy and palpation of the lig. iliolumbale (▶ https://doi.org/10.1007/000-csa)

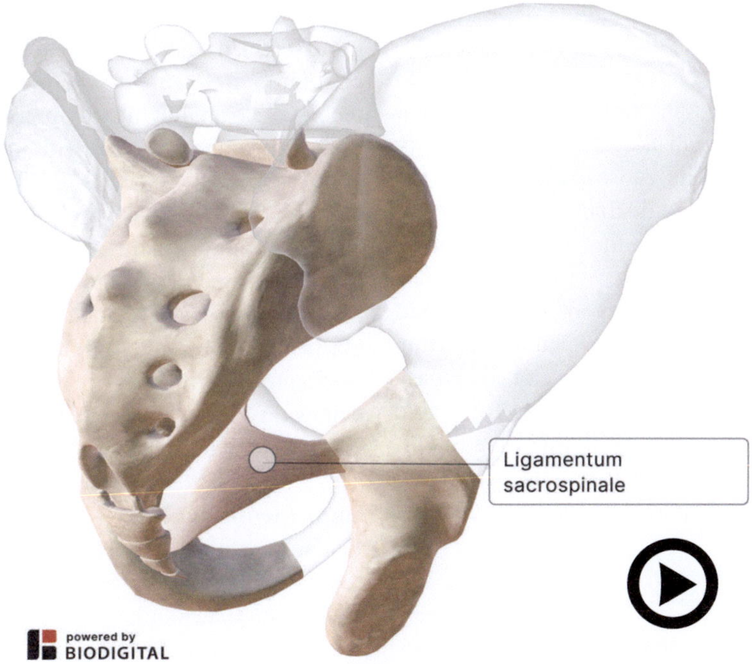

Fig. 4.2 Anatomy and palpation of the lig. sacrospinale (▶ https://doi.org/10.1007/000-cra)

Implementation Note

When palpating the sacrotuberal ligament, a gentle approach should be taken to avoid irritation of the pelvitrochanteric muscles (Fig. 4.3).

4.2.1.4 Palpation of the Inguinal Ligament

The inguinal ligament is formed by the lower edge of the aponeurosis of the transversus abdominis, obliquus externus abdominis and obliquus internus abdominis muscles and by

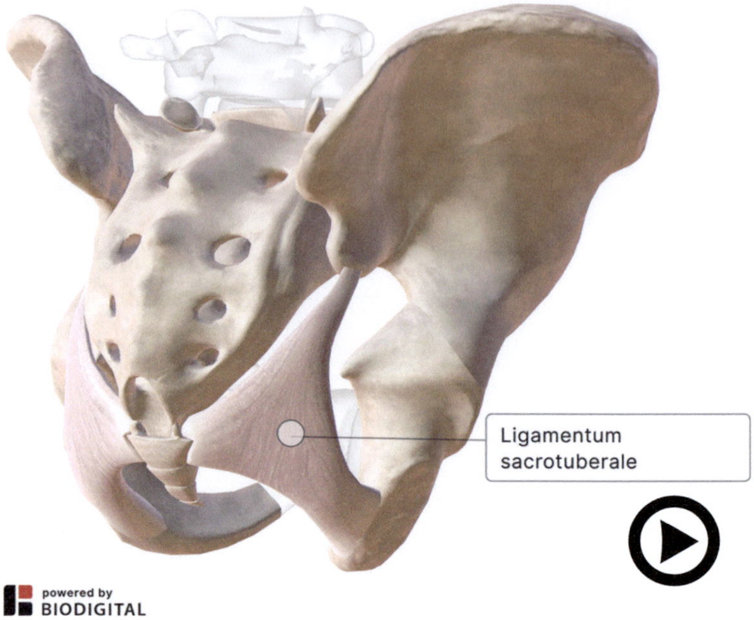

Fig. 4.3 Anatomy and palpation of the lig. sacrotuberale (▶ https://doi.org/10.1007/000-crb)

transverse fibres of the iliac fascia. Thus, myofascial structures of the abdomen meet those of the thigh and unite to form the inguinal ligament. It extends from the SIAS in a ventromedial direction and inserts at the pubic tubercle. In the central region, the arcus iliopectineus, which runs from the inguinal ligament to the pecten ossis pubis, separates the lacuna musculorum from the medially situated lacuna vasorum. Due to these anatomical conditions, it is important to be able to palpate this ligament. A starting position in the supine position is preferred, with the knee joints slightly supported. Flexion in the hip joint causes relaxation in the groin region, so that a more precise distinction can be made between the ligamentary and surrounding structure during palpation.

Starting from the SIAS, the fingertips of the index and middle fingers are placed flat in the caudomedial direction. Subsequently, palpation can be carried out on an imaginary connecting line in the direction of the symphysis. To be able to differentiate the ligament optimally, it is advisable to palpate transversely to the course of the ligament. As a fixed elastic structure, the inguinal ligament is clearly perceptible and can be followed to its base.

Implementation Note

Due to the anatomical proximity, palpation in the area of the lacuna vasorum may irritate the femoral artery or vein. In the area of the lacuna musculorum, both the femoral nerve and the iliopsoas muscle are closely related to the inguinal ligament. All the above-mentioned structures can react symptomatically if the intensity of palpation is too high, which is why tact is required here in the truest sense of the word (Fig. 4.4).

4.2.2 Palpation of the Ligaments at the Hip Joint

The art. coxae, which is mainly secured by bones, is additionally stabilised by ligaments. These collagen-fibre connective tissue structures, which are in depth close to the joint, are difficult to palpate. In addition to the ischiopubofemoral ligament and the transverse acetabular ligament, which are not directly palpable, parts of the iliofemoral ligament can be accessed with the fingertips.

4.2.2.1 Palpation of the Iliofemoral Ligament

The iliofemoral ligament is best palpated in the region of origin at the pelvis. To do this, first locate the SIAI with the fingertips and then palpate distolaterally in depth. A firm elastic structure can be felt in the direction of the greater trochanter. During passive internal rotation with combined extension in the hip joint, the parts under the finger tense, whereas they tend to relax during abduction.

Implementation Note

Palpation of this ligament proves to be very demanding and requires a high degree of sensitivity, as the fibres are in depth and there are also a large number of surrounding structures, such as the rectus femoris muscle. Therefore, only one stimulation is possible (Fig. 4.5).

4.2.3 Palpation of the Ligaments of the Knee Joint

The transportable hinge joint is mainly stabilised by ligaments. Some ligaments can be palpated by the practitioner,

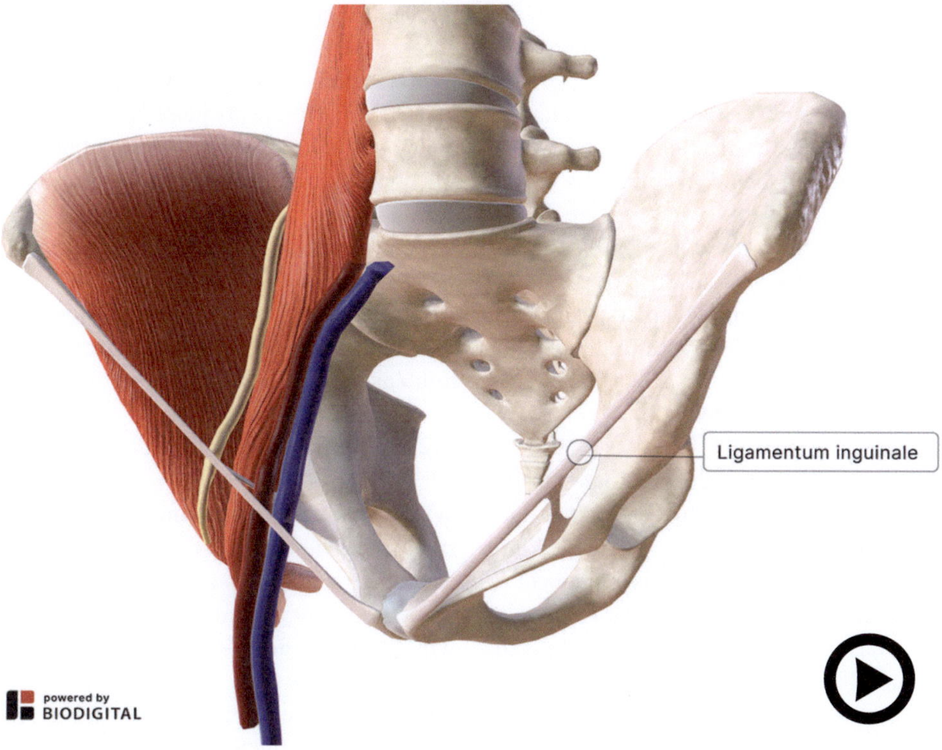

Fig. 4.4 Anatomy and palpation of the lig. inguinale (▶ https://doi.org/10.1007/000-crc)

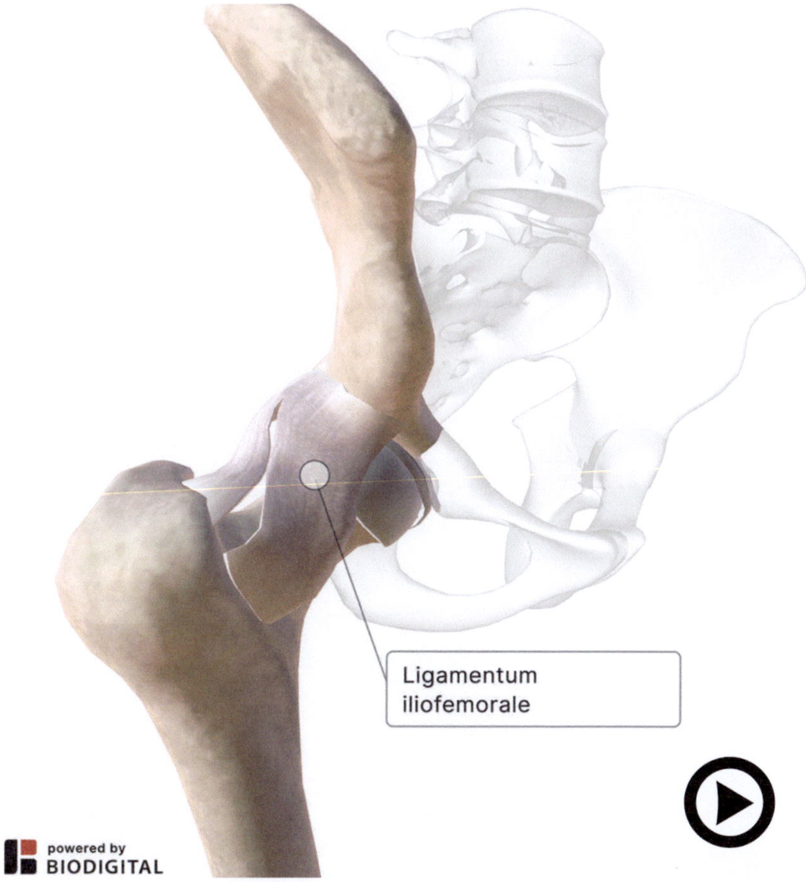

Fig. 4.5 Anatomy and palpation of the lig. iliofemorale (▶ https://doi.org/10.1007/000-crd)

while others cannot. In addition to the cruciate ligament, the transversum genus ligament, the meniscofemoral ligaments and the popliteum arcuatum and obliquum ligament, which cannot be palpated, ligaments such as the medial and lateral collateral ligaments and the patella ligament can be felt. It should be noted that the person being examined is in the supine or lateral position so that the structures are easily accessible. High loads as well as the considerable prevalence of injuries reflect the enormous relevance of palpation in the knee region [3]. In the following chapters, palpation of the ligaments of the art. genus is described in detail.

4.2.3.1 Palpation of the Tibial Collateral Ligament

The stabilisation of the articular genus against forces in the direction of valgisation is mainly realised by the internal ligament. The tibial collateral ligament, which can be divided into a deep anterior and a superficial posterior part, is a ligament of about 4 cm wide and 20 cm long [4]. Beginning at the medial femoral epicondyle, it runs steeply distally, splits off to form the medial meniscus and then inserts below the medial tibial condyle. In the insertion area, the bursa anserina is embedded, which minimises friction between the pes anserinus superficialis and the lig. collaterale tibiale. The medial ligament is a collagen-fibrous structure that is often affected in lower limb injuries [5]. For this reason, it is extremely important to be able to palpate the fibrous courses to draw conclusions about the integrity. The superficial position and few corresponding structures in the area of the inner ligament allow optimal palpatory access. The patient is placed in a supine position, and the knee joint is slightly flexed. The epicondylus medialis femoris is first located with the steeply placed fingertips. Then palpate distally, and notice a flat structure. When palpating across the course of the ligament, the collagenous fibres can be distinguished from surrounding tissue. With the described procedure, the ligament can be followed distally until its insertion.

Instructions for use:

To make palpation even more precise, the joint can be moved in extension and in valgisation during palpation. This tightens the ligament and makes it easier to define (Fig. 4.6).

4.2.3.2 Palpation of the Collateral Fibular Ligament

With a rather narrow, roundish shape, the external ligament runs from the epicondylus lateralis femoris distally to the caput fibulae. This position leads to a stabilising function compared to a varicosity of the art. genus. The ligament, which is more delicate than the inner ligament, can be easily palpated as it is only slightly covered by other structures. From the supine position, the head of the fibula is first visited via the fingertips and then palpated in the proximal direction. If the knee joint is slightly flexed, the rounded shape transverse to the course is best palpated. If the articular genus is moved in extension, the collateral fibular ligament can be better differentiated from the surrounding tissue.

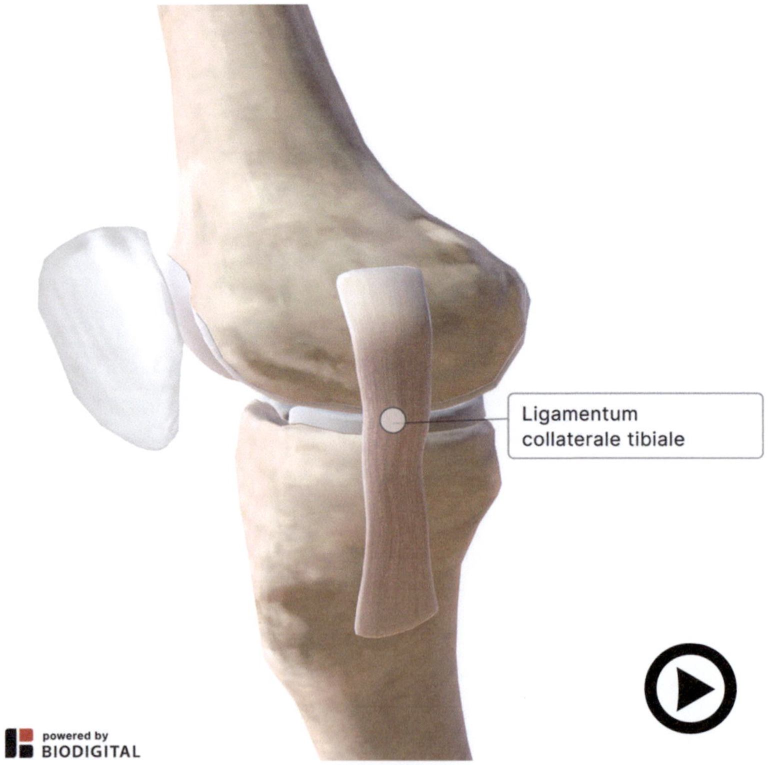

Fig. 4.6 Anatomy and palpation of the lig. collaterale tibiale (▶ https://doi.org/10.1007/000-cre)

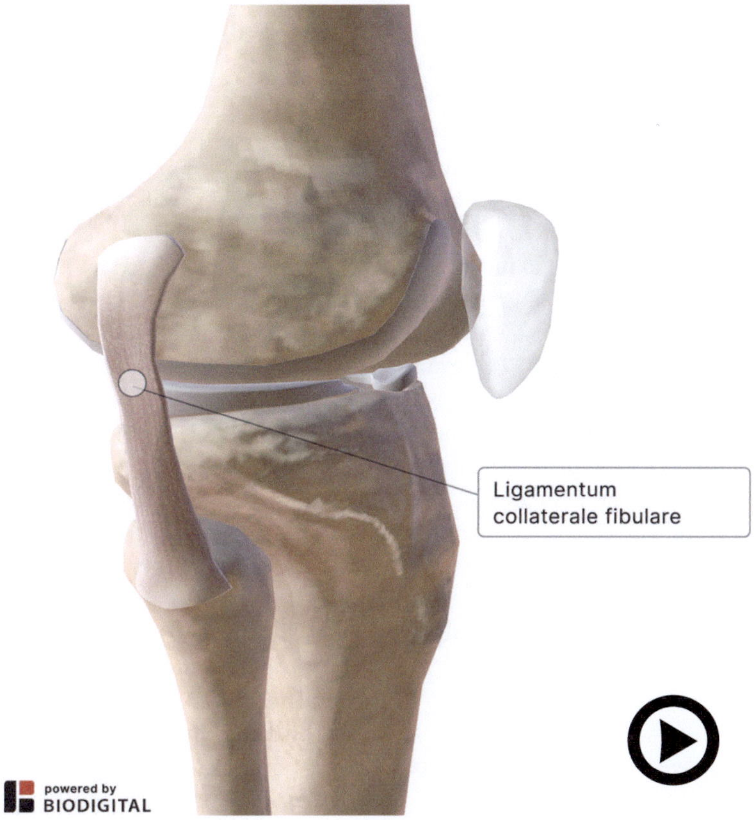

Fig. 4.7 Anatomy and palpation of the lig. collaterale fibulare (▶ https://doi.org/10.1007/000-crf)

Implementation Note
The caput fibulae can easily be confused with the lateral condyle of the tibia. Care should therefore be taken to palpate this area precisely (Fig. 4.7).

4.2.3.3 Palpation of the Patella Ligament

The connection between the tendon of the quadriceps femoris and its insertion at the tibial tuberosity is ensured by the patella ligament. This ligament, which can often be detected visually, is very superficial and can therefore be easily palpated. For this purpose, the client is in the supine position. Starting at the apex of the patella, the fingertips, which are placed on the surface, move distally and reach the patellar ligament directly. The firm elastic structure can be felt even better transversely to the course of the fibres. The ligament then ends at the tibial tuberosity, which becomes present as an osseous elevation. An active movement in extension initially causes a contraction of the quadriceps femoris muscle, which secondarily leads to a significant increase in tension of the patellar ligament.

Implementation Note
The patella ligament is most clearly felt in 90° flexion with additional isometric tension of the quadricepos femoris muscle (Fig. 4.8).

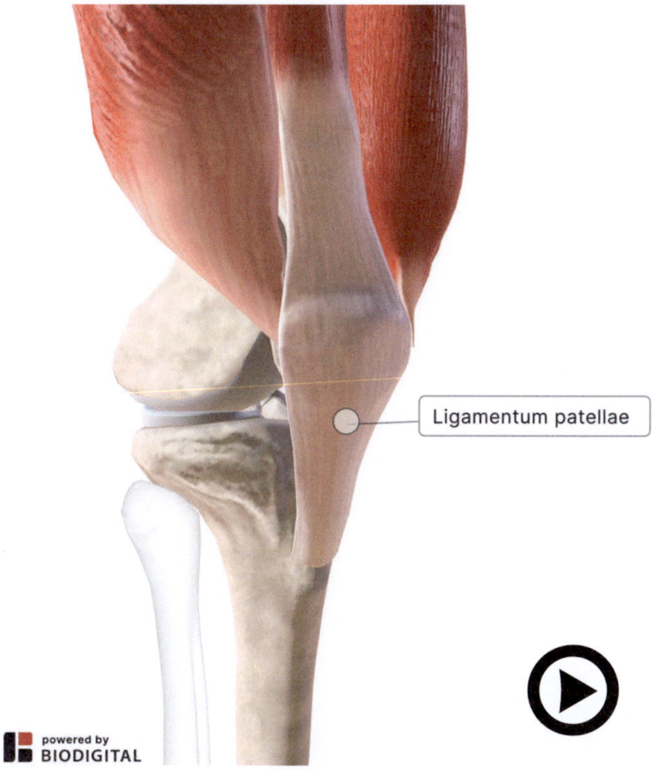

Fig. 4.8 Anatomy and palpation of the lig. patellae (▶ https://doi.org/10.1007/000-crg)

4.2.3.4 Palpation of the Menisci

The two menisci form the reinforcement of the concavity of the tibial plateau in relation to the convex femoral condyles. As elastically deformable fibrocartilage, they move on the tibia. While the medial meniscus has less freedom of movement of a few millimetres due to its contact with the medial ligament and slides anteriorly during internal rotation, the lateral meniscus can move to a greater extent and must move posteriorly during the same rotation [6]. If the tibia moves in external rotation, the sliding directions of the menisci are opposite. This knowledge is useful for palpation. The examiner is in the supine position, while at the same time both knee joints are flexed 90°. Starting from the apex patellae of the knee joint to be examined, the clinician palpates laterally or medially. The steeply positioned palpating fingers are now in the femorotibial joint space and are thus in contact with the anterior horns of both menisci. If the examiner moves the lower leg from a 90° flexion position into internal or external rotation, both menisci will shift dynamically perceptibly on the tibial plateau in an anteroposterior direction.

Implementation Note

As the respective meniscus moves anteriorly, it is most accessible to palpation (Fig. 4.9).

4.2.4 Palpation of the Ligaments of the Foot

The foot, which can be divided into tarsus, metatarsus and antetarsus, forms a biomechanically functional unit. All 26 bones (excluding the sesamoid bone) must harmonise with each other so that individual, everyday loads can be carried out. These numerous bones are connected to each other by joints, which are to a large extent massively stabilised by ligaments. These rather short ligaments lie superficially and are accessible to palpation from the dorsal side. For optimal palpation of the ligaments, the client is placed in a supine position.

4.2.4.1 Palpation of the External Ankle Ligaments

In injuries to the lower extremity, the talocrural articularis with the associated periarticular structures is often involved [7]. Especially when twisting in inversion (plantar flexion + supination), the external ligaments experience a strong stress situation.

Starting from the supine or optional lateral position, the lateral malleolus is first felt with the fingertips. Then only one fingertip (middle or index finger) is used to feel the course of the respective ligament, as the ligaments are very narrow.

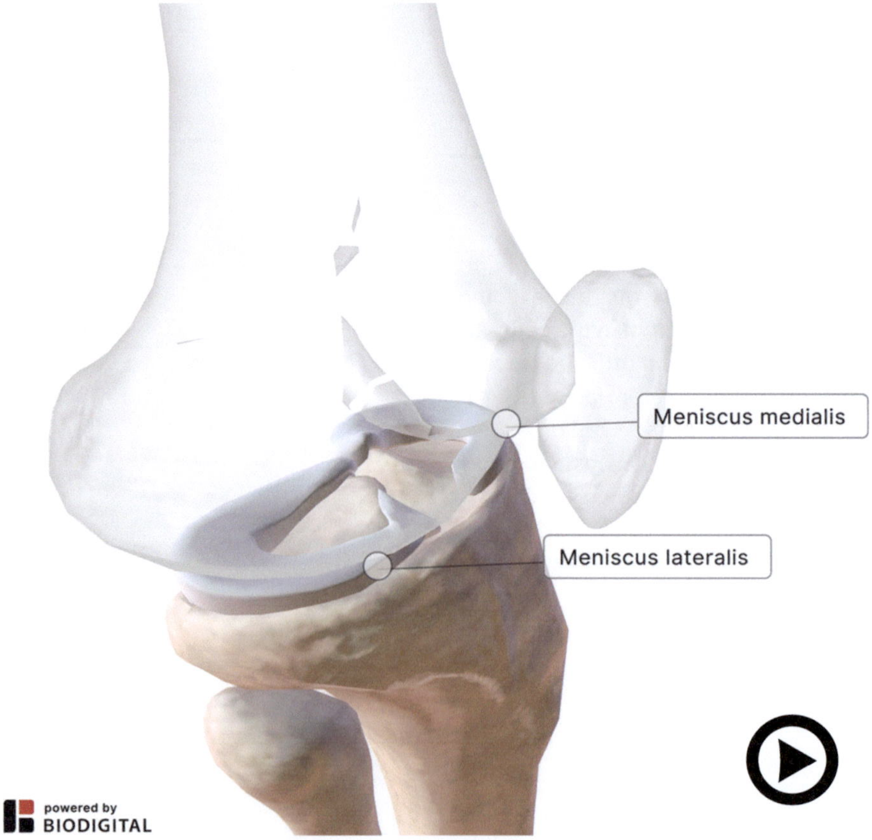

Fig. 4.9 Anatomy and palpation of the menisci of the knee joint (▶ https://doi.org/10.1007/000-crh)

The anterior fibulotalar ligament is found directly in the first depression when the fingertip moves distally and slightly anteriorly from the starting point towards the talus. During a combination movement in plantar flexion and supination, there is a perceptible development of tension in the anterior fibulotalar ligament. The taut ligament comes towards the palpation finger, resulting in better differentiation from the surrounding tissue.

Moving distally from the lateral malleolus, the palpation finger goes directly to the fibulocalcaneal ligament, which is also felt in the depression directly towards the calcaneus. In order to differentiate this ligament from surrounding structures, pure supination is set in the lower ankle joint. Another part of the fork ligament is the lig. fibulotalare posterius. Starting from the lateral malleolus, palpation is performed posteriorly in the direction of the Achilles tendon. The ligament is felt directly at the bony end of the fibula. With dorsal extension and supination, it increases its state of tension and appears under the finger.

Implementation Note

Inversion trauma is common in the upper ankle joint and can cause painful areas in the region of the external ligaments. For this reason, palpation should be accentuated at points but nevertheless started gently at first (Fig. 4.10).

4.2.4.2 Palpation of the Inner Ligaments of the Ankle Joint

The deltoid ligament is divided into four parts that globally limit pronation and thus stabilise the ankle joints. The starting point of all parts is the medial malleolus. Starting from this point, the individual ligaments are palpated. The anterior part is formed by the pars tibionaviculare and the pars tibiotalare anterius.

The palpation finger leaving the bony edge in the direction of the dorsum of the foot feels a firm elastic structure directly in the first depression. Both parts take almost the same course. It is therefore difficult to distinguish them from each other. A combination movement in plantar flexion and pronation causes an increase in tension in the tibionavicular ligament and the tibiotalar anterior ligament. The practitioner can take advantage of this fact during palpation. When palpating distally in extension of the medial malleolus, stimulation is applied to the tibiocalcaneal ligament. The tibiocalcaneal ligament increases its tension during isolated pronation. If the examiner palpates posteriorly from the medial malleolus towards the Achilles tendon, it is possible to palpate the posterior tibial plateau. In the depression, which can be felt after the posterior edge of the bone, the fixed elastic structure can be palpated. The quality of palpation increases during pronation with coupled dorsal extension.

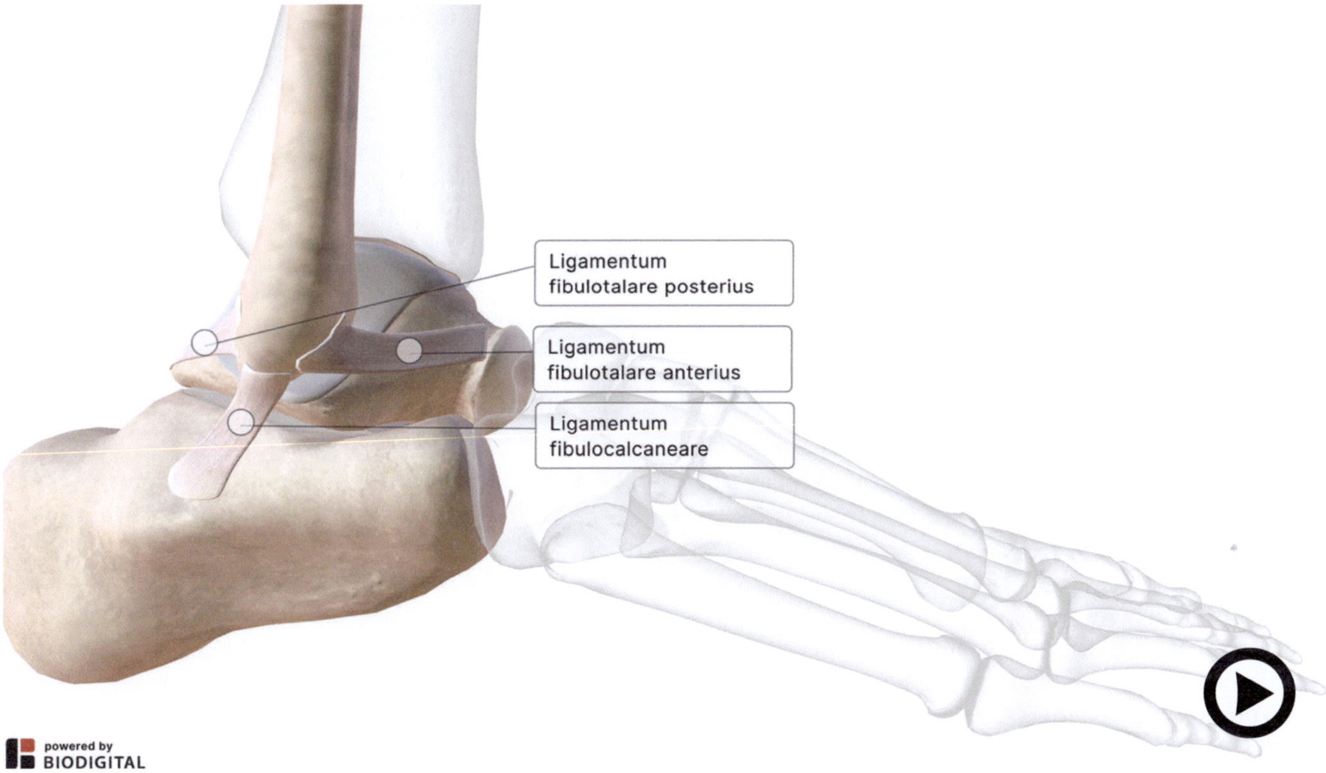

Fig. 4.10 Anatomy and palpation of the external ligaments of the ankle (▶ https://doi.org/10.1007/000-crj)

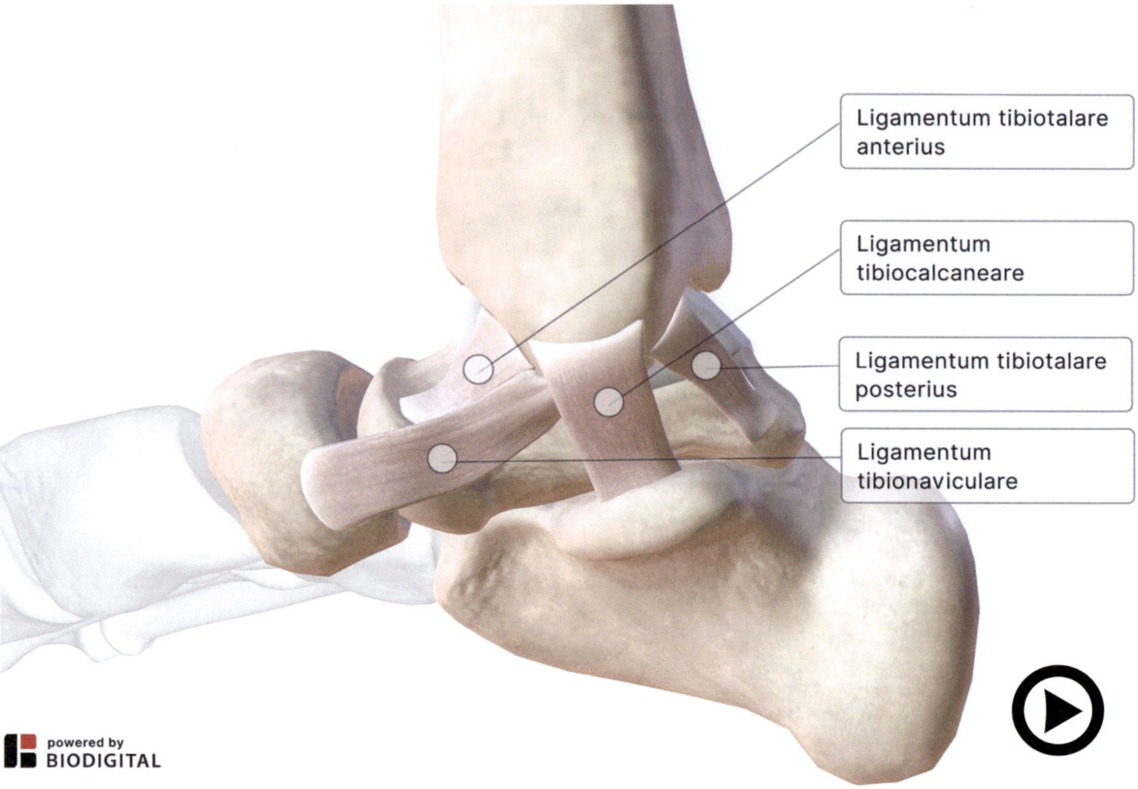

Fig. 4.11 Anatomy and palpation of the internal ligaments of the ankle (▶ https://doi.org/10.1007/000-crk)

Implementation Note
Especially after pronation trauma of the ankle joints, the inner ligaments of the deltoid ligament may be irritated and react painfully to palpation. Therefore, gentle palpation should first be performed in this region (Fig. 4.11).

4.2.4.3 Palpation of the Bifurcate Ligament

As a connecting device between the calcaneus and the os cuboideum or os naviculare, the bifurcate ligament can be felt dorsally on the surface. The calcaneocuboid ligament, the lateral part of Chopart's ligament, is best felt by first palpating the cuboid bone and then moving towards the calcaneus. In the joint space between the two bones, the rather small ligament will be felt in the middle part. The upper part of the bifurcate ligament, which is the calcaneonavicular ligament, is difficult to feel because soft tissue is located above the palpation area.

Implementation Note
As the bifurcate ligament is often affected after supine or inversion trauma, pressure dolences can often occur in this region during palpation (Fig. 4.12).

4.2.4.4 Palpation of the Plantar Aponeurosis

The plantar surface of the foot is formed via the aponeurosis plantaris, which radiates into the plantar fascia. This region of the foot is best accessed via the prone position, while the corresponding knee joint is set in 90° flexion. The plantar fascia can now be examined precisely with the palpation fingers, as it is located rather superficially. It extends from the calcaneus distally and opens at the joint capsules of the metatarsophalangeal joints. With dorsal extension, the tension of the plantar aponeurosis increases, while it relaxes with plantar flexion of the toes.

Implementation Note
Due to various foot deformities, which are common, the plantar aponeurosis may be under increased tension and thus react symptomatically during palpation (Fig. 4.13).

4.2.4.5 Palpation of the Intermediate Ligaments in the Tarsus, Metatarsus and Antetarsus

All bones in the foot are connected to each other by ligaments. Amphiarthroses exist in the areas of the tarsus and metatarsus and in the transition between the two, which are stabilised by tight intertarsal and intermetatarsal ligaments. Access to these is only realised via the dorsum of the foot in the form of stimulation. The individual joint spaces, which are spanned by the corresponding ligaments, are used for orientation. The structures are palpated from the supine position with the steeply placed fingertips of the index or middle finger. In the distal area of the foot, especially the interpha-

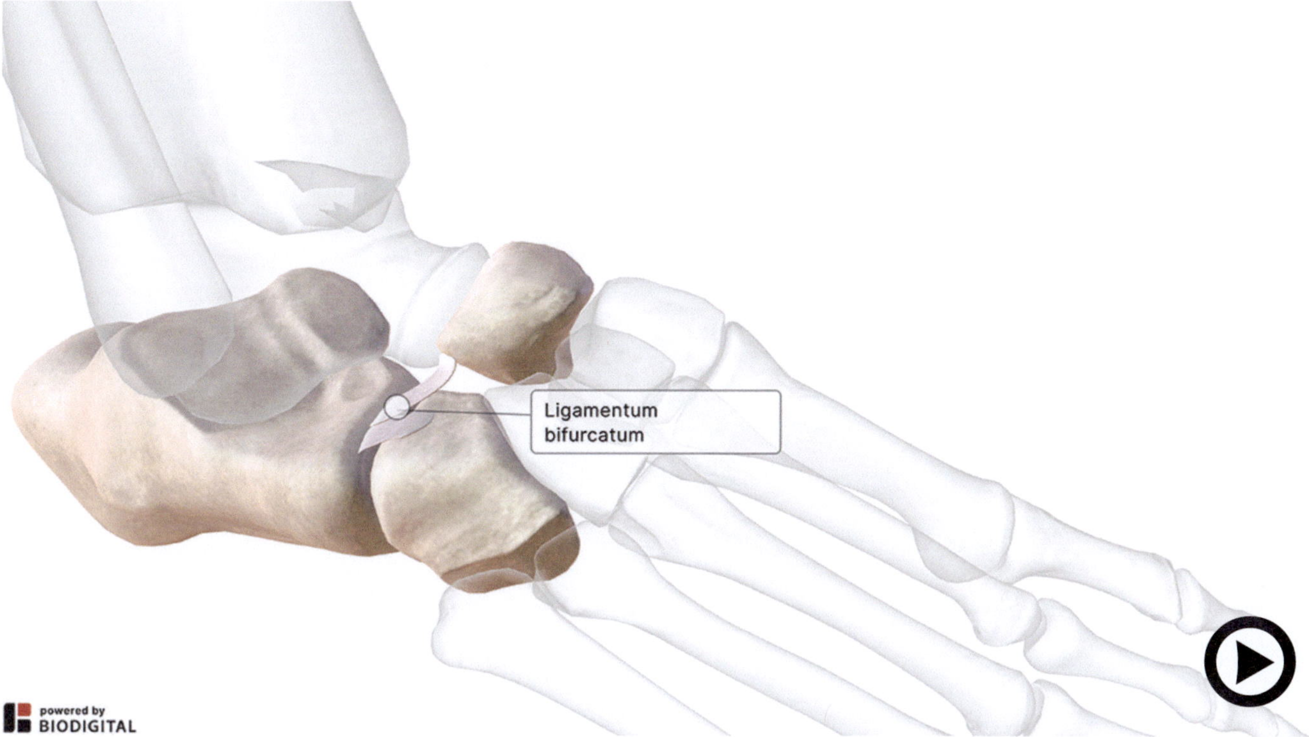

Fig. 4.12 Anatomy and palpation of the lig. bifurcatum (▶ https://doi.org/10.1007/000-crm)

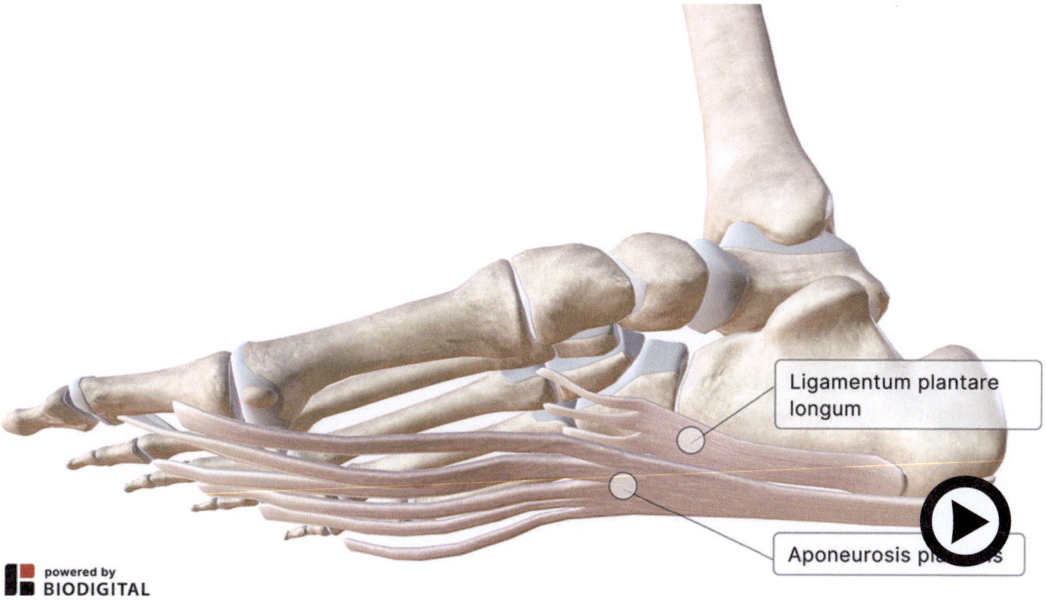

Fig. 4.13 Anatomy and palpation of the lig. plantare longum (▶ https://doi.org/10.1007/000-crn)

langeal joints of the antetarsus, the ligamenta collaterialia can be grasped laterally and medially of the joints by stimulation. As there is a very close relationship between the capsule and the ligament in this area, precise differentiation is challenging.

Implementation Note

The ligaments in the area of the tarsus, metatarsus and antetarsus are very difficult to feel. It is therefore of great importance to know the anatomical position precisely in advance to hit the position with the palpation fingers (Fig. 4.14).

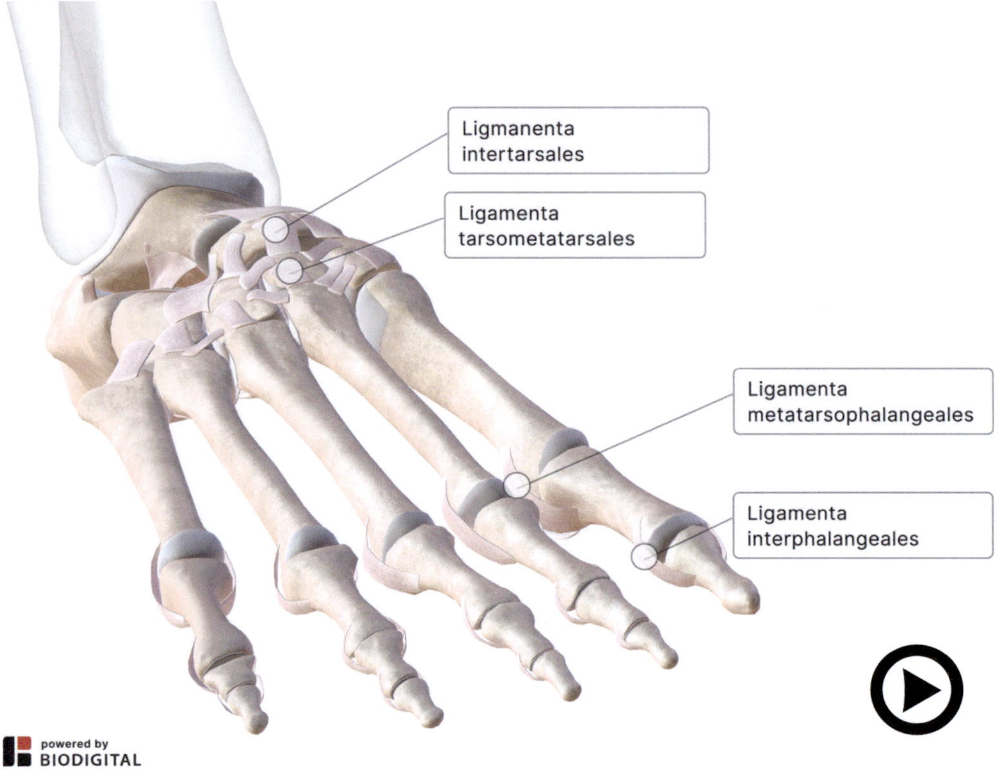

Fig. 4.14 Anatomy and palpation of the ligg. im tarsus, metatarsus und antetarsus (▶ https://doi.org/10.1007/000-crp)

4.3 Palpation of the Ligaments of the Spine

The human spine is built according to the tensegrity model. Bones that are stable in bending, together with ligaments, muscles and tendons that are stable in stretching, create a tension-belt mechanism that is stable in itself. Because of this division, the region of the columna vertebralis is robust and at the same time functionally flexible and can cope with everyday demands. To gain the necessary strength in each segment, most of the ligaments of the spine tend to be located in depth, which does not allow palpation. However, some ligaments are accessible and are described in the following chapters. The recommended starting position for this is the sitting or supine position.

4.3.1 Palpation of the Supraspinal Ligaments

From the sitting position, the proc. spinosus of C7 is first visited with the fingertips. Since the most caudal vertebra of the cervical spine has a prominent spinous process, it is easy to palpate it. For better differentiation, an extension of the cervical spine can be performed, in which the proc. spinosus of C6 is shifted anteriorly, whereas C7 retains its position. Starting from the spinous process of C7, continuous caudal palpation is then performed with moderate pressure in the anterior direction. After each spinous process, a small depression is created which is covered by a firm elastic structure. These structures, which are stretched during a flexion movement in the spine, represent the supraspinal ligaments. They extend continuously from one proc. spinosus to the underlying proc. spinosus and thus cover the entire spinal column from the dorsal side.

Implementation Note
A better possibility of differentiation is possible via a flexion component of the spine (Fig. 4.15).

4.3.2 Palpation of the Nuchae Ligament

Palpation of the easily accessible nuchal ligament begins at the protuberantia occipitalis externa at the back of the head while the client is positioned in the sitting position. Starting from this point, palpation is made caudally until a firm cord of tissue is felt between the parts of the erector spinae muscle. The cervical spine then assumes flexion. During this

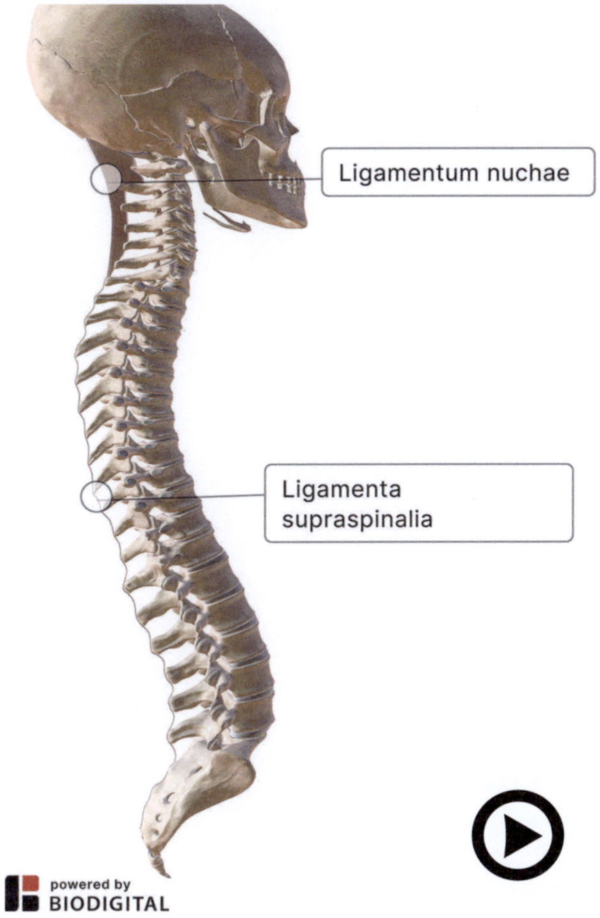

Fig. 4.15 Anatomy and palpation of the lig. supraspinalia (▶ https://doi.org/10.1007/000-crq)

movement, the nuchae ligament tenses and becomes clearly palpable as a firm elastic structure. Palpation can then be performed on the ligament with the fingertips up to the proc. spinosus of C7. The ligament then merges into the supraspinal ligament.

Implementation Note
The movement of the cervical spine in flexion should be performed slowly so that the ligament can be grasped in its entire structure (Fig. 4.16).

4.3.3 Palpation of the Sternocostal Ligament

The sternocostal ligaments are best felt in the supine or sitting position. Ribs I–VII, which are true ribs connected to the sternum, are connected to it via the sternocostal ligaments. Starting from the sternum, the fingertips, which are laid flat, are moved to the right or left in the direction of a rib and, at each articulated transition, encounter the respective incisura costalis, which can be felt as a small raised area. In this region is the corresponding sternocostal ligament of the respective rib, which, however, is difficult to differentiate from the surrounding tissue. Therefore, when palpating these ligaments, the focus is on stimulation.

Implementation Note
Due to the demanding sensation, it is necessary to know the exact anatomical location (Fig. 4.17).

4.4 Ligaments of the Upper Extremity

While the ligaments of the lower extremity are elementary for human locomotion, the ligaments of the upper extremity have another important task, namely they stabilise everyday movements in the shoulder girdle and the arms. This area of the body is also constructed according to the tensegrity model, so that form-stable bodies are created from an unstable bone framework via the tension-belt mechanism of firm-elastic ligaments, tendons and muscles. An important stabilising function is assigned to the ligaments, which are located close to the joints and ensure that movements proceed smoothly. It is therefore important to know about the position and function of the ligaments, to palpate them and then to be able to assess the state of tension. This chapter describes the location of the palpable ligaments and presents techniques for ligamentary palpation. The starting position of the client will vary between sitting, supine and prone.

4.4.1 Palpation of the Ligaments of the Shoulder Girdle and Shoulder Joint

The shoulder girdle as well as the shoulder joint realise the coarse adjustment of the arm so that a fine and targeted movement of the hand is biomechanically possible. Furthermore, there is a close connection between the shoulder girdle and the shoulder joint, as they are mutually dependent. If the humeroscapular joint is moved, the shoulder girdle must have a certain degree of mobility at the same time; otherwise, the final degree of movement cannot be achieved [8]. Five joints can be counted as part of this entire region, which are stabilised by ligaments. Some of them can be palpated. The exact procedure is described in the following chapters for the palpable ligaments. The client is in the supine or sitting position.

4.4.1.1 Palpation of the Interclavicular Ligament

The curvilinear ligament that connects both clavicles and is in contact with the manubrium sterni becomes accessible for palpation via the incisura jugularis. The palpating fingers contact the most cranial part of the manubrium from ventrally and move further cephaladward with moderate pres-

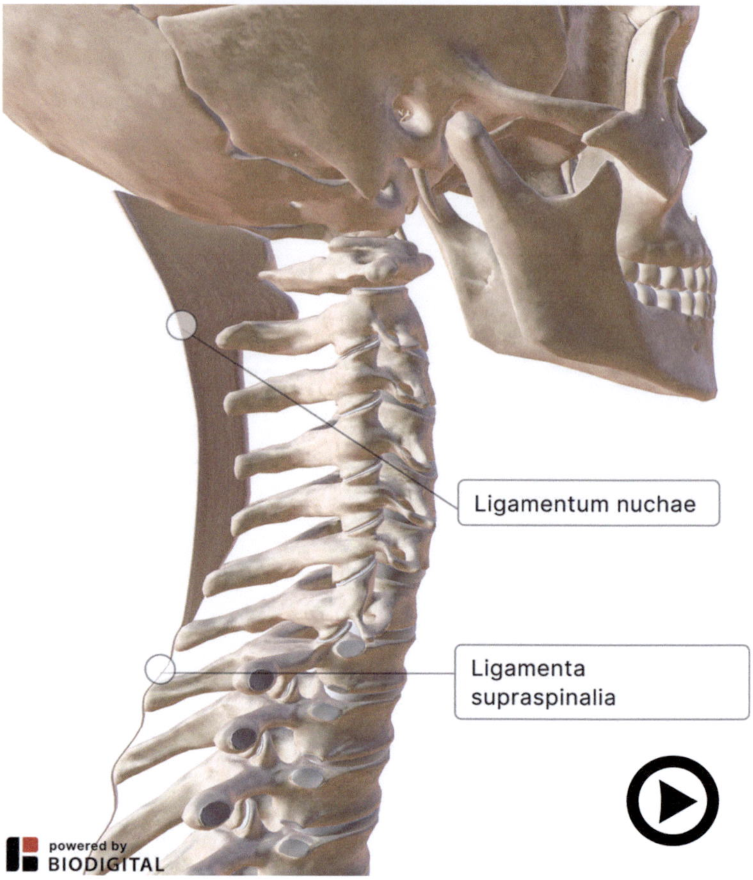

Fig. 4.16 Anatomy and palpation of the lig. nuchae (▶ https://doi.org/10.1007/000-crr)

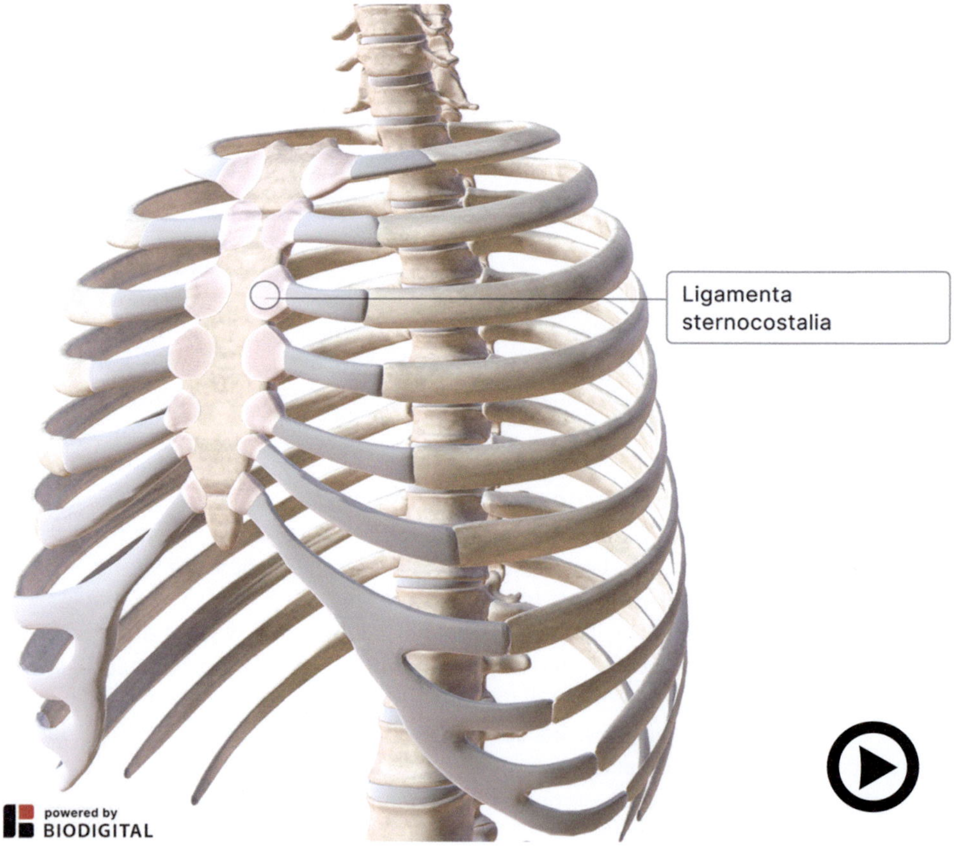

Fig. 4.17 Anatomy and palpation of the lig. sternocostalia (▶ https://doi.org/10.1007/000-crs)

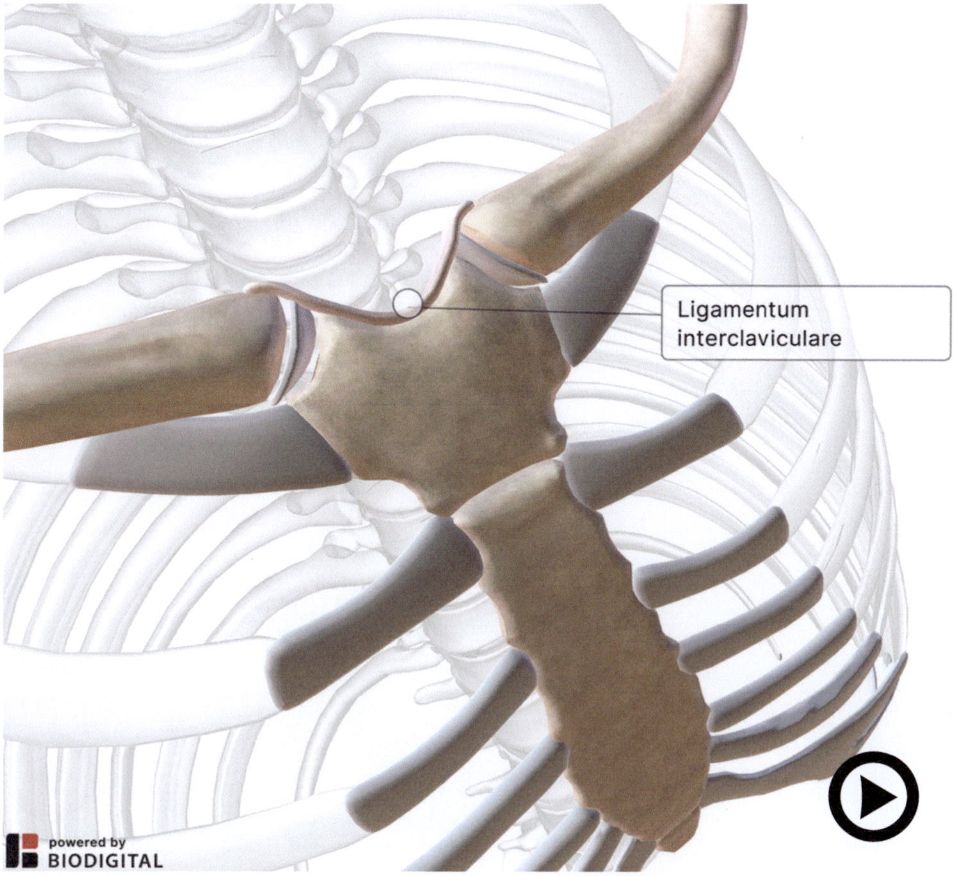

Fig. 4.18 Anatomy and palpation of the lig. interclaviculare (▶ https://doi.org/10.1007/000-crt)

sure. The first point of contact is directly in the first depression of the jugular fossa, which is located between the extremitates sternales of the two clavicles. From there, the steeply placed fingertip is placed from cranial towards caudal directly on the upper edge of the incisura jugularis. In this region is the interclavicular ligament, which is difficult to differentiate from surrounding tissues because of its direct connection to the bone.

Implementation Note
The jugular fossa is a very sensitive region that can quickly develop unpleasant sensations when pressure is applied. Because of this, caution and a gentle approach are recommended during palpation (Fig. 4.18).

4.4.1.2 Palpation of the Sternoclavicular Ligament

The flat ligament that connects the clavicle to the sternum via the SCG can be divided into an anterior and a posterior part. While the posterior part cannot be felt, the anterior part of the stabilising ligament can be palpated. As soon as the client has found his starting position in the sitting or supine position, the fingertips are placed centrally, flat on the clavicle. Then, with moderate pressure, palpate medially towards the manubrium until a clear break in the bony structure becomes apparent. This gap is the joint space of the art. sternoclavicularis and the starting point of ligamentary palpation. Directly in the region of the joint is the capsule and the sternoclavicular anterior ligament. Due to the bony proximity and the direct connection to the capsule, it is difficult to distinguish the ligamentous structures from the surrounding structures. A precise knowledge of the anatomical position is therefore a basic requirement.

Implementation Note
The structure of the ligament is rather flat and localised directly on the bone. In addition, parts of the sternocleidomastoid muscle lie above it, which is why pressure dolences often occur during palpation (Fig. 4.19).

4.4.1.3 Palpation of the Coracoclavicular Ligament

This ligament, which connects the clavicle with the proc. coracoideus, is best palpated from the starting position in the supine position or optionally in the sitting position with the arm in a passive position. It mainly provides stability for the ACG and is divided into two parts, the trapezoideum ligament and the conoideum ligament. The proc. coracoideus of

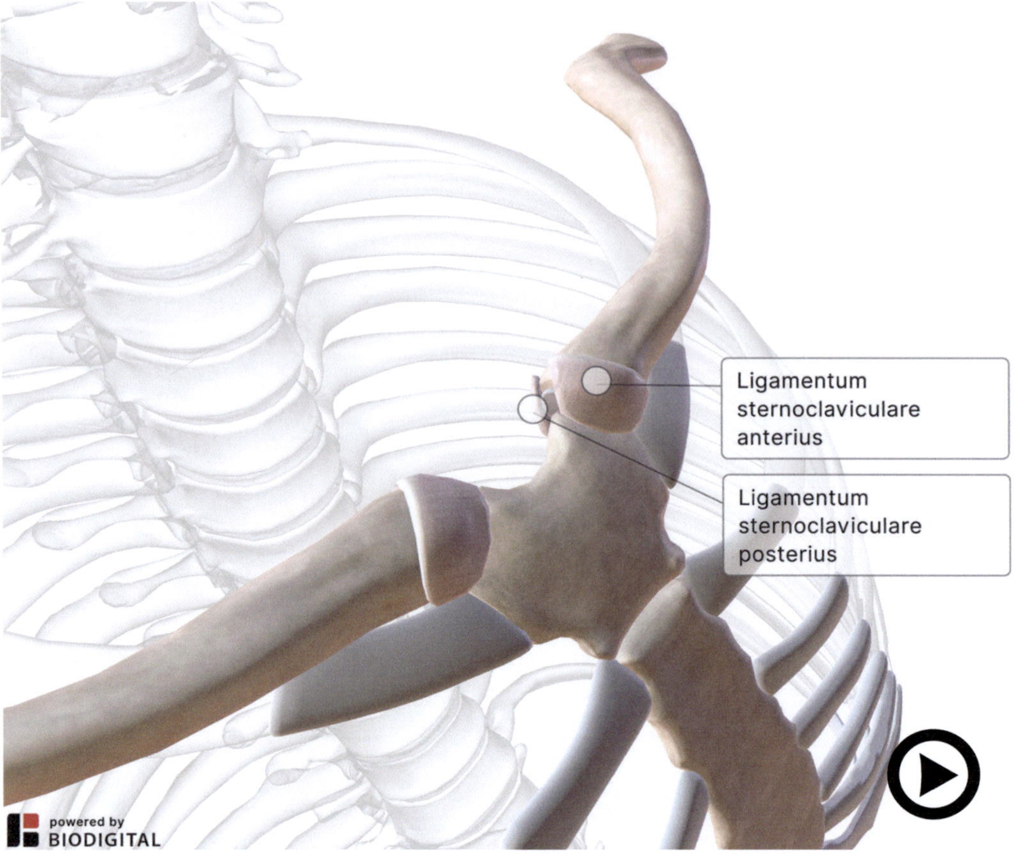

Fig. 4.19 Anatomy and palpation of the lig. sternoclaviculare (▶ https://doi.org/10.1007/000-crv)

the scapula is chosen as the starting point for palpation. The steeply positioned fingertip moves cranially and enters directly into a depression. In the groove, which is lined with soft tissue, a firm-elastic structure can be felt with increased pressure. The palpation finger is now directly on the anterior part of the coracoclavicular ligament, the trapezoideum ligament. The ligament behind it only leads to an increase in the firm-elastic sensation. It requires precise knowledge of the anatomical position of the ligament so that correct stimulation is possible.

Implementation Note
This region should be done gently at first and then slowly going deeper; otherwise, protective tensions may occur which make palpation difficult (Fig. 4.20).

4.4.1.4 Palpation of the Acromioclavicular Ligament

The clavicle articulates at its lateral end with the shoulder height. This gives rise to the art. acromioclavicularis. This flat joint is stabilised by a capsule and two ligaments, the palpably accessible lig. acromioclaviculare superius and the lig. acromioclaviculare inferius. For palpation, which is initiated via the clavicle, the starting position can be individually selected so that the arm is passively stabilised. The index and middle fingers are placed flat and palpated laterally on the clavicle until a slight elevation is felt. In this region is the joint space of the ACG and above it the lig. acromioclaviculare superius. Because of the direct proximity to the capsule as well as to the bone and the only slight degree of movement in the joint itself, direct palpation is difficult. Good anatomical knowledge is therefore the basis for stimulation.

Implementation Note
Due to the myofascial influence of the trapezius pars descendens muscle and the deltoid muscle, pressure dolences can occur frequently in the region of the acromioclavicular ligament (Fig. 4.21).

4.4.1.5 Palpation of the Glenohumeral Ligament

The ligament, which runs between the glenoid cavity and the humeral head and serves to stabilise external rotation, can be divided into a superior, a medial oblique and an inferioventral and inferiodorsal part. Between the two inferior parts is the axillary recess, which is tightened as a reserve fold of the shoulder joint capsule during final abduction.

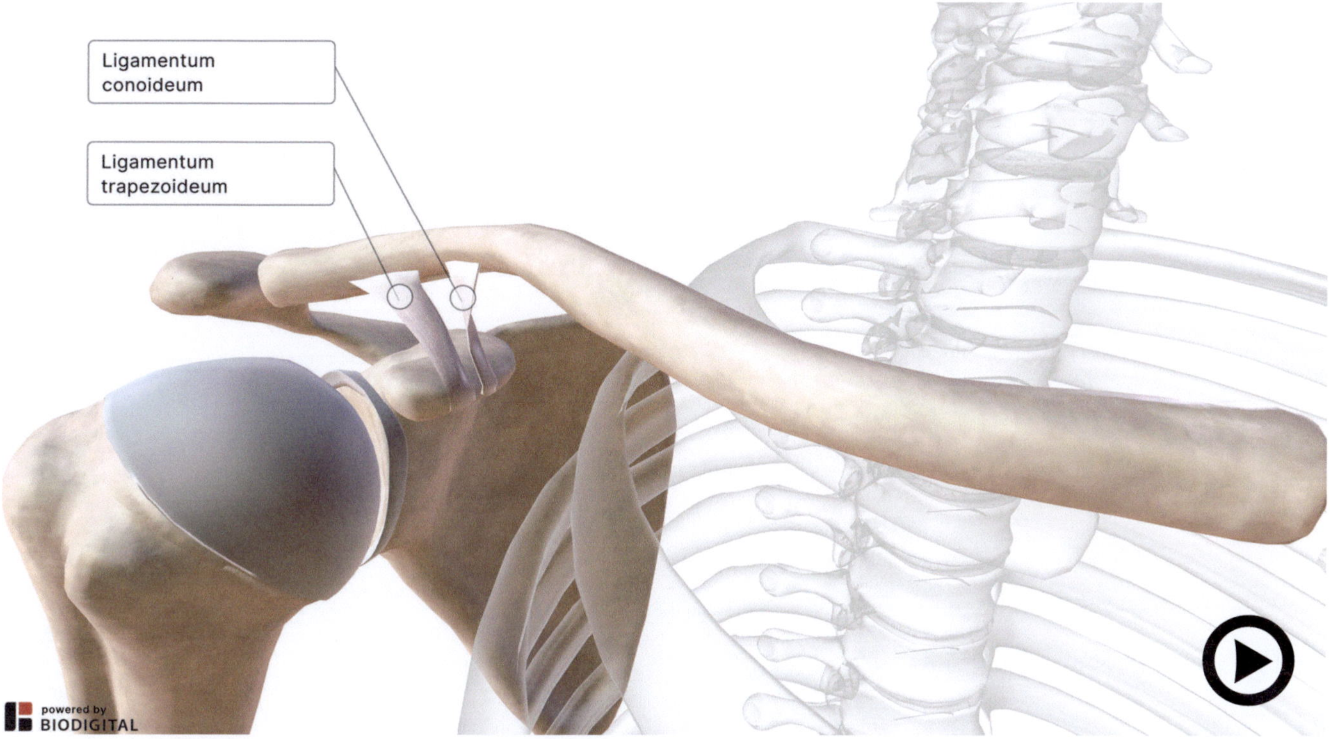

Fig. 4.20 Anatomy and palpation of the lig. coracoclaviculare (▶ https://doi.org/10.1007/000-crw)

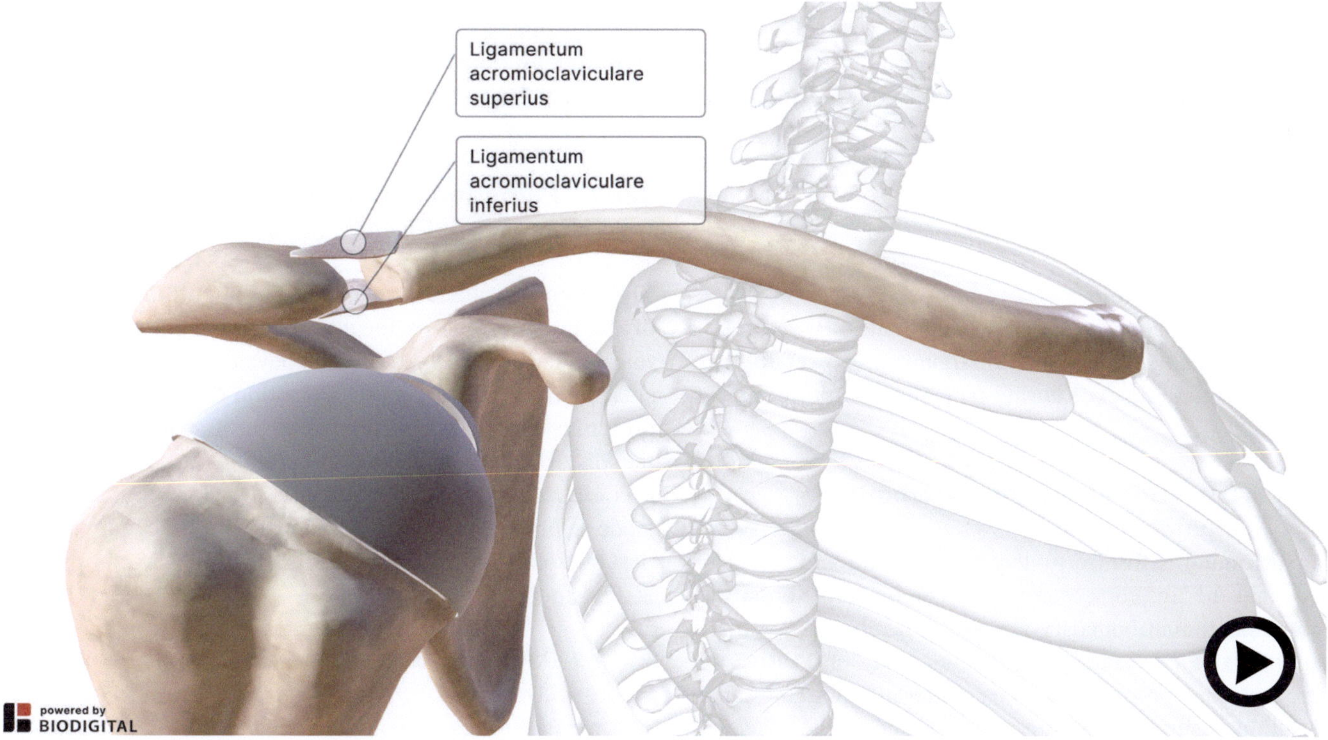

Fig. 4.21 Anatomy and palpation of the lig. acromioclaviculare (▶ https://doi.org/10.1007/000-crx)

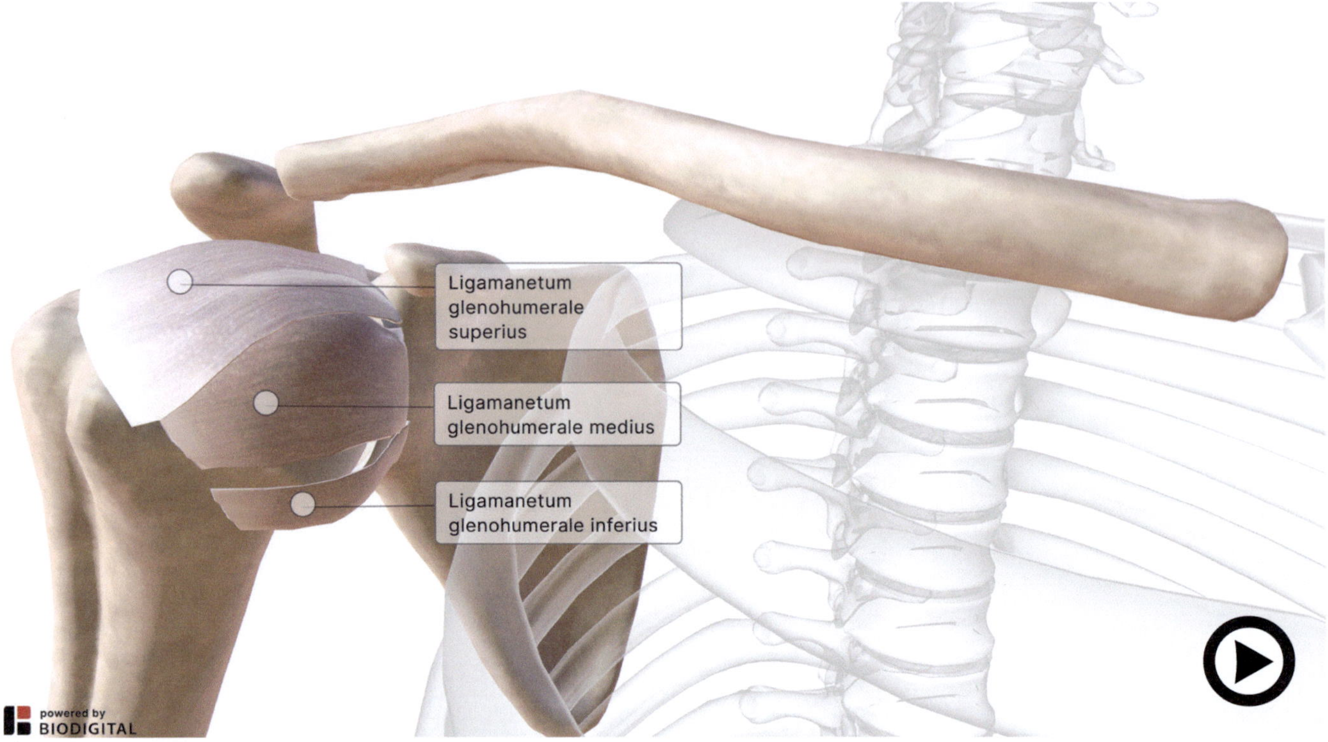

Fig. 4.22 Anatomy and palpation of the lig. glenohumeralia (▶ https://doi.org/10.1007/000-cry)

Every fibre part of the ligament is covered by muscles. Therefore, a maximum of stimulation but no direct palpation of the ligament is possible. To reach the anterior parts of the ligament, the patient is asked to lie on his back. Then, starting from the tuberculum minus humeri, palpation is carried out slightly medially. Dorsal pressure is then applied at the level of the glenohumeral joint space to stimulate the ligamentous structures.

Implementation Note
Symptomatic palpation does not automatically indicate a negatively changed glenohumeral ligament. Especially here, the myofascial influence during palpation should be considered (Fig. 4.22).

4.4.1.6 Palpation of the Coracoacromial Ligament

The acromion is formed by the acromion, the proc. coracoideus and the lig. coracoacromiale. The humeral fornix thus forms the cranial boundary for the humeral caput so that it cannot luxate headwards. The ligament plays a decisive role here and can be provided with palpation stimuli in the supine or sitting position via the steeply positioned long finger berries. To do this, the fingers are first placed on the proc. coracoideus. Then the bony reference point is left in a lateral direction, and a slight depression is felt. A moderate dorsal thrust can be used to apply a stimulus to the ligamentous structure.

Implementation Note
The arm should be positioned passively. This minimises the myofascial influences of the coracobrachialis and pectoralis minor muscles as far as possible (Fig. 4.23).

4.4.2 Palpation of the Ligamenta at the Elbow Joint

The articulatio cubiti is an important joint for the movements of the arm. It consists locally of three and functionally of four joints (see Sect. 3.6), which have a well-structured capsular ligamentous apparatus. Palpation of these ligaments is difficult because many muscles of the forearm originate in the distal humerus and run superficial to the ligaments. Precise knowledge of the position is therefore of great importance, along with good positioning. The procedure for the best possible stimulation of the ligaments of the elbow joints is described below.

4.4.2.1 Palpation of the Ulnar Collateral Ligament

The medially located collateral ligament, which makes an important contribution to the stability of the elbow joint, is divided into three parts, which counteract valgisation. They run from the epicondylus medialis humeri to the incisura trochlearis. Starting from the epicondylus medialis humeri,

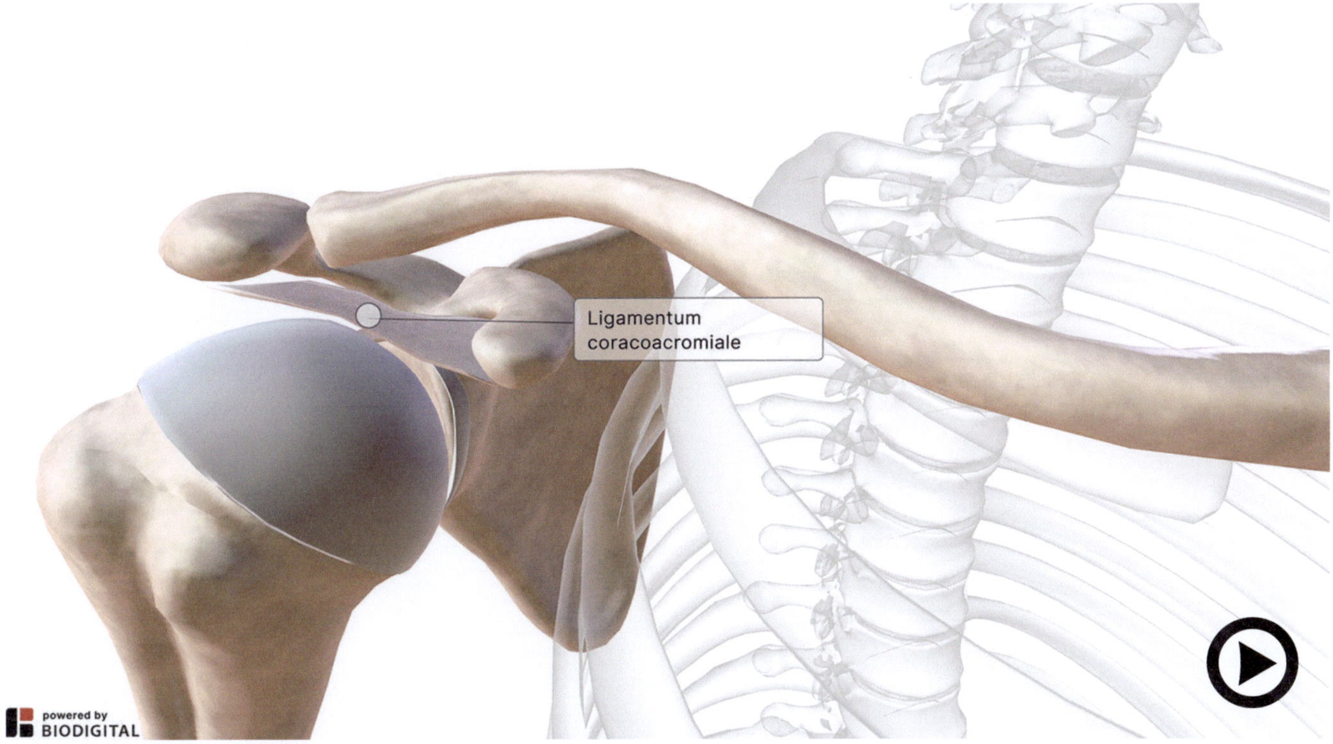

Fig. 4.23 Anatomy and palpation of the lig. coracoacromiale (▶ https://doi.org/10.1007/000-crz)

palpation begins with the palpation finger in a steep position. First, the arm of the person being palpated is placed in the 0-position. The finger moves from the bony reference point in the direction of the olecranon and falls directly into an easily perceptible depression. The arm is now slowly bent while remaining in the depression. A firm-elastic structure is felt under the finger during the movement. This is the posterior part of the ulnar collateral ligament. Directly distal to this palpation point runs the transverse part, which is difficult to detect, but can also be perceived as a firm-elastic structure. Directly anterior to the medial humeral epicondyle, there is also a depression in which the anterior part of the ligament is located. As this part lies directly above the humerus and ulna in depth and numerous soft tissue structures of the wrist and finger flexors run above it, palpation is difficult to realise.

For better differentiation, the ligament can be distinguished from surrounding muscle tendons by means of targeted finger flexor contraction. An exact anatomical position is a basic requirement for this.

Implementation Note

In epicondylopathia medialis humeri, also called golfer's elbow, there is an ingrowth of blood vessels and free nerve endings in the affected tendons [9]. Pain may be felt on palpation of the ligament for the above reason. Therefore, caution should be exercised (Fig. 4.24).

4.4.2.2 Palpation of the Radial Collateral Ligament

On the lateral side of the forearm, at the transition from the lateral humeral epicondyle to the proximal radius, is the radial collateral ligament. It radiates into the anulare radii ligament, thus limiting varus stress and significantly supporting the capsule in its function. The short, tight ligament, which is part of the lateral collateral ligament complex, is often fused with the superficial forearm extensors, which makes direct palpation difficult [10].

The palpation starts at the epicondylus lateralis humeri, which is visited with moderate pressure of the index or middle finger. The arm is in an extended starting position for this. The lateral side is then palpated distally in the direction of the caput radii. As soon as a depression is felt on the bony edge of the lateral humeral epicondyle, the finger stops, and the elbow is moved slightly into flexion. After about 30°, a fixed-elastic structure can be felt directly in the joint space. These fibres are those of the radial collateral ligament.

Implementation Note

In lateral humeral epicondylopathy, also known as tennis elbow, the lateral capsular ligamentous apparatus is frequently affected in addition to the extensor muscles [11]. A pain indication on palpation is possible for the above-mentioned reason. Therefore, caution should be exercised (Fig. 4.25).

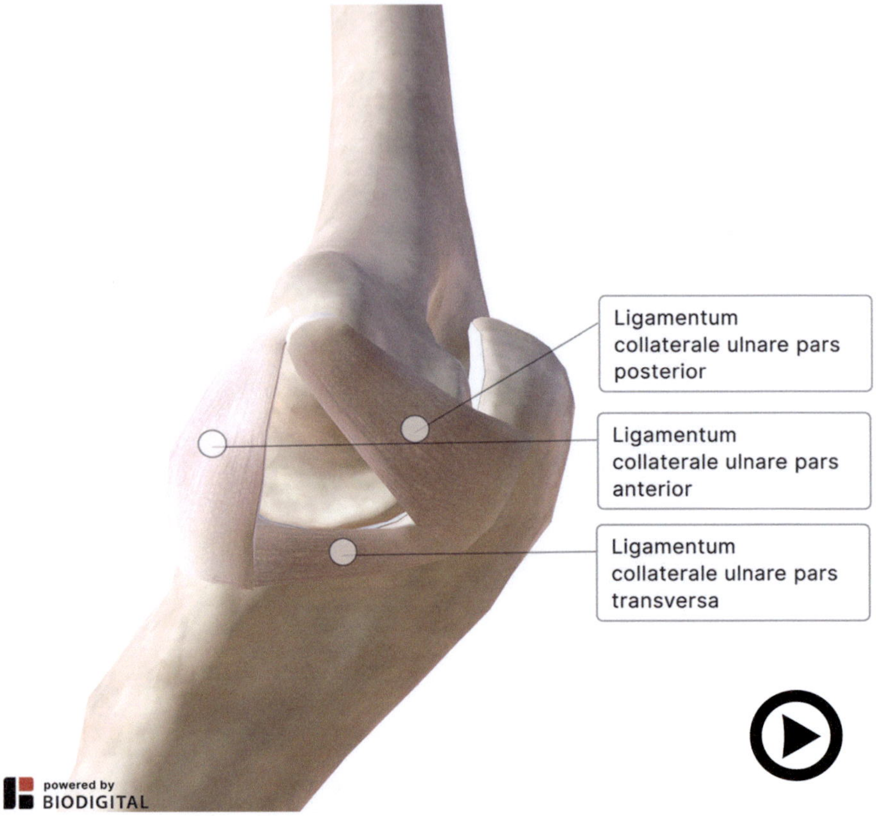

Fig. 4.24 Anatomy and palpation of the lig. collaterale ulnare (▶ https://doi.org/10.1007/000-cs0)

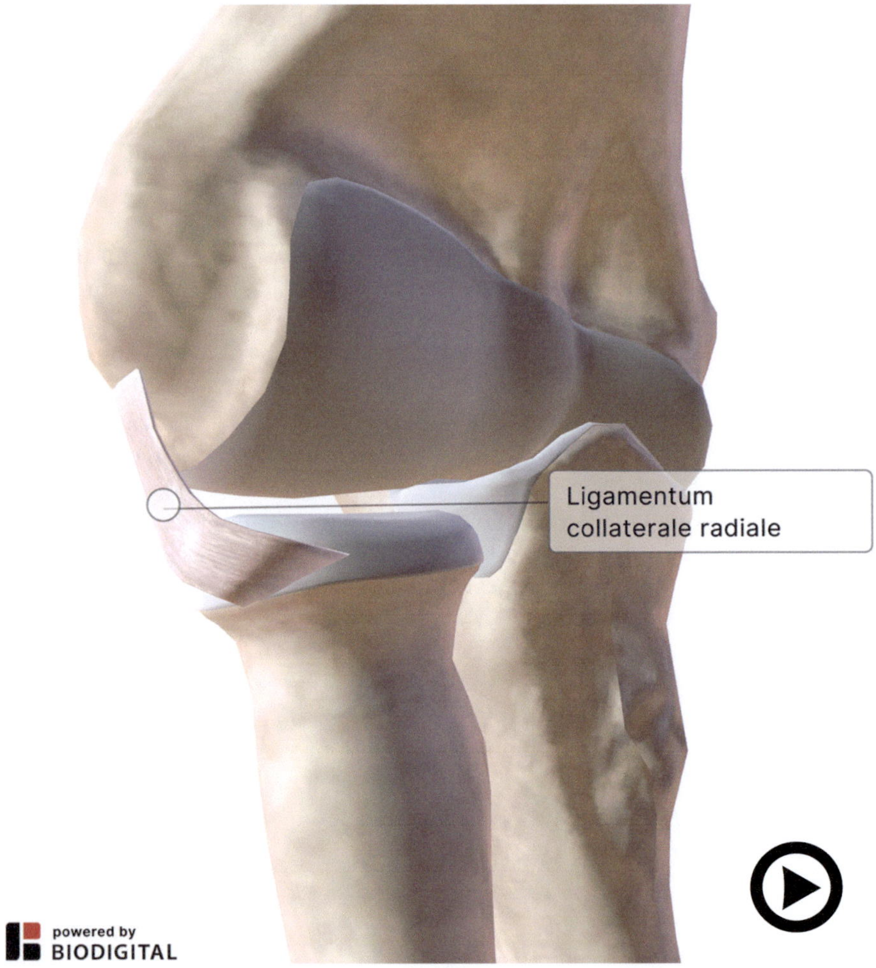

Fig. 4.25 Anatomy and palpation of the lig. collaterale radiale (▶ https://doi.org/10.1007/000-cs1)

4.4.3 Palpation of the Ligaments on the Hand

True to the tensegrity model, the instrument of the instruments consists of bones that are stable in bending and which complete the traction-belt mechanism via ligaments, muscles and tendons that are stable in stretching.

The joints of the hand are spanned in their entirety by ligaments.

As a large proportion of the articular connections are amphiarthroses, palpation of the ligaments proves challenging as little range of motion is possible. A palmar and dorsal approach to palpation is possible. In addition, translatory motion impulses will be necessary to locate ligamentous structures. A good knowledge of the anatomical position is of great importance, as it is difficult to differentiate them from the surrounding tissue due to the large number of ligaments. In addition, numerous other structures such as tendons and other soft tissues make palpation very difficult. For this reason, care should be taken to position the hand passively so that the back or palm of the hand is exposed.

The following chapters present the selection of palpable ligaments of the hand.

4.4.3.1 Palpation of the Palmar Aponeurosis

The palmar fascia complex, which is the distal extension of the palmaris longus and brevis muscle, consists of dense fibrous connective tissue, is superficially localised and is therefore very accessible by palpation. The aponeurosis is important for the gripping function as well as the protection of the underlying structures.

A palmar approach is intended for palpation, so the hand should be positioned accordingly. The index or middle finger is placed in the middle at the level of the proximal carpus row from the palmar side with the fingertips. The client then performs an active grasping movement, which is stopped about halfway through. By means of this isometric tension, the aponeurosis is clearly felt above the individual metacarpal spaces as a firm-elastic structure.

Implementation Note

When Dupuytren's disease is diagnosed, hypertonic pressure-dolent areas are occasionally found in the area of the palmar aponeurosis [12] (Fig. 4.26).

4.4.3.2 Palpation of the Retinaculum Musculorum Flexorum and the Lig. Carpi Palmare

The spatial proximity of these two structures causes the common palpation of the transverse fibres. While the carpi palmare ligament is located somewhat more superficially and proximally, the retinaculum musculorum flexorum is located somewhat more distally in depth and forms the palmar

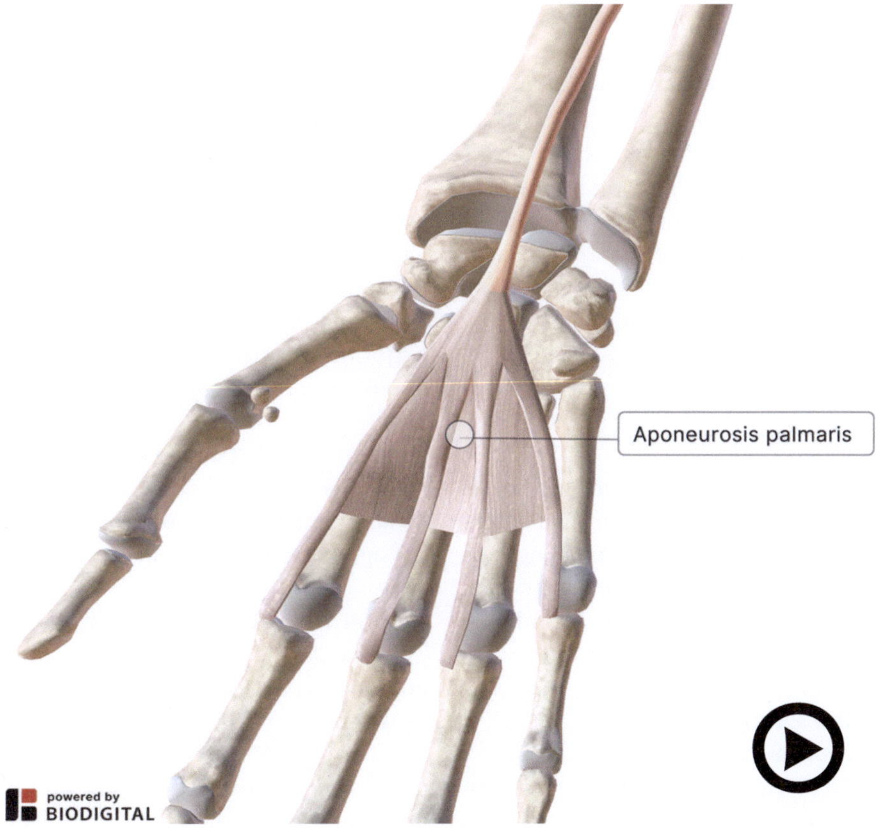

Fig. 4.26 Anatomy and palpation of the aponeurosis palmaris (▶ https://doi.org/10.1007/000-cs2)

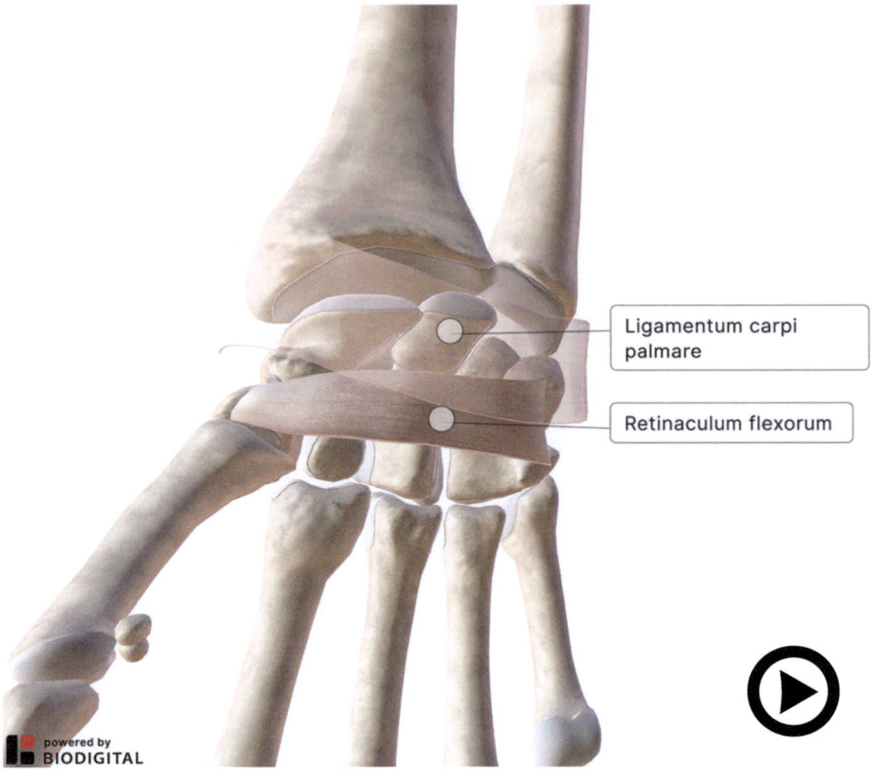

Fig. 4.27 Anatomy and palpation of the retinaculum flexorum et Lig. carpi palmare (▶ https://doi.org/10.1007/000-cs3)

boundary of the carpal tunnel. Like a sweatband, both structures fix the flexor tendons of the hand in close proximity to the bones. Thus, a direct palpatory demarcation from other soft tissues is difficult.

Palpation begins at the os pisiforme, which is first visited palmar to the os triquetrum. Then the steeply positioned palpation finger moves in a medial direction until it leaves the bony edge and exerts moderate pressure in a dorsal direction. A firm-elastic structure becomes palpable, the retinaculum musculorum flexorum. This extends to the os trapezium.

Somewhat more proximal but also running transversely, there is the lig. carpi palmare transversum, which, however, is only moderately palpable, as it is rather thin and can hardly be differentiated from surrounding fibres.

Implementation Note

The retinaculum musculorum flexorum covers the carpal tunnel and is therefore partly responsible for any carpal tunnel syndrome due to its contact with the corresponding flexors and the median nerve [13]. If paresthesia occurs during palpation, the pressure should be reduced accordingly (Fig. 4.27).

4.4.3.3 Palpation of the Palmar and Dorsal Radioulnar Ligaments

The ulna and radius are connected distally by short taut ligaments so that the necessary stability can be built up. Both ligaments belong to the triangular fibrocartilaginous complex and are tightened during supination so that they can limit this direction of movement. The close relationship to the bone and the numerous soft tissues in this region make the ligaments difficult to palpate. It is advisable to grasp the distal ulna at the level of the ulnar styloid with the pincer grip and then move it translationally palmar and dorsal to the fixed radius. The palpation fingers should make gentle contact with the palmar and dorsal joint space. During the translatory movement to the dorsal, a small, firm-elastic structure in the dorsal joint space can be felt. These fibres are those of the dorsal radioulnar ligament. The same procedure can be performed palmarly, although palmarly the quality of palpation is severely compromised due to surrounding tissues.

Implementation Note

Precise anatomical knowledge of the position of both ligaments is imperative, as the quality of palpation in this area is not optimal due to periarticular structures (Fig. 4.28).

4.4.3.4 Palpation of the Ulnocarpal Ligaments

The ulnocarpal ligament complex is formed by various structures and serves to stabilise the wrist in the direction of radial abduction. On the ulnar side, a distinction can be made between a palmar region, which includes the ulnocarpal ligament, and a dorsal region with the ulnar collateral carpal ligament. Because of the direct relationship to soft tissues in

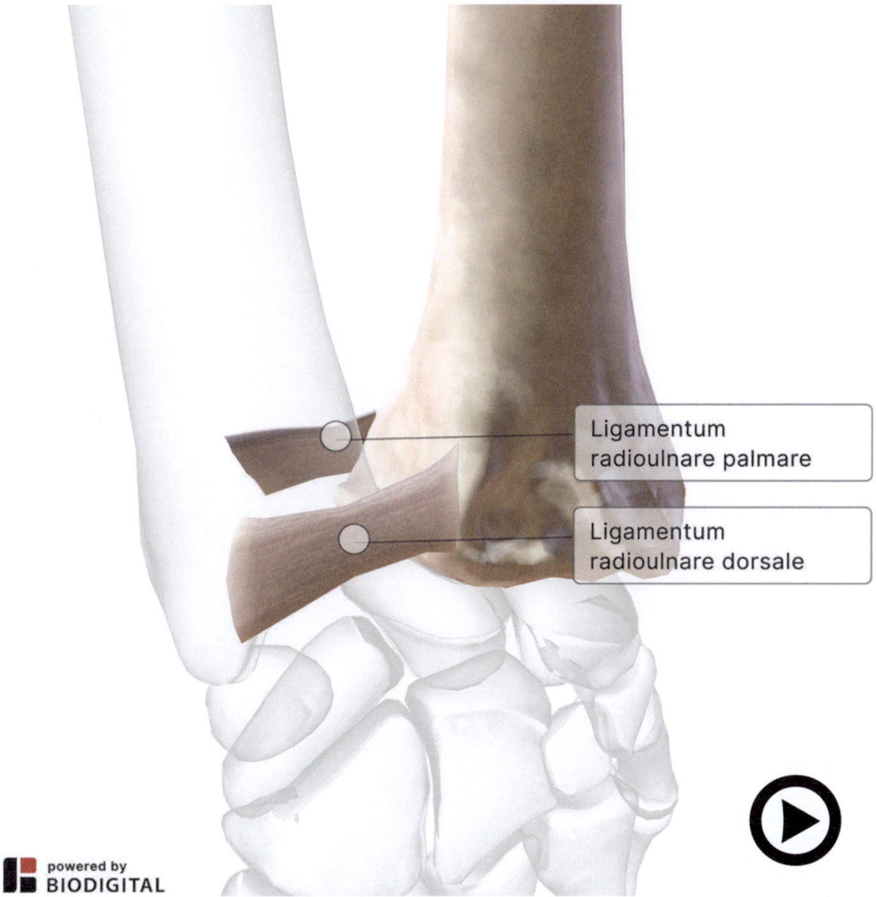

Fig. 4.28 Anatomy and palpation of the lig. radioulnare palmare et dorsale (▶ https://doi.org/10.1007/000-cs4)

this region, palpation should be carried out as follows and requires some sensitivity.

The os triquetrum is fixed in a pincer grip so that the thumb and index finger contact the joint space and the articular disc from the dorsal and palmar sides, respectively. Then a translatory movement impulse is carried out in the dorsal direction, during which the firm-elastic ulnar carpal ligament is felt in the joint space. During the translatory movement towards the palmar side, the ulnocarpal ligament becomes slightly palpable during the same procedure.

Further ligaments from this complex are not palpable.

Implementation Note

While palpation of the dorsal parts of the ligamentous complex is much more palpable, the palmar parts are covered by soft tissue, making palpation difficult (Fig. 4.29).

4.4.3.5 Palpation of the Radiocarpal Ligaments

The radiocarpal ligament complex is formed by numerous structures and serves to stabilise the wrist in the direction of ulnar abduction. On the radial side, a distinction can be made between a palmar area, which includes the radiocarpal ligament, and a lateral area with the collateral carpi radial ligament. Because of the direct relationship to numerous soft tissues in this region, palpation should be carried out as follows and requires sensitivity.

The os scaphoideum is fixed in a pincer grip coming from the radial direction, so that the thumb and index finger have contact with the joint space to the radius from the dorsal and palmar sides, respectively. Then a translatory movement impulse is carried out in the dorsal direction, during which the fixed elastic carpi radial ligament is felt in the joint space. During the translatory movement towards the palmar side, the radiocarpal ligament can be felt slightly.

Further ligaments from this complex are not palpable.

Implementation Note

While palpation of the lateral portions of the ligamentous complex are clearly palpable, the palmar portions are covered by soft tissue, making palpation difficult (Fig. 4.30).

4.4.3.6 Palpation of the Carpometacarpal Ligaments

The connecting ligaments between the carpus and metacarpus each extend from one bone of the distal carpal row to its opposite metacarpal from dorsal and palmar. Direct palpa-

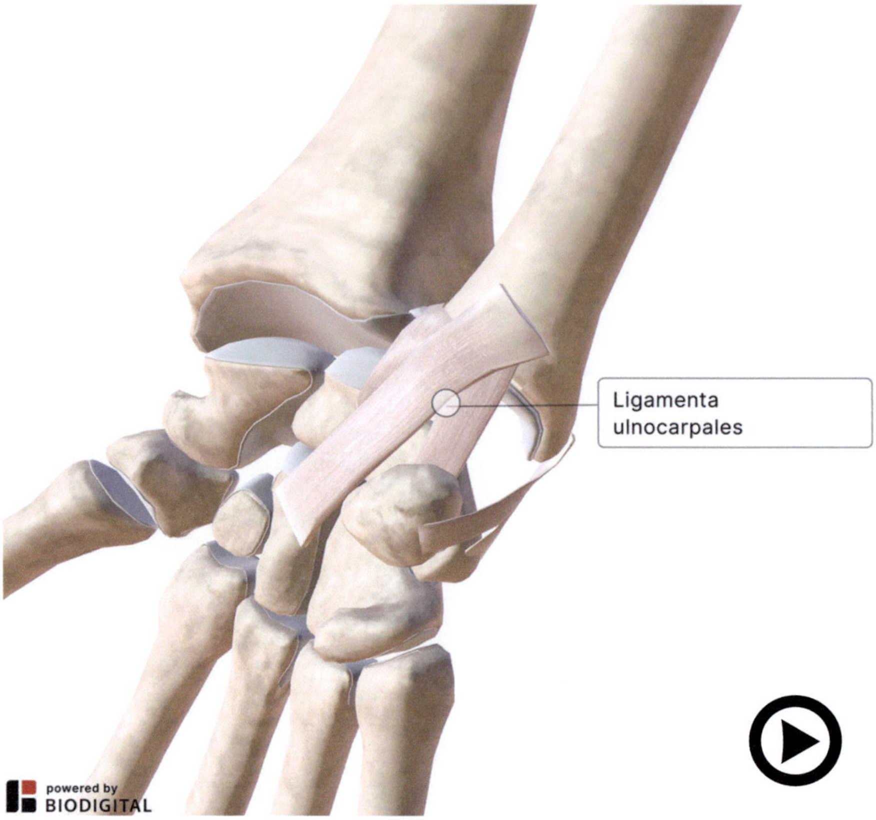

Fig. 4.29 Anatomy and palpation of the ligg. ulnocarpales (▶ https://doi.org/10.1007/000-cs5)

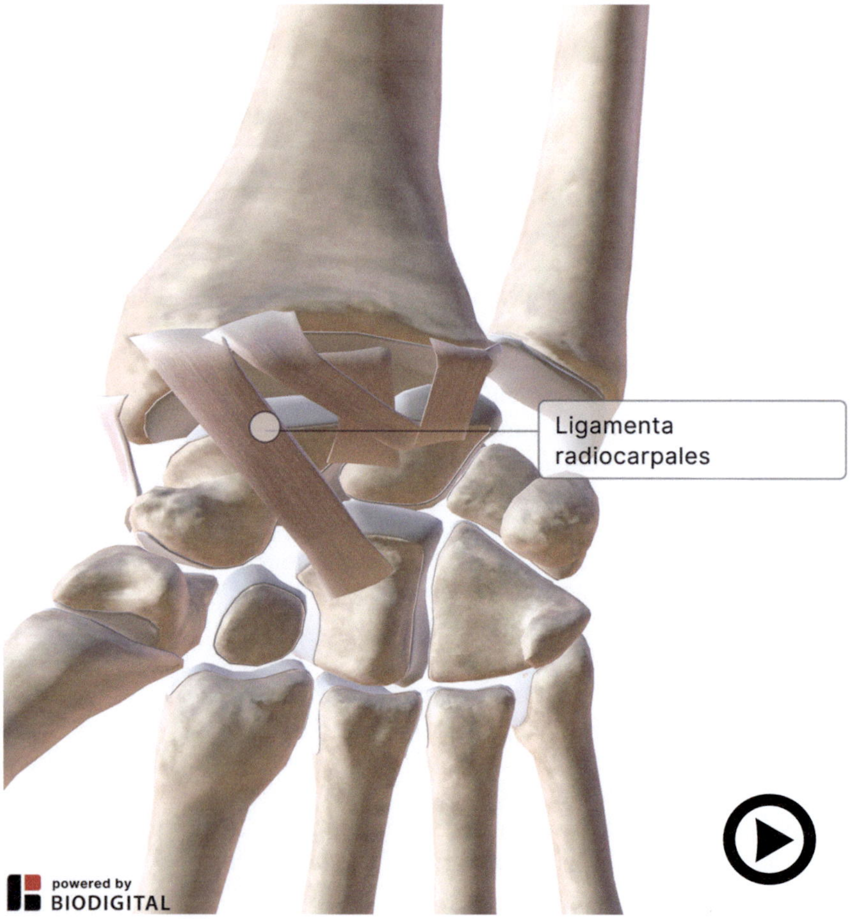

Fig. 4.30 Anatomy and palpation of the ligg. radiocarpales (▶ https://doi.org/10.1007/000-cs6)

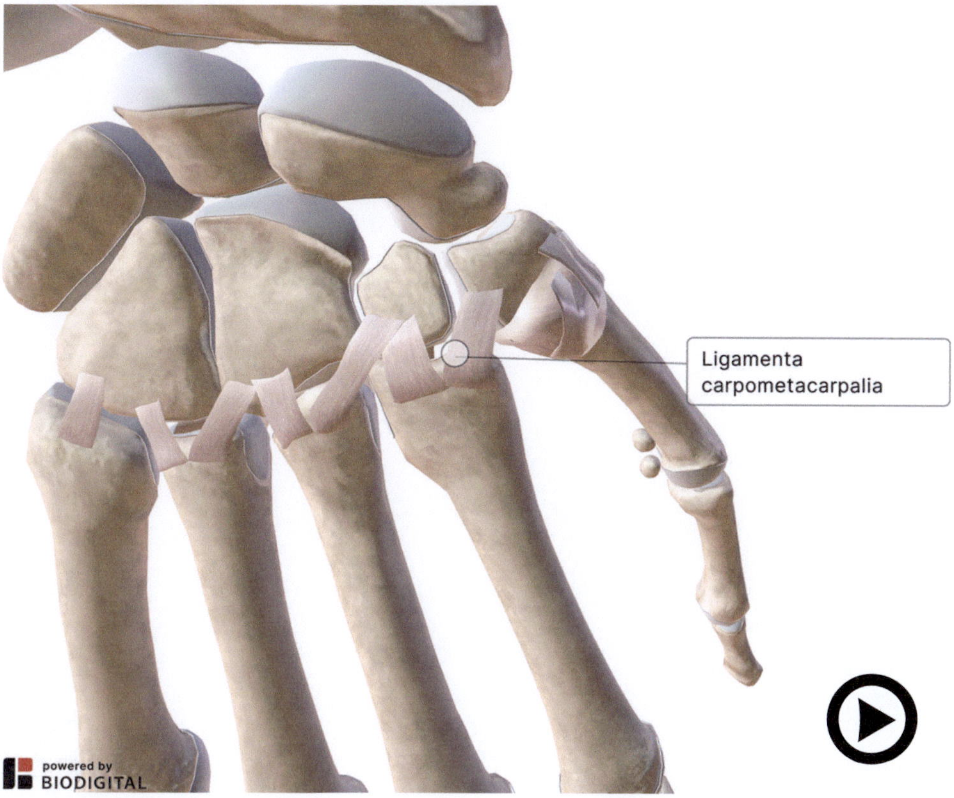

Fig. 4.31 Anatomy and palpation of the ligg. carpometacarpalia (▶ https://doi.org/10.1007/000-cs7)

tion of the ligaments is difficult because the amphiarthroses allow little movement, and numerous tendons and soft tissues cover the region. It is only possible to use the pincer grip, which is taken proximally at the base of a metacarpal, to move the joint translationally to be able to record ligamentous structures in the joint space. While the dorsal parts of the hand are more likely to be felt during a dorsal translatory movement, palmar parts cannot be palpated.

Implementation Note

Palpation in this area is hardly valid. Only with precise anatomical knowledge can a stimulus be applied directly to the corresponding ligament (Fig. 4.31).

4.4.3.7 Palpation of the Metacarpophalangeal Radial and Ulnar Ligaments II and V

There are ligaments on each side of the metacarpophalangeal joints which, together with the capsule, can limit the directions of movement. Direct palpation is only possible of the collateral ligaments in the second metacarpophalangeal joint from the radial side and in the fifth metacarpophalangeal joint from the ulnar side.

For the former band, the right thumb is placed in the joint space of the left art. metacarpophalangeales II coming from radial, and the client's index finger is embraced with the whole hand. Then the embraced index finger is moved in the direction of ulnar abduction until a firm-elastic structure is felt under the thumb. The palpable fibres are parts of the radial collateral ligament of the second metacarpophalangeal joint. For the radial collateral ligament of the right metacarpophalangeal joint, the left thumb or hand is used for palpation.

The ulnar collateral ligament of the fifth metacarpophalangeal joint is palpated with the index finger. For this purpose, the right index finger is placed ulnar to the joint space of the left art. metacarpophalangealis V, and then the little finger is grasped with the remaining fingers of the palpation hand. The ulnar collateral ligament can be located by means of a traction coupled with a radial reduction. Due to the overlying structures, palpation is rather difficult.

Implementation Note

The palpation quality can be enhanced if the corresponding finger is set in traction (Fig. 4.32).

4.4.3.8 Palpation of the Annular Ligament

The annular ligaments, which are located palmar, fix the flexor tendons of the fingers to the bone so that they can perform palmar flexion. The annular ligaments can be divided into five parts (A1–A5) and extend over almost the entire course of the flexor digitorum profundus muscle. While A1, A3 and A5 are located at the level of the joints (MCP, PIP,

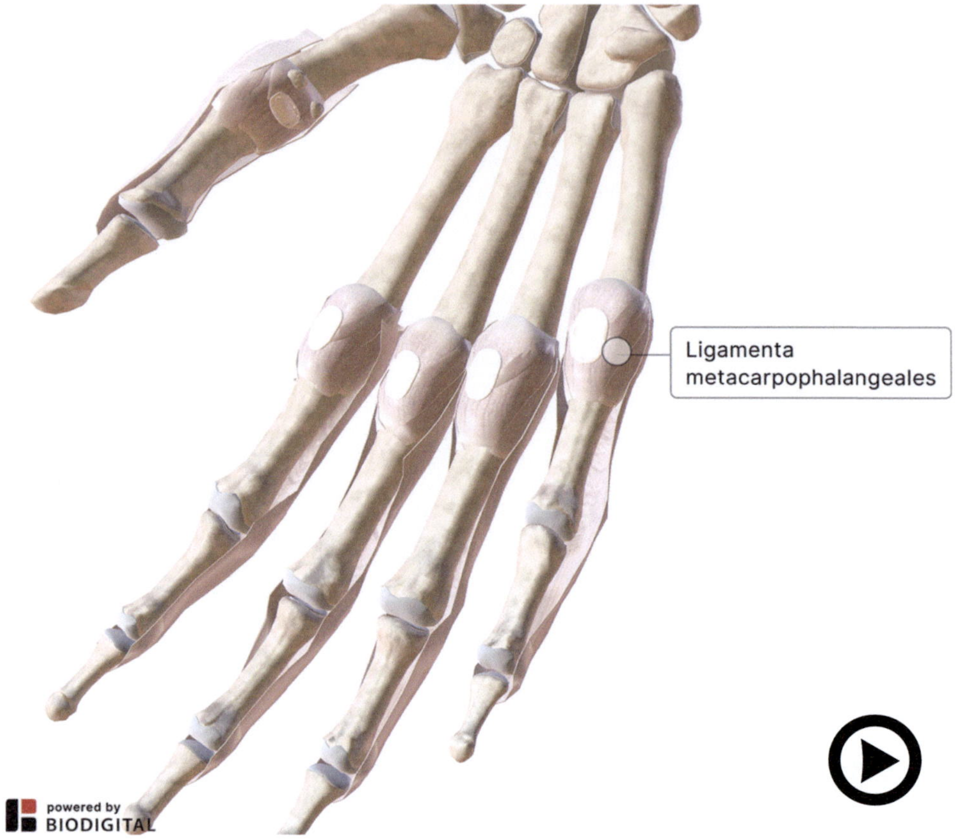

Fig. 4.32 Anatomy and palpation of the ligg. metacarpophalangeales radiales et ulnares (▶ https://doi.org/10.1007/000-cs8)

DIP) and therefore cannot be directly palpated, A2 and A4 are in the palmar course of the proximal and medial phalanx. Direct palpation is difficult. Nevertheless, the ligaments can be stimulated because they are located directly under the skin.

In order to access those ligamentous structures, the index fingertip is placed centrally on the proximal or medial phalanx of the palmar and an isometric contraction of the fingers in flexion is adopted by the client until the tendon is clearly felt under the palpating finger. Then, with moderate tension, the tendon is moved radially or ulnarly. This tensions the parts of the annular A2 and A4 ligaments, which can be felt as a fixed-elastic structure on the tendon wheels.

Implementation Note

To better feel fibres of the ligaments, the held contraction can be done in different angular positions so that the tendons become more prominent (Fig. 4.33).

4.4.3.9 Palpation of the Collateral Interphalangeal Ligaments

The collateral ligaments of the interphalangeal joints are in close contact with the respective capsule and are therefore difficult to differentiate from other fibres. A possible approach can be made by means of the index finger at the level of the respective joint space from radial or ulnar. While the finger lies between the phalanges, a movement impulse is initiated in the direction of radial or ulnar reduction. This causes a slight opening movement in the hinge joints, which puts the fibres of the corresponding collateral ligaments under increased tension.

Implementation Note

During palpation, not only the ligament is felt, but also large parts of the capsule. Therefore, it is difficult to locate the exact fibres of the respective ligament (Fig. 4.34).

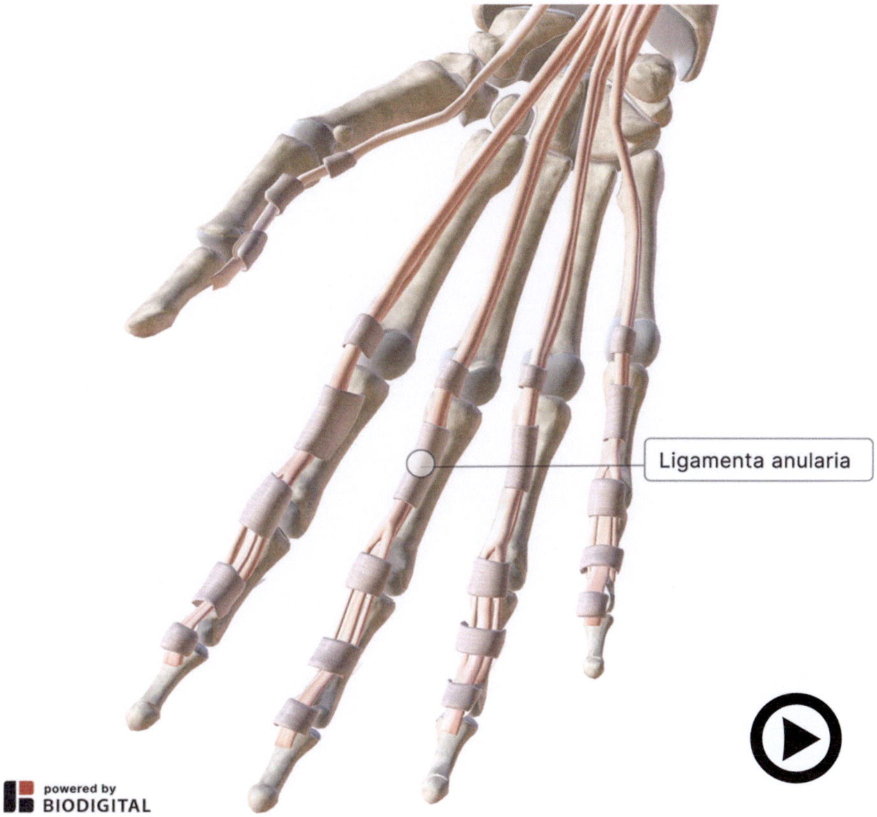

Fig. 4.33 Anatomy and palpation of the ligg. anularia (▶ https://doi.org/10.1007/000-cs9)

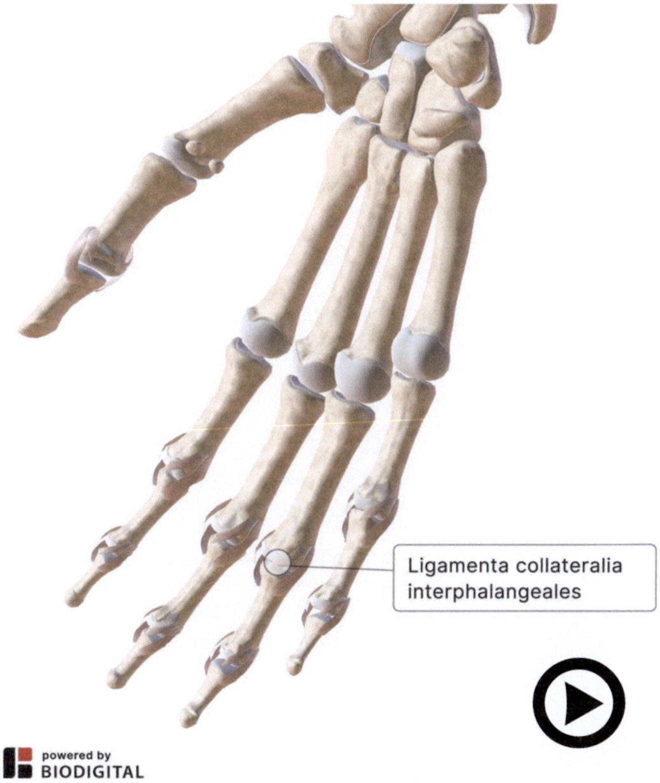

Fig. 4.34 Anatomy and palpation of the ligg. collateralia interphalangeales (▶ https://doi.org/10.1007/000-cr9)

4.5 Palpation of the Lateral Temporomandibular Ligament

The ligament extends cranially from the arcus zygomaticus caudally to the lateral and dorsal side of the collum mandibulae. Its function is to limit the movements of the mandible.

To palpate the lateral temporomandibular ligament, the zygomatic arc is visited first. The zygomatic arc is then followed occipitally in the direction of the external acoustic meatus. About one transverse finger before reaching it, the palpation finger is moved caudally. It is now on the fibres of the lateral temporomandibular ligament. The ligament can now be traced caudally to the collum mandibulare.

Implementation Note

Opening and closing the temporomandibular joint cause a movement of the caput mandibulae, which can be felt very well under the palpation finger. This makes it easier for the practitioner to find the ligament (Fig. 4.35).

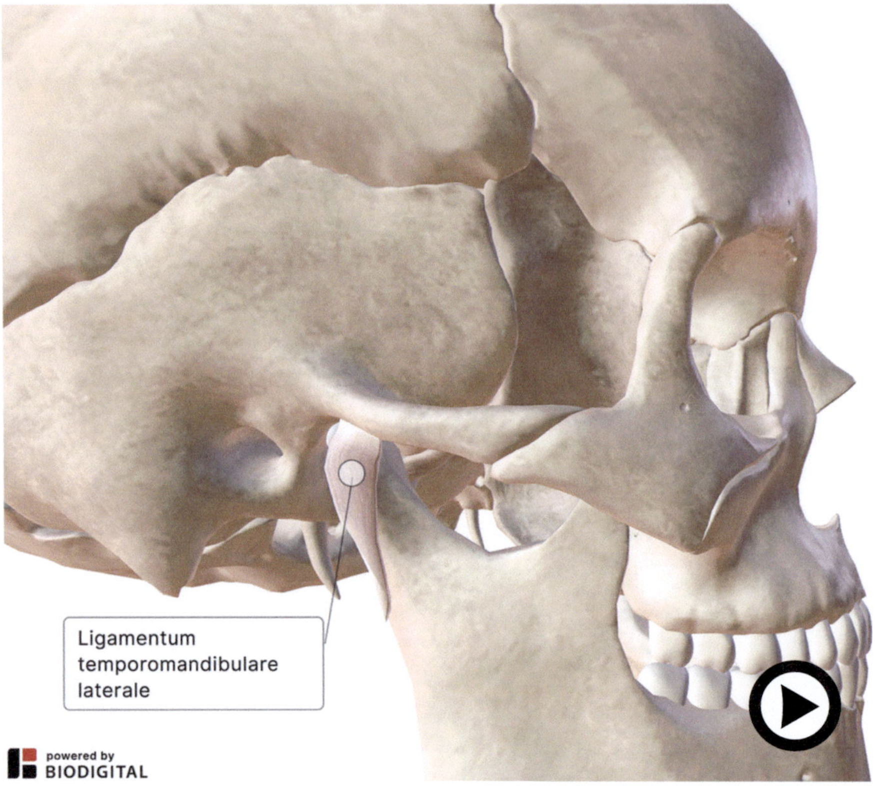

Fig. 4.35 Anatomy and palpation of the lig. temporomandibulare laterale (▶ https://doi.org/10.1007/000-csb)

References

1. Varma, S., Orgel, J., & Schieber, J. (2016, July 12). Nanomechanics of type I collagen. *Biophysical Journal, 111*(1), 50–56. https://doi.org/10.1016/j.bpj.2016.05.038
2. Heineck, J., Liebscher, T., & Zwipp, H. (2001). Abrissfraktur der Basis des Os metatarsale V. *Operative Orthopädie und Traumatologie, 13*, 151–158. https://doi.org/10.1007/PL00002279
3. Steinmetz, R., McDonald, M., Tkach, S., Hamilton, J., Heigle, G., Hollabaugh, K., et al. (2020, June 10). Prevalence of ligamentous knee injuries in pedestrian versus motor vehicle accidents. *BMC Musculoskeletal Disorders, 21*(1), 369. https://doi.org/10.1186/s12891-020-03397-w
4. LaPrade, R., Engebretsen, A., Ly, T., Johansen, S., Wentorf, F., & Engebretsen, L. (2007, September). The anatomy of the medial part of the knee. *The Journal of Bone and Joint Surgery American Volume, 89*(9), 2000–2010. https://doi.org/10.2106/JBJS.F.01176
5. Bollier, M., & Smith, P. (2014, October). Anterior cruciate ligament and medial collateral ligament injuries. *The Journal of Knee Surgery, 27*(5), 359–368. https://doi.org/10.1055/s-0034-1381961
6. Dürselen, L., & Freutel, M. (2015). Biomechanik des Meniskus. *Orthopädie und Unfallchirurgie up2date, 10*(3), 215–227. https://doi.org/10.1055/s-0041-101820
7. Doherty, C., Delahunt, E., Caulfield, B., Hertel, J., Ryan, J., & Bleakley, C. (2014, January). The incidence and prevalence of ankle sprain injury: A systematic review and meta-analysis of prospective epidemiological studies. *Sports Medicine, 44*(1), 123–140. https://doi.org/10.1007/s40279-013-0102-5
8. Lee, D. (1993). Biomechanics of the thorax: A clinical mode of in vivo function. *Journal of Manual & Manipulative Therapy, 1*(1), 13–21. https://doi.org/10.1179/106698193791069771
9. Hoogvliet, P., Randsdorp, M., Dingemanse, R., Koes, B., & Huisstede, B. (2013, Novemeber). Does effectiveness of exercise therapy and mobilisation techniques offer guidance for the treatment of lateral and medial epicondylitis? A systematic review. *British Journal of Sports Medicine*, *47*(17), 1112–1119. https://doi.org/10.1136/bjsports-2012-091990
10. Hackl, M., Bercher, M., Wegmann, K., Müller, L., & Dargel, J. (2016, July). Functional anatomy of the lateral collateral ligament of the elbow. *Archives of Orthopaedic and Trauma Surgery, 136*(7), 1031–1037. https://doi.org/10.1007/s00402-016-2479-8
11. Paksoy, A., Laver, L., Tok, O., Ayhan, C., & Kocaoglu, B. (2021, June). Arthroscopic lateral capsule resection is enough for the management of lateral epicondylitis. *Knee Surgery, Sports Traumatology, Arthroscopy, 29*(6), 2000–2005. https://doi.org/10.1007/s00167-020-06255-3
12. Turesson, C. (2018, August). The role of hand therapy in Dupuytren disease. *Hand Clinics, 34*(3), 395–401. https://doi.org/10.1016/j.hcl.2018.03.008
13. Lee, S., Hwang, S., An, Y., & Choy, W. (2020, August). The influence of transverse carpal ligament thickness on treatment decisions for idiopathic mild to moderate carpal tunnel syndrome. *Annals of Plastic Surgery, 85*(2), 127–134. https://doi.org/10.1097/SAP.0000000000002386

Palpation of the Musculature

5

Contents

Supplementary Information The online version contains supplementary material available at https://doi.org/10.1007/978-3-662-69186-1_5. The videos can be accessed individually by clicking the DOI link in the accompanying figure caption or by scanning this link with the SN More Media App.

R. Bauer, S. Wolfram, *Atlas of Palpation*, https://doi.org/10.1007/978-3-662-69186-1_5

5.1 Basics of Muscle Palpation

The active system of the human organism is characterised by over 650 muscles with approx. 250 million muscle fibres and generally comprises approx. 40% of the total body mass [1]. Each muscle performs its individual movement task, so that the body as a whole can move both grossly and finely motorically. Everyday activities can only be realised through the targeted tensioning of the contractile elements, as joints are mobilised thanks to these structures. The musculature is composed of smooth, striated musculature and special cardiac musculature. While the smooth musculature, which is predominantly located in the organ systems, is for the most part not suitable for direct palpation, the focus in this chapter falls on the striated skeletal musculature. Each joint is covered by skeletal muscles, which can be divided into muscle origin, muscle belly and muscle insertion. A tendon exists at the origo and insertio, respectively, which establishes direct contact with the bone via the transition zone. Thus, the venter is enclosed centrally. The muscle belly, which is usually best felt on palpation, can be divided into different components. The smallest functional unit, with a length of up to 3.8 μm, is the sarcomere, which consists of myosin, actin, titin, desmin and nebulin [2]. Many sarcomeres in series form a myofibril, which is encased by the endomysium. Many myofibrils form a muscle fibre, which in turn is surrounded by the perimysium internum. Several muscle fibres form a primary bundle, and several primary bundles consequently form a secondary bundle. Secondary bundles are encircled by the perimysium externum. All these bundles are enclosed by the epimysium or muscle fascia and thus form the outer edge, which experiences the pressure of the finger during palpation after the individual skin layers.

For palpation, it is important to know the anatomy of the muscle. Knowledge of the region of origin or insertion is very important. If these regions are moved away from each other, the muscle is stretched and takes on a higher tension; it thus becomes firmer to the touch. If the origo and insertio are moved towards each other actively or against resistance, the muscle contracts and increases in tension. Increases in tone can be helpful in locating the muscle to differentiate it from the surrounding tissue. For this reason, muscles are first palpated in a passively approximated starting position in the course and then tensed in their function to make them more precisely accessible. The palpation sensation is rather soft during passivity and becomes firmer with the contraction of the muscle. The exact procedure is described precisely in the individual chapters.

An important clinical sign that can generally be considered for all muscles is the "mushy sign." The "mushy sign" occurs when fluid accumulates in the muscle. This is often the case after trauma and can be indicative of a muscular injury. Another clinical abnormality that can occur during palpation is a radiating sensation to a specific region as soon as the muscle is felt in depth. For this reason, gentle contact is recommended at first.

5.2 Musculature in the Pelvic/Hip Joint Region

The human pelvis absorbs forces from the upper and lower extremities as well as the trunk and distributes them accordingly. In terms of the tensegrity model, the statics of the pelvis are influenced by numerous structures, including the musculature. Due to the elementary role of the pelvis, it is important to know the position and function of the individual muscles and to be able to palpate them. A changed state of tension of these structures affects the entire statics and can therefore also influence the distribution of forces in the whole body. The hip joint is closely related to the pelvis, as numerous muscles in the pelvic region pass over the hip joint and find their attachment at the femur. For this reason, this chapter presents palpation of the flexors, extensors, external and internal rotators, and abductors and adductors of the hip joint and the pelvic floor muscles. It is advisable to first choose an approximate position to relax the respective muscle and then to differentiate the structure from the surrounding tissue with the help of the contraction and the associated increase in tone. It is recommended to perform the procedure with the fingertips of the index and middle fingers.

5.2.1 Palpation of the Iliac Muscle

One part of the iliopsoas muscle is formed by the iliacus muscle, which originates in the iliac fossa, passes under the inguinal ligament through the lacuna musculorum and attaches to the lesser trochanter of the femur. The hip flexor portion is innervated by direct branches from the lumbar plexus from segments L1–L4 and by the femoral nerve. In addition to its main function of flexion in the hip joint, it can perform external rotation and adduction synergistically. A change in the tension of this muscle is often due to permanent sitting in everyday life and at the same time forms a reason which increases the priority of being able to feel this muscle together with its tone [3].

Palpation of the iliacus muscle takes place in the supine position with the legs passively positioned or elevated, so that there is about 70–90° flexion in the hip joint. The head is slightly supported so that there is no potential tension on the abdominal wall. The practitioner stands to the side of the patient and contacts the contralateral crista iliaca in the anterior region with the steeply positioned fingertips. If the fingers are then guided in a medial direction, they fall directly into a depression lined with soft tissue. If pressure is now applied in a laterocaudal direction, the fingertips directly hit the area of origin of the iliac muscle. The course of the muscle can then be followed caudomedially. During palpation, the inguinal ligament is felt as a transverse structure. After this region, the lacuna musculorum, the iliacus muscle joins the psoas major muscle and becomes one muscle. The insertion can be palpated proxomedially on the lesser trochanter of the femur with the fingers. A clearer palpation sensation can be made by the client moving his hip joint slightly actively in flexion.

Implementation Note

Palpation of the iliacus muscle should be gentle, as the structure can often be pressure-dolent in its area of origin.

Furthermore, palpation of the insertion region is difficult because numerous muscles from the adductor region lie above the lesser trochanter (Fig. 5.1).

5.2.2 Palpation of the Psoas Major and Minor Muscles

A portion of the iliopsoas muscle is shaped by the psoas major and minor muscles. The region of origin of the superficial portions of the greater hip flexor extends from the 12th thoracic vertebral body to the 4th lumbar vertebral body and the intervertebral discs in between. The deep-lying tendons of origin are located at the processi costales of the lumbar spine. The greater psoas muscle is innervated by direct branches from the lumbar plexus from segments L1–L4 and the femoral nerve. The psoas minor muscle, which is inconstant, originates from the 12th thoracic and 1st lumbar vertebrae and is controlled by direct branches of the lumbar nerves I–III [4]. Both muscles have a similar distal course. The lesser psoas muscle attaches to the iliopectineal arc of the inguinal ligament, while the greater psoas muscle passes underneath it to the lesser trochanter of the femur. Therefore, they are not differentially illuminated during palpation.

In addition to the main function of flexion in the hip joint, the psoas major muscle can synergistically perform adduction as well as external rotation and some fibres, depending on the position, internal rotation. Due to its origins, it can also move the lumbar spine into equilateral lateral flexion, reciprocal rotation and flexion. A negative change in this muscle is often due to permanent sitting in everyday life and at the same time is an important reason to be able to feel this muscle and its tone.

Palpation of the psoas major and minor muscles is performed with the patient in the supine position with the legs passively positioned or elevated so that there is about 70–90° flexion of the hip joint. The head is placed slightly underneath so that there is no potential tension on the abdominal wall. The palpator stands to the side of the client and makes contact with the homolateral SIAS. Starting from this reference point, three transverse fingers of the patient are mea-

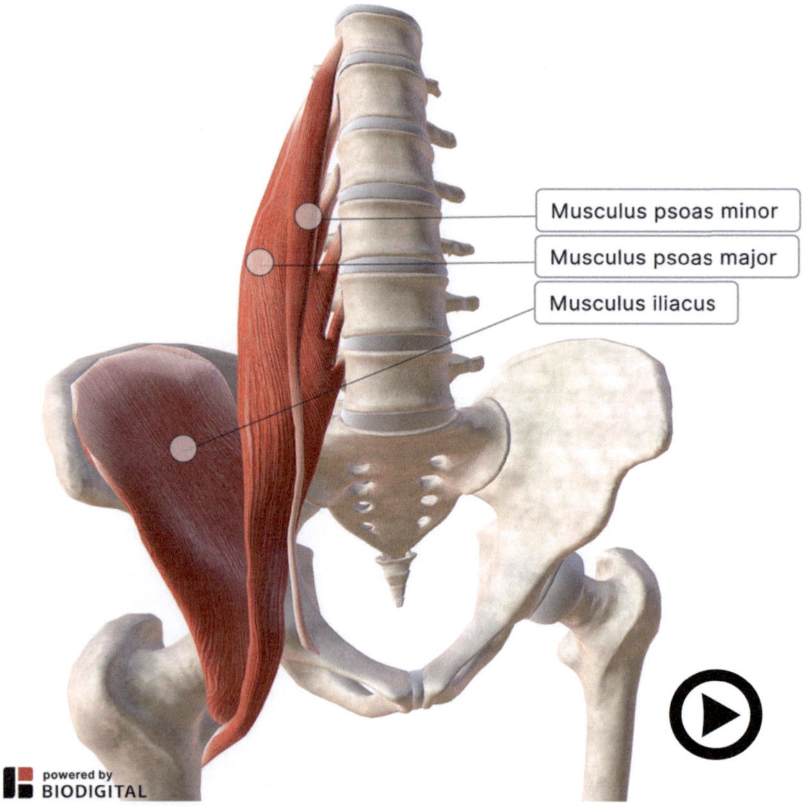

Fig. 5.1 Anatomy and palpation of the M. iliacus (▶ https://doi.org/10.1007/000-csc)

sured cranially and three transverse fingers medially in the direction of the umbilicus. At this point, the steeply placed index fingers of the palpation hands are placed side by side along the body. In addition, both middle and ring fingers can be applied so that both hands can palpate the course of the muscle with three fingers each.

In order to grasp the psoas major and minor, the palpation fingers are glided dorsomedially, obliquely in the direction of the spine, until an elastic resistance is felt. The client is then asked to move the hip joint slightly into flexion so that the muscle contracts and can be felt as a firm cord. This tension makes it possible to differentiate the muscle from surrounding tissue. The muscle belly can then be felt caudally into the lacuna musculorum. It is important to remember that many soft tissues, such as the intestinal loop, are located between the palpation fingers and the muscle to be palpated.

The insertion can be felt proxomedially on the lesser trochanter of the thigh with the fingers. A clearer palpation sensation can be obtained by the client moving his hip joint slightly actively in flexion.

Implementation Note

Palpation of the psoas major and minor should be performed gently, as the structure can often react pressure-dolent in its course. The left side in particular should initially be tapped with little pressure, as the aorta pars abdominales is located in this region. It can be felt through the characteristic pulse wave.

Furthermore, palpation of the insertion region is difficult because numerous muscles from the adductor region lie above the lesser trochanter (Fig. 5.2).

5.2.3 Palpation of the Sartorius Muscle

The sartorius muscle is located anteriorly on the thigh and shows an oblique course from the SIAS to the pes anserinus superficialis in the area of the proxomedial tibia. It is therefore a double-joint muscle and can actively support a movement in flexion, external rotation and abduction in the hip joint and a movement in internal rotation and flexion in the knee joint. The sartorius muscle is innervated via the femoral nerve from segments L2–L4.

For palpation, the client is placed in a supine position with the knee joint slightly underneath.

Palpation starts at the bony reference point of the SIAS, which is also the region of muscle origin. The practitioner standing sideways places the middle fingertip steeply on the homolateral SIAS and mentally forms an oblique line running distomedially. This line reflects the course of the muscle and forms the palpatory point of attack. The palpating middle finger

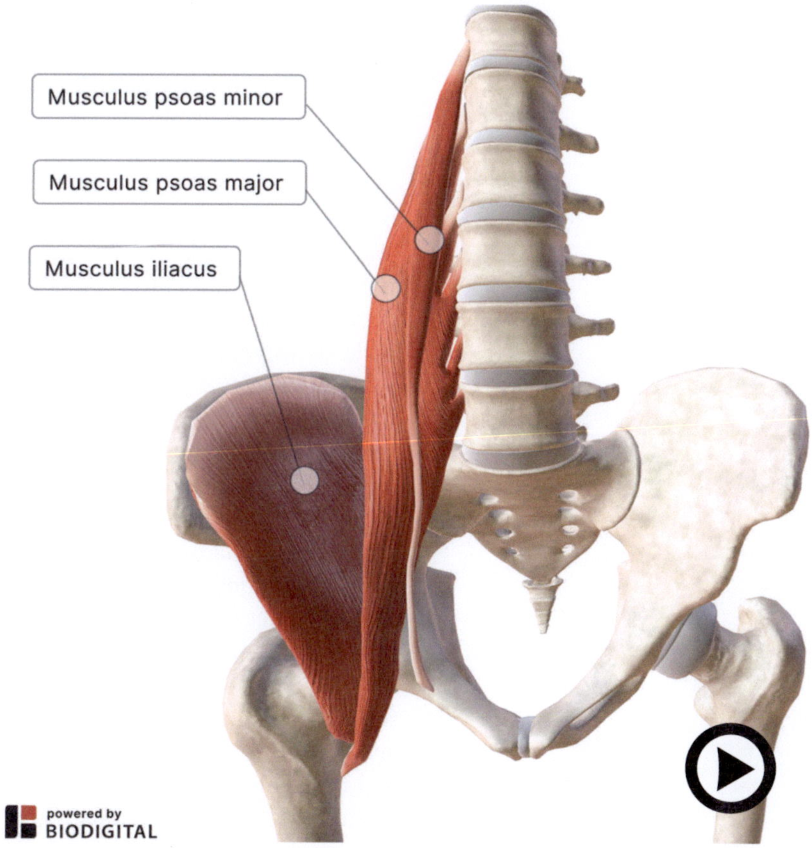

Fig. 5.2 Anatomy and palpation of the M. psoas major et minor (▶ https://doi.org/10.1007/000-csd)

will move distally on this oblique line. The index and ring finger applied at the same time can differentiate the sartorius muscle from the surrounding tissue, as both limit the cord at its edges.

Implementation Note

Although the sartorius muscle is very superficially localised, it only shows a small surface area of contact, which makes palpation in its course difficult to some extent. Especially in the distal area, the adductors can influence the palpation sensation. By actively moving the client's knee joint in internal rotation and flexion, the resulting contraction of the sartorius muscle can clarify the palpation result (Fig. 5.3).

5.2.4 Palpation of the Gluteus Maximus Muscle

The gluteus maximus with its extensive area of origin in the regions ala ossis ilii, dorsal side of the os sacrum, os coccygis as well as lig. sacrotuberale and fascia thoracolumbalis is localised superficially and therefore very easy to grasp. In its lateral course, it tapers and finally inserts with the proximal attachments to the iliotibial tract and with the distal attachment to the gluteal tuberosity of the femur. Through innervation via the inferior gluteal nerve from the sacral plexus with segments L5–S3, the gluteus maximus muscle can perform extension and external rotation in the hip joint. Furthermore, the cranial parts support abduction, while the caudal parts synergistically support adduction of the art. coxae.

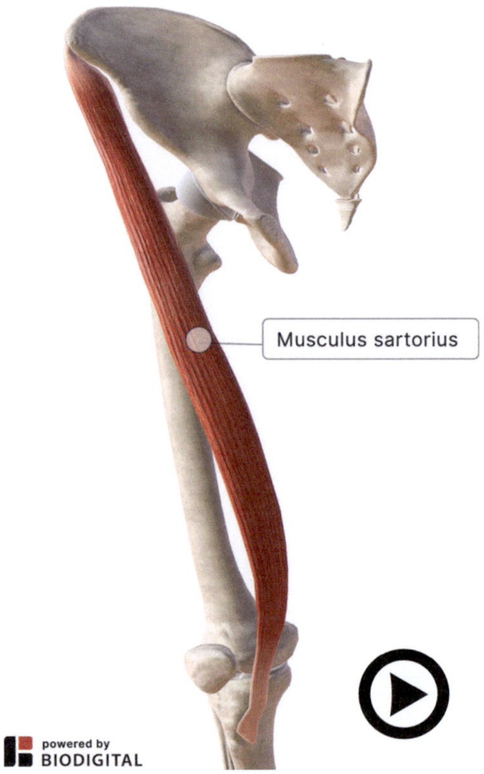

Fig. 5.3 Anatomy and palpation of the M. satorius (▶ https://doi.org/10.1007/000-cse)

For palpation, the person to be palpated is in the prone position while the clinician stands laterally and makes contact with the os sacrum and the SIPS. For this purpose, the heel of the hand is placed on the sacrum in the region of origin in such a way that the fingers point to the contralateral side in the direction of the iliotibial tract. The hand is placed flat and thus has contact with the entire muscle belly. The client is then asked to move the whole leg in a long or short lever in the direction of extension in the hip joint. The contraction makes the course of the muscle clearly perceptible, so that individual regions of the muscle can then be examined more closely with the placed fingertips. The insertion region can be felt proximally on the iliotibial tract (Sect. 5.3.9) and distodorsally on the gluteal tuberosity of the femur.

Implementation Note

The gluteal fascia, located above the gluteus maximus muscle, often causes painful conditions. Because of this frequent sensitisation, a rather gentle approach is recommended at first (Fig. 5.4).

5.2.5 Palpation of the Gluteus Medius and Gluteus Minimus Muscles

The middle and small gluteal muscles play an important role in stabilising the pelvis in the middle stance phase during the single-leg stance. They can do this, among other things, when the innervation via the superior gluteal nerve from segments L4–S1 functions harmoniously. In addition to stabilising the pelvis in the frontal plane, both muscles are largely responsible for abduction in the hip joint. In addition, the ventral parts of the gluteus medius can support internal rotation and flexion, while the dorsal parts work synergistically in external rotation and extension in the hip joint. In addition to these commonalities, there are small differences in palpation, which is why the gluteus medius muscle is discussed first.

While the patient is lying prone, the fingertips of the palpating hand contact the contralateral iliac crest. While in the dorsal third the gluteus maximus overhangs the gluteus medius, making precise palpation difficult, the palpator has good access to it in the medial and anterior thirds of the upper edge of the ilium. Starting from this region, the fingertips of the index and middle fingers move distolaterally until they leave the bony edge. They directly meet the region of origin of the m. gluteus medius at the ala ossis ilii between the linea glutea anterior and posterior. Starting from the origo, the fingertips are placed in the direction of the greater trochanter, where the muscle is attached. For an exact differentiation, the client, who is in the prone position, should stretch in the direction of abduction to achieve a contraction of the muscle.

The gluteus minimus muscle is completely covered by the gluteus medius muscle and is therefore difficult to reach with the

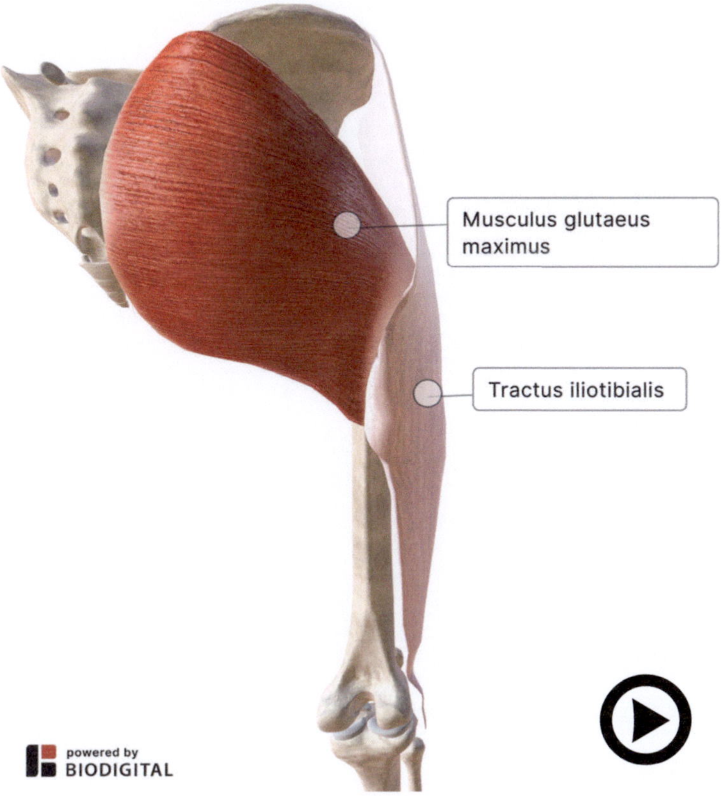

Fig. 5.4 Anatomy and palpation of the M. glutaeus maximus (▶ https://doi.org/10.1007/000-csf)

fingertips. With its region of origin at the ala ossis ilii between the linea glutealis inferior and linea glutealis anterior, it lies in depth. The palpation can be done in a similar way but starting about three transverse fingers caudal to the iliac crest. Then the fingertips are placed steeply and begin to gently palpate the depth. There must be no contraction of the muscle; otherwise, the fingertips would not reach the necessary depth. At depth, a stimulus can be applied to the gluteus minimus muscle.

The small gluteal muscle also inserts at the greater trochanter, which is very easy to grasp laterally on the thigh.

Implementation Note
If negative changes are present, both muscles may react with a transferred pain to the lateral side of the leg (Fig. 5.5).

5.2.6 Palpation of the Piriformis Muscle

The pear-shaped muscle, named for its course, is located dorsally on the pelvis. It starts at the facies pelvica of the os sacrum in the anterior region lateral to the foramina sacralia I–IV. Starting from the area of origin, it runs laterally and thus divides the foramen ischiadicum majus into a supra- and infrapiriform part. It then attaches to the greater trochanter or the trochanteric fossa of the femur. By innervating direct branches from the sacral plexus of segments L5–S2 and parts of the sciatic nerve, it can move the hip joint in external rotation and abduction. In addition, it provides cushioning for the sciatic nerve and can support internal rotation of the hip joint from 80 degrees of flexion.

When palpating the muscle, the client is positioned in the prone position while the palpator stands on the ipsilateral side. As the gluteus maximus muscle covers the piriformis muscle, the steeply positioned fingertips must first palpate through the gluteus maximus muscle in depth before the structure can be identified. There are two ways to stimulate the pear-shaped muscle belly.

For the first variant, a triangle is created mentally from the corner points SIPS, tuber ischiadicum and trochanter major, and the centre of the triangle is determined by the side bisectors. This centre of the triangle lies directly on the muscle belly of the piriformis muscle.

A second variation builds on anatomical positional relationships in relation to the client's hand. For this, the practitioner first compares his hand with the patient's hand in terms of the length of the hand from the ball to the distal end of the middle finger. Then, with the patient in the prone position, the practitioner's distal hand is placed with the ball of the hand on the tuber ischiadicum of the homolateral side. The fingers are placed on the buttocks pointing cranially. The cranial hand of the practitioner standing to the side seeks contact with the greater trochanter with the ball of the hand and then places

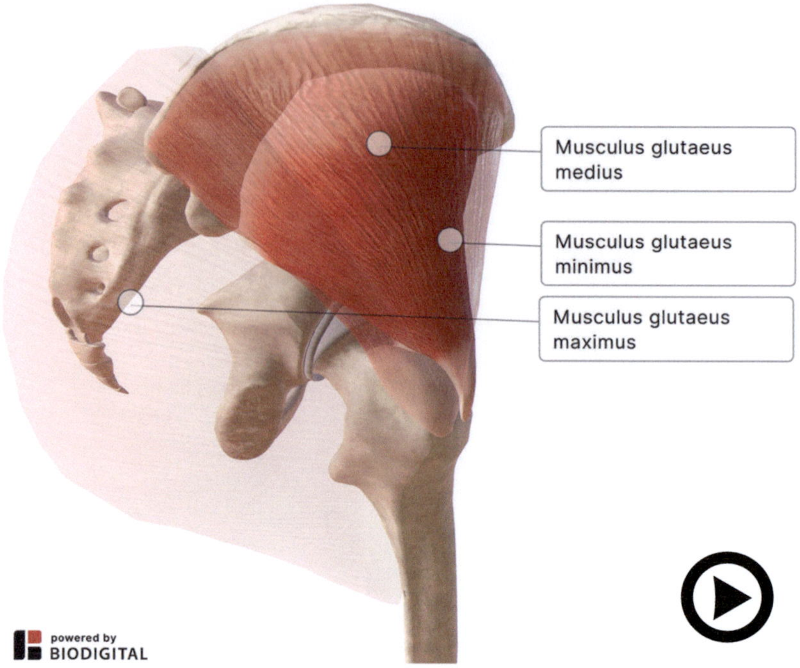

Fig. 5.5 Anatomy and palpation of the M. glutaeus medius et minimus (▶ https://doi.org/10.1007/000-csg)

the fingers pointing medially on the buttocks. An intersection of both middle fingers is created directly on the muscle belly of the piriformis muscle. It should be noted that the intersection of the client's middle fingers is to be used, which is why the length of the hand was compared in advance.

Both variants lead to the palpation point, which is then used to palpate the piriformis muscle in depth with the fingertips steeply positioned. As soon as the fingers of the cranial palpation hand have made contact through the gluteus maximus muscle, a contraction is initiated via the muscle function to make the palpation more precise. For this, the client flexes his homolateral knee joint and is then asked to move the hip joint into external rotation. The practitioner gives resistance to the medial malleolus with the distal hand and at the same time feels with the cranial hand that the piriformis muscle increases its state of tension.

Implementation Note

During palpation, the client may indicate pressure-induced, pressure-sensitive areas, which may also radiate distally into the leg when pressure is applied. In many cases, this distal radiation is due to irritation of the sciatic nerve [5] (Fig. 5.6).

5.2.7 Palpation of the Pectineus Muscle

The pectoralis muscle, which is assigned to the adductor group because of its position and function, originates in the ramus superior ossis pubis and runs from the pecten ossis pubis to the tuberculum pubicum. Its rather short caudolateral course ends in the linea pectinea and the linea aspera of the femur. The innervation via the obturator nerve and the femoral nerve from segments L2–L4 enables it to perform adduction, external rotation and flexion in the hip joint.

To palpate the muscle, first place the client in the supine position so that the clinician can make contact with the homolateral superior pubic branch with the fingertips of the index and middle fingers. Starting from the pubic tuberosity, palpation is made caudolaterally until the finger leaves the hard-appearing bone and enters soft tissue. A stimulus is applied directly to the muscle belly of the pectineus muscle. A contraction in adduction can be used to differentiate from surrounding structures.

Implementation Note

Palpation in this region should be done gently at first, as it is very intimate on the one hand and can often be pressure-dolent on the other. It is recommended to establish a clear transparency for the client regarding the location of the muscle (Fig. 5.7).

5.2.8 Palpation of the Adductor Longus Muscle

The long adductor, which is located on the inner side of the thigh, runs near the symphysis from the ramus superior ossis pubis obliquely laterodistally until it finds its attachment in the medial third of the linea aspera of the dorsal femur. It is innervated by the obturator nerve from segments L2–L4 and, due to its anatomical position, can move the hip joint in adduction, external rotation and flexion.

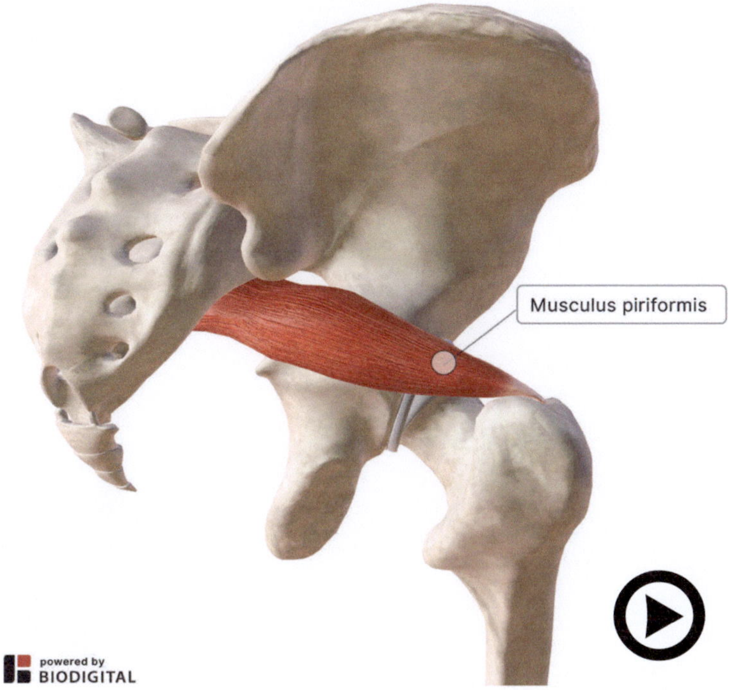

Fig. 5.6 Anatomy and palpation of the M. piriformis (▶ https://doi.org/10.1007/000-csh)

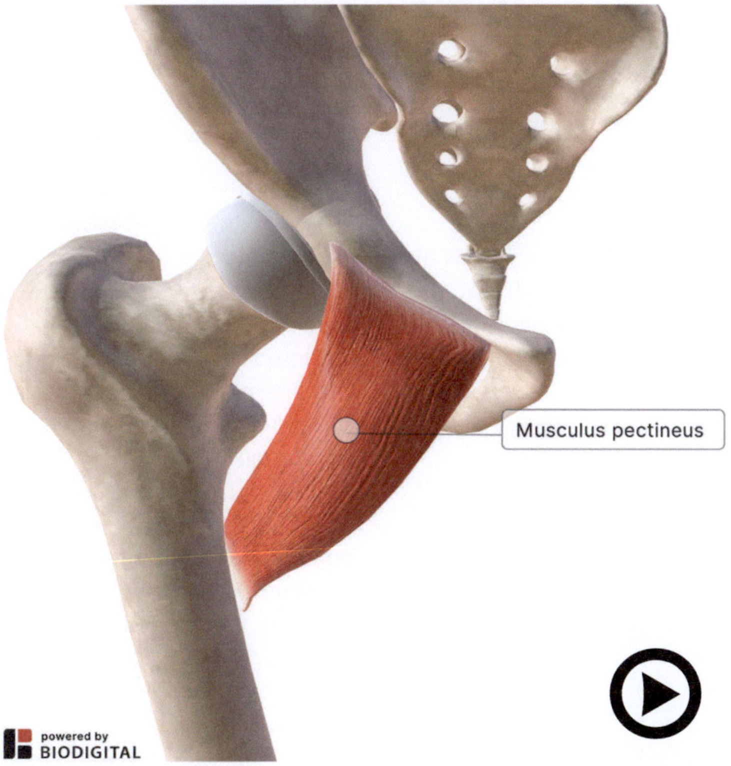

Fig. 5.7 Anatomy and palpation of the M. pectineus (▶ https://doi.org/10.1007/000-csj)

For palpation, with the client placed in the supine position with the knee joints underneath, the index or middle finger first contacts the homolateral pubic tubercle. Starting from this bony reference point, palpation is made distally and slightly laterally until the finger is immersed in soft tissue. The index or middle fingertip is located just distal to the pectineus muscle and directly on the belly of the adductor longus muscle. By contracting in adduction, this muscle can be differentiated from nearby parts of the quadriceps femoris muscle and felt laterodistally as it progresses.

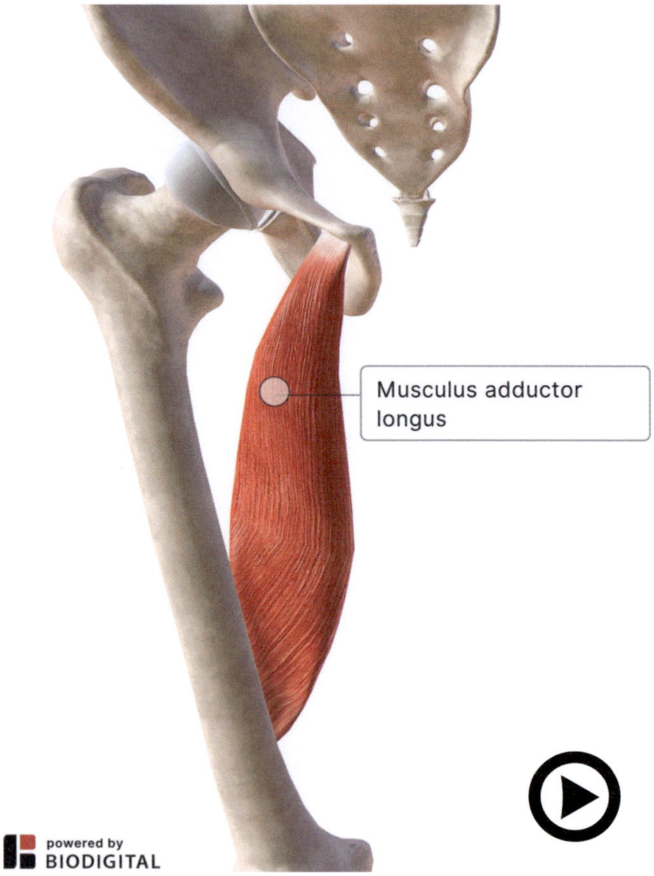

Fig. 5.8 Anatomy and palpation of the M. adductor longus (▶ https://doi.org/10.1007/000-csk)

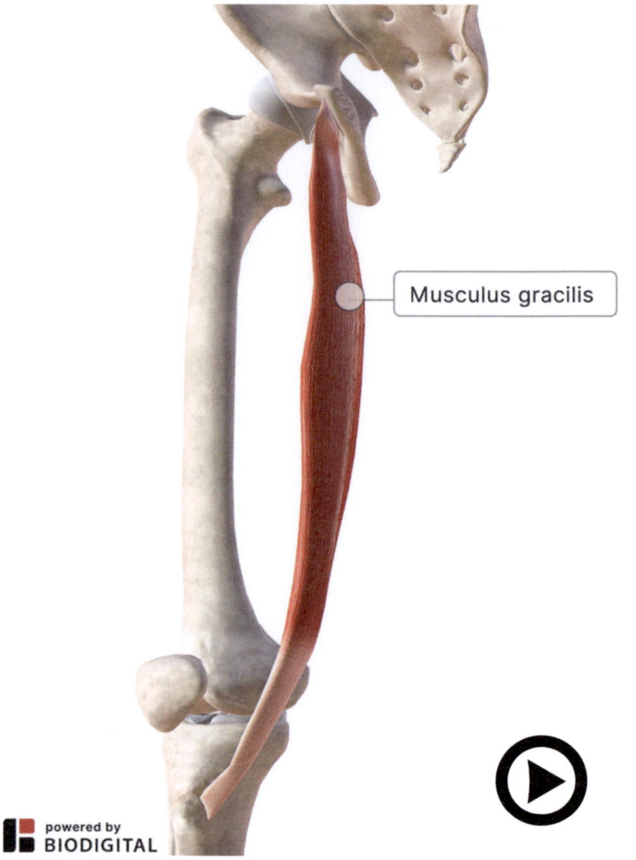

Fig. 5.9 Anatomy and palpation of the M. gracilis (▶ https://doi.org/10.1007/000-csm)

Implementation Note

The adductor longus muscle is crossed by the sartorius muscle in the middle of its course and is overlapped by the vastus medialis muscle after this intersection. Palpation is therefore very good in the proximal third, while it should be differentiated in the further course of the muscle by means of a targeted contraction (Fig. 5.8).

5.2.9 Palpation of the Gracilis Muscle

The slender muscle, which is superficially located on the inner side of the thigh, is counted among the adductors and is also the only double-jointed muscle of this group. It originates near the symphysis at the ramus inferior ossis pubis and then runs steeply along the inner side of the thigh distally towards the knee joint, where it finds its insertion at the pes anserinus superficialis together with the sartorius and semitendinosus muscles. Innervation via the obturator nerve from segments L2–L4 enables the gracilis muscle to move the hip joint in the direction of adduction, flexion and internal rotation and the knee joint in internal rotation.

The palpation of this muscle is achieved through a medial approach with the client in a lateral position with his back to the practitioner. The lower leg is slightly flexed at the knee joint, while the upper leg is extended at the hip and knee joints and positioned underneath. The fingertips are positioned steeply anteroproximally at the close of the thigh of the lower leg. It is important to stay anterior to the adductor magnus muscle, which is located directly in the middle of the inner side and posterior to the gracilis muscle. Then the fingertips move steeply distally onto the muscle belly. From the middle of the course, the adductor magnus muscle is overlapped by the posterior semimembranosus muscle, which enables the palpator to differentiate the gracilis muscle from surrounding tissue by means of a contraction in adduction. In addition, an active dynamic movement in knee flexion can take place, which causes the semimembranosus muscle to contract and thus increases the precession of the palpation of the gracilis muscle.

Both muscle bellies are directly next to each other so that accurate palpation is easily possible. The tendon can then be traced medially at the knee joint with the index finger.

Implementation Note

The inner thigh is often very sensitive and intimate, which requires a gentle and transparent approach to the client (Fig. 5.9).

5.2.10 Palpation of the Adductor Brevis Muscle

The deep-lying small hip joint adductor is located anterioproximally on the thigh and is covered distodorsolaterally by the pectineus muscle and the adductor longus muscle. The insertion of the muscle occurs in the dorsal region of the femur via the linea aspera in the proximal third. Functionally, it supports adduction and flexion in the hip joint. From a flexion of 80°, it in turn has an extensor effect in the hip joint. The small adductor receives innervation via the obturator nerve from segments L2–L4.

During palpation, which takes place in the supine position, the therapist is guided by the homolateral pectineus muscle and the adductor longus muscle. When the fingers are on the pectineus muscle, they move distally along the femoral artery about two transverse fingers. They then fall into a small depression that is bordered distally by the edge of the adductor longus muscle. In this depression, the steeply positioned fingertips apply pressure in depth and thus stimulate the adductor brevis muscle.

Implementation Note

Due to the anatomical position and the covering musculature, direct stimulation of the muscle is only possible in a small area (Fig. 5.10).

5.2.11 Palpation of the Adductor Magnus and Minimus Muscle

The large adductor is located on the inner side of the thigh and can be palpated very well in the proximal third. It has a broad origo at the ramus inferior ossis pubis, which extends to the tuber ischiadicum and then runs steeply distally until it inserts with proximal fibres into the labium mediale of the linea aspera and with distal fibres at the tuberculum adductorium. Functionally, it is responsible for adduction and synergistic extension in the hip joint. In addition, proximal fibres can move external rotation and distal fibres can move the hip joint back into internal rotation in an inflected position from external rotation. For this contraction, the adductor magnus muscle receives its innervation via the obturator nerve from segments L2–L4 and the tibial nerve from segments L4–L5.

For palpation of the muscle, the client is placed in a lateral position with his back to the therapist. While the lower leg is extended, the upper leg is flexed at the knee and hip joints. The palpator contacts the adductor magnus muscle with the fingertips directly proxomedial to the thigh joint of the lower leg. As the muscle lies superficially and is not covered by any muscles in the proximal third, direct contact with the tissue is possible. If the fingertips continue to palpate distally on the muscle belly, halfway through it becomes noticeable that a structure coming from anteriorly (m. gracilis) and a structure

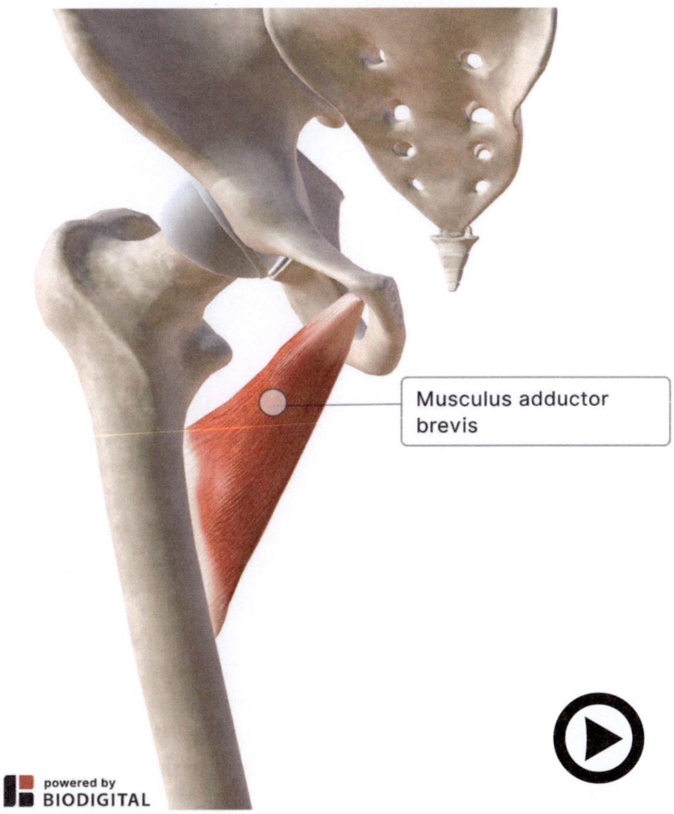

Fig. 5.10 Anatomy and palpation of the M. adductor brevis (▶ https://doi.org/10.1007/000-csn)

coming from posteriorly (m. semimembranosus) strongly influence the palpation result. In the distal end of the adductor magnus muscle, access with the fingertips is possible again at the adductor tuberosity of the medial epicondyle of the femur.

As a proximal split, the adductor minimus runs obliquely distolaterally from the ramus inferior ossis pubis and inserts dorsally in the upper third of the linea aspera of the femur. It is covered by the ischiocrural musculature and the gluteus maximus muscle.

Functionally, it supports adduction and external rotation in the hip joint. It receives innervation via the obturator nerve from segments L2–L4.

The stimulation of the muscle belly can be achieved through a dorsal approach. For this purpose, the patient is in the prone position while the therapist stands laterally at the level of the thighs. The fingertips are first applied to the biceps femoris muscle (see Sect. 5.3.7) and palpate proximally at the lateral edge. They then meet fibres of the gluteus maximus muscle in the gluteal region. Directly at the first encounter, the steeply positioned fingertips apply a stimulus in depth in the anterior direction. This stimulus is transmitted to the adductor brevis muscle, which extends almost to the inferior edge of the trochanter minor.

Implementation Note

During palpation in the proximal third, a contraction in adduction can increase the tactile sensation. The adductor minimus muscle can only be palpated by stimulation (Fig. 5.11).

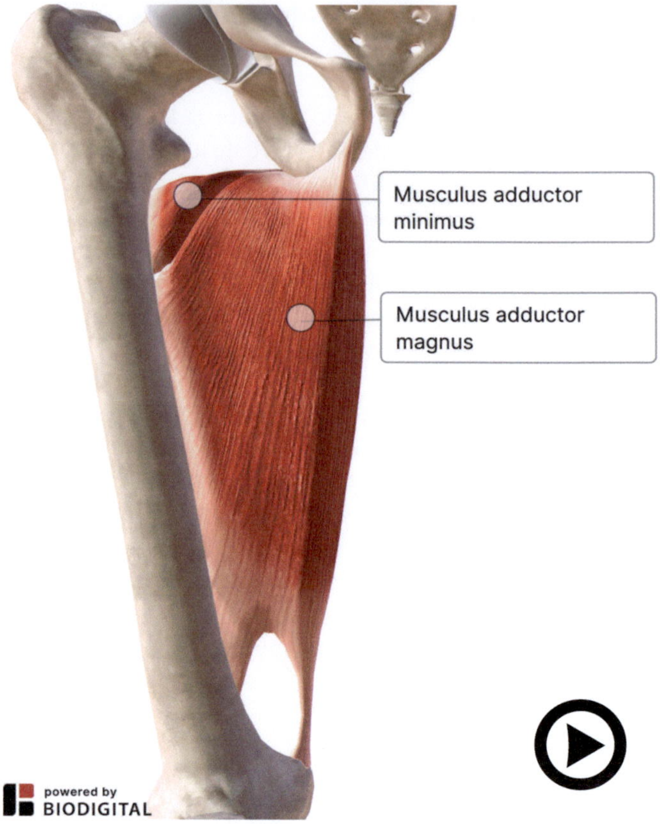

Fig. 5.11 Anatomy and palpation of the M. adductor magnus et minimus (▶ https://doi.org/10.1007/000-csp)

5.2.12 Palpation of the Mm. Gemelli, M. Obturatorius Internus and M. Quadratus Femoris

Below the gluteus maximus muscle and caudal to the piriformis muscle is the pelvitrochanteric musculature, which is also known by the abbreviation "GOGO" or more precisely "GOGOQ" musculature. Behind this name are the individual muscles with their initial letter in the order from cranial to caudal. Starting with the m. gemellus superior and the m. obturatorius internus, the m. gemellus inferior and the m. quadratus femoris follow. All four muscles are innervated via direct branches of the sacral plexus from segments L5–S2. The m. obturatorius externus is illuminated separately. The function of external rotation in the hip joint is common to all muscles. Due to the anatomical proximity of the four muscles to each other, palpation in combination is appropriate. Before this is described, the anatomy of the individual components of the pelvitrochanteric musculature will be examined in more detail.

The superior gemellus muscle, which originates in the spina ischiadica, runs horizontally to the lateral side, where it inserts via a common tendon with the internal obturator muscle on the greater trochanter and the trochanteric fossa of the femur. In addition to its external rotatory function, it can synergistically support adduction and extension in the hip joint. It can also be counted as part of the triceps coxae muscle group.

The internal obturator muscle, which is located directly caudal to the superior gemellus muscle and belongs to the triceps coxae muscle, has its origin at the posterior obturator membrane. It runs obliquely posterolaterally in the direction of the ischiadica minor, at the level of which it is deflected almost at right angles, passes through the ischiadicum minus foramen and inserts on the greater trochanter and the trochanteric fossa of the femur. In addition to its external rotatory function, it can support extension and adduction in the hip joint in the neutral position, while in the flexed position, it performs abduction synergistically. The muscle is innervated via the musculi obturatorii interni nerve.

The inferior gemellus muscle, which is the third component of the triceps coxae muscle, originates from the tuber ischiadicum of the ischii bone. From there, it runs horizontally to the side and inserts via a common tendon with the internal obturator muscle at the trochanteric fossa of the femur. In addition to its direct innervation from the branches of the sacral plexus, it is also controlled via the quadratic femoral nerve.

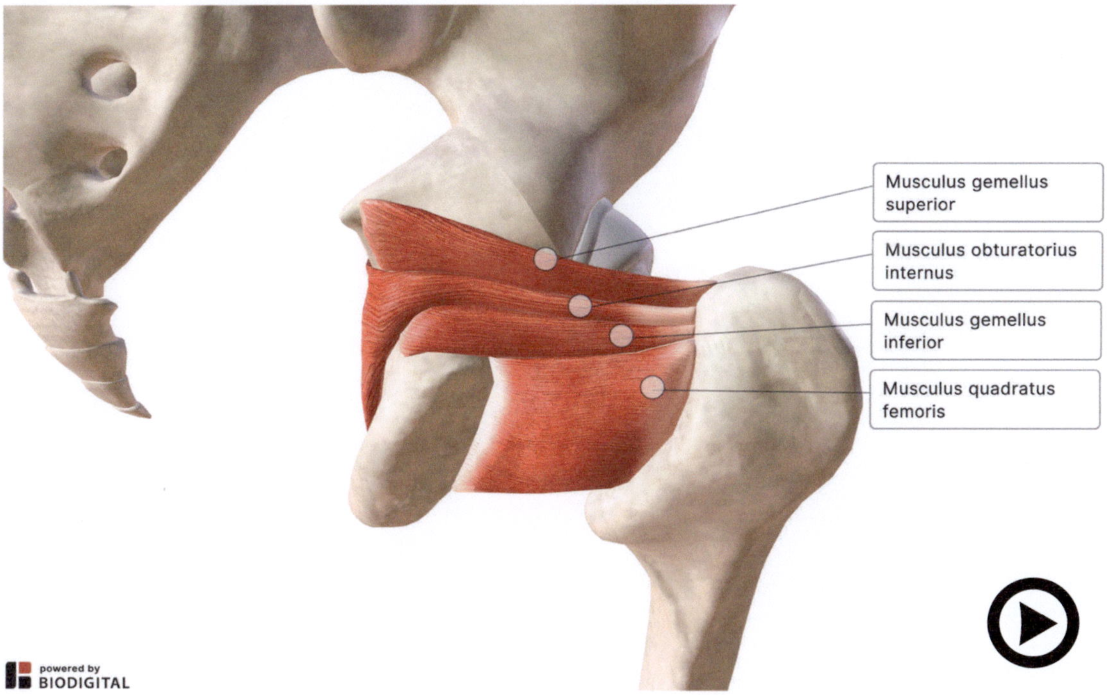

Fig. 5.12 Anatomy and palpation of the Mm. gemelli, M. obturatorius internus, M. quadratus femoris (▶ https://doi.org/10.1007/000-csq)

The quadratus femoris muscle, which is the most caudally located muscle of the pelvitrochanteric group, originates at the tuber ischiadicum, then runs caudolaterally and inserts at the crista intertrochanterica, posteriorly at the proximal femur. It is also innervated by the quadratic femoral nerve and can perform adduction in the hip joint synergistically. The quadratus femoris muscle is closely related to the adductor magnus muscle [6].

For palpation of the pelvitrochanteric muscles, the client is placed in the prone position while the clinician, standing sideways, contacts the homolateral side of the buttocks with the fingertips placed steeply. The piriformis muscle, described in Sect. 5.2.7, can be chosen as the starting point for contact. Starting from this reference point, the depth of the palpation is moved caudally by one transverse finger of the patient. It is important to compare the width of the client's fingers with your own beforehand to establish a relationship. The superior gemellus muscle follows caudally from the piriformis muscle, the internal obturator muscle one transverse finger further, followed by the inferior gemellus muscle offset by another transverse finger and the quadratus femoris muscle at the caudal end by another transverse finger. The four muscles can then be stimulated in their course from medial to lateral.

Implementation Note

All four muscles are covered by the gluteus maximus muscle, through which the palpation fingers must first glide. For this reason, palpation is challenging, as it is hardly possible to establish specific muscle tone via contraction to differentiate the "GOGQ muscles" (Fig. 5.12).

5.2.13 Palpation of the External Obturator Muscle

The external iliac sphincter, which originates on the anterior surface of the obturator membrane, runs posterolaterally and inserts on the trochanteric fossa of the femur. Via innervation by the obturator nerve, from segments L2–L4, it can move the hip joint into external rotation when contracted and synergistically support adduction.

Due to its superficial location, the external obturator muscle can be palpated via an anterior approach. For this purpose, the client is placed in a supine position with the knee joints underneath, while the palpator stands laterally and contacts the homolateral ramus superior ossis pubis with the fingertips. The fingertips then move caudally, leaving the bone and meeting soft tissue. In this region, they have to slide down between the pectineus and adductor longus muscles to reach the obturatius externus muscle.

It is recommended to first apply tension in hip joint adduction to feel the two muscle bellies. Then, at the moment of relaxation, the steeply positioned fingertips are used to feel further into the depths until they encounter a firm-elastic structure. This firm-elastic property is produced by the m. obturatorius externus and the underlying membrana obturatoria.

Implementation Note

Palpation in this region should be done gently at first, as it is very intimate on the one hand and can often be painful on the other. Sufficient transparency should be created in advance by educating the client (Fig. 5.13).

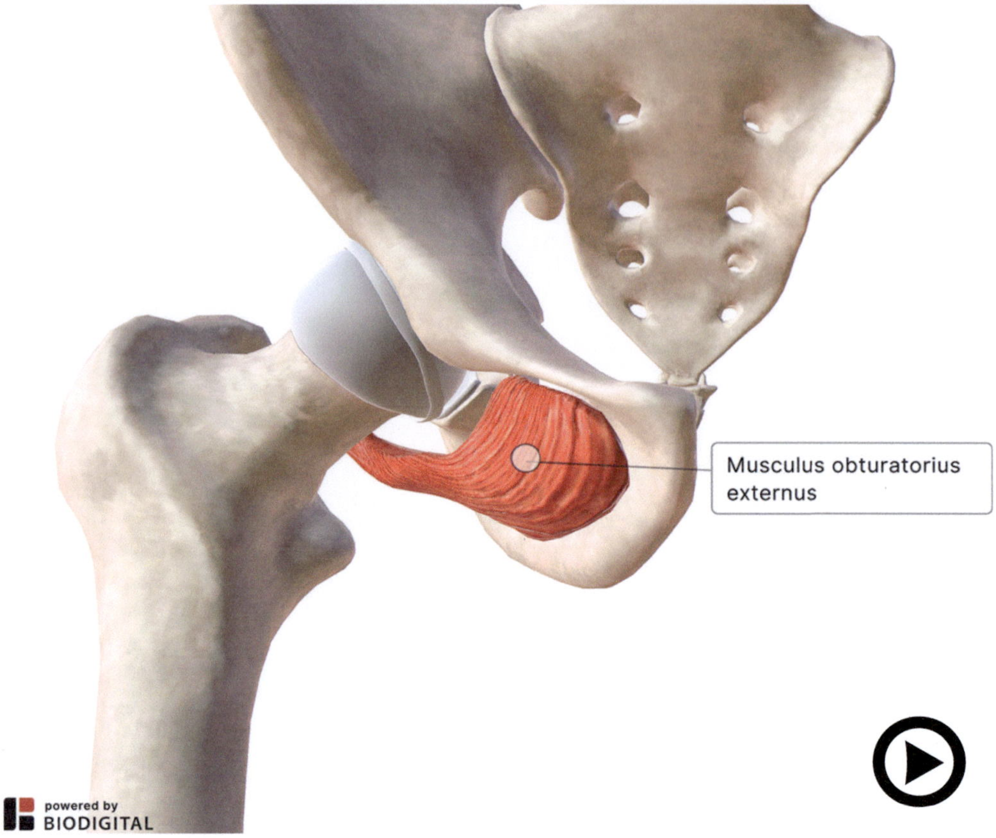

Fig. 5.13 Anatomy and palpation of the M. obturatorius externus (▶ https://doi.org/10.1007/000-csr)

5.2.14 Palpation of the Tensor Fasciae Latae Muscle

With its origin at the SIAS and its oblique course distolaterally into the tractus iliotibialis and the fascia lata, the tensor fasciae latae muscle is the strongest internal rotator of the hip joint. In addition to this main function, the muscle, which is innervated by the superior gluteal nerve from segments L4–L5, can also perform abduction and flexion in the art. coxae.

Due to its superficial position, the muscle can be felt very well from the supine position. To do this, first place the fingertips of the index and middle fingers on the homolateral SIAS. Then the client is asked to move the leg in the hip joint into an internal rotation. The clear contraction of this muscle allows its course to be grasped directly from the tense situation and at the same time differentiated from surrounding structures. After the contraction, the muscle can also be easily felt in its course in a relaxed state.

Implementation Note
As an internal rotator, the tensor fasciae latae muscle is the antagonist for the numerous external rotators in the hip joint. For this reason, as well as a frequent approach in flexion due to increased sitting in everyday life, the muscle can often react in a pressure-dolent manner when palpated (Fig. 5.14).

5.2.15 Palpation of the Pelvic Floor Muscles

The musculature in the pelvic floor area is an amalgamation of numerous muscles. While the pelvic diaphragm is formed by the levator ani muscle, the coccygeus muscle and the sphincter ani externus muscle, the urogenital diaphragm consists of the transversus perinei superficialis and profundus muscles. The entire pelvic floor is an important functional unit that resists strain from internal organs. In addition, it can influence the statics of the pelvis as well as the arterial, venous, and nervous supply of the lower extremity through excessive tension, which can result from an emotional background or too much physical strain, among other things. Palpation of the associated muscles is therefore recommended in order to find out the general tension relationship of the pelvic floor. However, not all muscles need to be palpated for this, which is not possible anyway due to the anatomical position.

For palpation, the client is in a relaxed supine position with the knee joints supported. The practitioner stands side-

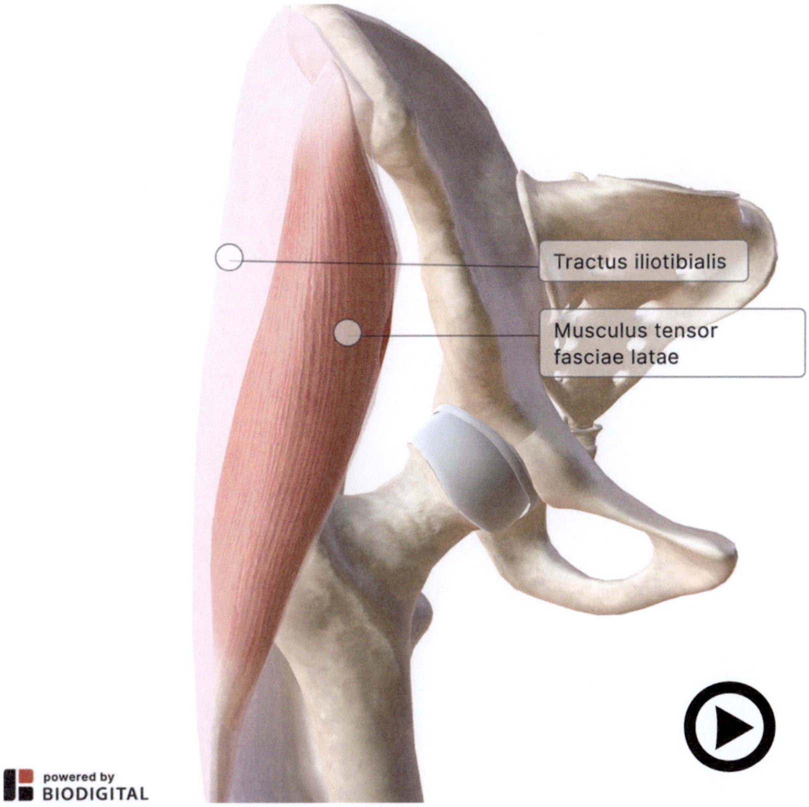

Fig. 5.14 Anatomy and palpation of the M. tensor fasciae latae (▶ https://doi.org/10.1007/000-css)

ways and contacts the contralateral tuber ischiadicum via an anterior approach with the index finger or optionally the thumb. Starting from the inner edge of the ischial tuberosity, palpation is then made in depth towards the symphysis at the inner edge of the ramus inferior ossis pubis. The palpating finger has direct contact with the ischiocavernosus muscle and the transversus perinei superficialis and profundus muscles. If the palpating fingers move posteriomedially from the ischiadic tuberosity, they come into direct contact with the iliococcygeus muscle, then medially with the pubococcygeus muscle and medially from this with the puborectalis muscle, which are part of the anterior levator muscle. Palpation can only detect a tension of the entire pelvic floor as a result, as it is hardly possible to differentiate the individual muscles from each other. The palpator can only apply a stimulus to the muscle complex to experience the overall tension.

To improve the quality of palpation, the client can induce tension in the pelvic floor by mentally actively holding back the urine.

Implementation Note
Palpation in this region should be done gently at first, as it is very intimate on the one hand and can often be accompanied by pain on the other. It is recommended to establish a clear transparency for the client regarding the position and function of the muscles in advance (Figs. 5.15 and 5.16).

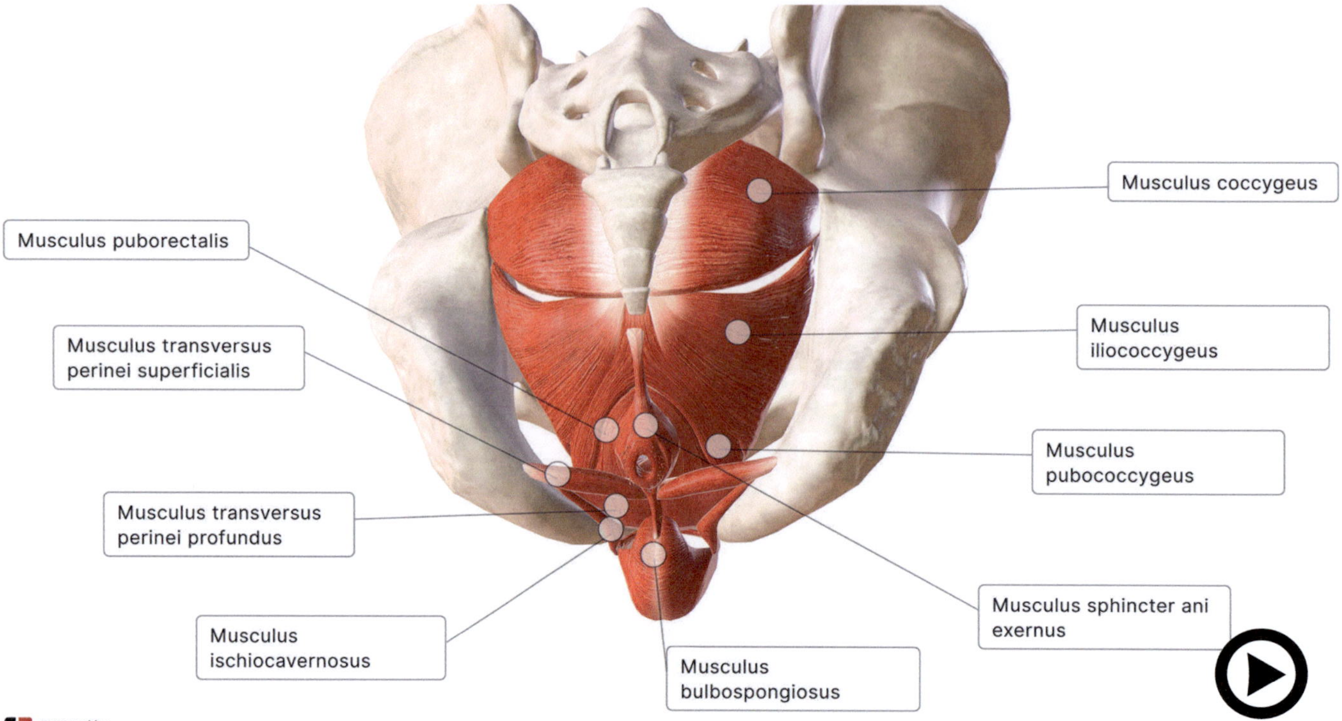

powered by BIODIGITAL

Fig. 5.15 Anatomy and palpation of the male pelvic floor muscles (▶ https://doi.org/10.1007/000-cst)

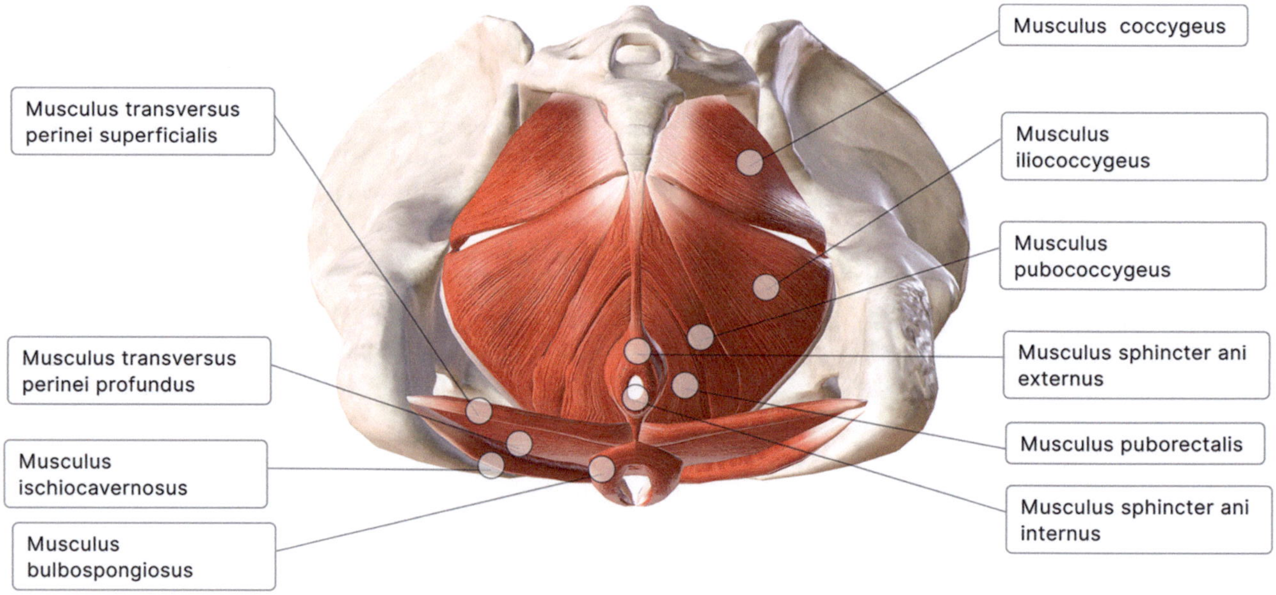

powered by BIODIGITAL

Fig. 5.16 Anatomy and palpation of the male pelvic floor muscles

5.3 Musculature in the Area of the Knee Joint

As a transportable hinge joint, the knee joint ensures mobility in flexion, extension as well as internal and external rotation. This mobility is mainly carried out by muscles located anteriorly, laterally and posteriorly on the thigh. The anterior quadriceps femoris consists of four parts and is the antagonist of the posterior ischiocrural muscle group, which is divided into three parts. Lateral to the thigh is the iliotibial tract, which also has an influence on the knee joint.

In addition to mobility, the knee joint must also provide the necessary stability, which leads to a high prevalence of injuries in this region. In 2013 alone, there were 230,441 inpatient hospitalisations due to knee injuries, and about 14% of all injuries can be attributed to the knee joint region [7]. Based on this high number, it is necessary to be able to palpate the musculature in the area of the knee joint in everyday practice. For palpation, the client is positioned in a supine or prone position so that the practitioner has good access to the structures.

5.3.1 Palpation of the Vastus Medialis Muscle

The inner part of the quadriceps femoris muscle is characterised by the vastus medialis muscle, which originates in the cranial part of the intertrochanteric line, caudally on the medial labium of the linea aspera to the medial supracondylar line. Via an oblique distomedial course, it is attached from the medial side to the patellar ligament and also to the tibial tuberosity. Through innervation by the femoral nerve from segments L2–L4, the muscle can fulfil its tasks as a knee joint extensor, patella stabiliser and anteriorisation of the menisci.

During palpation, the patient is positioned in the supine position with the knee joint underneath. The practitioner first places his hand flat on the inner side of the distal thigh and allows the knee joint to be actively stretched in extension. The inner edge of the vastus medialis muscle is then felt under the hand. Precise palpation can then be performed with the fingertips on the edges of the muscle and on the venter.

Implementation Note
The medial edge of the muscle forms a boundary to the hiatus adductorius, which carries the femoral artery and vein as well as the saphenous nerve as a branch of the femoral nerve and the descending genus artery. For this reason, the medial border should be felt carefully (Fig. 5.17).

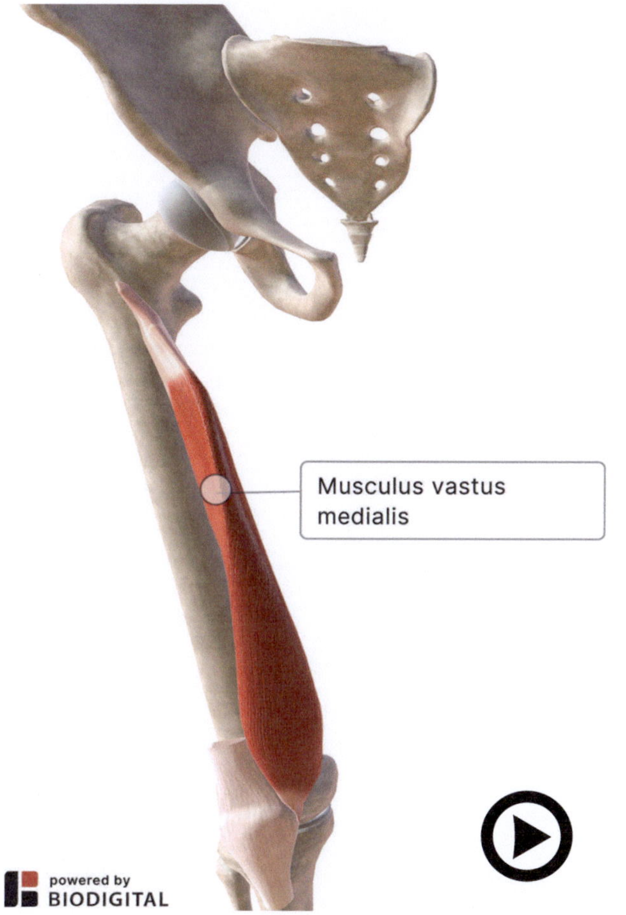

Fig. 5.17 Anatomy and palpation of the M. vastus medialis (▶ https://doi.org/10.1007/000-csv)

5.3.2 Palpation of the Vastus Intermedius Muscle

The middle part of the quadriceps femoris muscle, which originates on the anteroproximal femoral surface, runs steeply distally and is inserted via the patella ligament on the tibial tuberosity. Via innervation by the femoral nerve from segments L2–L4, the vastus intermedius can extend the knee joint and anteriorise the menisci.

The stimulation of the muscle belly is done with steeply positioned fingertips, which palpate through the rectus femoris muscle from anteriorly in the middle of the thigh. The client in the supine position can also perform an extension in the knee joint, which contracts the rectus femoris muscle in the middle of the thigh and thus ensures differentiation from the surrounding tissue.

Implementation Note
Due to its location directly under the rectus femoris muscle, direct palpation is not possible. The practitioner's goal is to

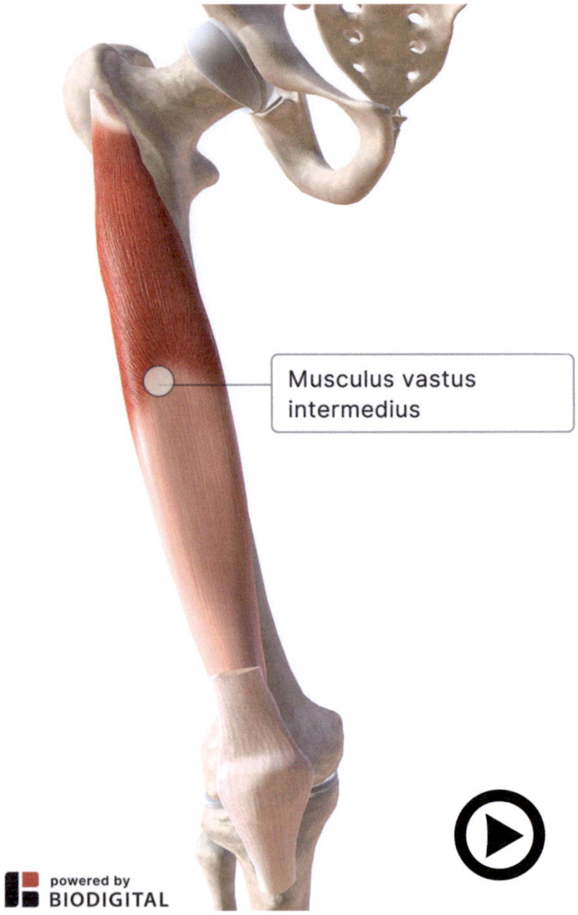

Fig. 5.18 Anatomy and palpation of the M. vastus intermedius (▶ https://doi.org/10.1007/000-csw)

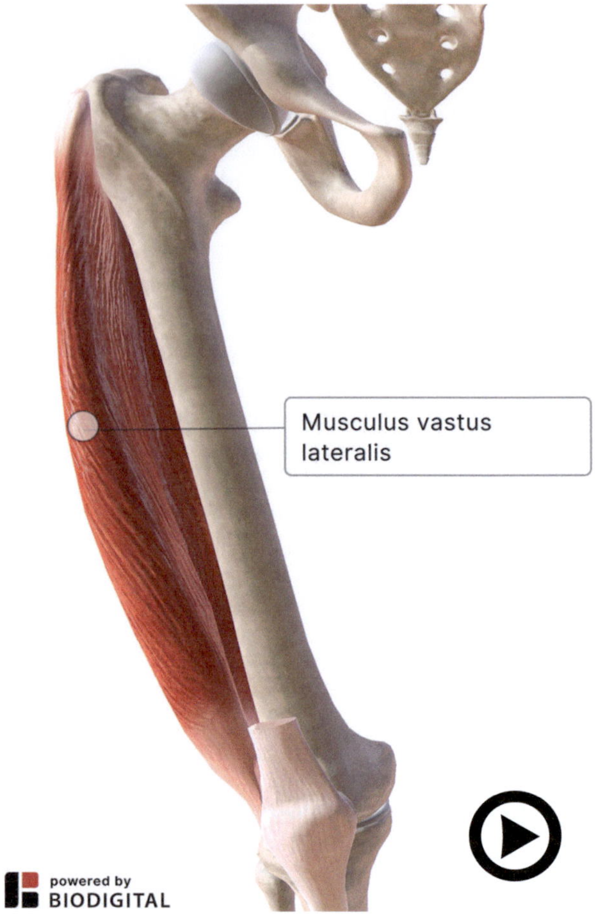

Fig. 5.19 Anatomy and palpation of the M. vastus lateralis (▶ https://doi.org/10.1007/000-csx)

stimulate the vastus medialis muscle with the described procedure (Fig. 5.18).

5.3.3 Palpation of the Vastus Lateralis Muscle

The external part of the quadriceps femoris muscle often has the largest mass of the four muscle bellies and is easily accessible by palpation via the lateral approach. It has a wide origin via an aponeurosis on the lateral labium of the linea aspera, on the lateral surface of the greater trochanter, on the linea intertrochanterica and via some fibres on the lateral septum intermusculare femoris. Its distomedial course towards the patella ends in the patella ligament and finally at the tibial tuberosity. The vastus lateralis is impelled by the femoral nerve, which controls it from segments L2–L4 and thus enables extension in the knee joint as well as lateralisation of the patella and anteriorisation of the menisci.

The clinician stands sideways for palpation and applies his hand distolaterally to the homolateral thigh of the supine patient. The client then activates the vastus lateralis muscle by extending the knee joint. Meanwhile, an increased tension can be felt under the hand. The edge of the vastus lateralis muscle is then located with the fingertips by defining the borders to surrounding structures with the fingertips during the contraction. Once these are defined, the muscle belly is felt in depth with the fingertips in a relaxed position.

Implementation Note
The vastus lateralis muscle is easily confused with the iliotibial tract, which is also located laterally on the thigh. The decontraction, in which the muscle tone decreases while the tractus iliotibialis retains its tension, can be used to differentiate between the structures (Fig. 5.19).

5.3.4 Palpation of the Rectus Femoris Muscle

Due to its superficial attachment, the vertical thigh muscle is very easy to feel and is a prime example of the palpation of muscles. The rectus femoris muscle, which originates with its caput rectum at the SIAI or with the caput reflexum at the upper edge of the acetabulum, lives up to its name and runs steeply distally until it inserts via the lig. patellae at the tibial tuberosity. It can initiate extension in the knee joint as well as anteriorisation of the menisci. Because it is located over two joints, it is also one of the hip joint flexors and thus supports the iliopsoas muscle. These numerous functions are made possible by the innervation of the femoral nerve, which controls the motor function of the region from segments L2–L4.

The practitioner stands on the homolateral side of the muscle to be examined.

From the supine position, the best way to feel the respective muscle belly is during activation. To do this, the clinician first places his flat hand mid-proximally on the thigh, has an extension performed in the knee joint and will feel a longitudinal muscle cord under the hand. This can then be outlined with the fingertips. After the contraction, the muscle belly is examined with the fingers steeply placed.

Implementation Note

In the case of injuries to the knee or hip joint and after operations in this region, the rectus femoris muscle can be hypertonic, while the remaining parts of the quadriceps femoris muscle are hypotonic. This phenomenon is due to the different distribution of the muscular fibre types (Fig. 5.20).

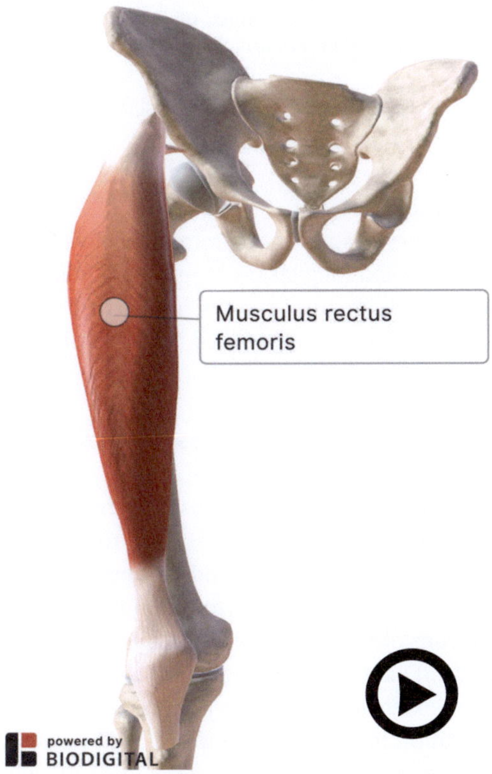

Fig. 5.20 Anatomy and palpation of the M. rectus femoris (▶ https://doi.org/10.1007/000-csy)

5.3.5 Palpation of the Semimembranosus Muscle

From the group of ischiocrural muscles posterior to the thigh, the semimembranosus muscle runs steeply caudomedially from the tuber ischiadicum and inserts at the pes anserinus profundus. The deep-lying goosefoot radiates via fibres to the condyle medialis tibiae, into the medial meniscus, into the dorsal knee joint capsule as well as into the fascia of the popliteus muscle and into the popliteum obliquum ligament. Through its innervation via the tibial nerve from segments L4–S3, the semimembranosus muscle can perform extension in the hip joint and flexion and internal rotation in the knee joint and also fixes the medial meniscus posteriorly.

For palpation, the client is in the prone position with the ankle joints slightly supported. The clinician stands sideways at the level of the knee joints and first places the flat hand medially in the hollow of the knee and actively flexes the knee. Two tendons are clearly felt under the hand, of which the medially located and rather straight one is that of the semimembranosus muscle. Under the held contraction, the index finger traces the tendon proximally and encounters a muscle belly that tends to be on the inner thigh. However, as the inner adductors are off, the muscle in tension can only be that of the ischiocrural muscle group. If the steeply positioned finger moves medially, it encounters the semitendinosus muscle directly after the muscle edge, which in turn shows a boundary with the biceps femoris muscle in the middle. Thus, the venter of the semimembranosus muscle is the most medial of all the parts of the ischiocrural muscle group.

Implementation Note

A common injury in sports is a strain in the posterior thigh as a result of a fast and long stride. If muscle fibres in the semimembranosus muscle are torn, this can be analysed via a "mushy sign" in the palpation of the relaxed muscle belly (Fig. 5.21).

5.3.6 Palpation of the Semitendinosus Muscle

This muscle takes its name from its long, well-defined attachment tendon, which is often used as a plastic for a cruciate ligament replacement, for example [8]. It arises from the caput commune together with the caput longum of the biceps femoris muscle at the tuber ischiadicum. In addition, it radiates with some fibres into the sacrotuberal ligament and can thus act on the sacral region through its tension. After a steep distomedial course, the semitendinosus muscle joins the gracilis and sartorius muscles in the superficial pes anserinus. It is innervated via the rami musculares of the tibial

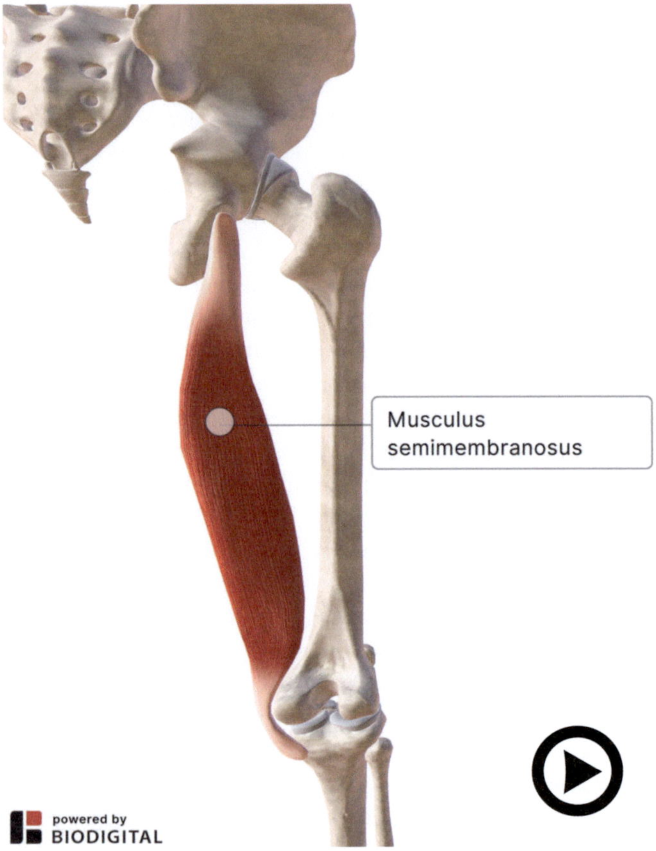

Fig. 5.21 Anatomy and palpation of the M. semimembranosus (▶ https://doi.org/10.1007/000-csz)

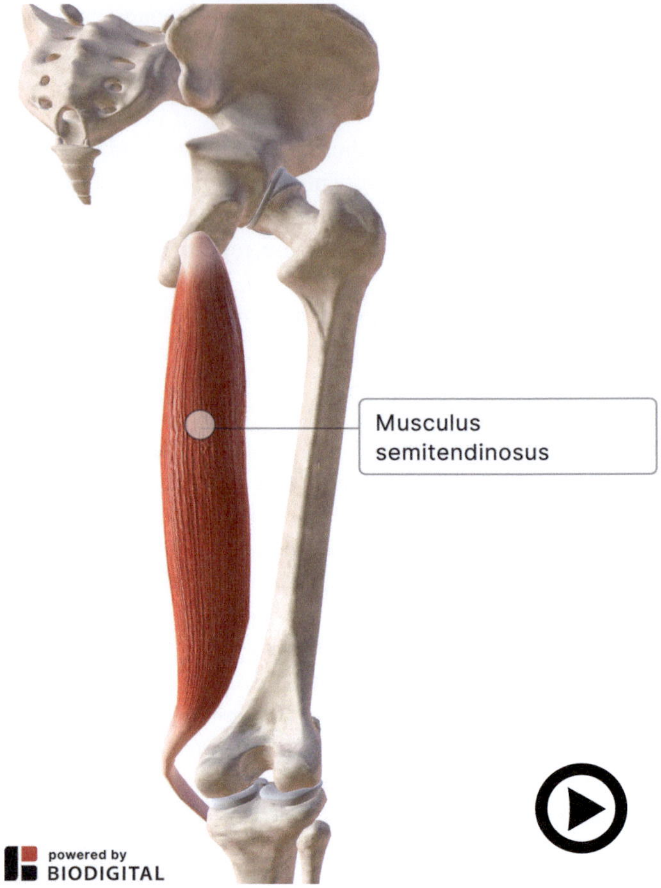

Fig. 5.22 Anatomy and palpation of the M. semitendinosus (▶ https://doi.org/10.1007/000-ct0)

nerve from segments L5–S2 and can functionally move the hip joint in extension and the knee joint, as a two-joint muscle, in flexion and internal rotation.

Palpation of the muscle, which can be started from two places, is performed in the prone position with the ankle joints underneath. In the first variant, the palpation fingers are placed medially in the popliteal fossa, and active flexion of the knee joint is performed. A tendon emerges prominently under the finger, which can be felt very well on the surface and can be traced far proximally. After the tendon is the muscle belly, which can be easily distinguished from the semimembranosus muscle medially and from the biceps femoris muscle laterally during contraction.

In the second palpation option, the clinician stands laterally at the level of the thigh and palpates directly in the middle of the posterior thigh with the steeply positioned fingertips of both fingers. In the meantime, he repeatedly makes small impulses in knee flexion in order to define a direct demarcation to the biceps femoris muscle, which is located more laterally.

The muscle belly can then be analysed in a relaxed starting position with the fingertips.

Implementation Note

A common injury in sports is a strain in the posterior thigh as a result of a fast and long stride. If muscle fibres in the semitendinosus muscle are torn, this can be analysed via a "mushy sign" in the palpation of the relaxed muscle belly (Fig. 5.22).

5.3.7 Palpation of the Biceps Femoris Muscle

The two-headed posterior thigh muscle, which is part of the ischiocrural musculature, originates from the tuber ischiadicum, the sacrotuberal ligament and the medial to distal surface of the linea aspera and the septum intermusculare femoris. It runs obliquely distolaterally and is inserted at the caput fibulae. Due to its location, the biceps femoris muscle can perform extension in the hip joint as well as flexion and external rotation in the knee joint. The action potentials for its contraction are received by the caput longum, which originates at the tuber ischiadicum, via the tibial nerve, whereas the caput breve, which finds its origin at the linea aspera, is innervated by the common fibular nerve. The spinal cord segments L5–S2 are the original information providers.

When palpating the biceps femoris, the patient is in the prone position, and the palpator stands laterally and contacts the flat hand in the contralateral popliteal fossa. The fingertips point laterally, and the client is asked to actively bend the knee joint. Meanwhile, a tendon is clearly felt under the hand, starting from the fibula head and running in a proximal direction. The fingertips follow the tendon and meet the muscle belly about a hand's width above the back of the knee. This can then also be felt in a decontracted position. A distinct groove can be felt in the medial area of the posterior thigh, which represents the transition to the semitendinosus muscle. In this way, the venter can also be differentiated from surrounding structures.

Implementation Note
A common injury in sports is a strain in the posterior thigh as a result of a fast and long stride. If muscle fibres in the biceps femoris muscle are torn, this can be analysed via a "mushy sign" in the palpation of the relaxed muscle belly (Fig. 5.23).

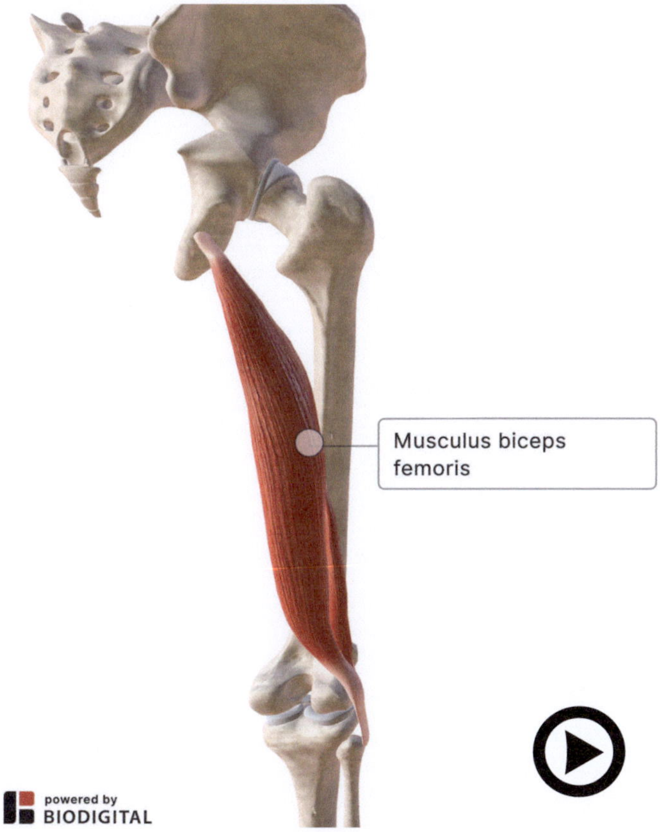

Fig. 5.23 Anatomy and palpation of the M. biceps femoris (▶ https://doi.org/10.1007/000-ct1)

5.3.8 Palpation of the Popliteal Muscle

True to its name, the popliteus muscle is located in the popliteal fossa. While it shows its origo at the condyle lateralis femoris and runs obliquely distomedially, it inserts over a large area that extends from the dorsal joint capsule over the planum popliteus tibiae to partially reach the middle of the lower leg at the facies posterior in the medial region of the tibia. The popliteus muscle is also called the capsular tensor. This describes one of its functions. In addition to this function, it can support internal rotation and flexion in the knee joint. It is innervated by the tibial nerve from segments L5–S2.

Palpation is performed in the prone position. The clinician stands at the side of the knee joint and first feels the caput fibulae from posteriorly over the contralateral popliteal fossa with the index fingertip. Starting from this point, the finger moves about three to four transverse fingers on a horizontal line medially and applies a pressure in depth towards the anterior at the end point. By actively tensing the lower leg in internal rotation, the muscle can be differentiated from the surrounding tissue. If the finger moves further distomedially towards the condyle medialis tibiae, it moves directly on the muscle belly. As the insertion is relatively broad, the clinician can also palpate distally from posteromedially along the medial edge of the tibia in order to appreciate the extensions of the popliteus muscle.

Implementation Note
Due to its location, the popliteus muscle is often exposed to increased stress in knee joint injuries, which can be perceived as hypertonicity and possibly also as a pressure-dolent area (Fig. 5.24).

5.3.9 Palpation of the Tractus Iliotibialis

The aponeurosis located laterally on the thigh forms the reinforcement of the fascia lata and receives its tendons of origin from the tensor fasciae latae muscle and the gluteus maximus and gluteus medius muscles. The steeply distal course allows the tractus iliotibialis to insert in the tuberculum of Gerdy at the condyle lateralis tibiae. Functionally, the tendon plate serves to stabilise against varus stress in stance and thus completes the traction-belt mechanism of the lower limb at the hip and knee joints.

Structural palpation is performed in the supine position with the knee slightly supported. The practitioner stands at the level of the knee joints and then contacts the lateral edge of the homolateral patella. Starting from this, palpation is performed laterally. In the course, firm connective tissue

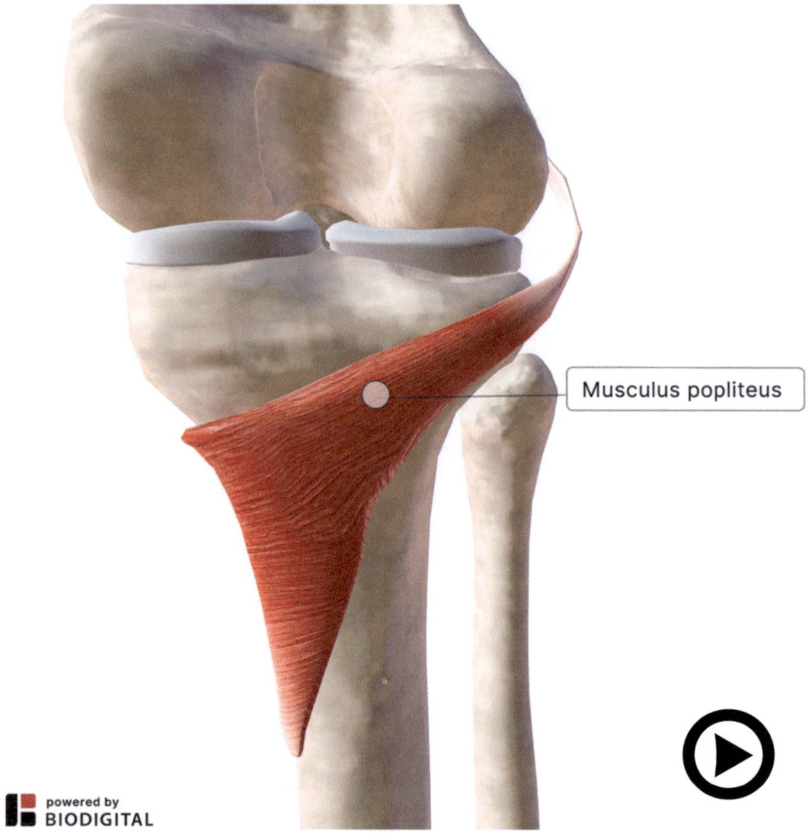

Fig. 5.24 Anatomy and palpation of the M. popliteus (▶ https://doi.org/10.1007/000-ct2)

fibres are felt. These fibres are the extensions of the iliotibial tract and are now traced proximally with the fingers. During proximal palpation, there is a widening of the initially narrow tendon. The aponeurosis extends over the entire lateral thigh and can be traced to the SIAS or crista iliaca. Differentiation is possible via active contraction in hip joint internal rotation, as here the tensor fasciae latae muscle places the tractus iliotibialis under tension.

Implementation Note
In iliotibial band syndrome, the tractus iliotibialis is irritated at its distal end and may appear painful on palpation (Fig. 5.25).

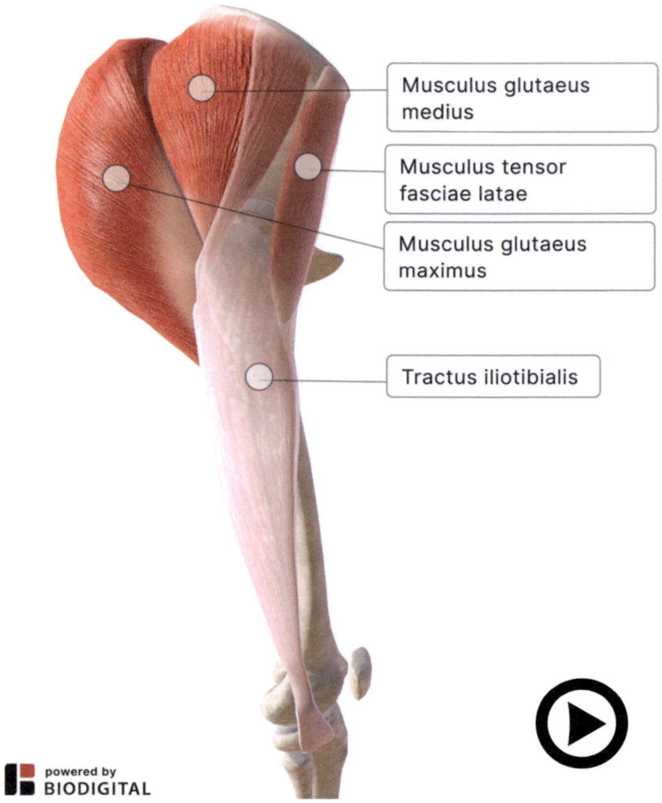

Fig. 5.25 Anatomy and palpation of the tractus iliotibialis (▶ https://doi.org/10.1007/000-ct3)

5.4 Musculature in the Area of the Lower Leg/Foot

Walking upright on two legs is an activity that appeared in human evolution about 2 million years ago. There is a possibility that the date given is even further in the past [9]. Some scientists place this development even further back in history. However, it is a fact that Australopithecus at that time had to adapt to environmental influences and started walking upright. This mode of locomotion ensured survival and was one of the main activities, covering 20–40 km daily. Walking itself is a biomechanical sensation. Due to the mechanised society, walking has regressed somewhat, so that nowadays only 10% of food calories have to be used for locomotion, whereas in 1900, it was about 90% [10]. "Sitting is the new smoking," says various headlines, describing a process in which numerous diseases can be traced back to a loss of movement. This makes it even more important to be able to precisely analyse the structures that make walking possible. These structures include the muscles of the lower leg and the foot. They stabilise the leg axis starting from the pes, which literally carries us through life. Starting from this highly complex biomechanical structure, ascending chains of cause and effect can arise that can have an influence on the entire statics of the human being. It is therefore essential to know the position and shape of the muscles in this region. These facts are described precisely in the following chapters so that accurate palpation is possible. Depending on the muscle, the starting position for palpation should be supine or prone.

5.4.1 Palpation of the Anterior Tibialis Muscle

The foot lift initiates the initial ground contact, where the foot touches the ground for the first time after the swing leg phase and thus allows the load of the body to meet the ground reaction force. Belonging to the pretibial muscle group, the tibialis anterior muscle originates from the facies lateralis tibiae in the upper two-thirds as well as from the membrana interossea cruris and the upper part of the fascia cruris superficialis. As a long, spindle-shaped muscle, it runs steeply distomedially and inserts on the medial and plantar surface of the medial cuneiform bone and on the base of the first metatarsal. Through its innervation via the profundal fibular nerve from segments L4–L5, it can realise dorsiflexion movements in the upper ankle joint and supination in the lower ankle joint. In addition, it is an important component of the stapes, which, together with the fibularis longus and tibialis posterior muscles, ensures stability in the ankle joints.

Palpation of the anterior tibialis muscle is done in the supine position with the knee joints slightly inferior. The therapist stands sideways facing the patient's head and contacts the homolateral margo anterior tibiae, in the middle of the lower leg, via the fingertips. Starting from the tibial crest, the finger berries move laterally where they meet directly with the muscle belly. If the foot is actively moved in dorsal extension in the upper ankle joint, a contraction of the foot lever is clearly noticeable, which allows a more precise differentiation. In a relaxed starting position, the entire muscle can then also be felt in depth.

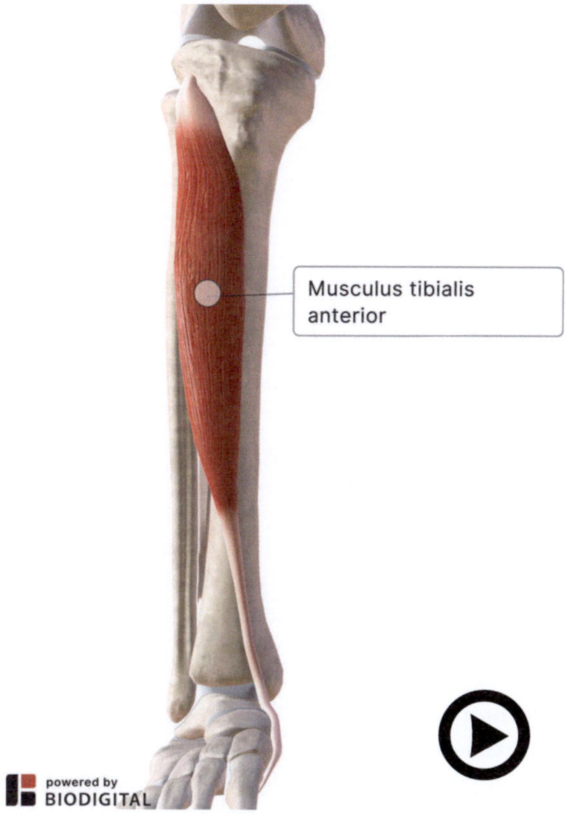

Fig. 5.26 Anatomy and palpation of the M. tibialis anterior (▶ https://doi.org/10.1007/000-ct4)

Implementation Note
The tibialis anterior muscle can react with pressure on palpation after high stress. In this case, we speak of so-called shin splints or tibial edge syndrome. Palpation should therefore be gentle at first. After trauma, there is also a risk of compartment syndrome (Fig. 5.26).

5.4.2 Palpation of the Extensor Hallucis Longus Muscle

The big toe extensor originates from the middle third of the facies medialis fibulae and the membrana interossea cruris and partly from the extensor digitorum longus muscle. It is covered in the proximal part by the anterior tibialis muscle, runs steeply distally to the dorsum of the foot, then crosses the anterior tibial artery obliquely distomedially and finally inserts in the dorsal aponeurosis and the base of the distal phalanx of the hallux. The only small muscle belly is enclosed by two long tendons and provides dorsiflexion in the upper ankle joint as well as in the proximal and interphalangeal joints of the big toe. In addition to these functions, which are made possible by innervation from the profundal fibular nerve from segments L4–L5, it can also support supination in the lower ankle joint.

For palpation, the patient is positioned in the supine position with the knee joints underneath. The therapist stands laterally in front of the bent leg and makes anterior contact with the talus or malleolus fork with the fingertips. Now the client is asked to move the big toe in extension so that the tendon of the extensor hallucis longus comes into view. The muscle can be felt proximally as well as distally with the help of the tendon, which becomes clear. It can finally be palpated to the distal phalanx with the fingertips.

Implementation Note
In the proximal region of the muscle, only stimulation is possible, i.e. no direct palpation, because the extensor hallucis longus muscle is covered by the tibialis anterior muscle and the extensor digitorum longus muscle. After trauma, there is also a risk of compartment syndrome (Fig. 5.27).

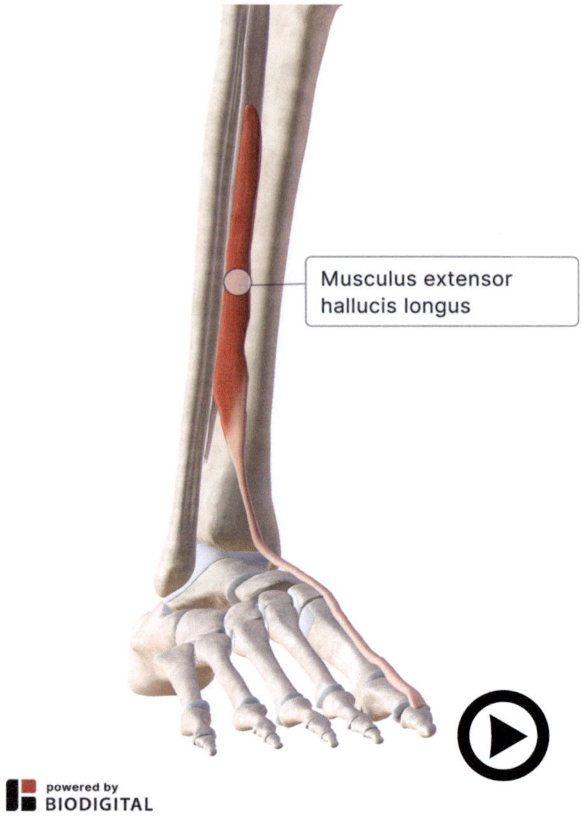

Fig. 5.27 Anatomy and palpation of the M. extensor hallucis longus (▶ https://doi.org/10.1007/000-ct5)

Implementation Note
As there are several muscles in the region of the lower leg that have similar functions, it is particularly important to differentiate the extensor digitorum longus muscle from other muscles by means of a separate contraction in dorsal extension of the toes II–V. After trauma, there is also a risk of compartment syndrome (Fig. 5.28).

5.4.3 Palpation of the Extensor Digitorum Longus Muscle

The long toe extensor, which belongs to the pretibial muscle group, has a broad origin at the lateral condyle of the tibia and at the caput fibulae, the margo anterior fibulae, the membrana interossea cruris and the septum intermusculare cruris. Its steep distal course ends in the dorsal aponeurosis of toes II–V and the respective distal phalanx. The extensor digitorum longus receives its innervation via the fibular profundus nerve, which enables dorsal extension in the upper ankle joint and in the II–V proximal and interphalangeal joints. In addition, it supports pronation in the lower ankle joint.

The extensor digitorum longus is palpated from the supine position with the knee joints underneath. The palm of the practitioner standing to the side contacts the area of the talus, and the client is asked to move the toes into dorsal extension. Here, the four tendons are clearly felt, which separate from the main tendon in this region. They can then be traced distally with the fingertips to the proximal phalanx II–V, whereas proximally they join to form a tendon and finally the muscle belly. The course of this can be felt with the steeply placed fingertips.

5.4.4 Palpation of the Fibularis Longus and Brevis Muscle

The fibular muscle group, which is an important component of the stapes, is also known by the obsolete name "peroneal muscle group" and is located laterally on the lower leg. The fibularis longus muscle and the fibularis brevis muscle form the main component and are supplemented by the fibularis tertius muscle, which appears only inconstantly as a splitting off the extensor digitorum longus muscle. The fibularis longus muscle, which originates at the caput fibulae, extends steeply distally and merges into a long tendon, which runs posterior to the lateral malleolus distoplantar and inserts at the medial os cuneiforme and the plantar metatarsal I. The fibularis longus muscle has a similar course. The fibularis

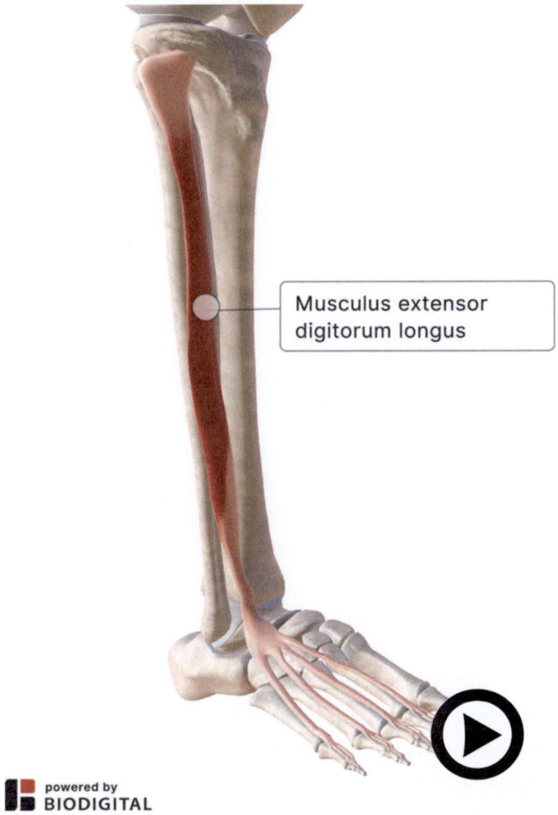

Fig. 5.28 Anatomy and palpation of the M. extensor digitorum longus (▶ https://doi.org/10.1007/000-ct6)

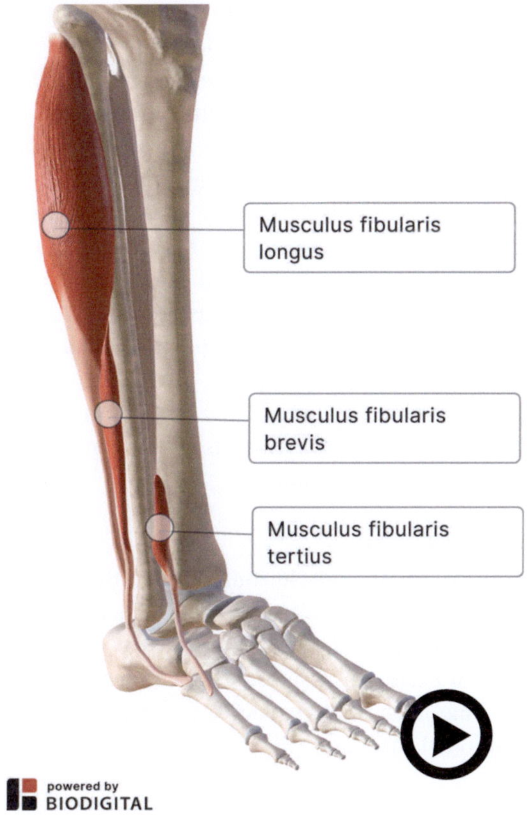

Fig. 5.29 Anatomy and palpation of the M. fibularis longus et brevis et tertius (▶ https://doi.org/10.1007/000-ct7)

brevis muscle follows a similar course, originating distally at the facies lateralis fibulae and the septum intermusculare cruris anterius and posterius. Its tendon also runs behind the lateral malleolus, but already attaches to the metatarsal V tuberosity. The inconstant fibularis tertius muscle, on the other hand, originates in the distal area of the facies lateralis fibulae and the membrana interossea cruris, runs distally in front of the malleolus lateralis as a splinter of the extensor digitorum longus muscle and inserts dorsally at the base of the metatarsal V. All three muscles move the ankle joints in plantar flexion and pronation. Active pronation is an important component in the development of the stapes. While the fibularis longus and brevis muscle receives its innervation through the superficial fibular nerve from the L5–S1 segments, the fibularis tertius muscle receives its action potentials through the profundal fibular nerve from the L5–S1 segments. Since the fibularis tertius muscle is absent in about 10.5% of people and shows variations in its structure, it is not described palpatorily in this chapter because, if it is present, it is automatically provided with a stimulus on palpation [11].

For feeling the fibular muscle group, a starting position in the supine or lateral position is recommended. The fingertips are applied steeply to the caput fibulae and, starting from this reference point, move distally along the fibula. Meanwhile, the client performs an active, dynamic pronation of the lower ankle joints. The contraction is clearly felt under the fingertips and can be perceived even more precisely by also assuming active plantar flexion. The fibular musculature can be felt throughout the fibula, with the fibularis longus muscle in the proximal area and the fibularis brevis and tertius muscle in the distal area.

Implementation Note

After long walks, this muscle can be irritated, which can lead to painful sensations on palpation (Fig. 5.29).

5.4.5 Palpation of the Posterior Tibialis Muscle

The posterior tibial muscle is often considered part of the stapes and extends obliquely distomedially from the posterior surface of the interosseous membrane, the adjacent surfaces of the tibia and fibula and the deep sheet of the fascia cruris. The relatively small muscle belly joins a tendon in the distal third of the lower leg, which passes through the tarsal tunnel directly behind the medial malleolus, changes direction and runs plantar. The insertion extends on the plantar side from the tuberositas ossis navicularis via the os cuneiforme mediale to the bases of the ossa metatarsalia II–IV. Via innervation by the tibial nerve from segments L4–S1, the posterior tibialis muscle can move the ankle joints in the direction of plantar flexion and supination.

Palpation of the muscle is only possible at its tendon directly on the medial malleolus, as it is covered in its region of origin by the gastrocnemius and soleus muscles. To do this, the index and middle fingertips are placed flat on the inner knuckle and a supination with plantar flexion is actively performed. During this inversion movement, a variably shaped tendon emerges, which lies directly on or immediately behind the medial malleolus. Palpation is best performed in the supine position.

Implementation Note
The posterior tibialis muscle runs through the tarsal tunnel with the flexor digitorum longus and flexor hallucis longus muscles, as well as with the posterior tibial artery and vein and the tibial nerve, and can cause tarsal tunnel syndrome if irritated. This leads to pain due to the compression of the aforementioned structures (Fig. 5.30).

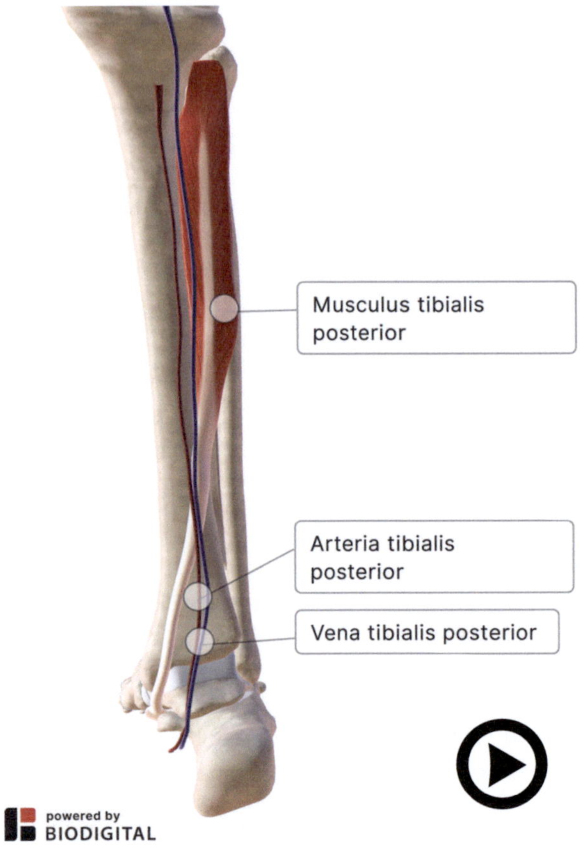

Fig. 5.30 Anatomy and palpation of the M. tibialis posterior (▶ https://doi.org/10.1007/000-ct8)

5.4.6 Palpation of the Flexor Hallucis Longus Muscle

The long big toe flexor belongs to the deep flexor group of the lower leg and originates from the posterior facies of the fibula, the interosseous membrane and the posterior intermuscular septum. In its steeply distal course, it is covered by the gastrocnemius and soleus muscles. The tendon of the flexor hallucis longus then runs behind the medial malleolus distally further underneath the sustentaculum tali through the sulcus tendinis musculi flexoris hallucis longi to the plantar and inserts at the base of the distal phalanx of the hallux. True to its name, it performs plantar flexion of the big toe in the interphalangeal as well as the metatarsophalangeal joint and supports plantar flexion in the upper ankle joint and supination in the USG. This is made possible by innervation through the posterior tibial nerve from segments L5–S1.

For palpation, the client is positioned in the supine position with the knee joints underneath. The therapist stands laterally at the level of the foot and applies the fingertips of the index and middle fingers centrally between the medial malleolus and the Achilles tendon. The client then actively performs plantar flexion of the big toe. This leads to a tensing of the muscle, which in turn is felt under the fingers. It is important that only the big toe moves, as the flexor digitorum longus muscle, whose tendon lies slightly anterior, and the tendon of the flexor hallucis longus muscle cross each other. They thus take a similar course. To ensure this, toes II–V can be fixed in dorsiflexion with the practitioner's other hand so that an isolated movement of the hallux occurs. In addition, the contraction impulse can be perceived in depth in the lower part of the middle third of the facies posterior fibularis. For this, the fingertips are steeply positioned and a dynamic movement of the big toe is actively performed.

Implementation Note
The flexor hallucis longus muscle runs through the tarsal tunnel with the flexor digitorum longus muscle and the posterior tibialis muscle, as well as with the posterior tibial artery and vein and the tibial nerve, and can cause tarsal tunnel syndrome if irritated. This leads to pain due to the compression of the aforementioned structures (Fig. 5.31).

5.4.7 Palpation of the Flexor Digitorum Longus Muscle

The long toe flexor belongs to the posterior deep lower leg musculature and has its origins at the posterior facies and the medial margo of the tibia. It runs steeply distally, posterior to the medial malleolus to below the sustentaculum tali through the tarsal tunnel, and inserts plantarly at the terminal phalan-

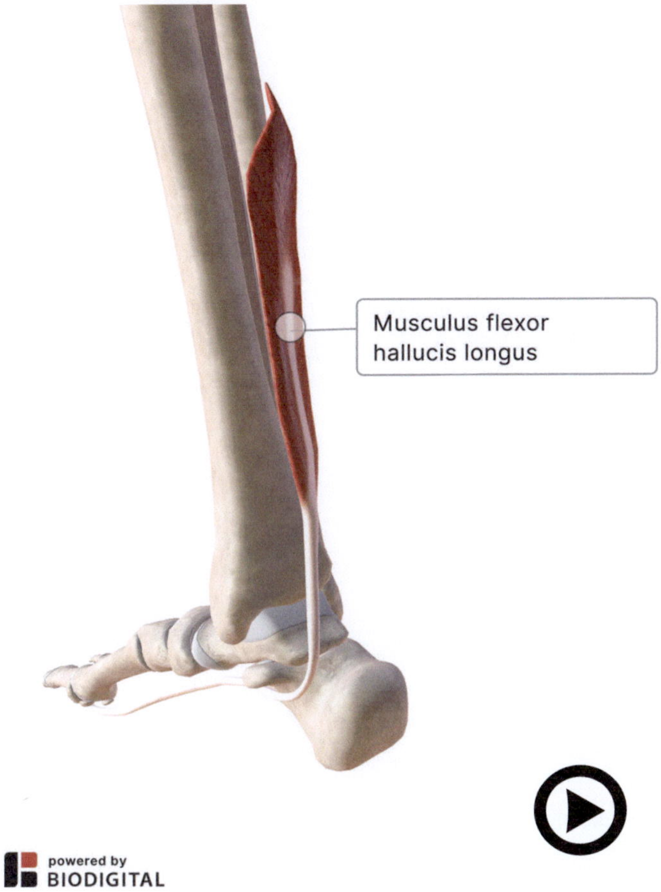

Fig. 5.31 Anatomy and palpation of the M. flexor hallucis longus (▶ https://doi.org/10.1007/000-ct9)

ges of toes II–V. In its insertion area, the flexor digitorum longus serves as the origin of the lumbrical pedis muscles. It also performs plantar flexion in the proximal and interphalangeal joints of toes II–V and in the upper ankle joint. It can realise these functions through its innervation via the tibial nerve from segments S1–S2.

For palpation of the muscle, the patient is to be positioned in the supine position with the knee joints underneath. The therapist stands at the level of the foot and places the fingertips of the index and middle fingers in the middle between the medial malleolus and the Achilles tendon. The client then actively performs a plantar flexion of the toes II–V. This causes the muscle to tense, which the fingers can perceive on the tendon of the flexor digitorum longus muscle. It is important to note that only toes II–V move because the flexor hallucis longus muscle, whose tendon is slightly posterior, and the flexor digitorum longus tendon cross. They thus take a similar course. To ensure this, the big toe can also be passively fixed in dorsal extension with the therapist's other hand, so that only a movement of the toes II–V in flexion takes place. Activation of the tibialis anterior muscle, which fixes the entire foot in dorsiflexion, can also make the palpation result more precise.

In addition, the muscle belly can be heard posteromedially on the calf during repeated dynamic flexion. For this, the fingertips make contact in the middle of the margo medialis tibiae and move one transverse finger in the posteromedial direction. A repetitive contraction of the toes II–V in plantar flexion is then performed, which leads to a palpable impulse under the finger berries.

Implementation Note
The flexor digitorum longus muscle runs through the tarsal tunnel with the flexor hallucis longus muscle and the posterior tibialis muscle, as well as with the posterior tibial artery and vein and the tibial nerve, and can cause tarsal tunnel syndrome if irritated. This leads to pain due to the compression of the aforementioned structures (Fig. 5.32).

5.4.8 Palpation of the Soleus Muscle

The clod muscle is included in the triceps surae muscle together with the gastrocnemius and plantaris muscles. It has its origin at the posterior facies of the tibia, at the linea musculi solei and partly at the fibula. In its steep distal course, it is predominantly covered by the gastrocnemius muscle, which is why direct palpation is only possible at specific points. Its insertion is ensured by the Achilles tendon on the calcaneal tuberosity. It can perform plantar flexion in the upper ankle joint and supination in the lower ankle joint through innervation of the tibial nerve from segments S1–S2.

For palpation of the muscle, the person to be palpated is positioned in the prone position while the clinician stands laterally at the level of the lower leg. The crus is placed underneath so that an angular position of approx. 45° is achieved in the knee joint. This brings the gastrocnemius muscle closer so that it contracts less efficiently during plantar flexion. The steeply positioned fingertips are first positioned posteriorly on the caput fibulae and then move distally on the lateral surface. Meanwhile, the foot is actively tensed in plantar flexion so that a contraction is felt under the finger. It is important that only the foot and not the toes move into plantar flexion; otherwise, the flexor digitorum longus muscle could distort the palpation sensation. In addition to palpating the lateral border, the medial border of the soleus muscle can also be felt using a similar approach, starting from the medial condyle of the tibia. In addition to both methods, a stimulus can also be applied to the soleus muscle from the middle of the lower leg. In this case, the longitudinal groove between the two heads of the gastrocnemius is searched for with the fingertips in the middle of the lower leg and then palpated in depth. Here, a direct stimulus is exerted on the clod muscle, as the gastrocnemius muscle is in an approaching position due to the flexed position in the knee joint. The distal insertion can be perceived via the Achilles tendon, which runs posteriorly on the lower leg and is easily

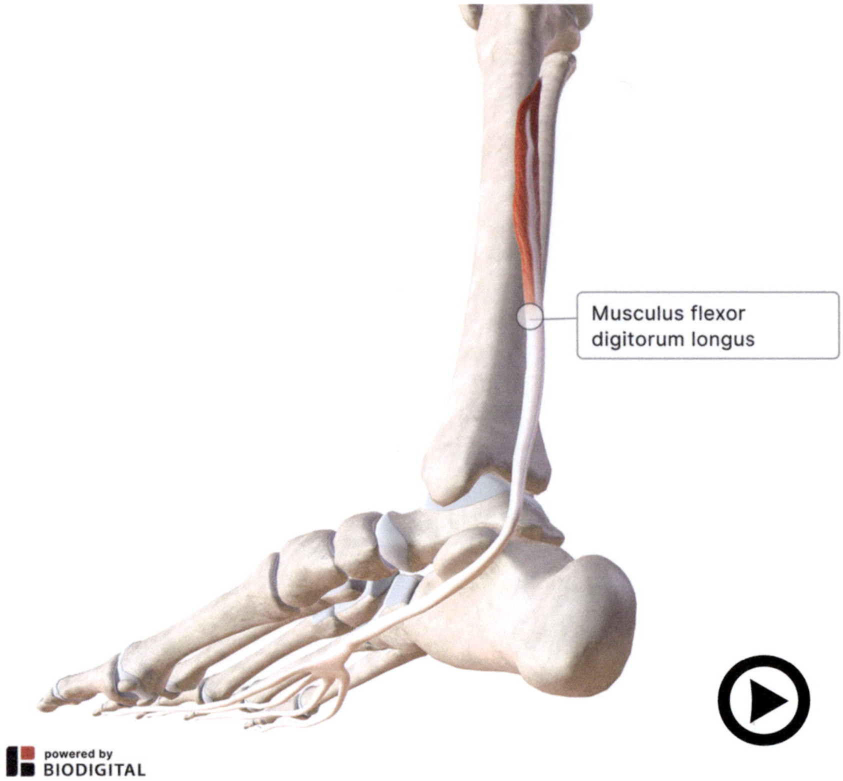

Fig. 5.32 Anatomy and palpation of the M. flexor digitorum longus (▶ https://doi.org/10.1007/000-cta)

palpable, and which appears directly behind the malleolus fork during plantar flexion.

Implementation Note
The soleus muscle can experience an increased degree of irritation after intense exertion or after contusions. In this case, clients report pain in the area of the Achilles tendon, calf and sometimes even homolateral sacroiliac joint (SIJ) (Fig. 5.33).

5.4.9 Palpation of the Gastrocnemius Muscle

The twin muscle, which is located posterior to the calf, forms a large part of the triceps surae muscle and forms the externally visible relief of the lower leg. The gastrocnemius muscle consists of two bellies, the medial part of which originates on the medial femoral condyle and the lateral part on the lateral femoral condyle. Both run steeply distally and end approximately in the middle third of the lower leg in the longitudinal Achilles tendon. The tendo calcanei then runs further distally and finds its insertion at the tuber calcanei. In addition to the main function of plantar flexion in the upper ankle joint, the gastrocnemius muscle can support flexion, as well as the medial part of internal rotation, lateral part of

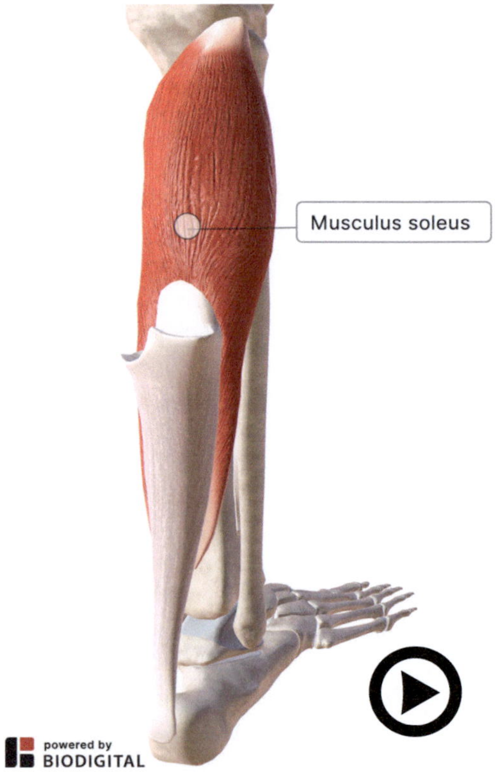

Fig. 5.33 Anatomy and palpation of the M. soleus (▶ https://doi.org/10.1007/000-ctb)

external rotation in the knee joint and supination in the USG. These motor functions result from innervation by the tibial nerve from segments S1–S2.

Due to its superficial position, this muscle is easy to palpate. While the client is positioned in the prone position, the palpator stands laterally at the level of the lower leg and places the hand flat on the proximal third of the homolateral calf. The palpator is asked to actively move the foot into plantar flexion in order to produce a noticeable contraction of the gastrocnemius muscle. The palm of the hand can first open the entire muscle so that selected regions such as muscle edges and muscle bellies can then be palpated with the fingertips. Directly in the middle of the proximal calf, a furrow can be felt with steeply placed fingers, which separates the lateral from the medial muscle belly.

Implementation Note

After contusions in the calf area or after sustained, repetitive strain, the muscle may react pressure-dolent on palpation (Fig. 5.34).

5.4.10 Palpation of the Plantar Muscle

Starting from the linea supracondylaris posterior at the lateral femoral condyle, the plantar muscle arises, which registers its muscle belly directly in the popliteal fossa and runs obliquely distomedially in a slender tendon after the popliteal fossa. It inserts over the Achilles tendon on the tuber calcanei and, due to its attachment, is synergistically responsible for flexion in the knee joint and plantar flexion in the upper ankle joint. In addition, it fulfils an important proprioceptive task, as it has a high density of receptors in relation to other muscles [12]. For this function, it is innervated by the tibial nerve from segments S1–S2.

Palpatory access can only be established in the popliteal fossa, as the plantar muscle is located posterior to the popliteal muscle but anterior to the gastrocnemius muscle. The client is positioned in the prone position with the ankle joints underneath, while the palpator, standing sideways, contacts the homolateral condyle lateralis femoris with the fingertips. The index fingertip then moves medially and is now proximal to the popliteus muscle and intermedial to the two heads of the gastrocnemius, directly in the centre of the popliteal fossa and on the plantar muscle. Stimulation is possible on the muscular structure, while sensation of the tendon is difficult due to the superimposed gastrocnemius muscle.

Implementation Note

The plantar muscle can show areas of tension in the muscle belly, which can appear pressured on palpation. In many cases, the client feels pain in the area of the back of the knee (Fig. 5.35).

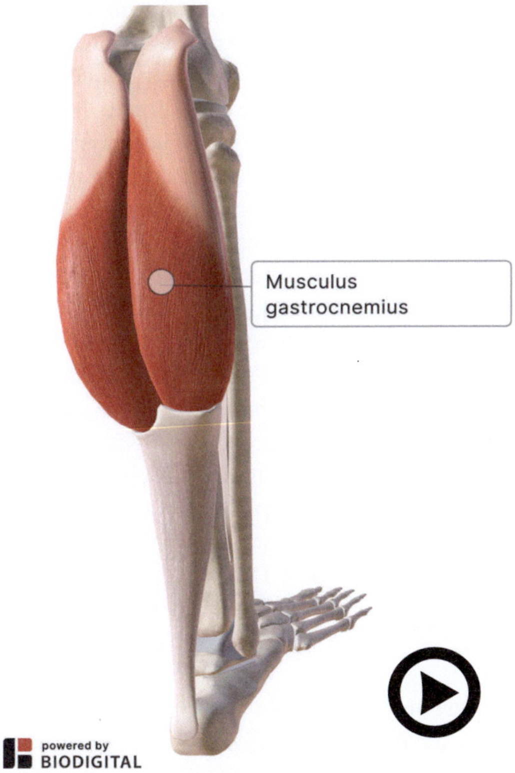

Fig. 5.34 Anatomy and palpation of the M. gastrocnemius (▶ https://doi.org/10.1007/000-ctc)

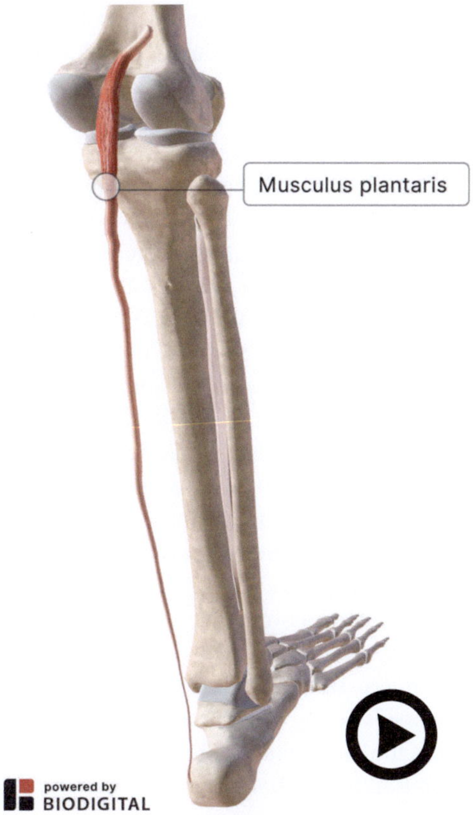

Fig. 5.35 Anatomy and palpation of the M. plantaris (▶ https://doi.org/10.1007/000-ctd)

5.5 Foot Musculature

The foot carries us through life. Every day, it adapts to the most varied ground conditions and footwear. This can be achieved by 28 bones and 21 muscles. This diversity makes the foot an adaptable instrument that enables walking, running, jumping and many other activities. Similar to the hand, the short foot muscles can also be divided into groups. There are the plantar and dorsal as well as the big and small toe ball muscles. In the following chapters, all 21 muscles are assigned to the respective groups and their anatomical position and function are described. The palpation process is also explained in terms of the groups mentioned.

For palpation, a starting position in the supine or prone position is recommended in order to be able to access the structures well.

5.5.1 Palpation of the Plantar Foot Musculature

The group of plantar muscles includes the m. quadratus plantae, the m. flexor digitorum brevis, the mm. interossei plantares pedis I–III and the Mm. lumbricales I–IV. All these muscles are accessible to plantar palpation. The preferred starting position is therefore prone with the knee joint bent 90°.

The two-headed quadratus plantae muscle originates on the plantar surface of the calcaneus. A caput mediale is distinguished from a caput laterale. The short muscle runs distally and opens directly into the tendon of the flexor digitorum longus muscle and therefore has the task of actively supporting it. The ability to act is made possible by innervation of the lateral plantar nerve from segments S1–S2.

The flexor digitorum longus is located in the sole of the foot. It originates plantarly at the calcaneus and then runs distally over a large area. In the course, it divides into four attachment tendons, which then divide again into two parts at the level of the metatarsophalangeal joints, in order to then attach to the respective medial or lateral edge of the corresponding middle phalanx. The resulting gap at the level of the metatarsophalangeal joints is needed as a passage point for the flexor digitorum longus muscle. Functionally, the flexor digitorum brevis muscle serves to flex the toes II–V in the metatarsophalangeal and proximal interphalangeal joints. The short foot muscle is innervated via the medial plantar nerve from segments L5–S2.

The mm. interossei plantares pedis are located medially on the metatarsals III–V. They originate at the base and the medial side of the ossa metatarsalia III–V, respectively. Their distal path ends at the medial side of the respective proximal phalanx and at the dorsal aponeuroses of the tendons of the extensor digitorum longus. Innervation via the lateral plantar nerve from segments S1–S2 allows the three muscle bellies to perform adduction and flexion in the III–V metatarsophalangeal joints and extension of the III–V metatarsophalangeal joints.

The four mm. lumbricales belong to the short foot muscles and are located in the area of the metatarsus. The origins of each belly are medial to the tendons of the flexor digitorum longus. Here, the first muscle begins with its origin on the medial side of the tendon of the second toe, and the second, third and fourth muscles originate from the medial and lateral sides of the two adjacent tendons, respectively. All four run distally along the metatarsals and insert on the dorsal aponeuroses of digiti II–V and on the tendon extensors of the extensor digitorum longus muscle. They are able to guide the metatarsophalangeal joints of the toes II–V into flexion. In addition, they can produce dorsiflexion in the middle and end joints and simultaneously move the splayed toes II–V into adduction. These functions are made possible by the medial plantar nerve for the lumbrical I–II muscles and the lateral plantar nerve for the lumbrical III–IV muscles. Both parts originate from the segments S1–S2.

For palpation of the plantar muscle group, the client is positioned in the prone position with the ankle joints underneath. The therapist stands directly to the side at the level of the feet and makes contact with the plantar calcaneus with the index and middle fingertip. The toes and foot should then be moved dynamically into dorsal extension. Here, the plantar aponeurosis is noticeably stretched under the fingers, whereupon the palpating fingers trace the structure heelward to the origin. Directly under the plantar aponeurosis at the level of the calcaneus and in the transition to the metatarsals is the flexor hallucis brevis muscle. The steeply placed fingertips feel the muscle in depth as soon as the patient moves the toes and foot in the direction of plantar flexion. As the quadratus plantae muscle is located further below the flexor hallucis brevis muscle, a plantar stimulus can only be applied at the level of the os cuboideum with the steeply positioned fingertips. The interossei plantares and lumbricales muscles can also only be stimulated. For this purpose, the fingertips of the index and middle fingers move into the space between the metatarsals II and V and can, when placed steeply, palpate the three interossei plantares muscles. The lumbrical muscles are located directly plantar to the metatarsals II–V and are thus accessed by bony palpation of the inferior bony surfaces with the fingertips. Direct palpation of these muscles is also not possible because numerous structures cover the muscles.

Implementation Note

Palpation in the plantar region of the calcaneus can be painful in the presence of a pronounced plantar calcaneal spur, as the continuum distortion penetrates the soft tissue (Fig. 5.36).

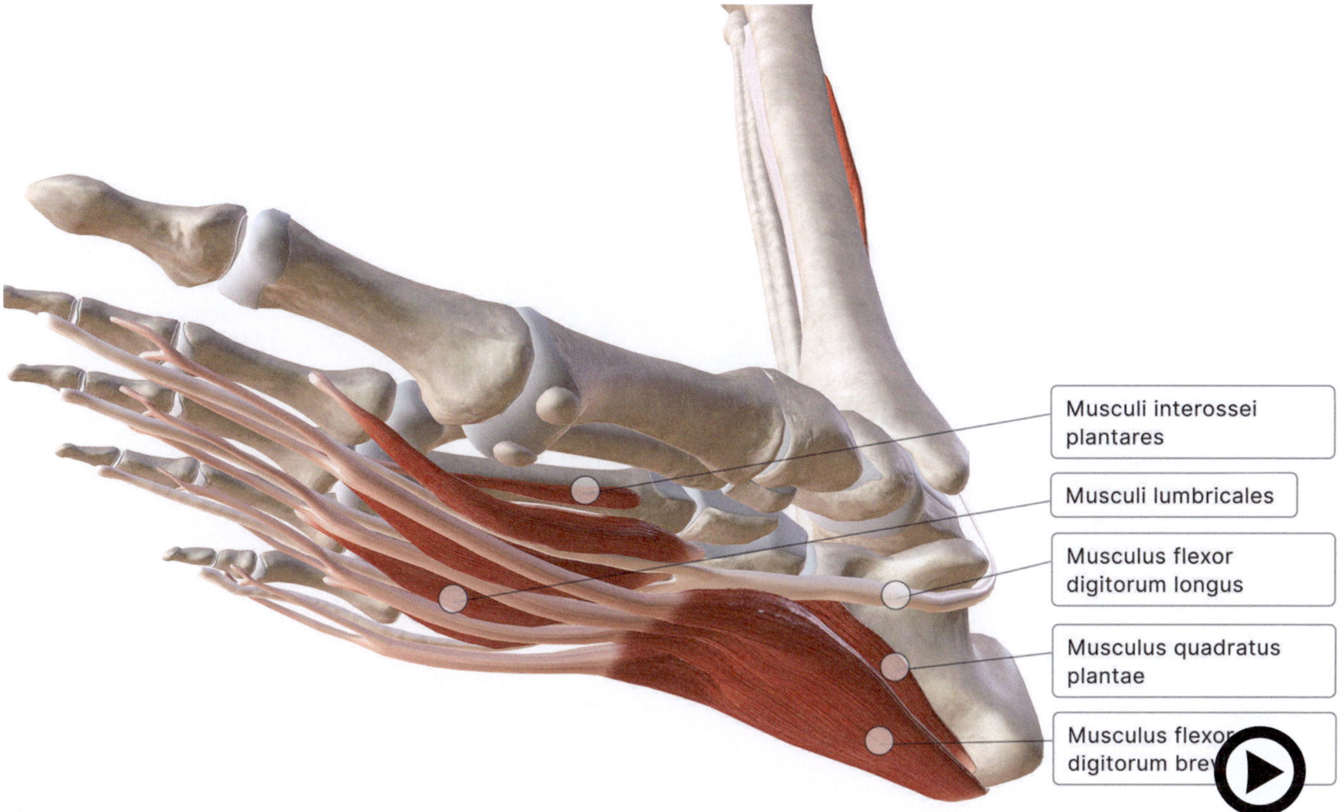

Fig. 5.36 Anatomy and palpation of the plantar foot muscles (▶ https://doi.org/10.1007/000-cte)

5.5.2 Palpation of the Short Hallux Foot Muscles

The group of short foot muscles at the ball of the big toe consists of the abductor hallucis, flexor hallucis brevis and adductor hallucis muscles. All three muscles are in close contact with the hallux and can move it. The big toe forms an important part of the functional longitudinal axis of the foot. This axis as well as the medial longitudinal arch of the foot and the rolling over the ball of the big toe are factors that are elementary for physiological gait. The palpatory approach is therefore important to be able to analyse the short foot musculature of the hallux.

The abductor hallucis muscle, which is the most proximal of the group, originates on the plantar medial surface of the medial process of the calcaneal tuberosity. It then runs plantar to distal and medial under the os naviculare and the os cuneiforme mediale and inserts in a long tendon medial to the proximal phalanx of the hallux and with some fibres in the joint capsule of the metatarsophalangeal joint. Through innervation via the medial plantar nerve from segments L5–S2, it can move the big toe in plantar flexion and abduction.

A little further distally, starting from the medial underside of the os cuboideum, the os cuneiforme mediale and intermedium as well as the tendon of the m. tibialis posterior, the lig. calcaneocuboideum and the lig. plantare longum, the m. flexor hallucis brevis extends along the metatarsale I distally. While the medial caput inserts via the medial sesamoid bone at the base of the proximal phalanx of the hallux and at the capsule of the MCP I, the lateral caput inserts via the lateral sesamoid bone at the base of the proximal phalanx of the hallux and at the capsule of the MCP I. The plantar flexion, which is common to both calcaneocuboideum and plantar ligament, extends distally. Plantar flexion, which both muscle bellies produce together in the art. metatarsophalangealis I, is innervated by the plantaris medialis nerve from segments L5–S1 for the caput mediale and by the plantaris lateralis nerve from segments S1–S2 for the caput laterale.

The adductor hallucis muscle, which is the most distal of this group, can be divided into a caput transversum and a caput obliquum. As the name suggests, the caput transversum runs transversely from the capsules and ligaments of MCPs III–V to the lateral side of the base of the proximal phalanx of the hallux and thus over the ball of the foot. The oblique caput obliquum arises in the regions of metatarsal bases II–IV and also attaches to the lateral side of the base of the proximal phalanx of the hallux. Both parts are innervated by the lateral plantar nerve and perform adduction in the metatarsophalangeal I articular.

Palpation is limited and is performed with the patient in the prone position. The clinician, standing sideways, applies the

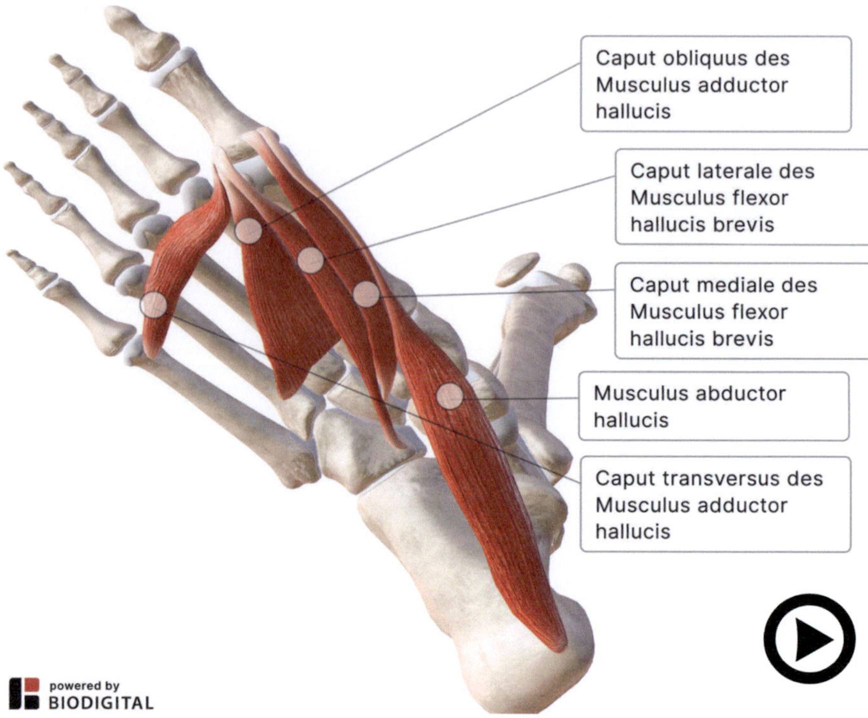

Fig. 5.37 Anatomy and palpation of the short foot muscles of the hallux (▶ https://doi.org/10.1007/000-ctf)

fingertips of the index and middle fingers, coming from the medial side, to the medial surface of the calcaneus about three transverse fingers distal to the medial malleolus. The patient then actively moves his big toe into abduction by spreading all toes. A clear contraction of the abductor hallucis muscle is felt under the fingers, as this muscle is located directly on the surface. The fingers then follow the muscle belly distally until they arrive at about the level of the base of metatarsal I from medial. Now the big toe is actively moved in the direction of flexion, which results in a noticeable contraction of the caput mediale of the flexor hallucis brevis muscle. The lateral caput and the adductor hallucis muscle cannot be palpated directly because the plantar aponeurosis and the lumbrical muscles are located plantar to the parts and therefore cover them. Only a stimulation via steeply positioned fingertips in the area of the respective caput of the ossa metatarsalia II–IV can lead to indirect contact with the muscle belly.

Implementation Note
The medial longitudinal arch of the foot, which is used as a guide for palpation of the abductor hallucis and flexor hallucis brevis muscles, can be sensitive to pressure in various foot deformities (Fig. 5.37).

5.5.3 Palpation of the Short Foot Muscles of the Digitus Minimus Pedis

In addition to the special musculature of the big toe, the lateral counterpart is the group of small toe muscles consisting of the abductor digiti minimi pedis, the flexor digiti minimi brevis pedis and the inconstant opponens digiti minimi pedis. The foot forms a total contact surface of about 100 cm^2 with the ground [13]. Thus, the muscles at the digitus minimus pedis make an important contribution regarding the lateral longitudinal arch of the foot and the individual movement of the little toe.

The muscle with the largest muscle belly in this group is the abductor digiti minimi pedis muscle. It originates at the medial and lateral tuberosity of the calcaneus and plantar at the metatarsal V and the plantar aponeurosis. Its steep distal course ends at the base of the proximal phalanx of the little toe and at the tuberositas ossis metatarsale V. The abductor digit minimi pedis can perform abduction and flexion in the metatarsophalangeal joint of the little toe via innervation by the plantaris lateralis nerve from segments S1–S2.

The flexor digiti minimi brevis muscle, which is located directly plantar to the metatarsal V, has its origin plantar to the base of the os metatarsale V and to the plantar long ligament and the tendon sheath of the peroneus longus muscle. It also runs distally and inserts at the base of the proximal phalanx of the little toe. The nerve supply, which also comes via the lateral plantar nerve from segments S1–S2, means that the muscle can move the metatarsophalangeal joint of the little toe in flexion and abduction during contraction.

The inconstant opponens digiti minimi pedis runs plantarly from the base of the metatarsal V and the plantar long ligament and tendon of the fibularis longus muscle distally and inserts on the lateral distal surface of the metatarsal V. It is innervated by the lateral plantar nerve from segments S1–S2 and is predominantly present for the traction-belt mechanism of the foot. In addition, it supports the opposition with the associated mobilisation of the metatarsal V.

Palpation of the muscles of the ball of the little toe is done from the prone position with the ankle joints underneath. The palpator stands sideways and first contacts the contralateral tuberosity ossis metatarsalis V via the fingertips. Starting from this bony reference point on the lateral edge of the foot, the fingertips move about one transverse finger to the plantar side and the patient is asked to spread his toes. A contraction of the abductor digiti minimi pedis muscle is felt, so that the muscle belly can be felt in the direction of the heel or the little toe.

For palpation of the flexor digiti minimi brevis pedis muscle, the homolateral metatarsal V is grasped centrally in the pincer grip between the thumb and index finger from the same starting position, so that the index finger rests plantarly and the thumb dorsally. The patient is then asked to perform flexion in the metatarsophalangeal joint of the little toe so that an increase in tone of the muscle under the index finger is felt. However, as the plantar aponeurosis covers parts of the muscle belly, direct palpation becomes difficult. However, stimulation is also possible through the aponeurosis.

The same applies to the inconstant opponens digit minimi pedis muscle. Its course is comparable to that of the flexor digiti minimi brevis muscle.

Implementation Note

With various foot deformities, palpation at the lateral edge of the foot can cause unpleasant sensations, which is why palpation should be started gently at first (Fig. 5.38).

5.5.4 Palpation of the Dorsal Short Foot Muscles

The initial contact with the ground, where the foot touches down heel first, is accompanied by a dorsal extension of the toes. For this gait phase, the foot toe lifters must be activated in order to be able to perform the movement. As part of this group, the short dorsal foot muscles are located on the dorsum of the tarsus and the metatarsus and are divided into three parts, the extensor digitorum brevis and extensor hallucis brevis muscles and the interossei dorsales pedis I–IV muscles.

The origin of the more lateral extensor digitorum brevis muscle is on the proximolateral surface of the calcaneus. It then runs distally in the form of three tendons, which radiate into the dorsal aponeurosis of toes II, III and IV. Innervation via the profundal fibular nerve from segments L5–S1 allows

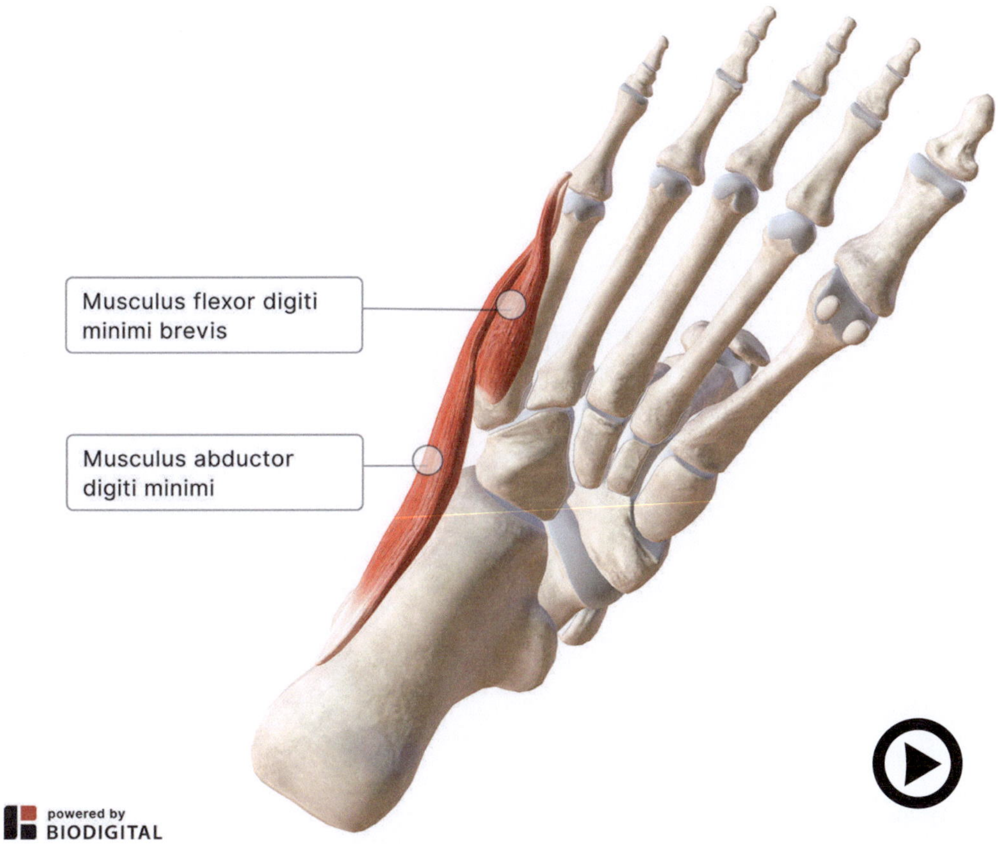

Fig. 5.38 Anatomy and palpation of the short foot musculature of the digitus minimus (▶ https://doi.org/10.1007/000-ctg)

the muscle to contract. This leads to a dorsal extension of the toes.

The extensor hallucis brevis muscle, which originates on the dorsal surface of the calcaneus, runs rather obliquely distomedially and inserts on the proximal phalanx and the dorsal aponeurosis of the hallux. Because of its similar course, the muscle is often described as the medial part of the extensor digitorum brevis muscle. It is also innervated via the profundal fibular nerve, from segments L5–S1, and is necessary for dorsal extension of the big toe.

The more intermetatarsal mm. interossei dorsales pedis I–IV extend distally between the metatarsals of two opposing bony surfaces and terminate in the proximal phalanx and the associated dorsal aponeurosis. Innervation via the lateral plantar nerve from segments S1–S2 allows abduction of toes III–IV away from the second toe, flexion of toes II–IV in the metatarsophalangeal joints and extension in the proximal and middle phalanges of toes II–IV.

Palpation of the dorsal short foot muscles is done in the supine position with the knee joints slightly underneath. The palpator makes dorsal contact with the os cuboideum with the index and middle fingertip and is now directly on the muscle belly of the extensor digitorum brevis. Through active dorsal extension of the toes, its venter becomes clearly visible through its contraction. This muscle is often already visible during contraction because it is localised superficially. Only the tendons of the extensor digitorum longus run above and must be distinguished from the short foot muscle by palpation.

Starting from the os cuboideum, the fingers move medially towards the os cuneiforme intermediale and are located directly on the muscle belly of the extensor hallucis brevis muscle. This muscle can also be differentiated more precisely from surrounding structures by a separate dorsal extension of the hallux. It is located rather superficially so that direct access to the muscle belly is possible.

For palpation of the mm. interossei dorsales pedis I–IV, the steeply placed long finger berries are placed dorsally in the four metatarsal spaces. A stimulus can be applied to the respective muscle belly in the middle third of the metatarsal bones.

Implementation Note

After inversion trauma, the region of origin of the extensor digitorum and extensor hallucis brevis muscles may be irritated, so palpation should be started gently (Fig. 5.39).

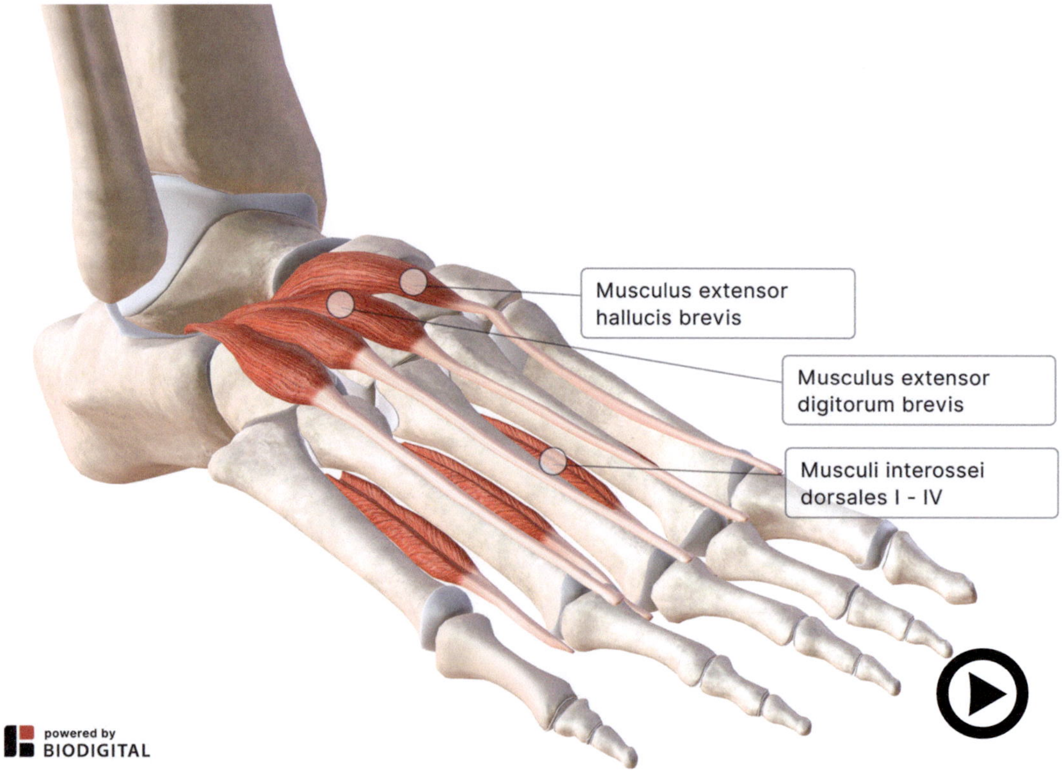

Fig. 5.39 Anatomy and palpation of the dorsal short foot musculature (▶ https://doi.org/10.1007/000-cth)

5.6 Musculature in the Trunk Area

The human being is built according to the tensegrity model in the sense of the tension-belt system. Unstable joint systems become dimensionally stable bodies via bones that are stable in bending and muscles, tendons and ligaments that are stable in stretching. The torso, with the associated spine and thorax, also reflects this system. In addition to the mobilising task, the trunk muscles have numerous other tasks, such as protecting the internal organs, harmonious locomotion and participation in the respiratory system. The trunk muscles can be divided into different groups. The following is an overview of the individual muscles. Subsequently, the palpation of the palpable structures is explained in detail in the following chapters.

In general, there is a division into trunk wall muscles in the narrower and broader sense, pelvic floor muscles and secondary migrated trunk muscles.

The torso wall musculature in the narrower sense includes the autochthonous back musculature, the prevertebral neck musculature and the thoracic and abdominal wall musculature.

The autochthonous back muscles are divided into a lateral and a medial tract. Within the lateral tract, there is the intertransverse system with the mm. levatores costarum and the mm. intertransversarii, the spinotransverse system with the m. splenius and the sacrospinal system with the m. longissimus and the m. iliocostalis.

The medial tract is divided into a transversospinal system, which includes the semispinalis, rotatores longi and brevi and multifidii muscles. In addition, the medial tract can be divided into a spinal system, which consists of the spinalis muscle and the interspinal muscles.

The short neck and head muscles are formed by the rectus capitis posterior minor and major muscles and the obliquus capitis superior and inferior muscles.

The prevertebral deep cervical muscles include the rectus capitis lateralis and anterior muscle and the longus colli and longus capitis muscles. As these muscles are located directly on the cervical vertebrae and numerous other structures cover them, they are not palpable and are only mentioned here for completeness.

The thoracic wall muscles are characterised by the mm. scaleni, the m. transversus thoracis as well as the mm. intercostales and mm. subcostales.

The abdominal muscles, which also belong to the trunk muscles in the narrower sense, are divided into a straight, an oblique and a deep part. The straight abdominal muscles include the rectus abdominis and the pyramidalis. The oblique abdominal muscles are formed by the transversus abdominis muscle and the obliquus externus and internus abdominis muscles. The quadratus lumborum muscle and the psoas major muscle, which were discussed in the section on the muscles of the hip joint (see Sect. 5.2.2), are assigned to the deep part.

The representative of the trunk wall musculature in the broader sense is the respiratory diaphragm with the pars sternalis, pars costalis and pars lumbalis.

The pelvic floor muscles, which as the most caudal structure have a connection to the trunk via the os coccygis, can be counted as trunk muscles but also as pelvic muscles. In this book, the muscles of the diaphragma pelvis and urogenitale are described in the section ter on the pelvic musculature (see Sect. 5.2.15).

Secondary migrated trunk muscles include the trunk rib muscles consisting of the serratus posterior inferior and superior muscles.

5.6.1 Palpation of the Autochthonous Back Muscles

The spinal musculature, literally formed on the spot and extending paravertebrally on the right and left sides of the spine, is collectively known as the erector spinae muscle and is divided into two parts, each with five muscles. This functional unit, which serves primarily to straighten the human body, forms an elementary part of the musculoskeletal system, is innervated directly by the dorsal rami of the spinal nerves and lies directly below the thoracolumbar fascia.

The lateral tract is composed of the levatores costarum, intertransversarii, splenius capitis and cervicis, longissimus and iliocostalis muscles. The medial tract is formed by the semispinalis, rotatores, multifidii, spinalis and interspinalis muscles. In some cases, the short neck muscles are also included, but these are listed separately in this book in Sect. 5.6.2.

Before the erector spinae muscle is explored as a whole structure, the anatomical course of the individual parts must be explained. For this purpose, we will start with the lateral tract.

The mm. levatores costarum are 12 paired rib elevator muscles and are divided into the mm. levatores costarum brevis and longi. The short parts originate at the procc. transversi of the 7th cervical vertebra and the 1st–11th thoracic vertebra and insert at the respective angulus costae of the next lower rib. The long parts follow a similar course starting from the procc. transversi of the 7th cervical vertebra and 1st–10th thoracic vertebra to the angulus costae of the next but one rib. Contrary to their name, they do not functionally lift the ribs, but instead provide extension in the case of bilateral contraction and ipsilateral flexion and slight contralateral rotation in the case of unilateral contraction.

The intertransverse muscles run from transverse vertebral process to transverse vertebral process, as can be seen in the structure name. They are classified into posterior and anterior cervical, thoracic and finally medial and lateral lumbar parts. They support the extension of the spine in the case of bilateral contraction and ipsilateral lateral flexion in the case of unilateral contraction.

The splenius muscle is divided into a pars capitis and a pars cervicis. The upper part is named after its connection to the skull, while the lower part is located in the cervical spine. Starting from the procc. spinosi of the 3rd–7th cervical and 1st–3rd thoracic vertebrae to the nuchae ligament, the splenius capitis muscle runs obliquely to the proc. mastoideus of the os temporale and to lateral parts of the linea nuchae superior. The splenius cervicis muscle, on the other hand, runs from the spinosus muscle of the 3rd–6th thoracic vertebrae to the posterior tuberosities of the transverse processes of the 1st–3rd cervical vertebrae. A bilateral contraction leads to an extension, i.e. a stretching of the cervical spine, whereas a unilateral contraction supports ipsilateral lateral flexion.

The longissimus muscle is, as its name suggests, the longest muscle in the erector spinae system. The muscle can be divided into a thoracic, cervical and a capital part. The thoracic part runs from the facies dorsalis of the os sacrum, the procc. spinosi of the lumbar spine and the procc. transversi of the lower thoracic spine to the procc. transversi of the lumbar spine, the procc. costales of the lumbar spine and to the 2nd–12th ribs between the angulus costae and the respective tuberculum costae. The longissimus cervicis muscle arises from the transverse processes of the 1st–6th thoracic vertebrae and inserts into the posterior tuberosities and the transverse processes of the 2nd–7th cervical vertebrae. The longissimus capitis muscle extends from the procc. transversi of the 4th–7th cervical vertebrae and the procc. transversi of the 1st–3rd thoracic vertebrae directly to the procc. mastoideus of the os temporale. Due to its location, the longissimus muscle can support the extension and lateral flexion of the spine in the respective regions. In addition, the muscle acts synergistically for expiration in the thoracic region and for equilateral rotation in the head region.

The iliocostalis muscle can be divided into three parts. The iliocostalis lumborum runs from the labium externum of the crista iliaca, the facies dorsalis of the os sacrum, the superficial leaf of the fascia thoracolumbalis and the spinous processes of the lumbar vertebrae to the angulus costae of the 5th or 6th to 12th rib, to the deep leaf of the fascia thoracolumbalis and to the procc. transversi of the upper lumbar spine. The iliocostalis thoracis muscle originates caudally at the angulus costae of the 7th–12th ribs and inserts cranially at the angulus costae of the 1st–6th ribs. The iliocostalis cervicis muscle originates at the costal angulus of the 3rd–7th ribs and attaches to the posterior tuberosity of the transverse process of the 4th–6th cervical vertebrae. Depending on the region, they support extension as well as ipsilateral lateral flexion. The iliocostalis muscle in particular also supports expiration, whereas the cervical part tends to help inspiration.

The semispinalis muscle, which belongs to the medial tract, is part of the transversospinal system and is only found in the thoracic and cervical spine. Viewed as a whole, it runs steeply from the transverse muscle and surrounding areas to the mediocranial and inserts six to seven vertebral levels higher on the spinosus muscle and the occipital bone. Since the most caudal muscle origin is located at the transverse process of Th12, the semispinalis muscle is divided into a pars thoracis, a pars cervicis and a pars capitis. When contracted on both sides, it causes extension of the cervical spine, straightening of the spine and stabilisation of the upper cervical joints. Unilateral contraction leads to rotation in the opposite direction with lateral flexion in the same direction.

The rotator muscles are predominantly pronounced in the thoracic spine and tend to be inconstant in the cervical and lumbar spine in humans. They extend from the proc. transversus to the proc. spinosus of the vertebra above. Only in the cervical spine does the respective proc. articularis form the origin. In the thoracic spine, there is a short and a long part, whereby the mm. rotatores longi only inserts two segments further cranially. True to their name, they perform a rotation to the opposite side and a lateral flexion to the same side during unilateral contraction. On both sides, they support the erection in extension.

The multifidii muscles are divided into a cervical, thoracic and lumbar or sacral part. In the thoracic region and the cervical spine, the muscle runs from the proc. transversus and the proc. articularis of the cervical spine to the proc. spinosus of the vertebra above. In the sacral region, the os sacrum, the sacrotuberal ligament and the crista iliaca form the surface of origin. While in the deep layer the attachments are located two vertebral bodies cranial to the proc. spinosus, the superficial bellies often skip up to five vertebral layers. The unilateral contraction achieves a rotation in the opposite direction and a lateral flexion in the same direction. The bilateral contraction, on the other hand, leads to an erection of the respective spinal segment.

The spinalis muscle gets its name from its course from the proc. spinosus to the proc. spinosus above it. With its thoracic, cervical and capital parts, the spinalis muscle extends from the third lumbar vertebra cranially to the occiput. Thus, the cervical parts insert at the linea nuchealis superior and inferior. Unilateral muscle activation leads to lateral flexion to the ipsilateral side and rotation to the contralateral side. The bilateral contraction causes the spine to straighten.

Following their name, the interspinous muscles extend between the procc. spinosi of the spinal column to the side of the spinous processes. They are divided into a cervical, a thoracic and a lumbar part, whereby the muscle bellies in the thoracic spine are inconstant. The most cranial origin is at C2, whereas the most caudal insertion is at the proc. spinosus of S1. The interspinous muscles also serve to straighten the spine.

The erector spinae muscle is felt as a composite of the lateral and medial tracts in the prone position. Two strands run paravertebrally from the os sacrum to the linea nuchae at the occiput. It should be noted that the long dorsal extensor is covered by the latissimus dorsi muscle in the lumbar and up to the middle thoracic spine and by the trapezius muscle from the middle thoracic spine to the occiput. However, as the large muscles are rather thin and move the shoulder girdle instead of the spine, palpatory differentiation is good. In addition, it should be noted that the erector spinae muscle has an oblique and step-like structure and that numerous muscles are in depth and are therefore not palpable. The following section describes the superficial muscles that can be stimulated during palpation.

Palpation begins at the os sacrum on the homolateral side. The palpation fingers contact the proc. spinosus of L5 and then move only one transverse finger width laterally. They are located directly on the lumbar parts of the erector spinae muscle. Strictly speaking, the finger berries lie on the m. longissimus and a further two transverse fingers laterally and then on the m. iliocostalis lumborum. These two muscle strands can be felt up to Th12 directly next to the spine. They then run obliquely craniolaterally. The muscle cord that connects directly from Th12 paravertebrally is that of the spinalis thoracis muscle. Lateral to this muscle, the semispinalis muscle joins it on the way to the cranial. From Th5–6, the longitudinal erector spinae muscle is formed by the splenius cervicis muscle. This can be felt again directly paravertebrally with the steeply erected long finger berries in the depth. Further laterally, the semispinalis thoracis muscle accompanies it until about Th2 and is then replaced by the semispinalis capitis muscle. From Th1, the splenius capitis muscle can be felt paravertebrally, which is then replaced by the semispinalis capitis muscle from C3. This then runs to the occiput. Laterally, the splenius capitis muscle is located on the head.

In general, an extension of the respective spinal region can be performed during palpation in order to better differentiate the cord of the long dorsal extensor from surrounding tissues.

Implementation Note

The erector spinae muscle is easily palpable on both sides about 3–4 transverse fingers lateral to the proc. spinosus. Further laterally, it is covered by surrounding structures (Fig. 5.40).

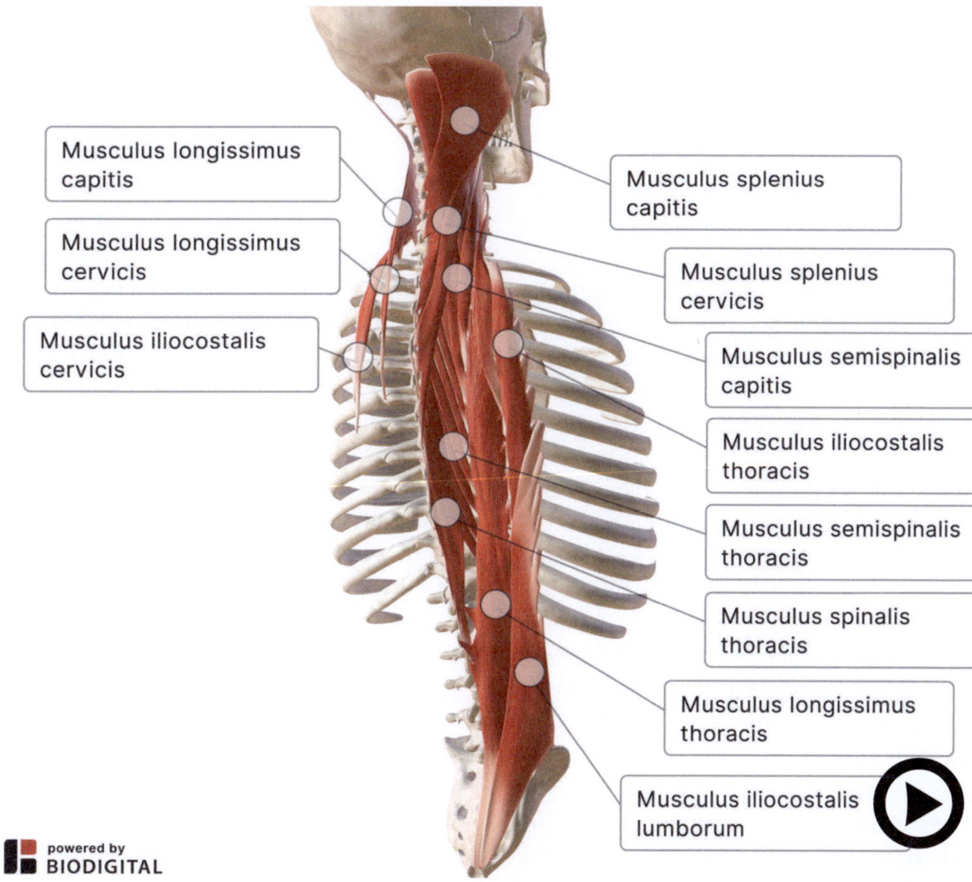

Fig. 5.40 Anatomy and palpation of the autochthonous back musculature (▶ https://doi.org/10.1007/000-ctj)

5.6.2 Palpation of the Short Neck Muscles

The skull has a central key function for humans. It not only houses the brain and numerous sensory organs, but also ensures orientation in space and targeted non-verbal communication. This orientation in space, but also the non-verbal transmission of stimuli, takes place via the smallest movements of the head, which are realised via small muscles. A fundamental part of this is attributed to the short neck muscles, which can also be described as a neck rosette. Four muscles at the transition between the upper cervical spine and the skull form this unit. These include the rectus capitis posterior minor and major muscles and the obliquus capitis inferior and superior muscles. All four muscles have a high density of receptors compared to other muscles [14]. The nuchae muscles receive their innervation via direct access from the rami posteriores of the spinal nerves and the suboccipital nerve from segment C1.

Palpation of the muscle group can only be done by stimulation, as the semispinalis capitis muscle covers it. During palpation, the respective bony reference points serve as orientation. First, the anatomical course is explained and then the palpation in union.

The rectus capitis posterior minor originates at the posterior tuberosity of the atlas and runs cranially to its insertion area, the inner third of the inferior linea nuchae. When contracted unilaterally, it can rotate the head ipsilaterally and tilt it sideways, whereas when contracted bilaterally, it performs an extension of the upper cervical joint.

The rectus capitis posterior major runs slightly obliquely from the proc. spinosus of the axis to the middle third of the linea nuchae inferior. It also performs ipsilateral rotation and lateral flexion during unilateral contraction and extension in the upper cervicals during bilateral contraction.

The oblique capitis inferior muscle originates from the spinosus muscle of the axis and inserts into the transversus muscle of the atlas. It therefore has no direct contact with the skull and can initiate rotation of the atlas to the ipsilateral side to allow functional displacement of the atlanto-occipital joints.

The obliquus capitis superior muscle, which like all other muscles of the neck rosette can be counted among the autochthonous muscles, runs obliquely from the proc. transversus of the atlas to the lateral third of the linea nuchae inferior. It inserts cranially of the insertion of the rectus capitis posterior major muscle and can support ipsilateral lateral flexion when contracted unilaterally and extension in the upper cervical joint when activated bilaterally.

The palpation of the short neck muscles is done in a compound while the client is in the supine position. The therapist sits behind the patient at the head end so that he can place the patient's skull in his hands. The posterior part of the os occipitale is held by the right and left heel of the hand, respectively, while the erect fingertips of the index, middle and ring fingers are applied to the right and left of the posterior tuberosity of the atlas, respectively. It is important to ensure that the head is in a neutral position or in a slight, passive extension and that the flexed fingertips point anteriorly in extension. A stimulus can then be applied to the short neck muscles in depth. Immediately to the right and left of the midline, the fingers meet the rectus capitis posterior minor muscle, one transverse finger laterally and then the rectus capitis posterior major muscle and again about one transverse finger laterally the obliquus capitis superior muscle. If the finger berries move one transverse finger laterally from the spinous process of the axis, they meet the obliquus capitis inferior muscle directly. In general, it should be remembered that directly under the fingers, there are first parts of the trapezius pars descendens muscle and then the semispinalis capitis muscle, before the short neck muscles, directly on the spine, that receive the stimulus from the fingers.

Implementation Note
Due to the strong sensitive wiring, the short head muscles can quickly build up hypertonus, which can lead to tension headaches (Fig. 5.41).

5.6.3 Palpation of the Scalenus Muscles

The staircase muscles, which are part of the deep neck musculature, are divided into an anterior, a medial and a posterior part. Their anatomical proximity to nerve and vascular roads describes the conciseness of the palpation of these three paired structures. Their location in the lateral cervical region means that the anterior scalenus muscle, together with the sternocleidomastoid muscle and the first rib, forms the anterior scalenus gap, which uses the subclavian vein as a passage point. The middle scalenus gap is formed by the scalenus anterior muscle, the scalenus medius muscle and the first rib. The subclavian artery runs through this and also fibres of the brachial plexus.

The scalenus anterior muscle traces its course from the tubercles anteriora of the procc. transversi of the third to sixth cervical vertebrae to the tuberculum musculi scaleni anterioris in the middle of the corpus of the homolateral first rib.

The posterior scalenus gap is formed by the scalenus medius muscle, the scalenus posterior muscle and the first two ribs. It should be noted that there are different definitions of the scalenus gap depending on the literature [15].

The scalenus medius muscle originates in the posterior tuberosities of the procc. transversi of the third to seventh

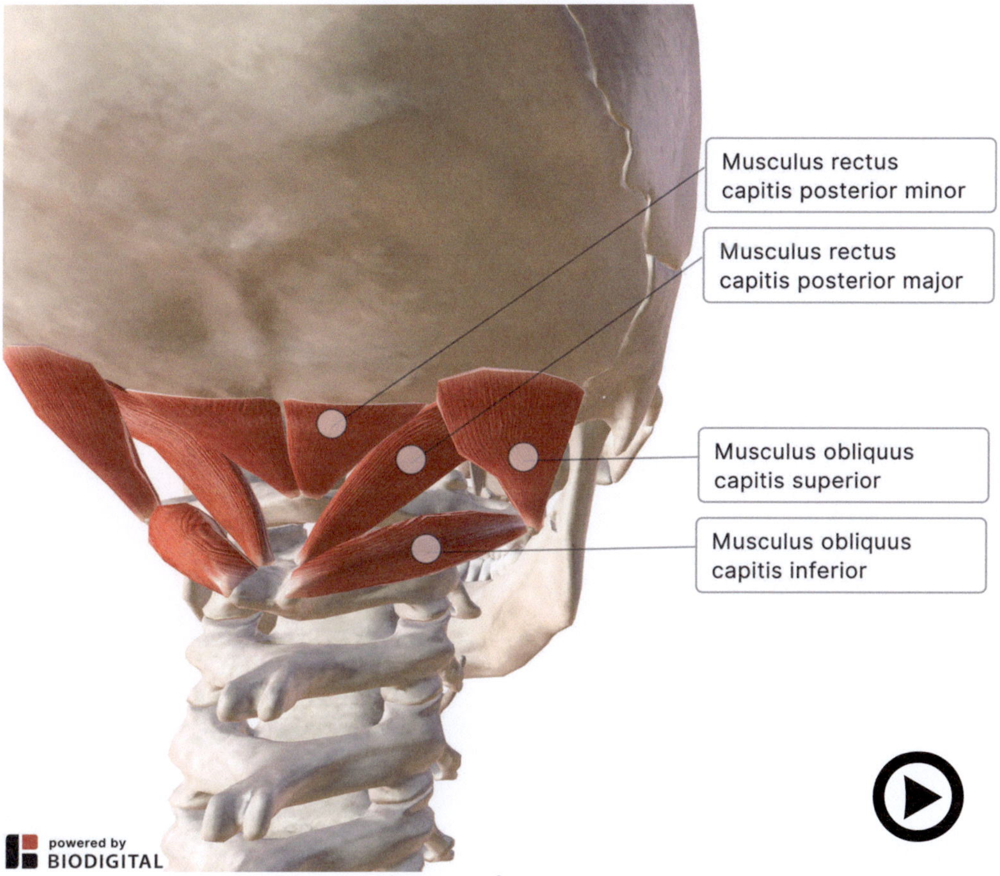

Fig. 5.41 Anatomy and palpation of the short neck musculature (▶ https://doi.org/10.1007/000-ctk)

cervical vertebrae. It inserts dorsally of the scalenus anterior at the middle part of the corpus of the first rib posterior to the sulcus arteriae subclaviae.

The scalenus posterior muscle arises from the posterior tuberosities of the procc. transversi of the fifth to seventh cervical vertebrae and runs caudolaterally to the outer surfaces of the second and occasionally to the third rib.

All three parts are innervated via direct nerve branches from the cervical plexus and the brachial plexus from segments C3–C6 and support ipsilateral lateral flexion when contracted unilaterally. When the muscles are activated on both sides, they lift the thorax and thus support breathing.

The scaleni muscles are palpated from the supine position. The head is placed slightly underneath, and the therapist stands sideways at the level of the rib cage facing the client's neck. The patient actively turns the head away from the therapist so that the sternocleidomastoid muscle contracts. The fingertips of the index and middle fingers make contact in the middle third of the head turner. The head is then moved back, and the muscles are slightly approached in lateral flexion to the same side. A groove, which demarcates the trapezius pars descendens muscle, can then be perceived at the posterior edge of the muscle. The steeply positioned fingertips move into this groove and palpate downwards. They are now directly on the scalenus medius muscle. In a relaxed starting position, a stimulus can be applied to the scalenus anterior muscle anterior to this structure. The posterior scalenus muscle is completely covered by the descending trapezius muscle, which makes it difficult to feel the muscle. Only a stimulus from the posterior edge of the scalenus medius muscle in a dorsal direction can be applied to the structure.

Implementation Note

Due to the described proximity to nerve and vascular pathways, palpation of the scaleni muscles must be gentle, as otherwise protective tensions can negatively influence the palpation result. In addition, the scaleni muscles can be responsible for pain transmitted to the upper extremity (Fig. 5.42).

5.6.4 Palpation of the Intercostal Muscles

The intercostal muscles, as the name suggests, stretch between the ribs and thus complete the thorax via the traction-belt mechanism, which protects the heart and lungs.

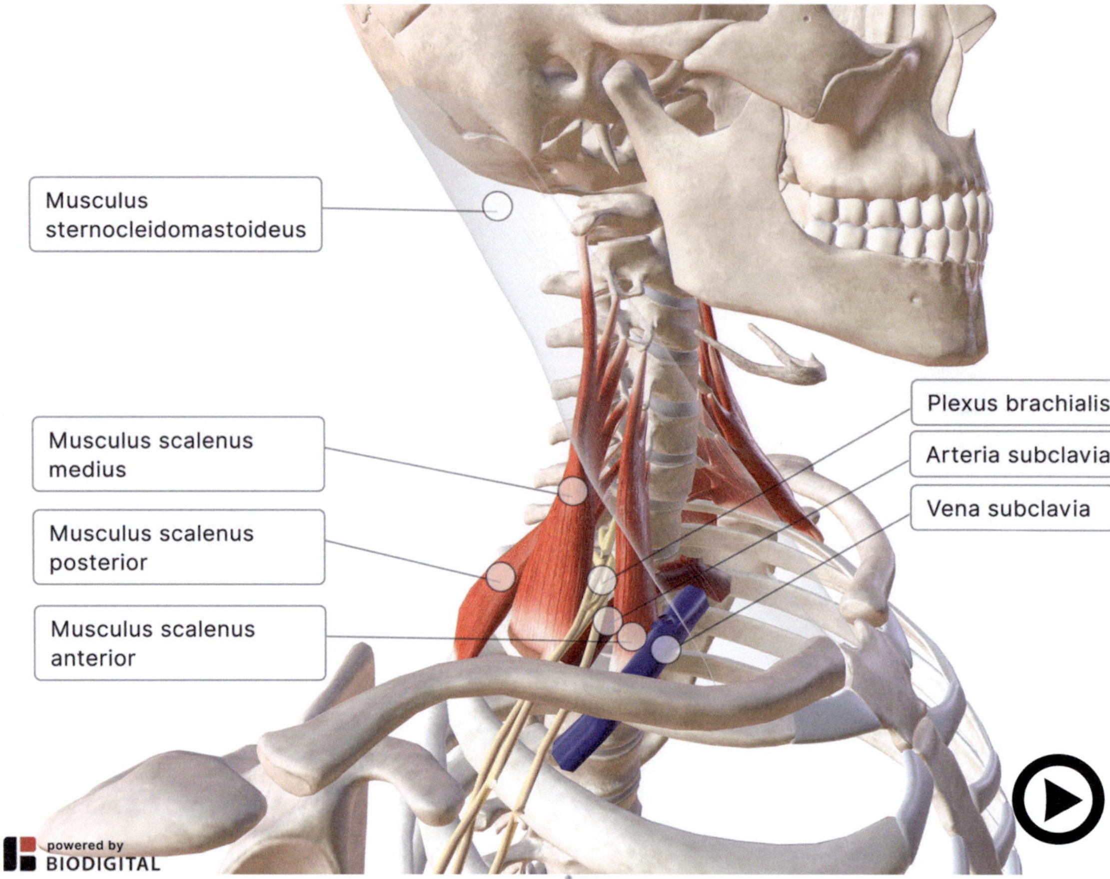

Fig. 5.42 Anatomy and palpation of the Mm. scaleni (▶ https://doi.org/10.1007/000-ctm)

At the same time, they also serve to keep the thorax mobile by moving the ribs in the direction of inhalation and exhalation. Three muscle groups can be found in each intercostal space. In addition to the mm. intercostales externi, the mm. intercostales interni and intimi also exist. The muscles receive their nerve supply via the intercostal nerves 1–11 from the segments of the same name.

The external intercostal muscles run diagonally from dorsocranial to ventrocaudal from rib to rib. They originate at the lower edge of the 1st–11th rib and insert at the upper edges of the next lower ribs 2–12. They extend from the tuberculum costae to the transition from bone to cartilage tissue and support inspiration.

The internal intercostal muscles run diagonally from dorsocaudal to ventrocranial from rib to rib and thus cross the external intercostal muscles. They originate at the upper edge of the 2nd–12th ribs and insert at the lower edges of the next higher ribs 1–11. They extend from the tuberculum costae to the transition from bone to cartilage tissue and support expiration. In a special case, muscle fibres can skip a rib. These fibres are listed in their entirety as mm. subcostales.

The mm. intercostales intimi represent a deep division of the mm. intercostales interni. The respective intercostal nerve and the intercostal artery are the separating structures of both muscle groups. The course and function are identical.

For palpation from the supine or lateral position, it is important to remember that the thorax is covered by the obliquus externus abdominis muscle in the caudal region and the pectoralis major and minor muscles in the cranial region. In the dorsocaudal region, the latissimus dorsi muscle and dorsocranially the teres major muscle and the scapula with the serratus anterior muscle will influence palpation. Despite this initial situation, a direct stimulus can be applied to the intercostal muscles in the intercostal spaces. For palpation, the ribs are first felt in the middle or anterior third with the index and middle fingers as the starting point. Then the fingers move to a higher or lower intercostal space and feel in depth. The stimulus produced initially hits the mm. intercostales externi and then reaches the mm. intercostales interni in depth. Depending on the region, the intercostal muscles can thus be felt with the fingertips.

Implementation Note
The intercostal nerves run in the intercostal spaces, which are influenced by the intercostal muscles and can be sensitive to palpation. Palpation should therefore be gentle at first (Fig. 5.43).

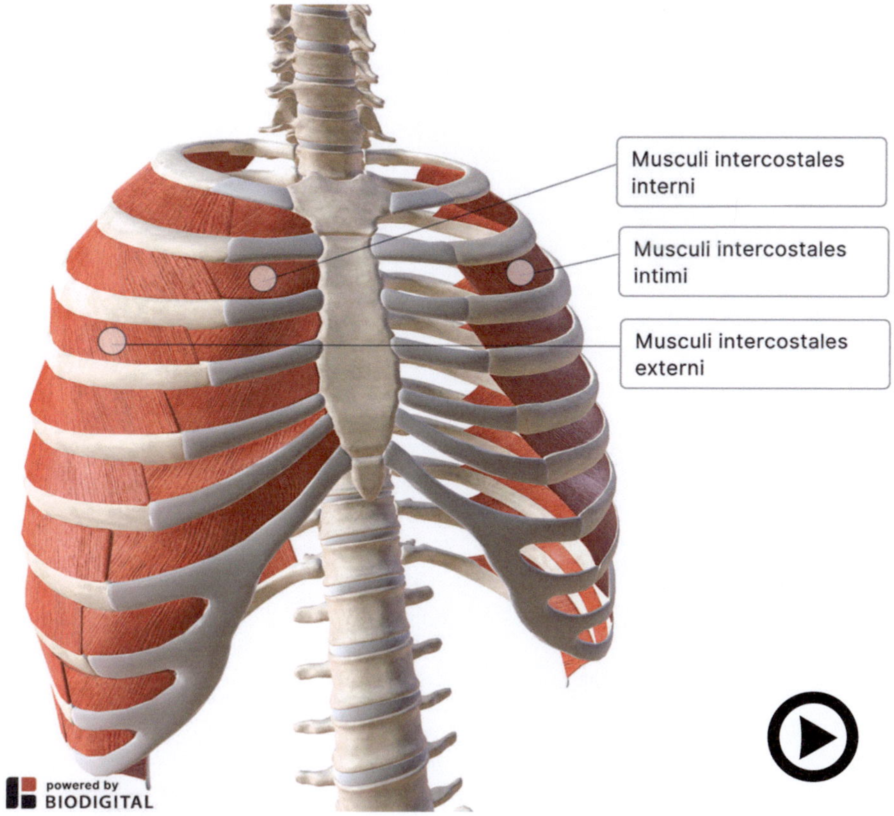

Fig. 5.43 Anatomy and palpation of the Mm. intercostales (▶ https://doi.org/10.1007/000-ctn)

5.6.5 Palpation of the Rectus Abdominis and Pyramidalis Muscles

Known as the "six-pack", the straight abdominal muscle is paired, ventral to the abdomen, and gets its nickname from its three to four intermediate tendons, which divide the muscle into individual segments. The vertically running muscle traces its origin to the anterior surface of the cartilages of the 5th–7th ribs. Some fibres are also fused with the costoxiphoid ligament and the proc. xiphoideus of the sternum. Both muscle strands then run steeply caudally to the right and left of the linea alba and insert at the ramus superior ossis pubis and at structures close to the symphysis. The rectus abdominis muscle is surrounded by the rectus sheath both ventrally and dorsally. It is innervated by the anterior branches of the thoracic 5–12 nerves and the associated intercostal nerves and by the lumbar 1–2 nerves. It flexes the trunk and increases the tension of the abdominal wall, which is essential for abdominal compression and thus for deep exhalation.

The individual segments of the rectus abdominis muscle are palpated from the supine position with the head underneath and the legs underneath or resting, so that the abdominal wall is relaxed. It should be noted in advance that the parallel running abdominal muscle is covered by the obliquus externus abdominis muscle, by the obliquus internus abdominis muscle and partially by the transversus abdominis muscle through their superficial aponeuroses. However, as the superficial muscles are rather thin, it is quite possible to feel the rectus abdominis muscle. Depending on the patient's body fat content, the individual segments are already visually recognisable in the inspection, so that the region of palpation becomes directly clear.

The fingertips of the index and middle fingers are placed about two transverse fingers to the right and left of the navel. The client is then asked to raise the upper body slightly with the head flexed. Already at the start of the movement, a clear tension of the caudal abdominal muscle areas becomes apparent. The entire muscle can be felt by moving the fingertips cranially up to the level of the proc. xiphoideus. In the caudal region, directly above the symphysis, an additional stimulus is applied during palpation to the pyramidalis muscle, which tenses the linea alba and is not present in a small proportion of people [16]. It runs in pairs from the pubic tubercle obliquely craniomedially and inserts into the linea alba. It is innervated by the 12th thoracic nerve, the 1st lumbar nerve and the subcostal nerve.

Implementation Note

The term "six-pack" should not distract from the fact that the muscle is divided into eight to ten segments. Usually six are visible, but at least eight are noticeable (Fig. 5.44).

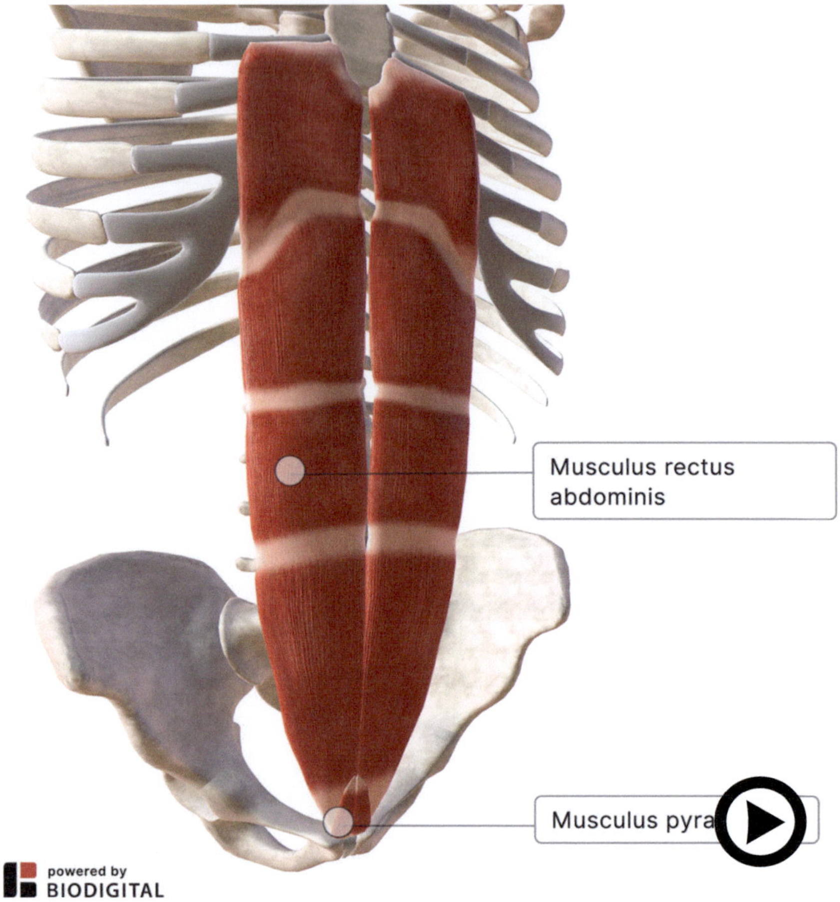

Fig. 5.44 Anatomy and palpation of the M. rectus abdominis (▶ https://doi.org/10.1007/000-ctp)

5.6.6 Palpation of the Transversus Abdominis Muscle

The transverse abdominal muscle has an extensive origin that extends from the inner surfaces of the 7th–10th costal cartilages and the 11th and 12th ribs via the fascia thoracolumbalis to the crista iliaca as well as the SIAS and the lig. inguinale. According to its name, it runs transversely towards the centre of the abdomen and inserts in the posterior leaflet of the rectus sheath, as well as in the linea alba. Together with fibres of the obliquus internus abdominis muscle, it also forms the cremaster muscle in males. In women, it radiates with some fibres into the lig. teres uteri. It is innervated via the intercostal nerves 5–12, the ilioinguinal nerve and the iliohypogastric nerve. Functionally, it constricts the abdominal organs when contracted on both sides and supports the abdominal press and thus expiration. The unilateral activation of the muscle leads to an equilateral trunk rotation.

Palpation is performed in the supine position on the contralateral side. It should be remembered in advance that the transversus abdominis muscle is located under the obliquus internus and externus abdominis muscles, which only allows stimulation of this structure. The finger berries first make contact with the tenth rib on the caudolateral thorax. Starting from this reference point, the fingers travel about three to four transverse fingers caudally and meet soft tissue directly. Now the patient is asked to perform a trunk rotation to the same side, which involves a contraction of the muscle and increases the quality of palpation.

Implementation Note
A lack of recruitment of the transversus abdominis muscle often manifests itself in hypotonicity. This can promote instability of the lumbar spine (Fig. 5.45).

5.6.7 Palpation of the Obliquus Externus and Internus Abdominis Muscles

The oblique abdominal muscles can be divided into an external and an internal part. The external obliquus externus abdominis originates on the outer surfaces of the 5th–12th ribs and runs divergently caudomedially. In its course, it crosses the fibres of the internal oblique abdominis muscle perpendicularly, which follows a craniomedial or crossing course. In addition, it forms the so-called Gerdy line anterolaterally on the trunk with the serrations of the serratus anterior muscle. At the base, it forms two extensions: the medial

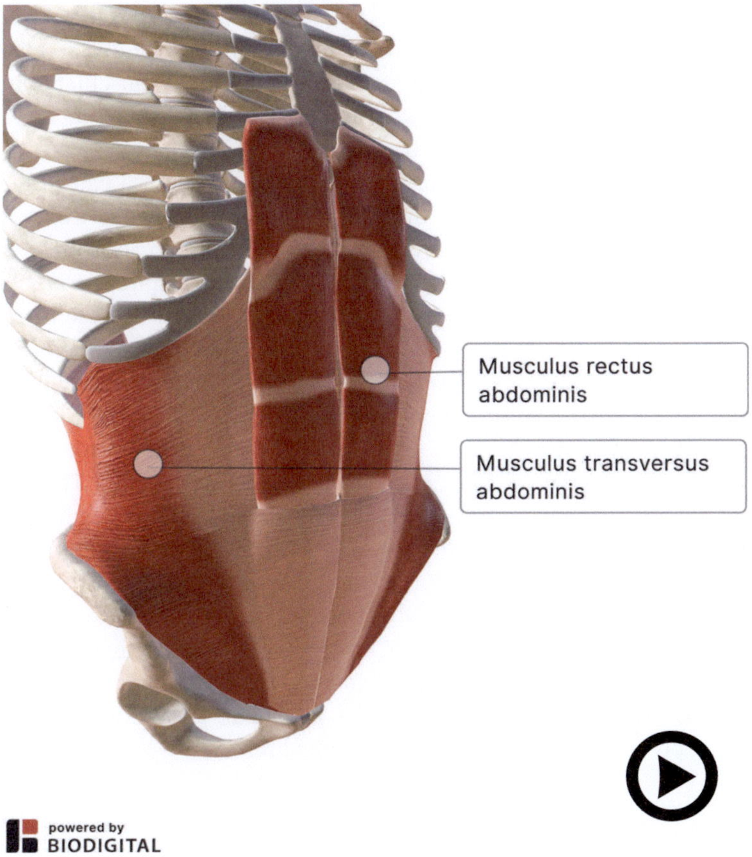

Fig. 5.45 Anatomy and palpation of the M. transversus abdominis (▶ https://doi.org/10.1007/000-ctq)

crus, which forms the rectus sheath and radiates into the linea alba, and the lateral crus, which inserts into the labium externum of the iliac crest, the inguinal ligament and the pubic tubercle. Between these two extensions, a small opening is formed, which forms the annulus inguinalis superficialis, the inguinal canal. The unilateral contraction of the obliquus externus abdominis leads to a reciprocal rotation of the trunk, which only works with an interaction of the obliquus internus abdominis of the contralateral side. In addition, it performs an ipsilateral flexion, which again can only take place in interaction with the obliquus internus abdominis muscle on the same side. The bilateral contraction leads to flexion of the trunk and dorsal tilt of the pelvis and supports the abdominal press during expiration.

The obliquus internus abdominis runs at a 90° angle crossing the external lateral abdominal muscle from the lamina profunda of the fascia thoracolumbalis, the linea intermedia of the crista iliaca as well as the lateral part of the lig. inguinale and the SIAS obliquely towards the mediocranial. It inserts at the 9th–12th costal cartilages, forms the posterior leaflet of the rectus sheath and radiates into the linea alba. Caudal fibres, together with parts of the transversus abdominis muscle, form the cremaster muscle in males. In women, fibres radiate into the lig. teres uteri. Unilateral contraction of the obliquus internus abdominis muscle leads to ipsilateral flexion, with joint tension of the obliquus externus abdominis muscle, and to rotation on both sides. With bilateral muscle activation, there is flexion of the trunk, elevation of the anterior pelvic edge and support of the abdominal press during expiration.

Both muscles are innervated via the anterior spinal nerves directly from the segments Th5–Th12 (external abdominis oblique muscle) and Th8–Th12 (internal abdominis oblique muscle) and the respective intercostal nerves. In addition, caudal parts are partially supplied by the iliohypogastric nerve, the genitofemoral nerve and the ilioinguinal nerve.

Palpation of the obliquus externus and internus abdominis muscles is done from the supine or lateral position with the head underneath and the knee joints in place or underneath. As both muscles are directly above each other, palpation often stimulates both structures. Differentiation can be made through muscle activation. While the fingertips are placed flat against the homolateral, anterior inferior costal arch, the patient is asked to move the equilateral shoulder in the direction of the opposite knee joint. Via this active rotation, the equilateral obliquus externus abdominis muscle and the contralateral obliquus internus abdominis muscle are tensed. This tension can be felt as a muscle loop in the course with the fingers. The external oblique abdominal muscle can also be stimulated anterolaterally on the trunk. For this, the serrated regions of origin of the serratus anterior muscle are located on ribs 4–9. They can be clearly felt on the lateral thorax, directly on the ribs, when the patient lifts the 90° anteverted arm in the direction of protraction from the support. Directly between the spikes are extensions of the obliquus externus abdominis muscle, which forms the Gerdy line in this region.

Implementation Note

In case of negative changes, the lateral abdominal muscles may transmit pain to the groin area and the area of the epigastric angle during palpation (Fig. 5.46).

5.6.8 Palpation of the Quadratus Lumborum Muscle

The quadratic lumbar muscle is part of the posterior deep abdominal musculature and is a continuation of the transversus abdominis muscle. It originates at the iliac crest and the iliolumbar ligament and runs steeply in a cranial direction. It inserts at the lower edge of the 12th rib and at the procc. costales from L1 to L4. The quadratus lumborum muscle is innervated via the muscular spines from the lumbar plexus and via the intercostal, subcostal and iliohypogastric nerves from segments Th12–L2. During a unilateral contraction, it pulls the 12th rib in a caudal direction and can perform an ipsilateral flexion of the trunk. When the thorax is fixed, it raises the lateral edge of the pelvis. In addition, it fixes the free ribs during expiration and thus supports the abdominal press. The bilateral muscle activation leads to a lordosis or extension of the lumbar spine.

Ventral to the muscle are the colon and kidney as well as the diaphragm and the iliopsoas muscle; therefore, palpatory access is possible from the dorsal side or alternatively from the prone position. The patient lies on his side facing the therapist, and the palpation fingers contact the homolateral 12th rib from the dorsal side. While the fingertips move about three to four transverse fingers caudally, the client tries to lift the upper body slightly off the support in the direction of lateral flexion. The pretension for this movement alone is sufficient to contract the muscle so that it can be palpated. The entire quadratus lumborum muscle can then be felt.

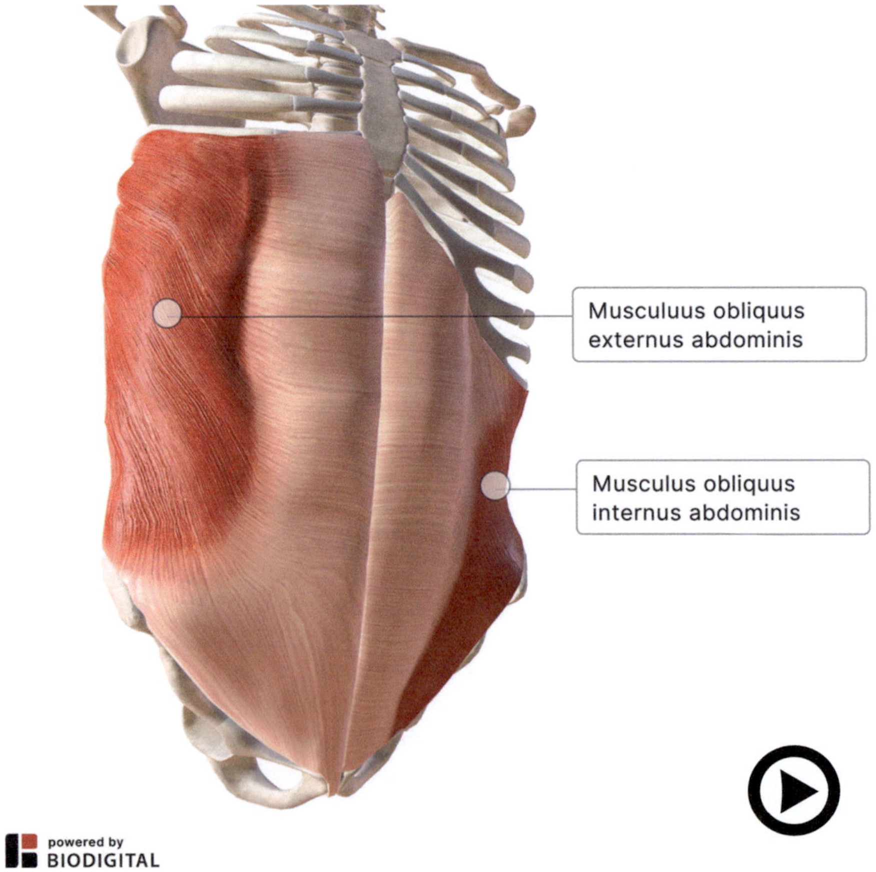

Fig. 5.46 Anatomy and palpation of the M. obliquus externus et internus abdominis (▶ https://doi.org/10.1007/000-ctr)

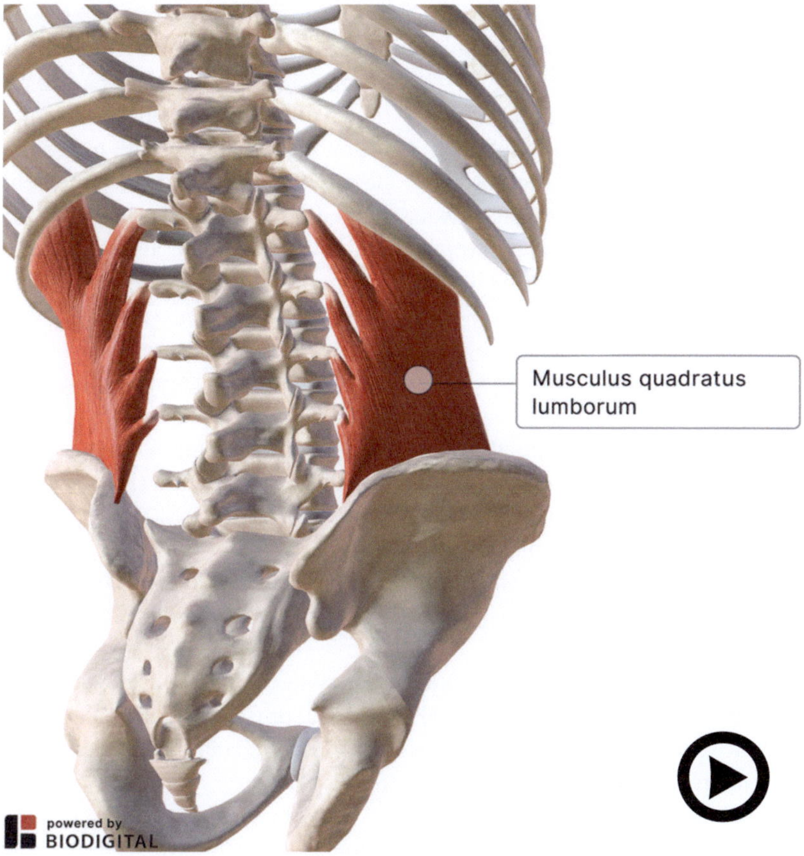

Fig. 5.47 Anatomy and palpation of the M. quadratus lumborum (▶ https://doi.org/10.1007/000-cts)

Implementation Note
If the quadratus lumborum muscle is overloaded, this can lead to painful conditions being transferred to the lumbar and abdominal areas (Fig. 5.47).

5.6.9 Palpation of the Respiratory Diaphragm

On average, humans take 25,000 breaths per day for gas exchange in order to provide oxygen for metabolism and to remove carbon dioxide as a metabolic end product. At about 500 mL of air per breath, this corresponds to about 12,500 L of air per day. This enormous task is mainly carried out by the respiratory diaphragm as the most important inspiratory muscle with the support of auxiliary respiratory muscles. Malfunctions such as side stitching and hiccups are also often due to this structure. The term diaphragm here stands for partition, as the diaphragm separates the thoracic cavity from the abdominal cavity in order to maintain pressure. This pressure valve function can affect the entire homeostasis of the body, as it is connected to numerous structures listed in this chapter. The diaphragm, which is about three to five millimetres thick, is described as a muscular plate and can be divided into several parts. In addition to the muscular parts, such as the pars sternalis, the pars costalis and the pars lumbalis with the crus laterale and the crus mediale dextrum and sinistrum, the central tendon, the centrum tendineum, exists in the middle of the diaphragm. The localisation of the respiratory diaphragm is clear from the naming of the parts. It extends from the back of the proc. xiphoideus over the cartilaginous regions of the lower costal arch of ribs 6–12 to the 1st–4th lumbar vertebrae and their adjacent intervertebral discs from ventral. All three parts radiate into the centrally located centrum tendineum. In addition, it interlocks with parts of the transversus abdominis muscle and has contact points with the medial lumbocostal arc, which thereby forms the psoas arcade via the medial arcuate ligament and the quadratus arcade via the lateral arcuate ligament. Between the pars lumbalis and the pars costalis, there is a muscle-free zone known as the Bochdalek cleft. The diaphragm continues to be directly connected to the pericardium via the phrenopericardiac ligament and extends to the fifth intercostal space on the left half of the thorax, while the highest point on the right side is at the fourth intercostal space.

In addition to the numerous junctions, the respiratory diaphragm has important perforations through which elementary structures pass from the thorax into the abdomen or vice versa. These include the oesophagus, the inferior vena cava, the aorta, the thoracic duct, the vagus nerve and the phrenic nerve. Furthermore, rather small structures pass through the partition wall, such as the left superior epigastric artery and vein in Larrey's cleft (trigonum sternocostale sinistrum), the right superior epigastric artery and vein in Morgagni's hole (trigonum sternocostale dextrum), the azygos and hemiazygos veins, the major and minor splanchnic nerve and the border cord of the sympathetic nervous system. All these structures can be influenced by the tone of the diaphragm.

The extensive innervation of the muscle and tendon plate takes place via several nerves. These receive their information from the respiratory centre, which is located in the medulla oblongata.

Thus, the phrenic nerves from the segments C3–C5, the phrenic accessorii from the segments C5–C7 and the spinal nerves of the thoracic vertebral segments significantly control the function of the diaphragm. Breathing is therefore consciously voluntary but also unconsciously involuntary controllable by humans.

The main function described above, as the most important inspiratory muscle and thus guarantor of energy production and metabolism, is supplemented by numerous other functions. It contracts during inspiration and relaxes during expiration until it actively supports the abdominal press during the last part of the exhalation. It can shorten by about 20–30% and moves about 4–6 cm cranially and caudally during the breathing cycle [17]. Thus, the respiratory diaphragm exerts pressure on surrounding structures and therefore also serves to stimulate intestinal activity and bile excretion, supports blood return via a suction effect in the veins, supports crying and delivery and finally regulates the acid-base ratio in the body [18].

Both dysfunctions caused by negative postural patterns and emotional stress situations can increase the state of tone of the diaphragm, among many other factors. This tension can be perceived during palpation with the fingertips. For palpation, the patient is positioned in a supine position with the head underneath and the legs in a straight position. The therapist stands at the level of the thorax, facing cranially, and places both hands ventrolaterally on the homolateral ribcage, with the fingertips positioned slightly offset in the direction of the abdomen. While the patient breathes in a relaxed manner, the therapist begins to feel into the tissue by flexing the fingers slightly under the costal arch during exhalation. In doing so, the fingertips move directly behind the lower ribs. During inhalation, the therapist feels that the fingertips are exposed to increasing pressure due to the contraction. This stimulus is initially complied with until, during the following exhalation, the finger berries again move into the depths. This can be done on the entire lower ribcage. In this procedure, a direct stimulus is applied to the diaphragm. The same procedure can also be done in a sitting position while the therapist stands behind the client and the client leans.

Implementation Note

It is essential to palpate gently at first. Due to the numerous connections to the vegetative and visceral system, palpation can also produce unpleasant sensations such as pain, nausea or shortness of breath (Fig. 5.48).

5.6.10 Palpation of the Posterior Superior and Inferior Serratus Muscle

The posterior saw muscle can be counted as part of the spinocostal or trunk rib musculature. It is a rather flat, low-lying muscle which can be divided into a superior and an inferior part.

The posterior superior serratus muscle is covered by the trapezius pars transversus muscle and the rhomboid muscles. It originates via an aponeurosis at the procc. spinosi of the 6th and 7th cervical and 1st and 2nd thoracic vertebrae and at the lig. nuchae. The muscle runs laterocaudally in three to four serrations and inserts at the 2nd–5th ribs lateral to the angulus costae. Due to its location, it can support inspiration by raising the ribs when contracted.

The posterior inferior serratus muscle originates on the spinosi procc. from Th11 to L3 and on the thoracolumbar fascia and runs in four individual spikes in a craniolateral direction. It inserts at the lower edges of the 9th–12th ribs near the angulus costae and is covered by the latissimus dorsi muscle. When contracted unilaterally, the posterior inferior saw muscle can easily support ipsilateral trunk rotation. Bilateral contraction pulls the ribs dorsocaudally, which aids thoracic constriction and thus expiration. In addition, it gives the diaphragm a stable punctum fixum, which in turn counteracts the cranioventral pull of the diaphragm and thus also prevents thoracic constriction and indirectly supports inspiration. Synergistically, it performs an extension of the spine and contributes to its stabilisation.

The posterior serratus muscle is supplied with nerves via the anterior spinal nerves from the segments Th1–Th5 for the superior part and Th11–L2 for the inferior part.

Palpation of the posterior sawing muscles is done from the prone position.

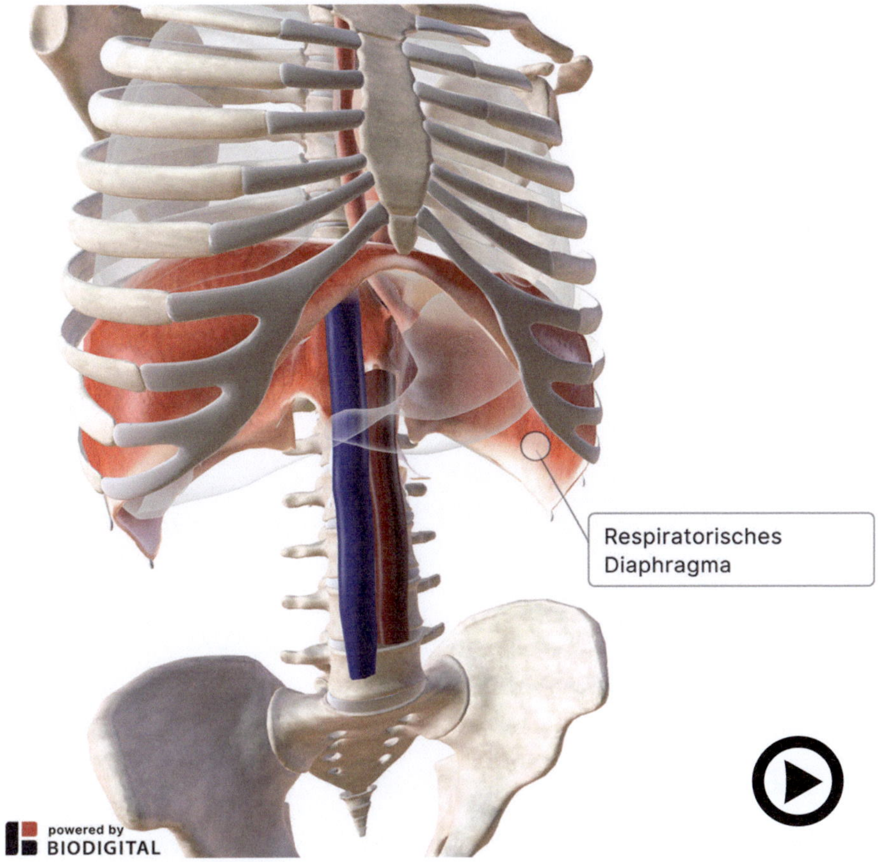

Fig. 5.48 Anatomy and palpation of the respiratory diaphragm (▶ https://doi.org/10.1007/000-ctt)

To palpate the upper part, the therapist stands sideways at the level of the rib cage and places the fingertips of the cranial hand on the prominent spinous process of C7 and the fingertips of the caudal hand on the cranial parts of the contralateral margo medialis scapulae. A line between the two hands describes the course of the muscle so that a targeted stimulus can be applied to the structure by moving the finger berries of the cranial hand towards the other hand. Due to the muscle surface of about four transverse fingers, the stimulus can also be applied to the structure starting from C7 about one transverse finger above and two transverse fingers below.

The inferior part can be accessed via the lower costal arch. The palpation fingers contact the contralateral 12th rib from the dorsal side and move horizontally towards the spine. In doing so, they meet the lower muscle belly of the serratus posterior inferior exactly in the middle of the path. A stimulus can then be applied to the flat muscle about three transverse fingers in the cranial direction. Another orientation can be established by connecting the two elbows. If both arms lie loosely along the body, a horizontal line is formed between them which intersects the spine at a certain height. At this height, the lower posterior saw muscle is located to the right and left of the proc. spinosus.

Implementation Note

Due to the superimposition of superficial muscles, the posterior superior and inferior serratus muscles are only accessible to palpation by stimulation in depth (Fig. 5.49).

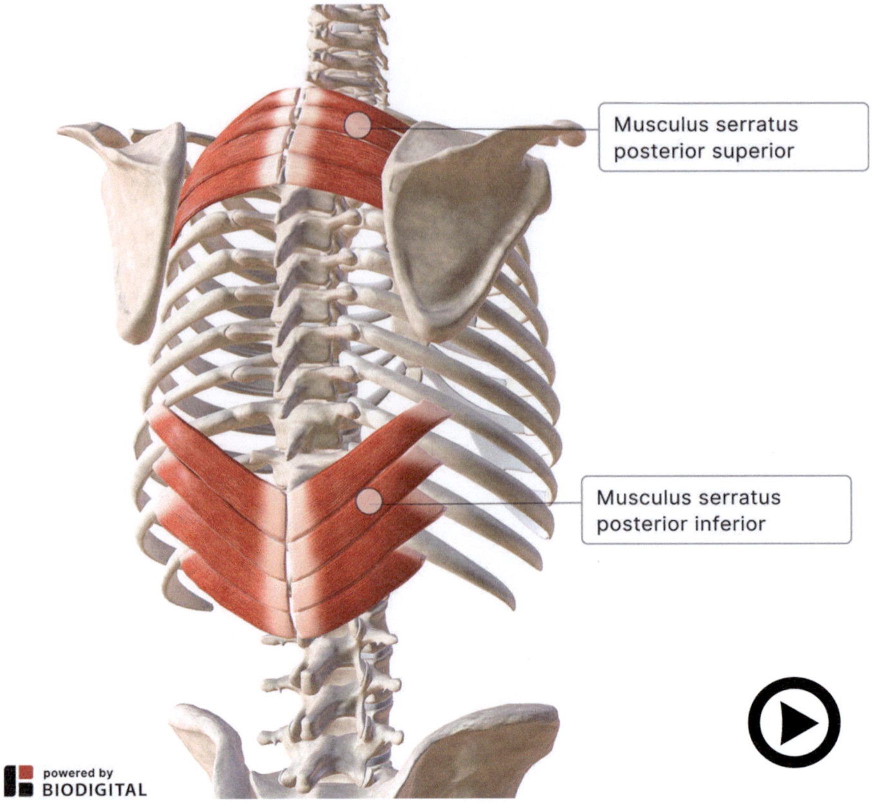

Fig. 5.49 Anatomy and palpation of the M. serratus posterior superior et inferior (▶ https://doi.org/10.1007/000-ctv)

5.7 Musculature in the Area of the Shoulder Girdle/Shoulder Joint

The most mobile joint in the body is the shoulder joint. The mobility of the shoulder girdle is indispensable for numerous everyday movements of the arms. This develops into a functional unit of the shoulder girdle and shoulder joint, in which the interaction can be realised via numerous muscles. In addition to the clavicle, the scapula, which can move on the thorax in a finely graduated manner via its suspension in muscle loops, plays an important role. This ensures the biomechanically important humeroscapular rhythm. In order for this unit to be able to meet the demands of everyday life, it is elementary to be able to palpate the muscular structures that can influence functionality and thus assess tone.

For palpation, it is suitable to position the patient in a sitting position with passively positioned arms. Alternatively, the prone, lateral or supine position can be chosen depending on the muscle. The palpable muscles, which are described individually in the following chapters in terms of position, function and palpation, include the levator scapulae muscle, the trapezius muscle, the sternocleidomastoid muscle, the rhomboideus major and minor muscles, the subclavius muscle, the pectoralis minor muscle and the serratus anterior muscle. The four rotator cuff muscles, the deltoid, latissimus dorsi, teres major and pectoralis major, and coracobrachialis muscles can also be palpated.

5.7.1 Palpation of the Scapular Levator Muscle

The Latin word "levare" translates into German as "to raise." The levator scapula muscle is therefore called the scapula lifter. This function is important to keep the scapula, in combination with other muscles, always perfectly aligned with the humerus. It can be counted among the secondary back muscles, but is functionally assigned to the shoulder girdle and is covered in the cranial part by the sternocleidomastoid and splenius capitis and cervicis muscles and in the caudal part by the trapezius pars descendens muscle. It connects the cervical spine with the shoulder girdle, as it extends obliquely caudolaterally from the procc. transversi of the 1st–2nd cervical vertebrae, as well as the tubercles posteriora of the procc. transversi of the 3rd–4th cervical vertebrae, to the angulus superior as well as to the spina scapulae and the upper edge of the margo medialis scapulae. The scapula elevator is innervated by the dorsal scapular nerve of the brachial plexus from segments C4–C5 and other fibres of the 3rd–5th cervical nerves from the cervical plexus. Functionally, it raises the scapula in a craniomedial direction and at the same time rotates it slightly. It also acts synergistically in the ipsilateral flexion of the cervical spine when the scapula is the punctum fixum.

In the middle part, the levator scapulae muscle is prominent in the lateral cervical region. There it is not overlaid by any muscle. This site is well suited for palpation, among other things, while the patient is positioned in the prone position or in a sitting position with the arm underneath. The anterior edge of the trapezius pars descendens muscle can first be felt by actively elevating the shoulder girdle. Secondly, the head is rotated to the opposite side, which allows the posterior border of the homolateral sternocleidomastoid muscle to be felt. Thirdly, the proc. spinosus of C4 is palpated, which only serves as an orientation line. If the steeply positioned fingertips now move between the anterior edge of the trapezius pars descendens muscle and the posterior edge of the sternocleidomastoid muscle at the level of C4 in the direction of the spine, they meet the levator scapulae muscle directly. This approach is suitable for the starting position in the sitting position.

In the prone position, the palpation fingers are first placed on the homolateral scapula, and the angulus superior scapulae is felt with the fingertips as the cranial tip of the margo medialis. Starting from this reference point, the fingers move in a craniomedial direction towards the cervical spine. The muscle cord of the levator scapulae muscle can best be palpated transversely from caudomedial to craniolateral.

Implementation Note

The levator scapulae muscle can transmit its pain to the neck, the homolateral shoulder region and also caudally along the margo medialis scapulae if there is a negative change (Fig. 5.50).

5.7.2 Palpation of the Trapezius Muscle

The trapezoidal hood muscle, which spans between the spine and the shoulder girdle, is counted among the secondary

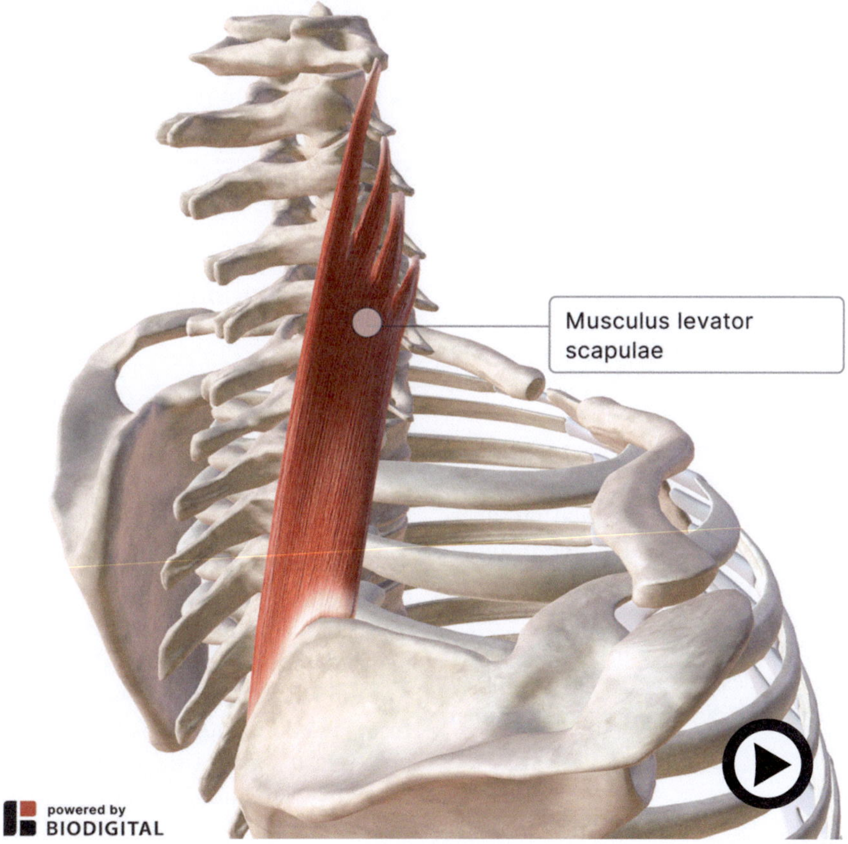

Fig. 5.50 Anatomy and palpation of the M. levator scapulae (▶ https://doi.org/10.1007/000-ctw)

back muscles and can be divided into a pars ascendens, pars transversa and pars descendens. However, the parts are not directly separable from each other, but merge smoothly.

The cranial descending pars originates from the superior nuchal line and the external occipital protuberance, as well as from the nuchal ligament and the spinosi procc. of all cervical vertebrae. It runs obliquely caudolaterally and inserts on the lateral third of the clavicle. It forms the dorsal border of the regio cervicalis lateralis and carries out the elevation in the shoulder girdle. In addition, it pulls the scapula obliquely craniomedially and rotates it outwards with the serratus anterior pars inferior muscle. The descending part can also perform a rotation of the head to the opposite side as well as an ipsilateral flexion of the cervical spine with a fixed shoulder girdle and unilateral contraction. The bilateral contraction can also support the dorsal extension of the cervical spine.

The horizontally running m. trapezius pars transversa arises via a tendon mirror at the level of the procc. spinosi of the 1st–4th thoracic vertebrae as well as at the lig. supraspinale and inserts at the acromion. It performs retraction in the shoulder girdle and displaces the scapula in a medial direction.

The ascending part of the hood muscle originates at the procc. spinosi of the 5th–12th thoracic vertebrae and at the lig. supraspinale. Following its craniolateral course, it inserts at the spina scapulae. Due to its course, it can perform a depression in the shoulder girdle and supports the descending part in the rotation of the scapula by moving it caudomedially.

All three parts fix the scapula to the thorax, making it a versatile articulating partner for the humerus.

The nervous supply for all three parts is realised via two accesses. The trapezius muscle is supplied motorically via the ramus externus of the accessorius nerve (XI cranial nerve) and proprioceptively via the ramus trapezius of the cervical plexus from segments C2–C4.

The superficially localised trapezius muscle can be easily palpated in the prone position and in the sitting position. If a triangle is formed between the external occipital protuberance, the spinosus of Th12 and the acromion, the resulting area describes the position of the trapezius muscle with its three parts. Each described pars can then be made palpable via its individual function in the shoulder girdle by means of the resulting contraction. The descending trapezius muscle can also be located by using the cranial pincer grip between the index finger and thumb.

Implementation Note

Due to everyday postural patterns, the trapezius pars descendens muscle tends to develop increased tension, which can react in a pressure-dolent manner during palpation, especially in the pincer grip. This can lead to pain being transmitted to the head area (Fig. 5.51).

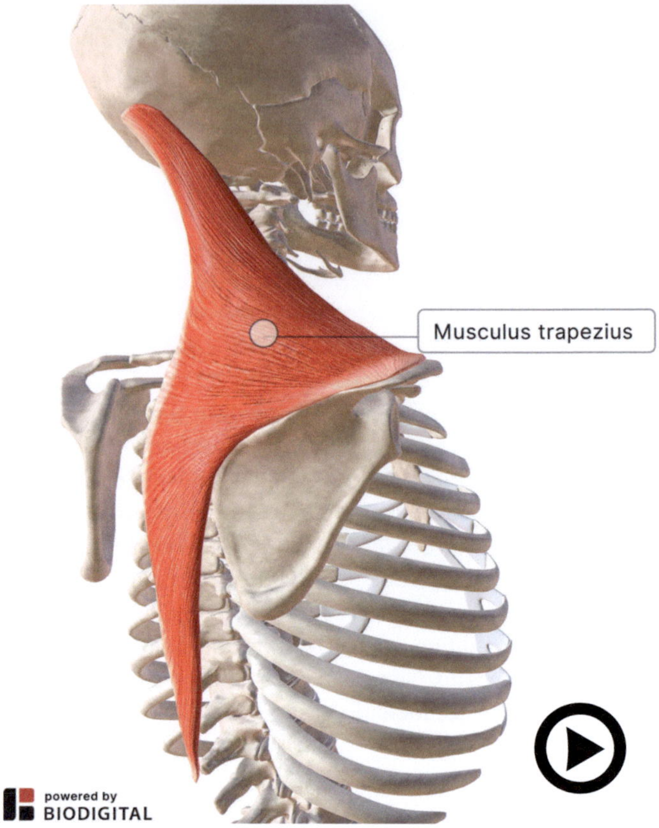

Fig. 5.51 Anatomy and palpation of the M. trapezius (▶ https://doi.org/10.1007/000-ctx)

5.7.3 Palpation of the Sternocleidomastoid Muscle

The muscle, whose name comes from its osseous attachment points, is called the head turner because of its function and belongs to the superficial layer of the neck musculature. The sternocleidomastoid muscle has two heads, the medial caput and the lateral caput. The caput mediale originates on the ventral craniolateral surface of the manubrium sterni and the caput laterale on the middle third of the anterior surface of the clavicle or the margo superior claviculae. Both parts run in the direction of the craniodorsal, shape the supraclavicular fossa in whose depth the vagus nerve is located and taper off from about the middle of the neck. The muscle inserts at the proc. mastoideus of the os temporale and with some fibres laterally at the linea nuchae superior of the os occipitale. The course of the head turner forms a dividing line both for the trigonum colli mediale or the regio cervicalis medialis and for the trigonum colli laterale or the regio cervicalis lateralis. Both sites are highly sensitive because, for example, the

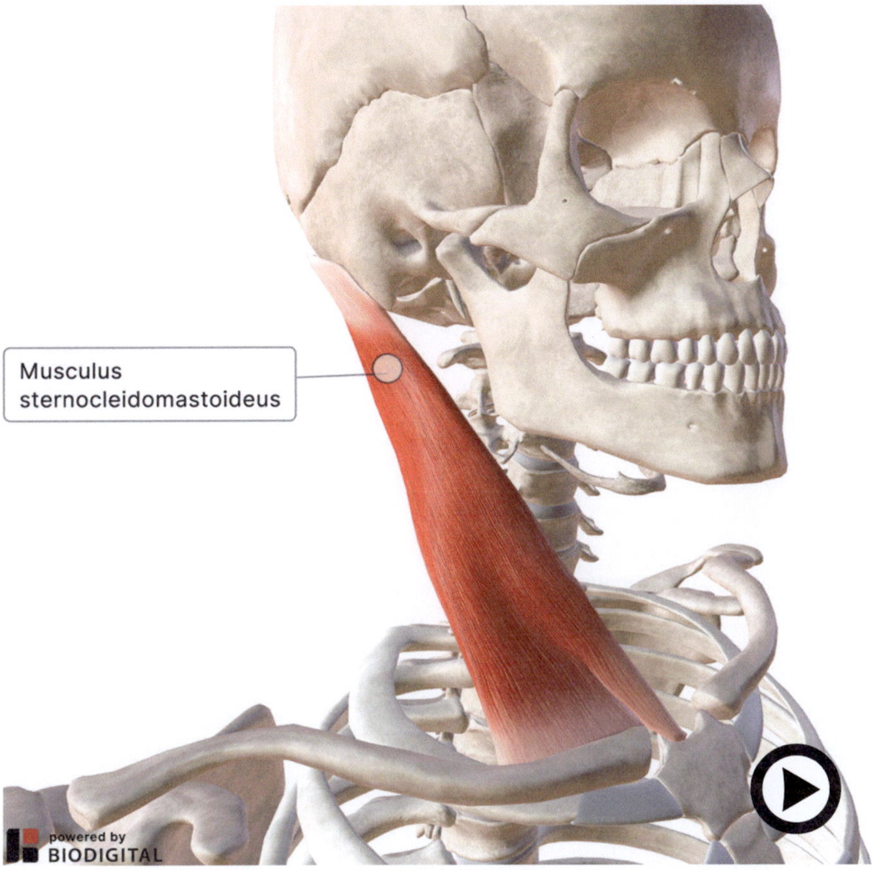

Fig. 5.52 Anatomy and palpation of the M. sternocleidomastoideus (▶ https://doi.org/10.1007/000-cty)

vagus nerve (10th cranial nerve), hypoglossal nerve (12th cranial nerve), accessorius nerve (11th cranial nerve) as well as arteries, veins, trachea and oesophagus are located in the former, and the accessorius nerve, parts of the cervical plexus as well as the subclavian artery and the jugular vein are located in the latter.

The sternocleidomastoid muscle is innervated by the accessorius nerve and by nerve branches of the cervical plexus from the C1–C4 segments. When actively contracted, it moves the head in ipsilateral flexion, in rotation to the contralateral side, in flexion with the head already flexed and in extension with the head extended. It also serves as an inspiratory respiratory muscle when the head is fixed.

Due to its superficial position, palpation can be carried out well in the supine position with the head underneath or in the sitting position. The therapist stands sideways to the patient and applies his fingers to the homolateral anterior surface of the manubrium. As soon as the patient performs an active head rotation to the opposite side, a clear contraction is felt over the tendon of origin. Subsequently, the entire course can be opened, initially over a large area with the fingertips. After an initial familiarisation phase on the part of the client, the quite intimate palpation in the neck area can also be carried out in a pincer grip. It is advisable to lay the head passively in order to be able to feel the structure in depth.

Implementation Note

Dysfunctions of the sternocleidomastoid muscle can manifest in transmitted pain to the head region (Fig. 5.52).

5.7.4 Palpation of the Major and Minor Rhomboid Muscles

The two rhomboid muscles, which belong to the middle layer of the secondary back muscles, connect the shoulder girdle with the spine and have a functional effect on it. While the major rhomboid muscle originates from the spinosi procc. of the 1st–4th thoracic vertebrae and the supraspinous ligament, the minor rhomboid muscle originates somewhat further cranially from the spinosi procc. of the 6th–7th cervical and 1st thoracic vertebrae and the nuchae ligament. Both have a similar rhombic course caudolaterally and insert at the margo medialis scapulae. Here, the large part starts below and the small part at the level of the spina scapulae. They therefore run directly parallel to each other. Both parts are innervated via the dorsal scapular nerve from the brachial plexus via segments C4–C6 and fix the scapula to the thorax. In addition, both pull the scapula craniomedially and thus support the scapular rotation, which is elementary for the joint functionality of the shoulder joint.

The rhomboid muscles are covered by the trapezius muscle and can therefore only be palpated indirectly by stimulation. After the person to be palpated has been positioned in the prone position, the therapist standing sideways makes contact with the proc. spinosus of C7, the vertebra prominens, with the steeply positioned fingertips of the cranial hand. The index finger berry of the caudal hand contacts the medial region of the spinae scapulae. The line arising between the two fingers forms the upper border of the rhomboid minor muscle. Moving caudally from this line, a contraction of both muscles can be induced by an active retraction movement. However, attention must be paid to the superficial trapezius muscle, which also performs a retraction, which is why only stimulation of the deeper rhomboid muscles is possible.

Implementation Note
The rhomboid muscles can cause transmissible pain in the area of the medial scapulae margo when negative changes occur (Fig. 5.53).

5.7.5 Palpation of the Subclavian Muscle

Below the clavicle is the short and rather narrow subclavian muscle, which is located deep behind the pectoralis major muscle. It originates from a short, strong tendon at the ventral corpus costae of the costa prima and its costal cartilage. The subclavian muscle then runs laterocranially in the subclavian muscle sulcus on the lower edge of the clavicle and inserts on the medial and lateral third of the underside of the clavicle. Innervation occurs via segments C5–C6 via the brachial plexus and ultimately via the subclavian nerve. Depending on the punctum fixum, the subclavian muscle caudalises the lateral third of the clavicle or elevates the first rib. It also protects the subclavian artery and vein as well as the brachial plexus and stabilises the SCG.

Palpation of the subclavian muscle is done from the supine position with the head underneath. The therapist, standing sideways, contacts the homolateral clavicle in the medial third with the fingertips. The fingers then move in a caudal direction and enter directly into a groove. In this groove, they meet the subclavian muscle directly. The muscle can then be followed in the direction of the manubrium sterni. Due to the overlapping of the pectoralis major muscle, only one stimulation is possible.

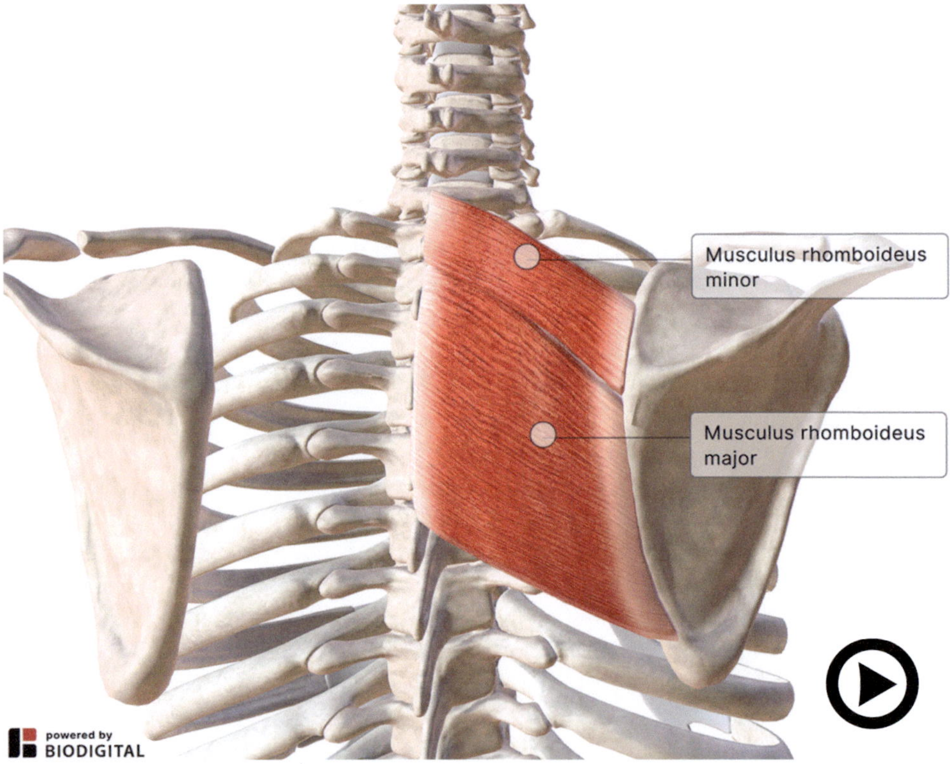

Fig. 5.53 Anatomy and palpation of the M. rhomboideus major et minor (▶ https://doi.org/10.1007/000-ctz)

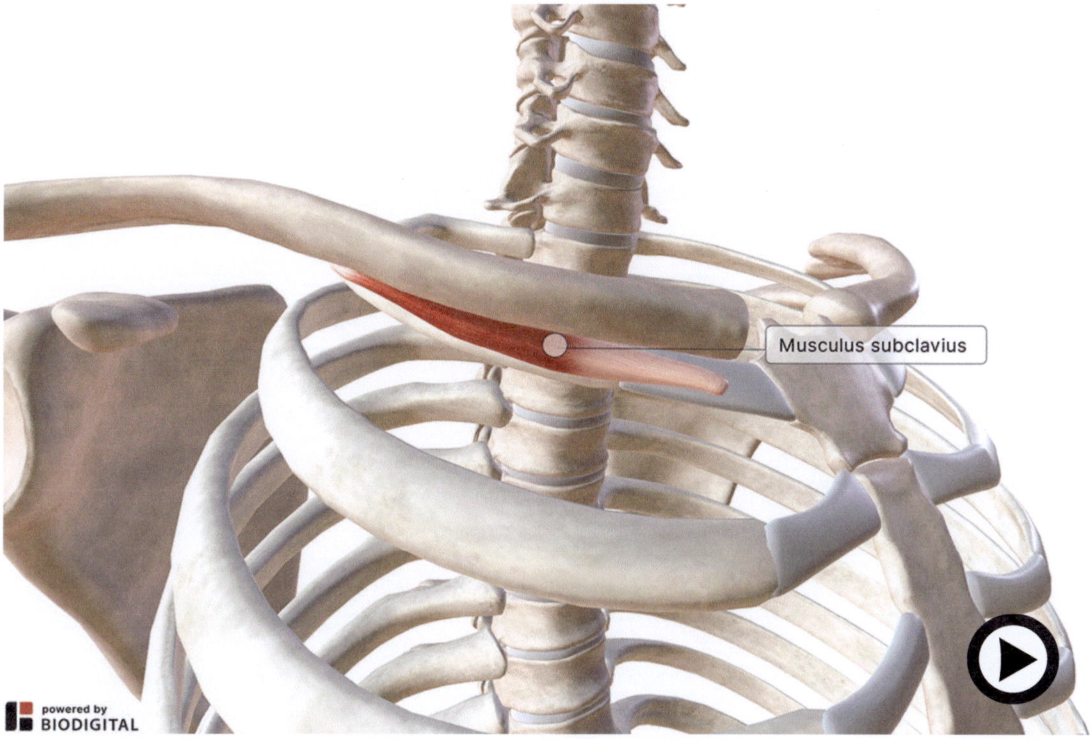

Fig. 5.54 Anatomy and palpation of the M. subclavius (▶ https://doi.org/10.1007/000-cv0)

Implementation Note
The application of pressure is also a stimulus to the nervous and vascular structures behind the subclavian muscle, which may be sensitive to pressure. A gentle approach is therefore recommended (Fig. 5.54).

5.7.6 Palpation of the Pectoralis Minor Muscle

The pectoralis minor is a thin, triangle-shaped muscle located under the pectoralis major muscle on the superolateral part of the thorax. It connects the shoulder girdle with the trunk, as it runs from the ventral corpus surfaces of the 3rd–5th ribs and the associated aponeuroses craniolaterally via a tapering tendon to the proc. coracoideus of the scapula. It is innervated by the medial pectoral nerve from segments C8–Th1 and the lateral pectoral nerve from segments C5–C7. The rather small muscle pulls the scapula caudomedially and thus supports the movement of the scapula, which is elementary for optimal movement in the shoulder joint. Furthermore, the pectoralis minor muscle participates together with the pectoralis major muscle as an auxiliary respiratory muscle.

For palpation of the pectoralis minor muscle, the patient is in a relaxed supine position. The therapist stands sideways and makes contact with the proc. coracoideus (see Sect. 2.8.2), which is located caudal to the lateral third of the clavicle, with the index and middle fingertip steeply placed. At this reference point, the finger meets the insertion tendon of the muscle. For the further course of the muscle, it is necessary to feel under the pectoralis major muscle. To do this, the patient actively abducts his homolateral arm to about 90° and performs a protraction with the same side of the shoulder girdle. The muscle edge of the pectoralis major muscle is felt ventrally on the shoulder in the direction of the axilla. This demarcation can be evoked even more clearly by horizontal adduction of the arm. The fingers to be palpated orientate themselves on the muscular edge of the pectoralis major muscle and move below it in depth along the ribs in the direction of the ventral thorax and the proc. coracoideus. The fingertips, which are now below the pectoralis major muscle, can create a stimulus on the pectoralis minor muscle with moderate pressure on the chest.

Implementation Note
When palpating the pectoralis minor, it is important to remember that there are nervous and vascular structures in the immediate vicinity that feed the upper limb. A gentle approach is therefore necessary (Fig. 5.55).

5.7.7 Palpation of the Serratus Anterior Muscle

The so-called boxer's or sawtooth muscle has its name because of its jagged origin on the ribs and its special char-

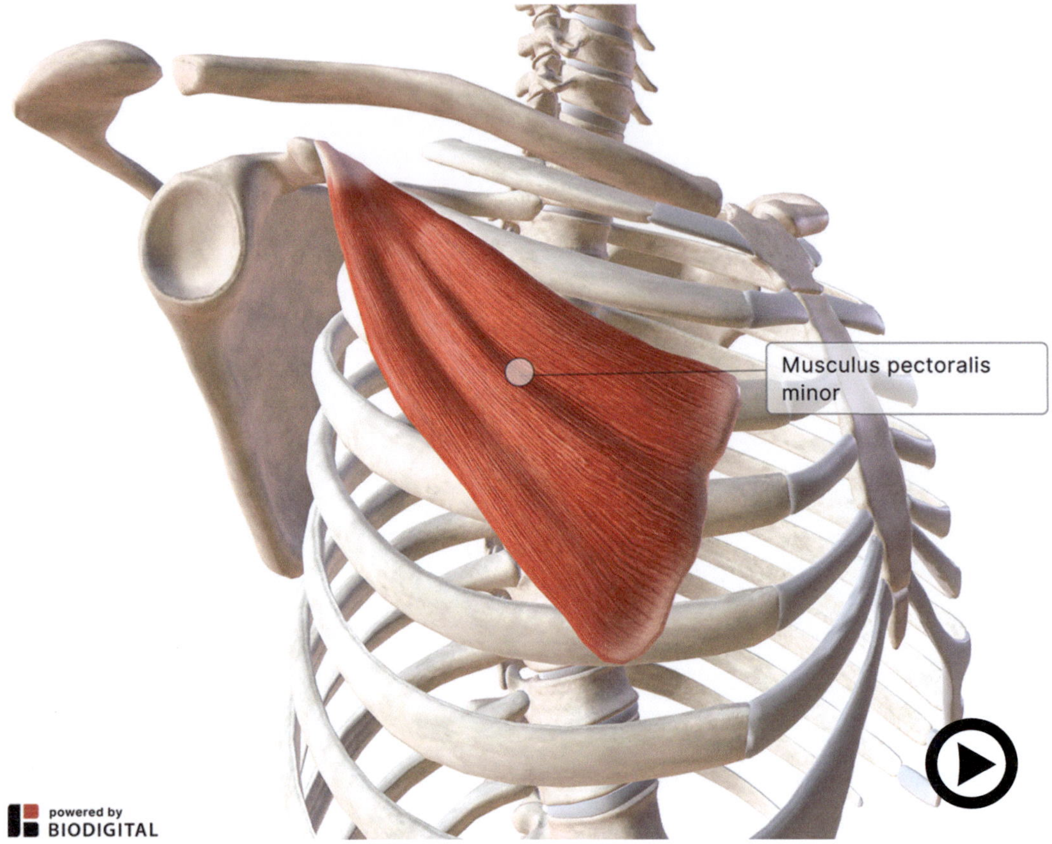

Fig. 5.55 Anatomy and palpation of the M. pectoralis minor (▶ https://doi.org/10.1007/000-cv1)

acteristics in athletes of this sport. It is divided into three parts, the pars superior, the pars intermedia and the pars inferior. The upper part runs from the corpus of the 1st–2nd ribs diagonally dorsally and inserts at the angulus superior of the scapula. The pars intermedia, which is the most pronounced, runs from the corpus of the 2nd–3rd ribs more horizontally to the margo medialis of the scapula. The lower part of the serratus anterior arises from the corpus of the 4th–9th ribs, runs obliquely dorsocranially and attaches to the margo medialis and the angulus inferior of the scapula. The pars inferior is the one that becomes visible in a good state of training. All origins form an abutment for the obliquus externus abdominis muscle and form the Gerdy line with it. The boxer muscle is innervated via the thoracic longus nerve from the brachial plexus via segments C5–C7. Due to its course, it can move the scapula on the thorax in such a way that it forms an optimal alignment with respect to the humerus. Thus, the upper part tends to perform an elevation of the scapula, whereas the middle and lower parts force a lateralisation. Protraction of the shoulder girdle and fixation of the scapula to the thorax are also made possible together with the rhomboid muscles. This increases the striking power of the arm if the muscle is well developed. In addition, it also contributes to the formation of the thoracic gliding surface and forms the medial wall of the axilla.

Palpation of the serratus anterior muscle is performed in the supine or lateral position. It should be noted that the superior pars is covered by the pectoralis major muscle and is therefore not directly suitable for palpation. The therapist stands to the side of the supine patient at the level of the rib-cage and places the fingertips of the index and middle fingers on the caudal end of the sternum. From this starting point, the fingers travel along the lower muscular edge of the opposite pectoralis major muscle laterally along the fifth rib. Just before they reach the arm lying at the side, the arm is actively moved by the patient to about 90° anteversion, and then the patient is asked to lift the arm with the shoulder girdle in the direction of protraction from the support. During this action, the serratus anterior muscle contracts and can be felt in its origin directly on the fifth rib under the fingers. Subsequently, the fingers can feel the further muscle bellies in the direction of the cranial and caudal ribs.

Implementation Note

If the patient performs an abduction of the overlying arm from the lateral position, the area is stretched and the muscle bellies directly on the ribs become more palpable (Fig. 5.56).

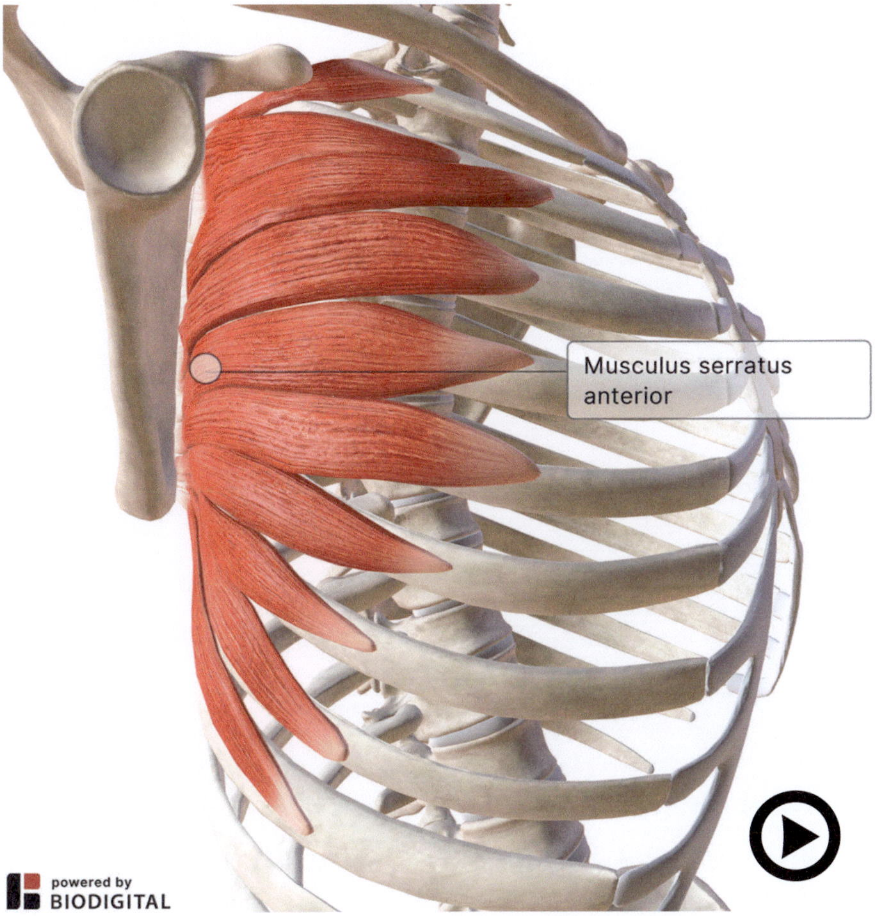

Fig. 5.56 Anatomy and palpation of the M. serratus anterior (▶ https://doi.org/10.1007/000-cv2)

5.7.8 Palpation of the Supraspinatus Muscle

The supraspinous muscle is part of the rotator cuff and belongs to the group of dorsal shoulder muscles. The rather narrow elongated muscle originates in the supraspinous fossa above the spina scapulae. The horizontal course ends at the tuberculum majus of the humerus and with some fibres at the capsule and the lig. transversum humeri. It is innervated via the suprascapular nerve from segments C4–C6 and is the initiator of abduction, which it performs together with the deltoid muscle [19]. It also performs external rotation, centres the caput humeri and tensions the shoulder joint capsule. Due to its course under the acromion, impingement situations can occur in the subacromial accessory joint, which can cause severe irritation of the muscle tendon.

The supraspinatus muscle is predominantly covered by the trapezius pars descendens muscle, which means that palpation is only possible in the sense of stimulation. For this purpose, the patient is in the prone or lateral position. In the first starting position, the therapist stands sideways and places the fingertips on the medial beginning of the spina scapulae of the homolateral side. Then the fingertips move slightly cranially and enter a depression, the supraspinous fossa. This is the origin of the supraspinous muscle, which can be stimulated cranially of the scapula in a lateral direction towards the acromion by palpation. If the patient is lying in a lateral position, the arm is placed along the body while the therapist stands at the head end of the client facing caudally. The fingers are applied to the acromion from the medial side in such a way that they make contact with the art. acromioclavicularis. If the steeply positioned fingers now feel directly in depth in the dorsomedial direction, they provide a direct stimulus to the muscle tendon of the supraspinatus muscle.

Implementation Note

Due to the anatomical position of the supraspinatus muscle, there can be frequent irritations and thus changes in tone and pressure dolences in the course of the muscle (Fig. 5.57).

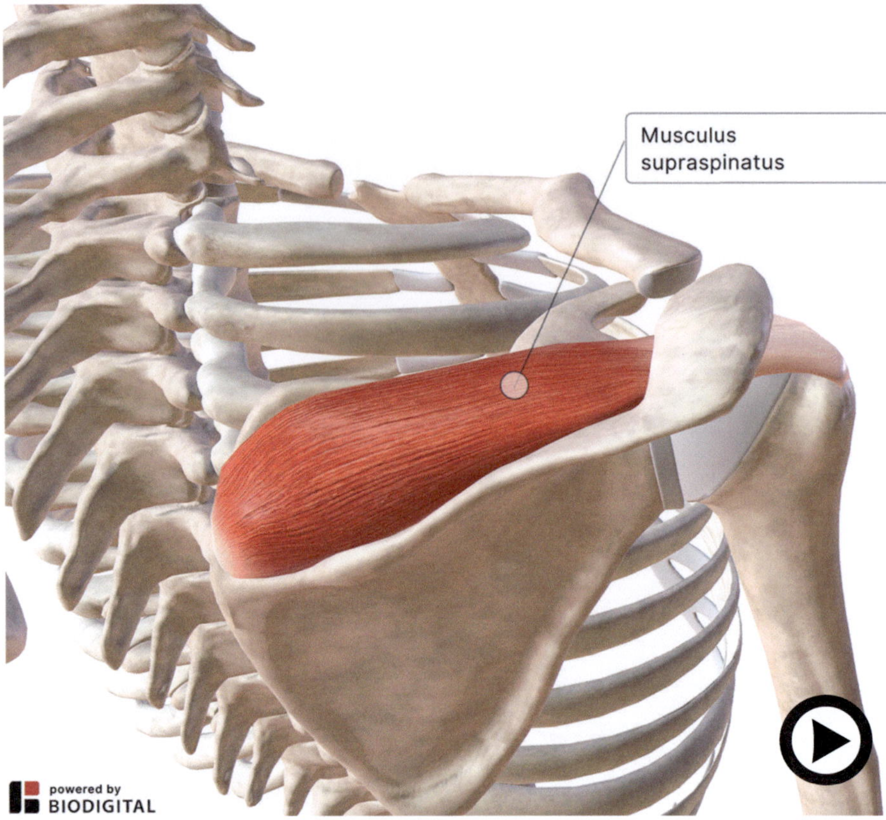

Fig. 5.57 Anatomy and palpation of the M. supraspinatus (▶ https://doi.org/10.1007/000-cv3)

5.7.9 Palpation of the Infraspinatus Muscle

The lower limb muscle has a triangular shape, is part of the rotator cuff and belongs to the group of dorsal shoulder muscles. Its large-surface origin is in the infraspinous fossa below the spina scapulae and partly at the facies infraspinata. The upper parts run rather horizontally, while the lower parts take a more craniolateral course. All sections taper into an attachment tendon that inserts at the greater tuberosity. The infraspinatus muscle is innervated via the suprascapular nerve from segments C4–C6 and accessory via the axillary nerve, which arises from the brachial plexus. In the rotator cuff group, it also ensures the centring of the caput humeri in the cavitas glenoidalis. From the neutral position, it supports abduction, whereas when the arm is abducted, it accompanies the return or adduction in the shoulder joint.

The stimulation is made possible by the steeply positioned fingertips which, starting from the medial spina scapulae, glide caudally into the infraspinous fossa and follow it laterally. Due to the overlapping of the trapezius and deltoid muscles, palpation is only possible through these structures.

Implementation Note

The infraspinatus muscle may be irritated after frequent and intense throwing movements, which can lead to increased pain sensations for the client when palpated (Fig. 5.58).

5.7.10 Palpation of the Minor Teres Muscle

The small round muscle is part of the rotator cuff and is counted as part of the dorsal shoulder musculature. The teres minor muscle follows a similar course to the infraspinatus muscle and originates from the middle third of the lateral scapula margo. Its oblique craniolateral course ends at the greater tuberosity of the humerus and the joint capsule. The weakest muscle of the rotator cuff receives its innervation through the axillary nerve from segments C4–C6 and largely supports the functions of the functional unit mentioned. It participates in adduction and retroversion of the arm, stabilises the shoulder joint and limits the medial and lateral axial gap. In addition, it supports the arthrokinematics by supporting the caudal glide of the caput humeri during abduction together with the latissimus dorsi muscle.

Palpation of the minor teres muscle is performed from the prone or optional lateral position. The therapist stands sideways and first makes contact with the inferior angulus of the scapula with the fingertips. Starting from this reference point, the fingers move cranially along the margo lateralis scapulae, crossing a muscular structure, the teres major muscle. After this first round structure, palpating further in the cranial direction, the next muscle fibres running craniolaterally appear. These are associated with the teres minor mus-

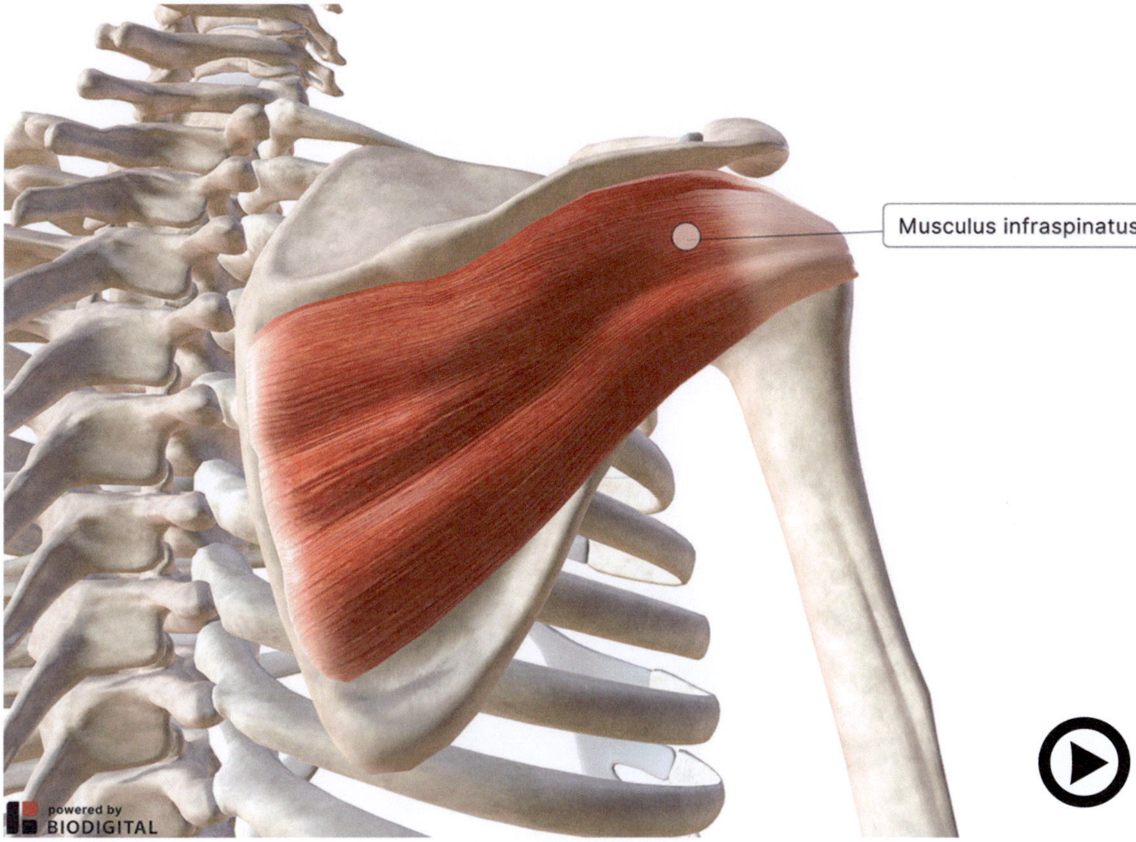

Fig. 5.58 Anatomy and palpation of the M. infraspinatus (▶ https://doi.org/10.1007/000-cv4)

cle. As the latter is covered by the deltoid muscle, a complete palpation is not possible.

Implementation Note
Due to its active involvement in everyday movements, it is not uncommon for dysfunction of the teres minor muscle to occur. This can lead to pain being transferred to the region of the shoulder joint (Fig. 5.59).

5.7.11 Palpation of the Subscapularis Muscle

The lower shoulder blade muscle is one of the four parts of the rotator cuff. It belongs to the group of ventral shoulder muscles. As the largest muscle of the rotator cuff, it finds its broad region of origin in the area of the subscapular fossa. Its fibres are horizontal in the superior parts and laterocranial in the inferior parts, so the muscle almost completely covers the ventral scapula. The tapered tendon inserts at the humeral tuberosity and with some fibres at the capsule of the shoulder joint. The subscapularis muscle is innervated by the subscapular nerve from segments C5–C8. It is an internal rotator of the shoulder joint, performs adduction of the raised arm and tensions the shoulder joint capsule. Furthermore, it contributes to the stabilisation and centralisation of the caput humeri and protects the joint from dislocation due to its broad attachment. In addition to these functions, together with the serratus anterior, it forms the thoracic gliding surface between the scapula and the thorax so that the latter can move on the thorax.

Palpation of the subscapularis muscle is performed from the prone or lateral position. If the patient is in prone position, the therapist stands sideways at thoracic level and places the client's homolateral arm on the back so that the back of the hand touches the os sacrum. Then the cranial hand grasps the homolateral shoulder from ventral and passively moves the shoulder girdle into retraction so that the scapula is slightly raised from the thorax. The caudal hand contacts the margo medialis scapulae via the fingertips. The fingers then slowly move under the scapula to make contact with the ventral surface of the scapula. Here they meet directly with the subclavian muscle.

If the patient is positioned in the lateral position, the overlying arm is passively placed behind the back. During this movement, the scapula is slightly lifted from the thorax, allowing palpatory access under the scapula. The therapist,

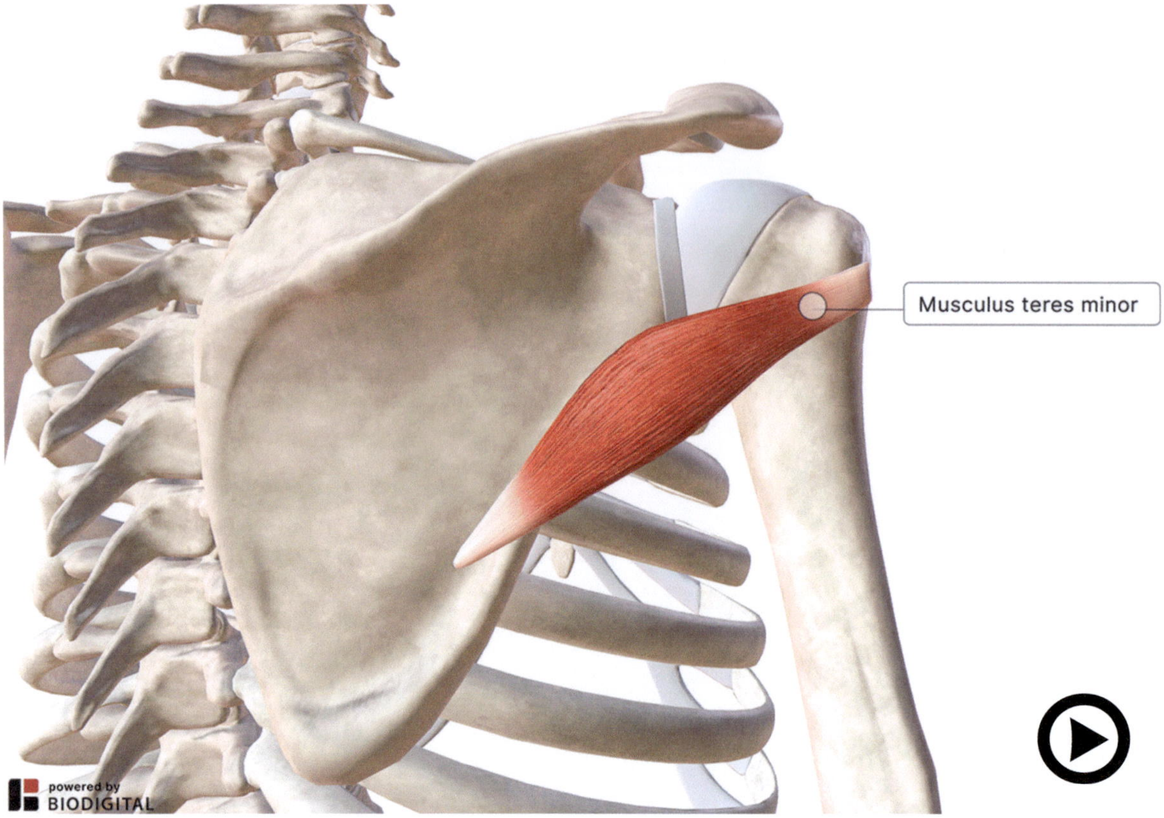

Fig. 5.59 Anatomy and palpation of the M. teres minor (▶ https://doi.org/10.1007/000-cv5)

standing at chest level, passively fixes the shoulder joint with the ventral hand and feels his way under the scapula with the fingertips of the dorsal hand in the region of the margo medialis. Here they meet directly with the origin of the subscapularis muscle.

Implementation Note
If the client is not able to relax his musculature extensively or if the scapula adheres too strongly over the sliding surface on the thorax, palpation under the scapula will prove difficult or not possible at first. In addition, the subscapularis muscle can transmit pain to the dorsal side of the shoulder joint and to the upper extremity in case of negative changes (Fig. 5.60).

5.7.12 Palpation of the Deltoid Muscle

The triangular deltoid muscle is part of the dorsal shoulder musculature and, from a biomechanical point of view, is a rolling muscle that significantly shapes the relief of the shoulder area. It wraps around the humeroscapularis from the ventral, lateral and dorsal sides. Anteriorly, there is the pars clavicularis, which originates on the lateral third of the clavicle; laterally, there is the pars acromialis, which adheres rather broadly to the acromion; and dorsally, there is the pars spinalis, which originates on the lateral third of the spina scapulae. While the anterior part has a dorsolateral and the posterior part a ventrolateral course, the acromial part draws steeply distally and inserts like the other two parts on the deltoid tuberosity. The deltoid muscle is innervated by the axillary nerve from segments C5–C6 and receives additional accessory control via the ventral branches of the thoracic nerves. Functionally, the pars clavicularis performs anteversion, adduction and internal rotation in the shoulder joint. The pars acromialis moves the shoulder joint in abduction during contraction and can support both anteversion with the pars clavicularis and retroversion with the pars spinalis proportionally. In addition, this part is responsible for the osteokinematic rolling of the humerus. The pars spinalis, on the other hand, performs retroversion, adduction and external rotation with the arm hanging. Both the pars clavicularis and the pars spinalis support abduction from 30° to 60° due to the inversion function.

The palpatory approach is considered very good because the deltoid muscle is superficial and not covered by any muscle. The client is positioned in a lateral position while the

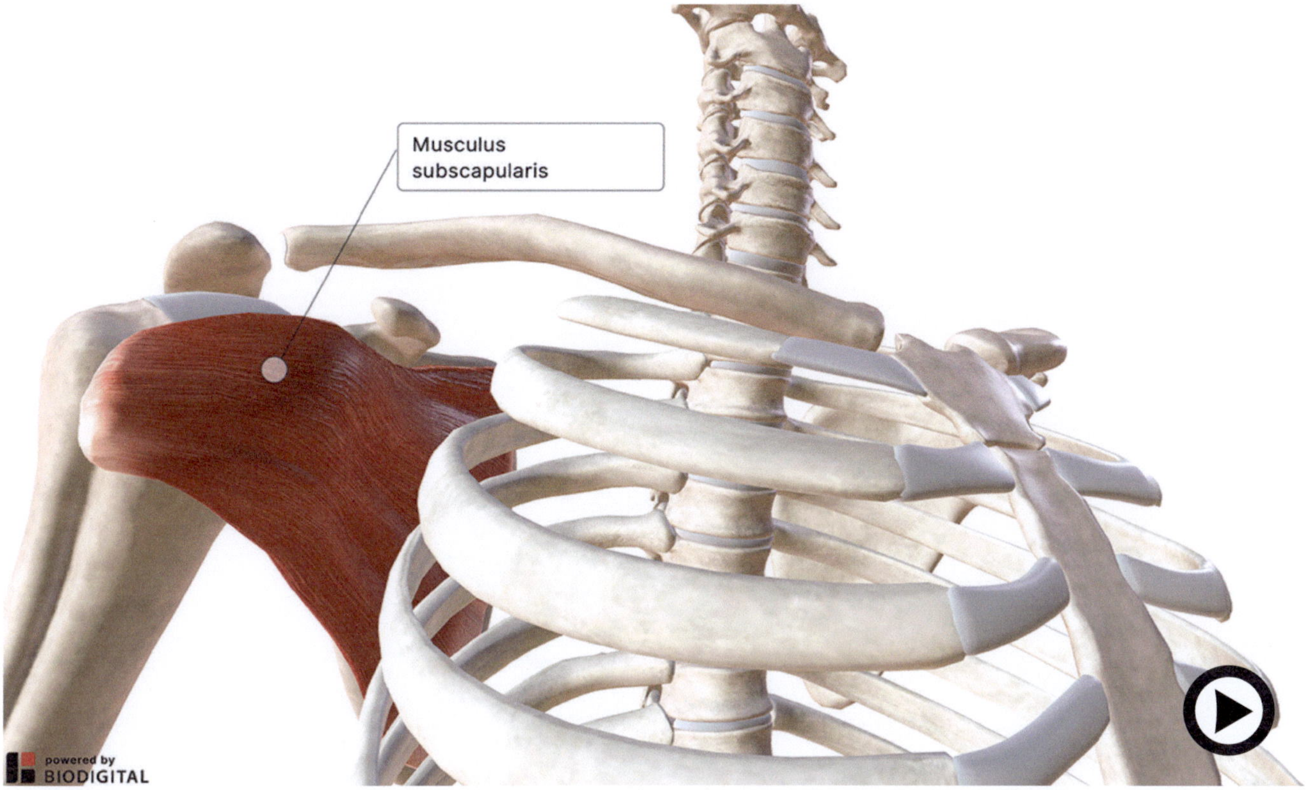

Fig. 5.60 Anatomy and palpation of the M. subscapularis (▶ https://doi.org/10.1007/000-cv6)

therapist stands at the level of the shoulder. First, the whole hand is placed flat on the shoulder, and the patient is asked to actively move his arm in abduction. This causes large parts of the deltoid muscle to contract so that an overview of the position can be obtained. Then the steeply placed fingertips can feel the edges of the muscle by moving from the deltoid tuberosity to the extremitas acromialis of the clavicle via shoulder height to the spina scapulae (see Sect. 2.8.2). Thus, all origins are palpated. The muscle bellies can also be reached by direct palpation in depth. It is suitable to place the arm passively along the body.

Implementation Note
Palpation can also be performed in the supine or lateral position. The deltoid muscle can transmit pain to the shoulder joint area (Fig. 5.61).

5.7.13 Palpation of the Latissimus Dorsi Muscle

The large, broad back muscle covers a large part of the back and shapes the V-shaped relief from the pelvis to the shoulders. The rather thin muscle is the largest of the human body in terms of area and can be divided into four parts that merge into one another.

The pars iliaca, which originates in the posterior third of the crista iliaca, runs craniolaterally and inserts into the crista tuberculi minoris and the sulcus intertubercularis.

The pars vertebralis originates at the procc. spinosi of the 7th–12th thoracic vertebrae as well as at the fascia thoracolumbalis and thus also at the spinous processes of the lumbar spine up to the first sacral proc. spinosus and the adjacent facies dorsalis ossis sacri. The portion runs craniolaterally and attaches to the crista tuberculi minoris and the sulcus intertubercularis.

The pars costalis, which has its origin at the 9th–12th ribs, runs laterocranially and also inserts at the crista tuberculi minoris and in the sulcus intertubercularis.

The rather inconstant pars scapularis has its origin at the angulus inferior scapulae, runs horizontally in a lateral direction and, like the other parts, attaches to the crista tuberculi minoris and the sulcus intertubercularis. The crossing attachment tendons lead to improved leverage and thus contribute to the economy of force application.

The latissimus dorsi muscle is innervated via the thoracodorsal nerve from segments C6–C8 and is also known as the apron truss muscle due to its function of internal rotation,

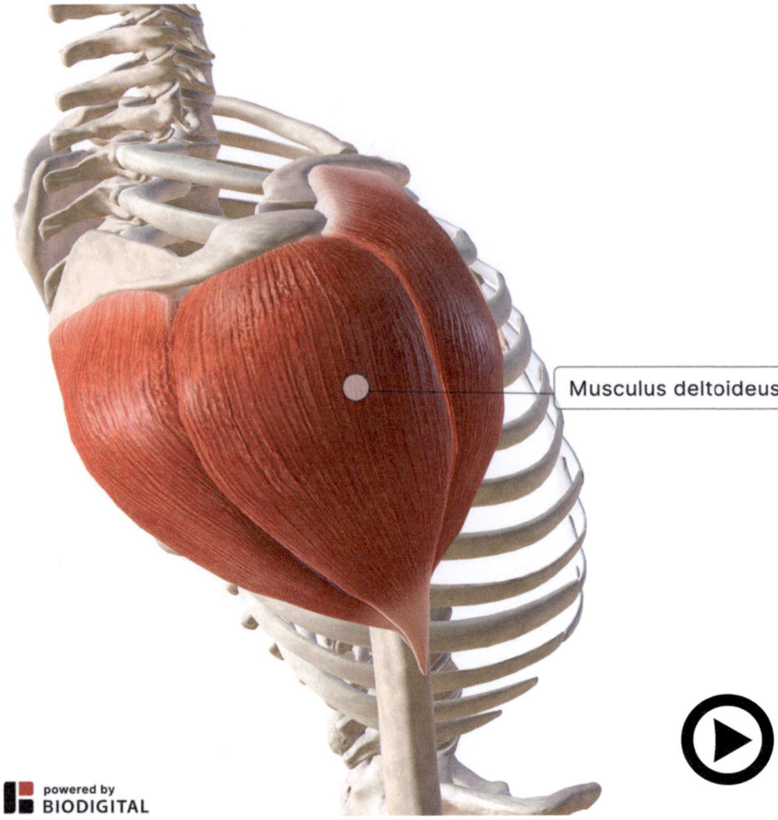

Fig. 5.61 Anatomy and palpation of the M. deltoideus (▶ https://doi.org/10.1007/000-cv7)

adduction and retroversion in the shoulder joint. In addition, it helps with coughing or forced breathing, forms the posterior axillary fold with the teres major muscle and pulls the upper body upwards during a pull-up when the arm is the punctum mobile. It forms the biomechanical antagonist to the deltoid muscle and, from an arthrokinematic point of view, serves for optimal caudal sliding of the caput humeri during abduction.

The superficial position of the latissimus dorsi muscle allows good palpation, which is done from the prone position. The therapist stands sideways and places both hands flat on the contralateral half of the torso. The patient is then asked to place the back of the hand of the contralateral arm on the os sacrum. This movement in adduction, internal rotation and retroversion in the shoulder joint will cause the muscle to contract and thus be very easy to feel. In a relaxed state, as soon as the arm is put back, the complete muscle belly can also be grasped in a pincer grip with one hand. The edges of the muscle are felt at the respective regions of origin with the raised fingertips.

Implementation Note

The latissimus dorsi muscle can cause pain transmitted to the area around the inferior scapular angulus of the homolateral side during palpation. In addition, changes in the muscle's state of tension can be transmitted to the thoracolumbar fascia due to the anatomical connection (Fig. 5.62).

5.7.14 Palpation of the Teres Major Muscle

The large round muscle is included in the dorsal shoulder musculature, but is not part of the rotator cuff as it does not radiate into the shoulder joint capsule. It originates at the inferior angulus of the scapula. The muscle is attached via a long tendon in the craniolateral region of the crista tuberculi minoris. This tendon is separated by a bursa from the tendon of the latissimus dorsi muscle, which follows a similar course. Innervation is provided by the subscapular nerve from segments C5–C8. It is also controlled by the thoracodorsal nerve and in rare cases by the axillary nerve. Functionally, it supports the latissimus dorsi muscle in terms of internal rotation, adduction and retroversion in the shoulder joint. If the scapula is the punctum mobile, the large round muscle moves the scapula in the direction of lateral rotation so that an optimal joint position can be established. In addition, it forms the medial and lateral axis gap and stabilises the shoulder joint.

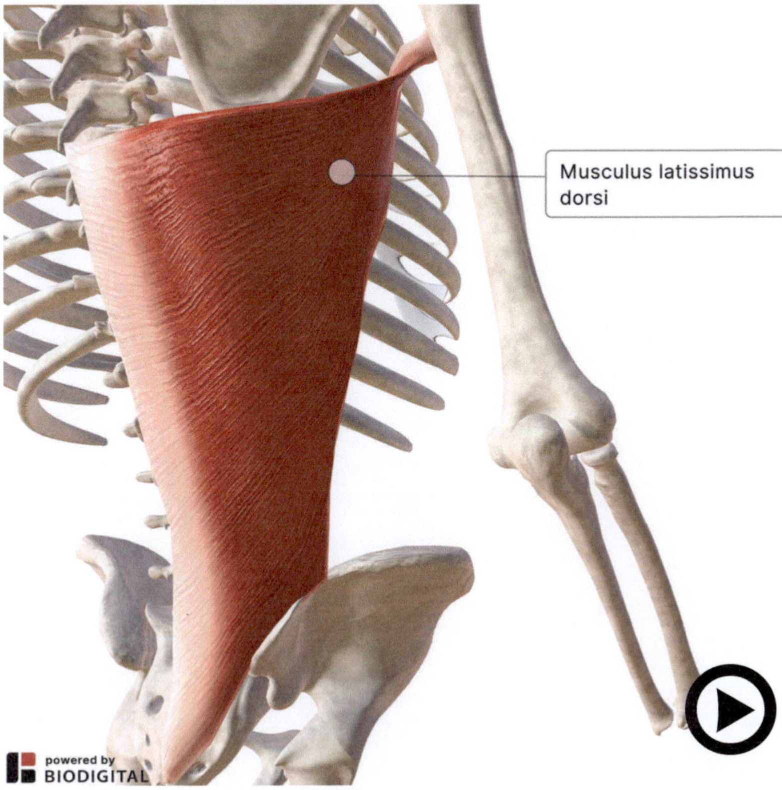

Fig. 5.62 Anatomy and palpation of the M. latissimus dorsi (▶ https://doi.org/10.1007/000-cv8)

Palpation of the teres major muscle is performed from the prone or optional lateral position. The therapist stands sideways and first contacts the inferior angulus of the scapula with the fingertips. Starting from this reference point, the fingers move cranially along the margo lateralis scapulae and directly cross a structure running slightly craniolaterally. This rounded structure is the teres major muscle, the course of which can be further felt with the fingertips.

Implementation Note

The teres major muscle is an elongated and rounded muscle that is easily overlooked during palpation. It is therefore important to feel directly the first resistance of that structure and to follow it in its course. The muscle can be responsible for transmitted pain to the dorsal shoulder area (Fig. 5.63).

5.7.15 Palpation of the Pectoralis Major Muscle

The pectoralis major muscle is located directly above the pectoralis minor muscle. This muscle connects the thorax, shoulder girdle and shoulder joint. It is located between the pectoralis fascia and the clavipectoralis fascia and can be divided into three parts.

The pars clavicularis, which originates on the medial half of the clavicle, runs laterocaudally and inserts distally on the crista tuberculi majoris via a flat tendon.

The pars sternocostalis records its origin on the homolateral side of the corpus sterni as well as the bony cartilage borders of the 2nd–7th ribs, runs rather horizontally and attaches via a flat tendon in the middle area of the crista tuberculi majoris.

The pars abdominis originates at the lamina anterior to the rectus sheath, runs in a craniolateral direction and forms its insertion at the crista tuberculi majoris in the proximal region. The pectoralis major muscle, which is innervated via the pectoralis medial nerve from segments C8–Th1 and the pectoralis lateral nerve from segments C5–C7, forms the infraclavicular fossa with the deltoid muscle and the clavicle, which ensures the passage of the cephalic vein. When the muscle contracts, it performs adduction and internal rotation in the shoulder joint. In addition, the pars clavicularis and the pars sternocostalis support the anteversion and together form the ventral wall of the axilla. When the arm is fixed, it also functions as an auxiliary inspiratory muscle.

Palpation of the large pectoral muscle is done from the supine position. The therapist stands sideways at the level of the client's head, facing caudally, and contacts the homolateral clavicle with the fingertips. The patient then moves his arm in 90° abduction with subsequent horizontal flexion. During this activity, the pectoralis major muscle contracts, which in turn can be perceived at the lower edge of the clavicle via the finger berries. Subsequently, the muscle edges can be followed in the direction medial to the clavicle, over the sternum to about the 7th rib. In addition, the insertion

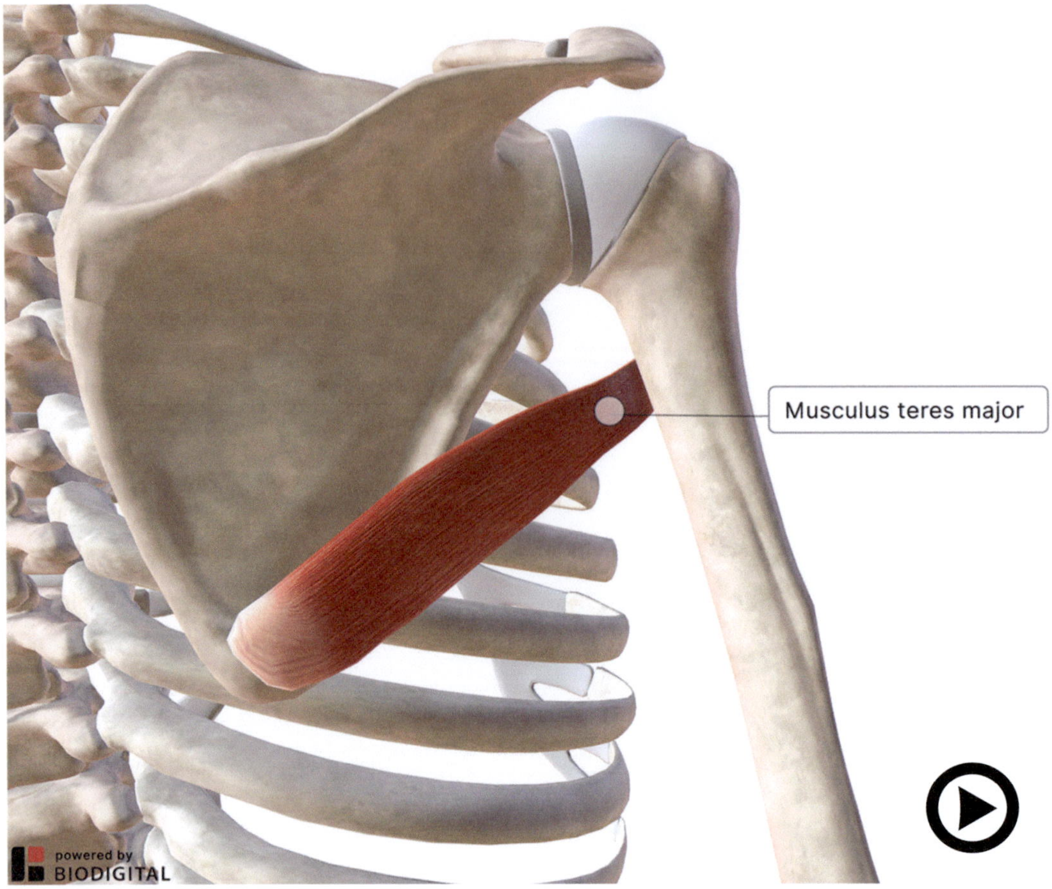

Fig. 5.63 Anatomy and palpation of the M. teres major (▶ https://doi.org/10.1007/000-cv9)

tendon can be clearly felt ventrally at the axilla in the transition to the arm during contraction. When the patient passively puts his arm down again, the muscle belly, which is localised superficially, can be examined with the fingertips.

Implementation Note
The pectoralis major muscle can cause referred pain to the chest and arm, giving the false clinical picture of angina (Fig. 5.64).

5.7.16 Palpation of the Coracobrachialis Muscle

The raven's beak upper arm muscle, which bears its name because of its course, is counted among the ventral group of shoulder muscles. Its origin is at the proc. coracoideus of the scapula together with the caput breve of the m. biceps brachii, with which it is also partially fused [20]. It runs steeply caudally and slightly lateroventrally and carries the neurovascular roads of the upper arm, which are formed from the brachial artery and vein as well as the radial, ulnar and median nerve. The coracobrachialis muscle attaches to the facies anterior of the humerus in extension of the crista tuberculi minoris. It is innervated via the musculocutaneous nerve from segments C5–C6. Based on the muscle's anatomy, it can functionally support anteversion, adduction and internal rotation in the shoulder joint and stabilise the humerus in the shoulder joint when contracted.

The stimulation of the coracobrachialis muscle is done from the supine position. The therapist stands sideways at abdominal level, and the client's arm is positioned slightly in abduction so that the axilla can be palpated. The fingertips of the hand facing the client are first applied to the brachial artery in the axilla on the homolateral side. For this purpose, the fingertips are placed proximally on the upper arm between the biceps brachii muscle (caput breve), the triceps brachii muscle (caput longum) and the proximal border, the latissimus dorsi muscle. A pulsating structure, the brachial artery, is in depth in the gap. Because the coracobrachialis muscle is located directly under the brachial artery, a direct stimulus can be applied to the structure in this region with the fingertips.

Implementation Note
The described nerve and vascular roads supply and dispose of the arm and should only be gently palpated (Fig. 5.65).

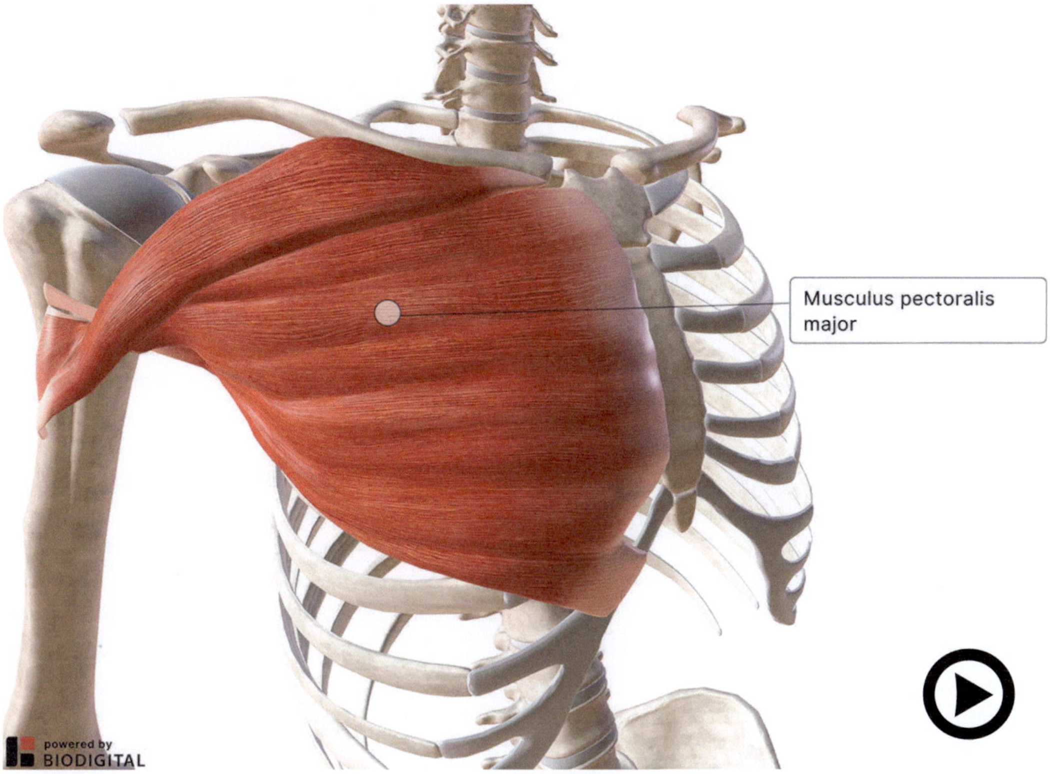

Fig. 5.64 Anatomy and palpation of the M. pectoralis major (▶ https://doi.org/10.1007/000-cva)

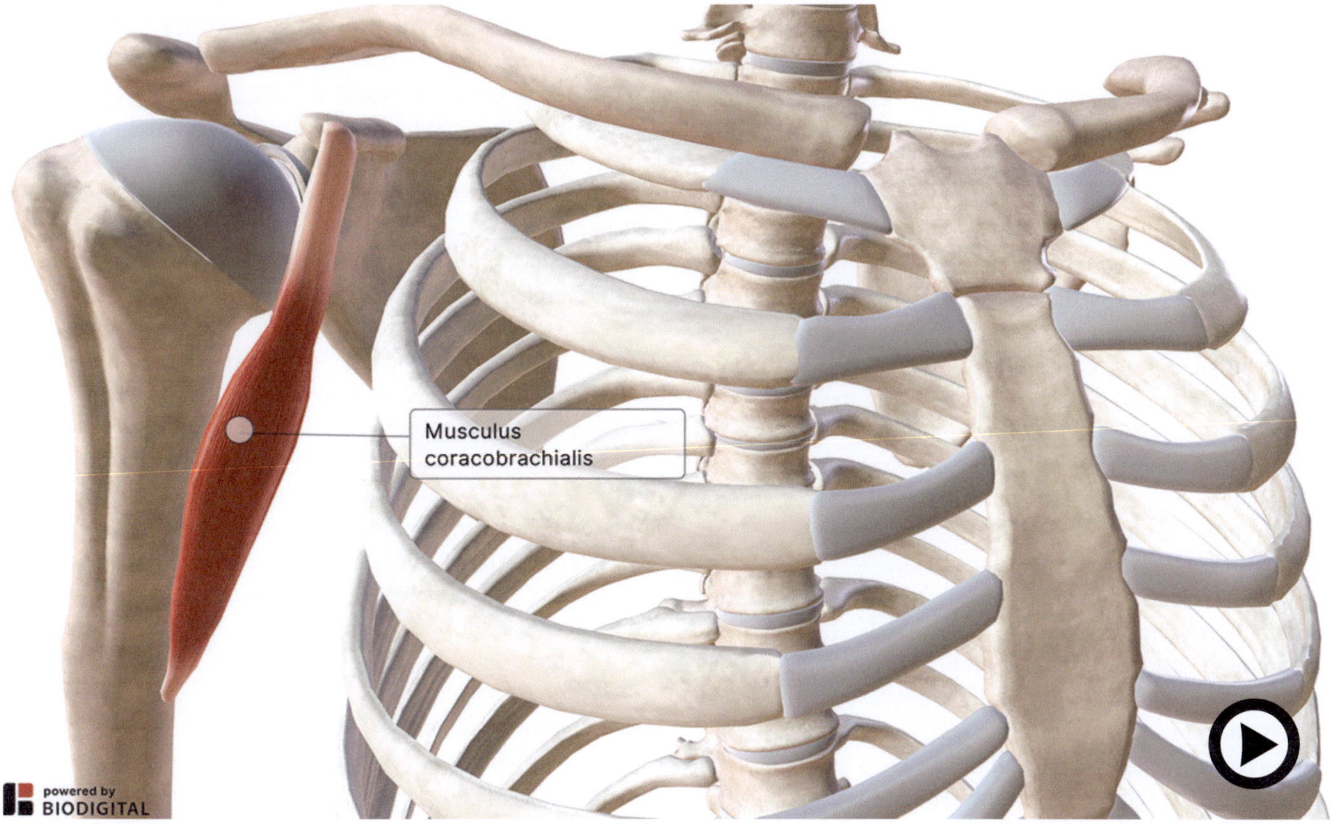

Fig. 5.65 Anatomy and palpation of the M. coracobrachialis (▶ https://doi.org/10.1007/000-cvb)

5.8 Musculature in the Area of the Elbow Joint

The mobility of the upper extremity plays an important role in coping with everyday activities. The elbow joints serve as length regulators and are thus able to position the hand perfectly. The mobility of the individual joints of the art. cubiti is ensured by its musculature. These include the triceps brachii and anconeus muscles, which are located posteriorly on the upper limb. These are completed by the biceps brachii and brachialis muscles, which are located anteriorly in the upper arm. The following sections describe the course and function of these muscles. In addition, individual palpation instructions are presented for each structure. Muscles that are also located in the area of the elbow joints but have their main influence in the area of the forearm or hand are discussed in Sects. 5.9 and 5.10.

5.8.1 Palpation of the Triceps Brachii Muscle

The three-headed humerus muscle is located on the back of the humerus and consequently consists of three parts. The caput longum, the caput mediale and the caput laterale together form the triceps brachii muscle, which is covered in its proximal part by the deltoid muscle. While the long head originates at the infraglenoid tuberosity, the fibres of the outer part begin at the lateral margo and the inner part at the medial margo of the dorsal facies of the humerus. All parts run steeply distally and insert at the olecranon of the ulna. The long tendon begins to develop from about the middle of the humerus. The attachment tendon radiates into the capsule of the elbow joint and is protected from excessive friction by the bursa subtendinea musculi triceps brachii. The triceps brachii muscle is mainly innervated by the radial nerve from segments C6–C8 and is therefore also the identifying muscle for segment C7. The caput longum has additional innervation from the axillary nerve. Due to the position of the muscle, it is mainly responsible for extension in the elbow joint. In addition, it stabilises the art. cubiti and cranialises the caput humeri in the cavitas glenoidale when carrying heavy loads. These functions, as well as those of retroversion and adduction in the shoulder joint, are carried out by the caput longum.

The superficial arm extensor is very easy to feel. For this, the patient is to be positioned in a prone or lateral position or in a sitting position, while the therapist stands to the side and makes contact with the back of the upper arm with the hand placed flat. The client is asked to actively extend the arm to the maximum at the elbow and to hold this position at the end. This causes the triceps brachii muscle to contract, which at this moment comes to light under the palm of the hand. The edges of the muscle can then be felt with the fingertips, whereby the medial caput is largely covered by the other two and can only be felt medially on the arm. Thus, the sensation is aimed more at the caput longum and the caput laterale, which in turn are covered by the deltoid muscle in the proximal part.

Implementation Note

In a good state of training, the triceps brachii muscle can already be recognised in the visual findings. This can make the subsequent palpation even easier (Fig. 5.66).

5.8.2 Palpation of the Anconeus Muscle

Joint capsules connect and protect the corresponding bony joint partners. In addition, they ensure sufficient production of synovial fluid, which supplies the joint with nutrients. The capsule must move dynamically during mobilisation of the joint and must not be trapped between the joint partners. To prevent this, muscles come into contact with the joint capsule. The anconeus muscle is one of these capsule tighteners, which is located posterior to the elbow. The small superficial triangular muscle originates at the lateral humeral epicondyle, the ulnar collateral ligament and the capsule and runs distomedially to the lateral side of the olecranon. Partial fibres also extend to the proximal part of the posterior surface of the ulna and to the capsule. It is innervated via the radial nerve from segments C7–Th1 and is functionally responsible for tensioning the capsule, as mentioned above. Furthermore, it supports extension in the elbow joint and guides the ulna during pronation movements in the radioulnar joints.

The superficial anconeus muscle can be palpated by stimulating the fingertips. For this purpose, the patient is in a prone or lateral position or in a sitting position and the therapist, standing at the side, makes contact with the olecranon of the ulna of the stretched arm with the index finger. Starting from this reference point, the finger moves one to two transverse fingers distally and one transverse finger laterally. It is now located directly in the middle between the ulnar edge and the proximal radioulnar art and thus directly on the anconeus muscle. A more precise differentiation can be made by actively tensing the arm into extension, whereupon the anconeus muscle contracts and can thus be felt even better.

Implementation Note

If the olecranon bursa is irritated, direct pressure over the fingertips may produce pain near the olecranon (Fig. 5.67).

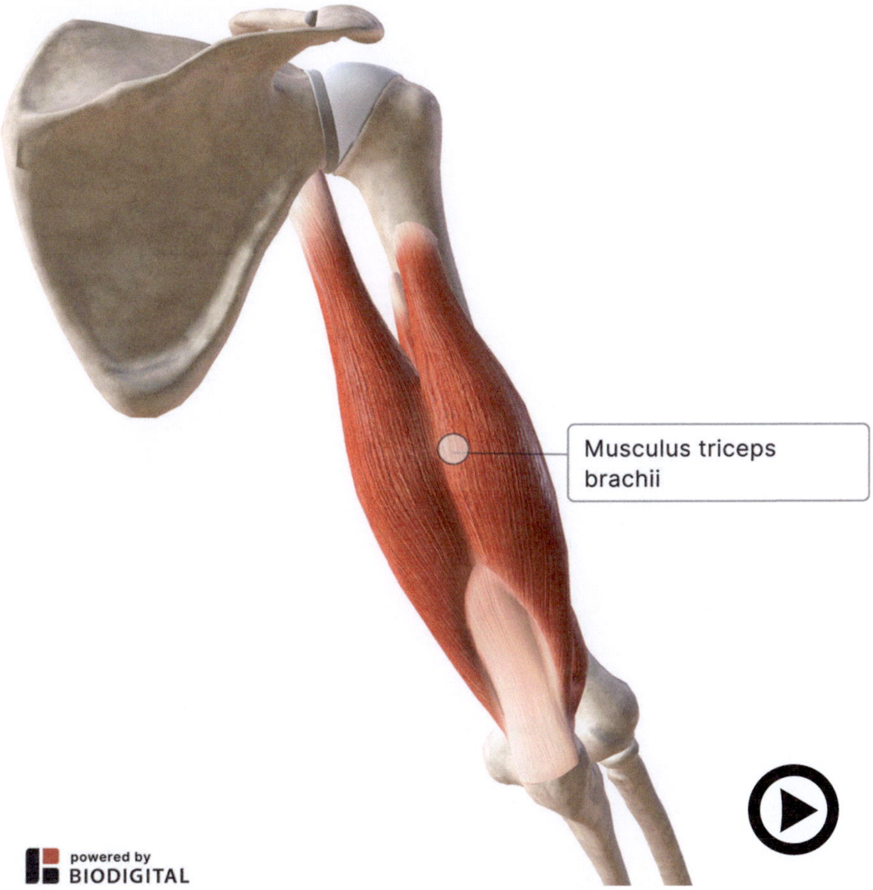

Fig. 5.66 Anatomy and palpation of the M. triceps brachii (▶ https://doi.org/10.1007/000-cvc)

5.8.3 Palpation of the Brachialis Muscle

An important flexor at the elbow is the brachialis muscle, which is located directly anterior to the humerus under the biceps brachii muscle. This rather broad muscle protrudes medially and laterally from the edge of the biceps brachii muscle and contributes a great deal to the muscle relief of the arm, even though it is not directly superficial. The humerus muscle originates at the facies anterior as well as the margo anterior of the humerus and at the septum intermusculare brachii mediale and laterale. The distally projecting broad muscle belly ends in a strong tendon, which inserts on the ulnar tuberosity as well as the anterior surface of the proc. coronoideus and part of the joint capsule. The nerve supply is provided by the musculocutaneous nerve and the radial nerve from segments C5–C7. Functionally, the brachialis muscle, as already mentioned at the beginning, ensures strong flexion in the elbow joint, as it only pulls across one joint. It also tightens the capsule anteriorly.

For palpation, the patient is positioned supine while the therapist stands sideways. The homolateral arm is positioned passively so that the hand rests on the abdomen. The therapist's distal hand grips the client's wrist, and the proximal hand is positioned with the palm anterior to the upper arm. Now the client is asked to perform flexion at the elbow joint against resistance so that the biceps brachii muscle is exposed under the proximal hand. Under this tension, the fingertips palpate the muscle edges from medial and lateral. After the resistance has been removed and the patient's arm is again in a passive position, the muscle belly of the biceps brachii muscle is moved medially or laterally so that the fingertips can palpate in the direction of the humerus. In depth, the stimulus is now applied to the brachialis muscle, which can be followed and felt up to its tendon attachment to the coronoid muscle of the ulna.

Implementation Note

As the ulnar nerve extends along the medial edge of the muscle and the radial nerve along the lateral edge, palpation should be started gently. Various radiating sensations in the direction of the thumb or side of the little finger may be due to nervous structures (Fig. 5.68).

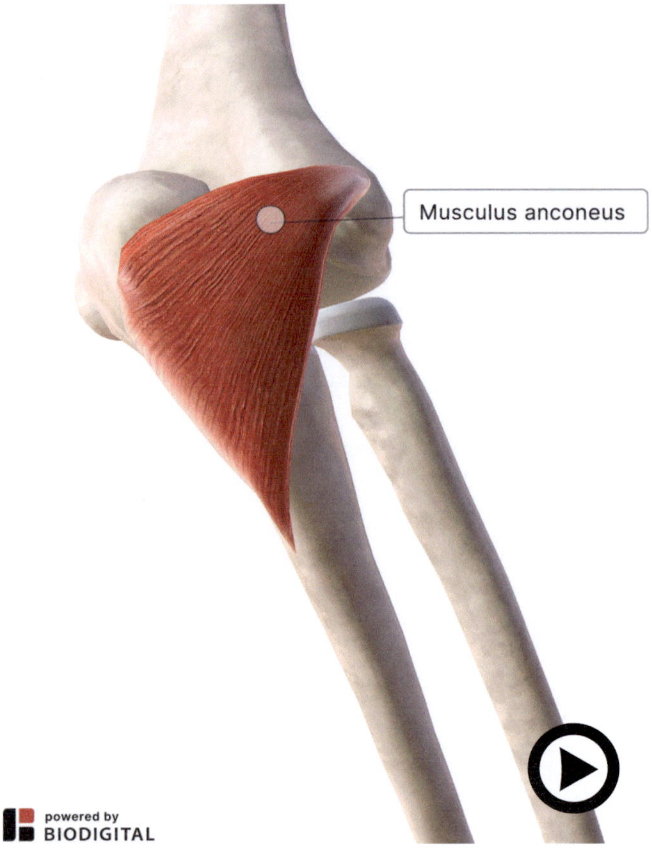

Fig. 5.67 Anatomy and palpation of the M. anconeus (▶ https://doi.org/10.1007/000-cvd)

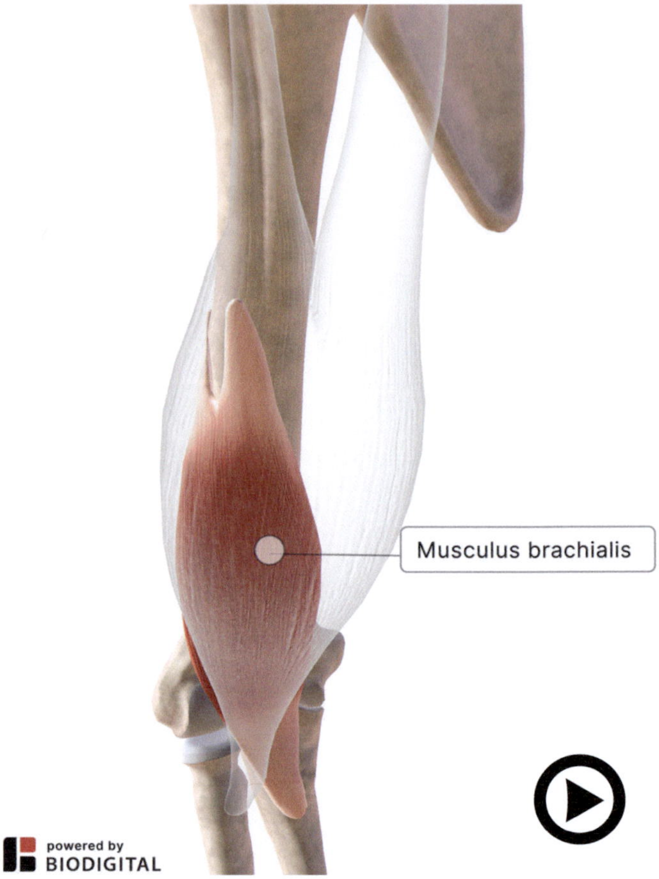

Fig. 5.68 Anatomy and palpation of the M. brachialis (▶ https://doi.org/10.1007/000-cve)

5.8.4 Palpation of the Biceps Brachii Muscle

The two-headed humerus muscle has two large, thick muscle bellies, which significantly shape the relief of the upper arm. The double-jointed muscle consists of a caput longum and a caput breve, is covered proximally by the deltoid muscle and in some cases has a caput tertium, which only originates on the humerus and then radiates into the muscle belly [21]. While the caput longum has its origin at the supraglenoid tuberosity, the caput breve originates at the proc. coracoideus of the scapula and is partially connected to the coracobrachialis muscle. Both run distally along the humerus, with the caput longum located laterally and the caput breve medially. Important in this context is the course of the long biceps tendon, which passes through the capsule into the sulcus intertubercularis within the vagina synovialis intertubercularis and under the lig. transversum humeri. Both muscle bellies open distally into a tendon, which inserts at the radial tuberosity or radiates into the aponeurosis musculi bicipitis, the so-called lacertus fibrosus of the forearm fascia. The biceps brachii muscle is innervated by the musculocutaneous nerve from segments C5–C7 and is therefore also the identifying muscle for segment C6. While the double-jointed muscle supports anteversion in the shoulder joint and the caput laterale supports abduction and internal rotation and the caput mediale supports adduction, it is responsible for flexion and supination in the elbow joint when the arm is flexed. In this context, the biceps brachii muscle is usually the strongest supinator alongside the supinator muscle [22].

Palpation of the two muscle heads is performed in the supine position with the therapist standing laterally at shoulder level. In order to feel the muscle belly, the fingertips are placed directly anteriorly in the middle of the upper arm and the client is asked to perform an active flexion in the elbow joint. The superficial biceps brachii muscle contracts noticeably. If a supination is performed in a flexed position at the same time, the palpation result can be made even more precise. The visible contraction also makes it easier to find the muscle. With precise palpation and dynamic contraction and relaxation of the muscle, even the longitudinal groove that separates the two abdomens can be felt.

The tendon of origin of the caput longum is palpated proximally on the humerus via the index finger berry. To do this, first locate the greater tuberosity (see Sect. 2.9). Starting from this reference point, the finger wanders in an anteromedial direction along the bone and will perceive a crossing,

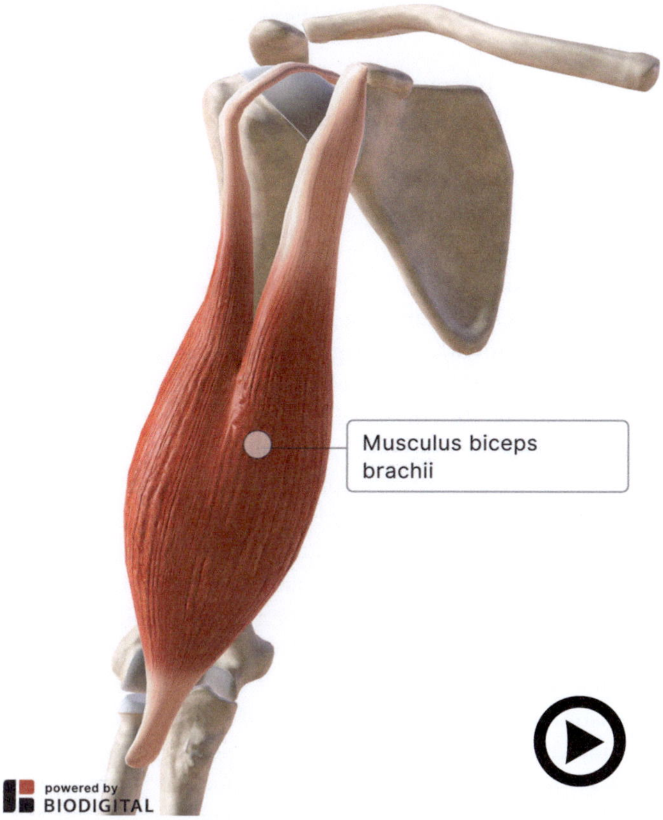

Fig. 5.69 Anatomy and palpation of the M. biceps brachii (▶ https://doi.org/10.1007/000-cvf)

lace-like structure if it runs horizontally. This tendon, located in the sulcus intertubercularis, is directly that of the caput longum of the biceps brachii muscle.

The insertion is determined by palpation by placing the index or middle finger centrally in the bend of the elbow and the patient actively performing flexion. Two tendons can be felt. The medial one is that of the brachialis muscle and leads to the proc. coronoideus, while the lateral tendon, that of the biceps brachii muscle, leads to the radial tuberosity. To feel this insertion, supination is performed with the elbow passively in flexion. This movement causes the radial tuberosity to move anteriorly so that the fingertips, which are steeply positioned in the crook of the elbow, are pushed out of this depression.

Implementation Note
Irritation of the long biceps tendon may cause pressure-soluble areas in the region of the intertubercular sulcus (Fig. 5.69).

5.9 Forearm Muscles

The antebrachium has a high number of muscles that control the precise and highly complex movements of the hand. For this fine adjustment, muscle groups are available that can be divided into a dorsal and ventral, respectively, superficial and deep, layer as well as a radial muscle group. In the following chapters, the individual groups are presented and the anatomical position as well as the sensation of the respective muscles in the complex is described. As the muscles are usually close together, direct and precise palpatory differentiation is difficult, which is why they are described in the grouping. Depending on the anatomy, the dorsal muscles are more likely to be palpated in the supine or sitting position. For the ventrally located muscles, the starting position in the prone or sitting position is recommended.

5.9.1 Palpation of the Dorsal Superficial Group

The group of dorsal superficial forearm muscles includes, in order from radial to ulnar, the extensor digitorum muscle, the extensor digiti minimi muscle and the extensor carpi ulnaris muscle. All three muscles originate at the condyle lateralis humeri, run obliquely distoulnar and are innervated via the radial nerve from segments C6–C8. Only the differentiated attachments allow for different functions of the muscles.

The flexor digitorum muscle inserts via the dorsal aponeurosis at the middle and distal phalanx of the digiti II–V and thus performs dorsal extension on the above-mentioned phalanges and associated proximal and interphalangeal joints. It also supports finger spreading and dorsal extension of the wrist and elbow joints.

The extensor digiti minimi muscle, as its name suggests, inserts via the dorsal aponeurosis on the proximal and distal phalanx of the little finger. Because of this insertion, it carries out the extension of the metacarpophalangeal joint and the interphalangeal joints of the little finger. In addition, it supports the abduction of the digitus V as well as the dorsal extension and ulnar abduction of the wrist and the extension of the elbow joints.

The extensor carpi ulnaris muscle, which is located furthest dorsally in this group, inserts at the base of the os metacarpale V and can thus perform ulnar abduction as well as extension in the wrist and extension of the elbow joints.

For palpation of the dorsal superficial muscle group, the patient is placed in a supine or sitting position with the art. cubiti slightly flexed. The therapist, standing sideways, first places the hand flatly in the proximal dorsal region of the forearm. The patient begins to dynamically perform a dorsal extension of the index finger, which leads to a noticeable contraction of the extensor digitorum muscle. If the patient performs the movement with the third, fourth and fifth fingers, the entire muscle belly can be felt. Palpation of the individual muscle cords is done with the finger berries raised, palpating the muscle distally to the dorsum of the hand. The extensor tendons, which begin at about the level of the wrist, are often already visible in advance. In order to feel the tendon dorsally on the phalanges, active dorsal extension of the fingers and palpation transverse to the course are necessary.

The same procedure is used to feel the extensor digiti minimi muscle, which connects ulnar to the extensor digitorum muscle. The muscle belly and the tendon can be located by moving the little finger over the fingertips.

For palpation of the extensor carpi ulnaris muscle, which connects ulnarward to the extensor digit minimi muscle, it is recommended to place the forearm passively on a support and with the elbow joint slightly flexed. The therapist applies his fingertips centrally on the ulnar edge while the patient performs an active ulnar abduction of the hand. During this movement, a contraction under the finger berries is directly perceptible, and the muscle can be felt in its course.

As all three muscles originate at the lateral humeral condyle, the origo can be felt by directly palpating the bony prominence. This is described in more detail in the section on bony palpation of the humerus (see Sect. 2.9).

Implementation Note

In the area of origin, overloading can lead to irritation known as epicondylopathia lateralis humeri or tennis elbow. Palpation in this region should therefore begin gently so as not to trigger over-irritation (Fig. 5.70).

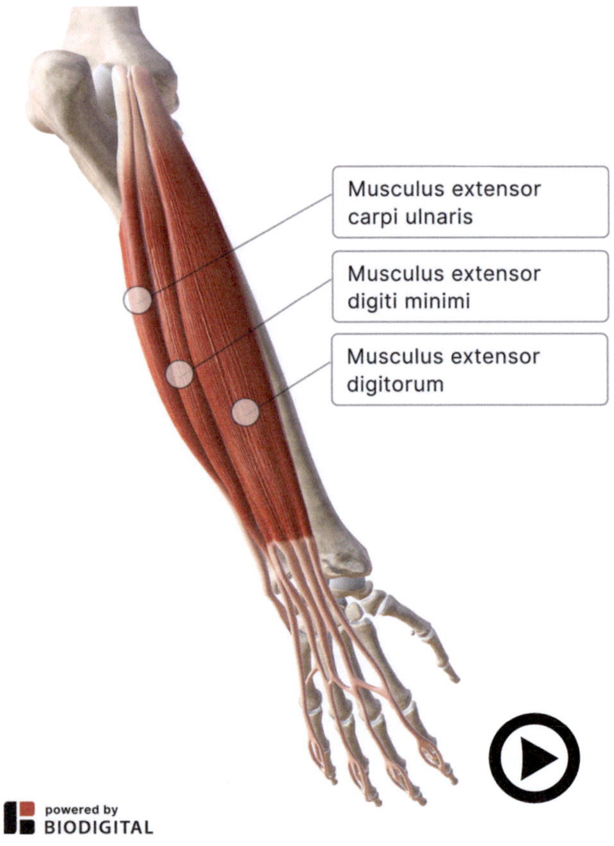

Fig. 5.70 Anatomy and palpation of the musculature of the dorsal surface group of the antebrachium (▶ https://doi.org/10.1007/000-cvg)

5.9.2 Palpation of the Dorsal Deep Group

The dorsal, deep forearm muscle group consists of the supinator muscle, the abductor pollicis longus muscle, the extensor pollicis brevis and longus muscle and the extensor indicis muscle. All the muscles in this group are innervated via the radial nerve from the brachial plexus with a segmental assignment of C5–C8. In this chapter, all the muscles are first presented compactly in their anatomical position and then palpated in their entirety as a group.

The supinator muscle originates as a so-called outward rotator at the lateral humeral epicondyle and at the radial collateral ligament, the annular ligament and the supinator muscle crest. It encases the radius in its course and inserts in its proximal third. In keeping with its name, it performs supination in the proximal radioulnaris.

The abductor pollicis longus, which originates at the dorsal facies of the radius, the ulna and at the end of the proximal third of the interosseous membrane, runs obliquely distoradially under the supinator muscle. It passes through the first tendon sheath compartment under the retinaculum extensorum and inserts at the base of the os metacarpale I and the os trapezium from the radial side. Functionally, it lives up to its name and performs abduction in the thumb saddle joint. In addition, it supports supination in the artt. radioulnares and radial abduction in the artt. radiocarpalis.

The extensor pollicis brevis arises in the distal third of the facies dorsalis radii and the membrana interossea antebrachii. It runs obliquely distoradially, passes through the first tendon sheath under the retinaculum extensorum and forms the radial border of the foveola radialis (tabatière) above the thumb saddle joint. It finds its insertion at the base of the proximal phalanx of the pollex via its insertion tendon, which crosses the radial artery. It performs extension in the metacarpophalangeal and saddle joints and supports radial abduction and extension in the wrist.

The extensor pollicis longus arises in the medial third of the ulna and the interosseous membrane antebrachii and follows a distoradial course comparable to that of the extensor pollicis brevis. In the third tendon sheath compartment, it passes under the retinaculum extensorum, then passes over the Lister's hump and forms the ulnar border of the tabatière. The insertion tendon crosses over, as does that of the extensor pollicis brevis muscle, but the radial artery attaches dorsally to the base of the distal phalanx of the pollex. Thus, the extensor pollicis longus can perform extension and radial abduction in the wrist, adduction in the thumb saddle joint and extension in the proximal and interphalangeal joints.

The extensor indicis muscle is a slender muscle with its origin in the distal area of the dorsal facies of the ulna and on the interosseous membrane. In the fourth tendon compartment, it runs obliquely distoradially under the retinaculum extensorum and inserts via a long tendon in the dorsal aponeurosis of the second finger. Due to its location, it performs extension in the wrist and the proximal, middle and distal joints of the second finger. In addition, it is responsible for adduction of the index towards the middle finger.

The palpatory exploration of the group of dorsal deep forearm muscles is done as in the order listed above, since the muscles from proximal to distal or radial to ulnar in this course are localised dorsally on the forearm. The patient is placed in a supine or sitting position. The therapist stands sideways and feels the structures on the homolateral side. Numerous muscles and tendons can be felt through the movements described at the beginning, but in some cases, only indirect stimulation of the structures listed is possible, as these are partly superimposed.

To palpate the supinator muscle, the thumb and index finger enclose the radius from the dorsal proximal third in a lumbrical grip. The contours of the muscle can then be perceived during active supination. The muscle is palpated in depth via the steeply placed fingertips. Starting from the distal end of the supinator muscle, the steeply positioned fingertips move one transverse finger in the direction of the ulna. The patient is then asked to move the thumb dynamically in the direction of abduction, against the resistance of the support. These movements, which take place around a radioulnar axis, will force the abductor pollicis longus muscle into a perceptible contraction. If the fingertips trace the muscle belly distally, it becomes increasingly palpable in the distal third, dorsal to the radius. Once in this area, the flatly placed fingertips move one transverse finger in the ulnar direction. The patient is asked to perform an extension of the thumb, which leads to a noticeable contraction of the extensor pollicis brevis muscle. The movement, which takes place around a dorsopalmar axis, guides the palpation fingers along the muscle tendon in a distoradial direction to an ascending tendon that forms the radial border of the tabatière. Starting from this tendon, directly one transverse finger in the ulnar direction, another tendon emerges during extension of the thumb. This is that of the extensor pollicis longus muscle and can be traced proximally over the fingertips. Here, too, a dynamic movement of the thumb in extension is useful to achieve a more precise feeling of palpation. Starting from the muscle belly of the extensor pollicis longus muscle in the distodorsal third of the radius, the fingertips again move one transverse finger in the ulnar direction and directly reach the extensor indicis muscle. This is felt during the active dynamic movement of the index finger in extension with the finger berries laid flat during the tendon towards the distal. It should be noted that the tendons of the extensor digitorum are also located in this region.

Implementation Note

In the case of tendovaginitis stenosans in the area of the forearm extensors, there may be increased pressure dolences in this region on palpation (Fig. 5.71).

5.9.3 Palpation of the Ventral Superficial Group

The superficial forearm muscles on the palm side are divided from radial to ulnar and consist of the pronator teres muscle, the flexor carpi radialis muscle, the palmaris longus muscle, the flexor digitorum superficialis muscle and the flexor carpi ulnaris muscle. All the muscles of this unit, except for the pronator teres muscle, perform palmar flexion in the wrist together and, except for the flexor carpi ulnaris muscle, are innervated by the median nerve from the brachial plexus through segments C6–Th1. The flexor carpi ulnaris receives its motor control via the ulnar nerve of the brachial plexus. While the anatomical description of the position is given compactly and individually for each muscle, the palpatory procedure with the patient in the supine or sitting position is described as a complex at the end of this chapter.

The flexor carpi radialis arises at the epicondylus medialis humeri and runs distoradially diagonally across the ulna. In the palm of the hand, it tangents the os scaphoideum and the os trapezium from the palm until it finds its insertion at the base of the os metacarpale II and partly III. In the elbow joints, it supports flexion and pronation, while in the wrist, it performs palmar flexion and radial abduction.

The humeral caput of the pronator teres arises from the medial humeral epicondyle, the antebrachial fascia and the intermuscular septum, while the ulnar caput originates from the ulnar coronoid muscle. Between these two heads, the median nerve runs in the so-called median tunnel, while the radial artery runs above it and the ulnar and brachial arteries run below the muscle. Due to its anatomy, it therefore forms the leading muscle for the median nerve. It inserts at the facies lateralis as well as the margo anterior in the medial area of the radius and, true to its name, performs flexion in the elbow joints and pronation in the artt. radioulnares.

The spindle-shaped palmaris longus muscle, which is inconstant, originates from the medial humeral epicondyle [23]. It first runs distally along the ulna, then crosses it in the direction of the radius in about the middle third of the bone, runs above the retinaculum flexorum and finally radiates into the palmar aponeurosis. In addition to synergistic flexion and pronation in the forearm, it performs palmar flexion of the wrists and simultaneously tenses the palmar aponeurosis.

The large flexor digitorum superficialis has three heads, each with a different origin. The humeral caput originates from the medial humeral epicondyle. The caput ulnare, on the other hand, originates from the proc. coronoideus of the ulna and the fascia antebrachii. The caput radiale originates from the radial tuberosity. All three muscle origins run distally under the retinaculum flexorum through the canalis carpalis and end in four end tendons, which split into two parts at the insertion, in each case laterally at the medial phalanxes II–V. Between this split, the caput radiale runs through the

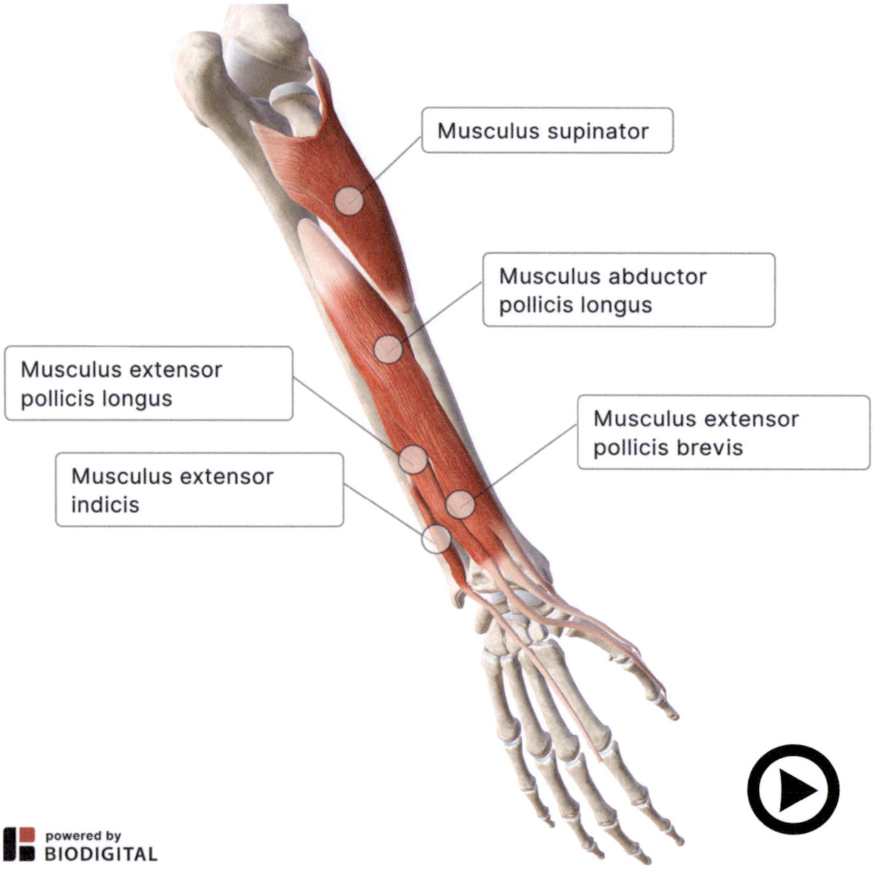

Fig. 5.71 Anatomy and palpation of the the musculature of the dorsal depth group of the antebrachium (▶ https://doi.org/10.1007/000-cvh)

tuberositas radii. The tendon of the flexor digitorum profundus runs between these splits. While the m. flexor digitorum superficialis performs flexion in the art. humeroulnare, it supports palmar flexion in the wrist as well as flexion of the fingers II–V in the proximal and proximal interphalangeal joint.

The most ulnar of the group, the flexor carpi ulnaris, arises via the caput humerale on the epicondylus medialis humeri and via the caput ulnare on the medial side of the ulnar olecranon. It runs distally along the ulna and guides the vena, arteria and ulnar nerve, thus representing their leading structure. The end tendon of the flexor carpi ulnaris runs above the retinaculum flexorum and inserts at the hamulus ossis hamati, the base of the metacarpal V and the os pisiforme. Due to its location, it can perform palmar flexion and ulnar abduction in the wrist.

When palpating this muscle group, with the patient seated or supine with forearms rotated into supination, the therapist standing to the side first applies his or her distal hand flat on the proximoulnar inner forearm surface. The patient is then asked to actively move his hand into palmar flexion, which leads to a noticeable contraction of the ventral superficial forearm muscles. Directly in the centre of this group, at the distal end of the proximal third of the ulna, the muscle belly of the flexor carpi radialis muscle becomes palpable as it lies superficial and partially covers surrounding muscles. If the already steeply erect fingertips move in a radial direction, a depression becomes noticeable at the edge of the muscle. The fingers remain in this depression, and while the patient performs pronation in the forearm, a contraction of the pronator teres muscle is made possible. If the fingers move from the starting point in the ulnar direction, the palmaris longus muscle, if present, joins after the palpable muscle edge. In the distal area of this muscle, the tendon can be felt and partly already recognised in the visual findings if it is present. To do this, the patient, with palmar flexed wrists, actively moves the tip of his thumb towards the tip of his little finger. The tendon of the palmaris longus palmar rises at the wrist. The tendon that is located directly radial to it is that of the flexor carpi radialis muscle. The steeply positioned fingertips feel along the palmaris longus muscle or, if not present, along the flexor carpi radialis muscle, approximately to the medial third of the forearm and again feel a depression in the ulnar direction. Directly in this depression, a stimulus can be applied to the flexor digitorum superficialis muscle, which is almost completely covered by the flexor carpi radialis muscle. This finger flexor can also be reached in the medial third of the forearm between the pronator teres muscle and the

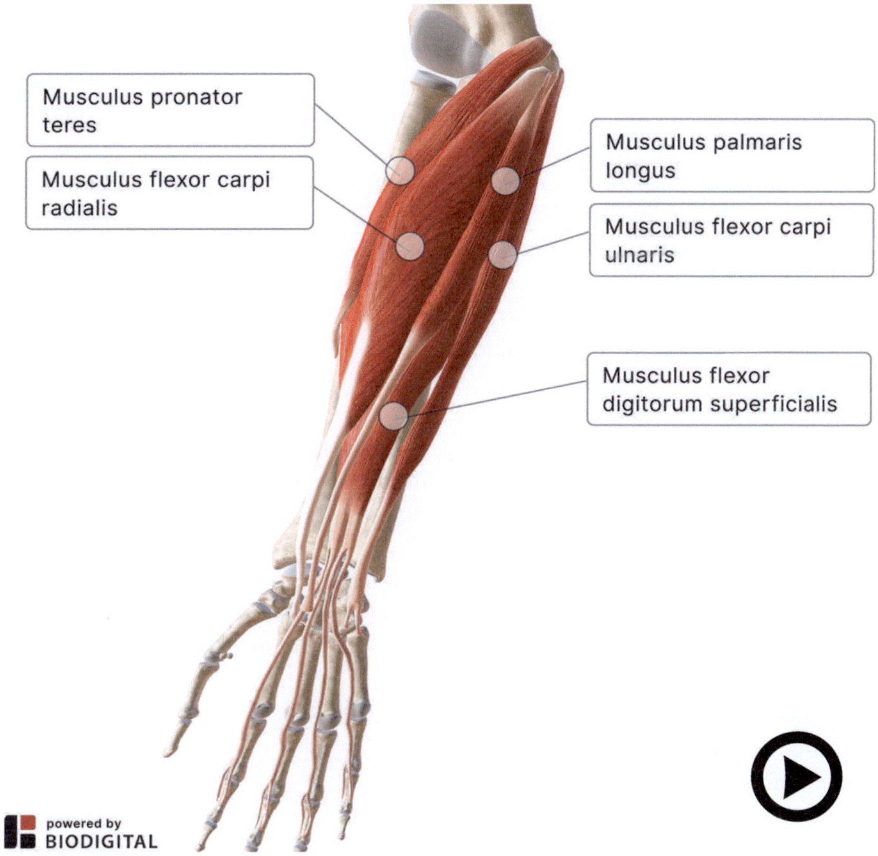

Fig. 5.72 Anatomy and palpation of the the musculature of the ventral surface group of the antebrachium (▶ https://doi.org/10.1007/000-cvj)

flexor carpi radialis muscle by applying a stimulus in depth. In addition, the tendons of the muscle become clearly perceptible and partly visible as soon as the patient actively moves the fingers II–V in flexion. With a dynamic change between contraction and decontraction, the muscle belly can already be inspected. For palpation of the flexor carpi ulnaris muscle, the fingertips are placed on the proximal ulnar forearm edge, and the patient is asked to perform ulnar abduction of the wrists. During this movement, the muscle will be revealed by contraction, and its course will be clearly palpable. Distally, its attachment tendon in the palmoulnar region of the wrist can be clearly grasped in a pincer grip.

Implementation Note
In acute epicondylopathia medialis humeri, or golfer's elbow, the region of origin may show increased sensitivity on palpation [24].

Due to the existing anatomical proximity, palpation of the pronator teres muscle can lead to irritation of the median nerve [25] (Fig. 5.72).

5.9.4 Palpation of the Ventral Deep Group

The flexor digitorum profundus, flexor pollicis longus and pronator quadratus muscles form the ventral deep forearm muscles. They are predominantly covered by the muscles from the superficial group and are therefore only sparsely accessible via stimulation. In the following, the muscles are first presented individually in their anatomical course, and instructions for palpation are given individually. The patient is in the sitting position with the arm in a passive position or optionally in the supine position.

The flexor digitorum profundus muscle originates as a deep finger flexor from the facies anterior to the proximal two-thirds of the ulna and the palmar membrana interossei antebrachii. The muscle belly is completely covered by the flexor digitorum superficialis muscle and extends distally along the ulna. The flexor digitorum profundus muscle divides into four end tendons that run under the retinaculum flexorum and insert palmately on the terminal phalanges of the 2nd–5th fingers. The innervation of the muscle by the median nerve and the ulnar nerve from the segments C7 to Th1 enables it to perform flexion in the wrist and the proximal, middle and distal joints of the fingers II–V.

For palpation of the flexor digitorum profundus, the therapist uses the ulnar artery as a guide, tracing it ventrally over the fingertips of the index and middle fingers, initially in the distal third of the ulna. Directly below the artery, a stimulus can be applied to the muscle belly with the fingertips steeply placed. Other areas of the muscle are covered by the flexor digitorum superficialis muscle and are therefore not directly palpable.

The flexor pollicis longus arises on the palmar side in the medial third of the facies anterior to the radius and the membrana interossea antebrachii. In its course, which follows the radius steeply distally, it is completely covered by the flexor digitorum superficialis muscle. The tendon of the muscle runs below the retinaculum flexorum through the carpal tunnel and inserts palmar sided at the distal phalanx of the thumb. The flexor pollicis longus muscle is innervated by the median nerve from segments C6–C8 and performs flexion and radial abduction in the wrists as well as opposition in the thumb saddle joint and flexion in the thumb metacarpophalangeal and terminal joints.

The palpatory approach for the flexor pollicis longus muscle can only be established in the distal region of the muscle. The palpator orients to the tendon of the flexor carpi radialis muscle, which clearly emerges during active flexion of the wrist, centrally and radially of the tendon of the palmaris longus muscle, if present. In this palmar region, the index fingertip is placed steeply between the two tendons in order to apply a direct stimulus to the flexor pollicis longus muscle in depth. The sensation of palpation can be enhanced by separate flexion of the thumb.

The pronator quadratus runs from the margo anterior of the ulna in the distal quarter transversely in a laterodistal direction to the radius, to which it inserts via the facies anterior in the distal quarter. The quadratic inward rotator lives up to its name by performing pronation in the artt. radioulnares due to its location and innervation via the median nerve from segments C7–Th1. In addition, it stabilises the distal radioulnar joint.

For palpation of the pronator quadratus muscle, the therapist orientates to the radial artery in the distal lateral quarter of the radius. The origin of the muscle is located directly ulnar to this artery and can be palpated by direct stimulation with the steeply positioned fingertips. If the pronator quadratus muscle is palpated further in the ulnar direction, numerous flexor tendons located in this region make palpation difficult.

Implementation Note

Due to the spatial proximity to the carpal tunnel as well as to the retinaculum flexorum, pressure dolences, especially in this region, can occur during palpation in the event of tendon irritation (Fig. 5.73).

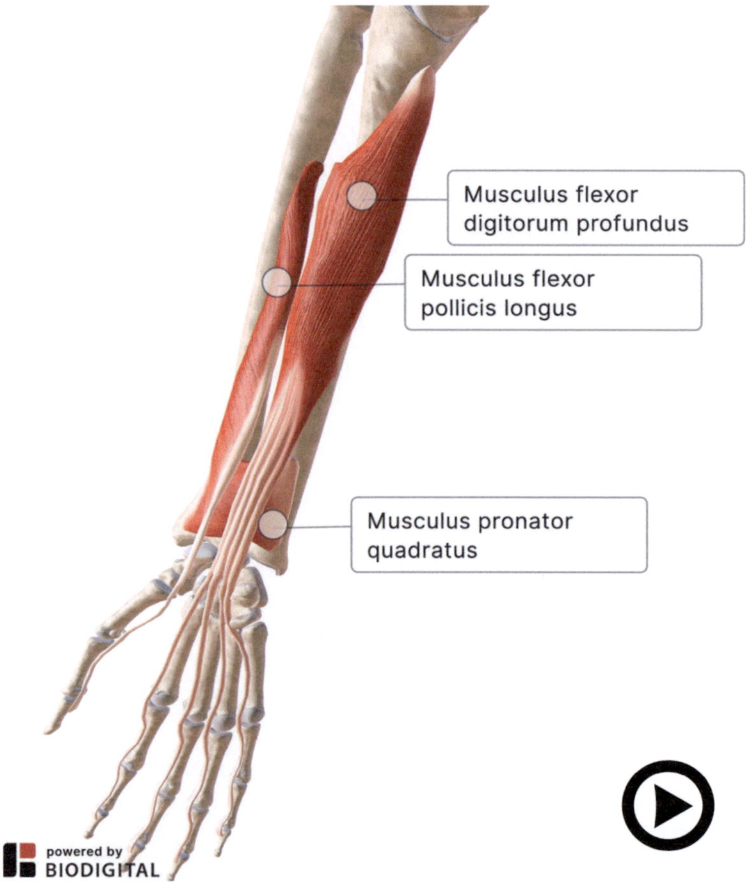

Fig. 5.73 Anatomy and palpation of the the musculature of the ventral depth group of the antebrachium (▶ https://doi.org/10.1007/000-cvk)

5.9.5 Palpation of the Radial Group

On the radial side of the forearm, the palpable muscle bellies of the brachioradialis and extensor carpi radialis longus and brevis muscles are in the proximal and medial thirds of the radius. The muscles mentioned are assigned to the radial group of forearm muscles and are presented below first separately in their anatomical course and then described as a group in relation to palpation. In addition to the common function of flexion in the art. cubiti, all muscles are innervated via the radial nerve from segments C5–C7.

The brachioradialis muscle originates from the distal third of the lateral humeral margo and the lateral brachial intermuscular septum. It extends distally along the radius and follows a similar course to the extensor carpi radialis longus muscle, finally inserting distally at the proc. styloideus radii. In addition to flexion in the elbow joint, it also performs pro- or supination in the artt. radioulnares, depending on the position of the joint.

The extensor carpi radialis longus arises at the facies lateralis of the distal humerus as well as the crista supracondylaris lateralis and the septum intermusculare laterale. In its course steeply distally and along the radius, the tendon is partially covered by the extensor carpi radialis brevis muscle. After its passage in the second tendon compartment below the retinaculum extensorum, the extensor carpi radialis longus muscle attaches dorsally to the base of the os metacarpale II. Due to its location, it also performs dorsal extension and radial abduction in the wrists in addition to flexion in the elbow joint.

With its origins at the epicondylus lateralis humeri, the lig. anulare radii and the lig. collaterale radii, the extensor carpi radialis brevis muscle is located furthest radially of this group. It also runs steeply distally along the radius, is partially overlapped proximally by the extensor carpi radialis longus muscle and runs under the retinaculum extensorum in the second tendon compartment to its insertion dorsally at the base of the os metacarpale III. Like its longer namesake, it also performs radial abduction and dorsal extension in the wrists in addition to flexion in the elbow joints.

Palpation of the radial group is performed in the sitting position with the arm passively positioned in 90° elbow flexion. The patient places his forearm on the support so that the thumb points upwards. The therapist then fixes the forearm distally while the patient tries to move his hand in the direction of the shoulder via elbow flexion. The brachioradialis muscle contracts, which can already be partially identified by the visual findings. The muscle belly can now be felt proximally in a pincer grip or by direct palpation of the fingertips, and its course can be developed distally. In the proximal area, the steeply positioned finger berries move laterally, fall into a depression after the brachioradialis muscle and are now directly on the muscle belly of the extensor carpi radialis longus muscle. As this muscle group is generally very superficial, palpation is clearly perceptible. An even more precise sensation of this muscle can be achieved by active radial abduction of the patient's hand on the pad. If the fingertips move about one transverse finger further in the radial direction, they meet directly with the muscle belly of the extensor carpi radialis brevis muscle, which is located at the outermost edge of the group and whose course can also be felt by radial abduction. As the extensor carpi radialis brevis muscle is partially covered proximally by its long fellow, it is often only palpable in the middle third.

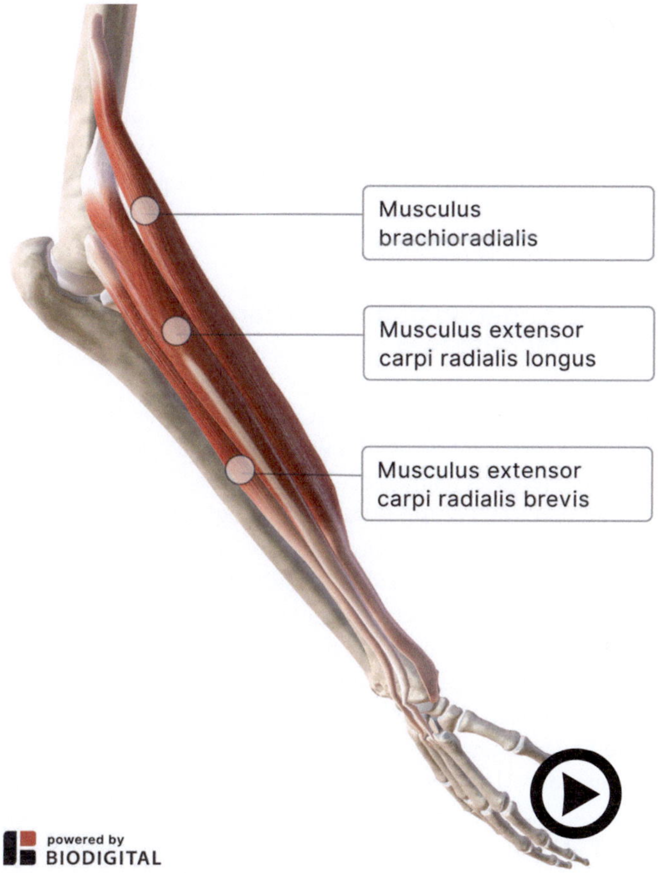

Fig. 5.74 Anatomy and palpation of the radial group (▶ https://doi.org/10.1007/000-cvm)

Implementation Note
In the case of acute lateral humeral epicondylopathy or tennis elbow, the region of origin may react with increased sensitivity on palpation (Fig. 5.74).

5.10 Hand Musculature

The "instrument of instruments," as the hand is often called, described in Sect. 3.7, can only produce the variety of movements via a highly complex system consisting of musculature. This muscular system, which controls the filigree motions, is subdivided into the group of metacarpal muscles and the thenar and hypothenar groups. In the following, the individual groups and their components are explained anatomically, and instructions for palpation are given. It is recommended to start with the client in a supine or sitting position.

5.10.1 Palpation of the Metacarpal Musculature

The palmar muscles located in the metacarpus have three members, the lumbricales I–IV, the interossei dorsales I–IV and the interossei palmares I–III.

The lumbrical muscles have their origins in the tendon of the flexor digitorum profundus muscle. The I and II muscles originate on the radial and volar sides of the tendons of the index and middle fingers, respectively, the III muscle originates from the tendons of the middle and ring fingers and the IV muscle originates from the tendons of the ring and little fingers. Muscle originates from the tendons of the ring and little finger. They run steeply distally and open into the dorsal aponeurosis of the second to fifth digits. Due to their location, they perform flexion in the proximal joints of fingers II–IV, whereas they initiate extension in the middle and distal joints. This enables innervation via the median nerve for the I and II muscles and innervation via the median nerve for the I and II muscles. This allows innervation via the median nerve for the I and II muscles and via the ulnar nerve for the III and IV muscles from segments C8–Th1, respectively.

The interossei dorsales I–IV, which fill the intermetacarpal space, are bicuspid and originate on the facing surfaces of the metacarpals in the proximal region. Thus, there are eight regions of origin, four interossei and four muscles extending distally. They insert into the dorsal aponeurosis of the II–IV fingers and at the base of the proximal phalanx of the same fingers. In this context, it is important to note that the second muscle draws from radial and ulnar to the middle finger, while the first extends to the index finger and the fourth to the ring finger. They are innervated via the ulnar nerve from segments C8–Th1 and perform flexion in proximal joints, whereas they assist extension in the middle and distal joints via the aponeurosis. In addition, they perform abduction of the II and IV fingers. They also abduct the second and fourth fingers away from the middle finger.

The interosseous palmar muscles I–III are only in contact with the index, ring and little fingers. They originate on the ulnar side of metacarpal II and the radial side of the IV and V metacarpals in the proximal region. The muscles run distally and insert into the dorsal aponeurosis and the respective proximal base of the same finger. They are innervated by the ulnar nerve from segments C8–Th1 and perform flexion in the respective proximal joints, whereas they act extensor in the middle and terminal joints. In addition, they perform adduction of the second, fourth and fourth fingers towards the middle finger.

Palpation of the metacarpal muscles is done as a group via a palmar approach. A stimulus is applied to the intermetacarpal spaces via the pincer grip with the thumb and index finger. This results in a stimulus being applied to the palmar musculature, which cannot be more precisely palpated. The fact that there is no part of the interosseous palmar muscles I–III in the space between D1 and D2 can be used as a means of differentiation (Fig. 5.75).

5.10.2 Palpation of the Thenar Muscle Group

The ball of the thumb is formed by the thenar muscle group, which consists of the abductor pollicis brevis muscle, the adductor pollicis muscle, the flexor pollicis brevis muscle and the opponens pollicis muscle. For humans, the thumb with all its movement possibilities plays an elementary role in everyday life. Not only is it very important for grasping, but it is also increasingly used for feeling. Another challenge arose with the introduction of the mobile phone. Here, it is used to write messages and perform other activities on the mobile phone. The filigree as well as powerful movements are realised via the muscles already mentioned, which are described below in their anatomical position and then developed as a group by palpation.

The abductor pollicis brevis muscle is located superficially and arises at the tuberculum ossis scaphoidei of the os scaphoideum and at the os trapezium of the palmar and retinaculum musculorum flexorum. In its distal course, along the palmar metacarpal I, it covers the flexor pollicis brevis muscle and the opponens pollicis muscle until it inserts via the radial sesamoid bone at the base of the proximal phalanx and proportionally at the joint capsule. By means of innervation via the median nerve from segments C6–C7, it performs abduction in the thumb saddle joint and thus also supports opposition, while it performs flexion in the metacarpophalangeal joint.

The adductor pollicis muscle can be divided into a transverse and an oblique caput. The transverse caput originates palmar at the metacarpal III, whereas the oblique caput originates palmar at the capitatum bone, the metacarpal bone base II, III and partly IV, and palmar partly at the hamate bone and the trapezium bone. Depending on the fibrous traction, both parts run in the direction of the proximal phalanx of the thumb and thus obliquely distoradially or horizontally radially. The most powerful muscle in the ball of the thumb inserts over the ulnar sesamoid bone at the base of the proximal phalanx of the pollex and is innervated by the ulnar

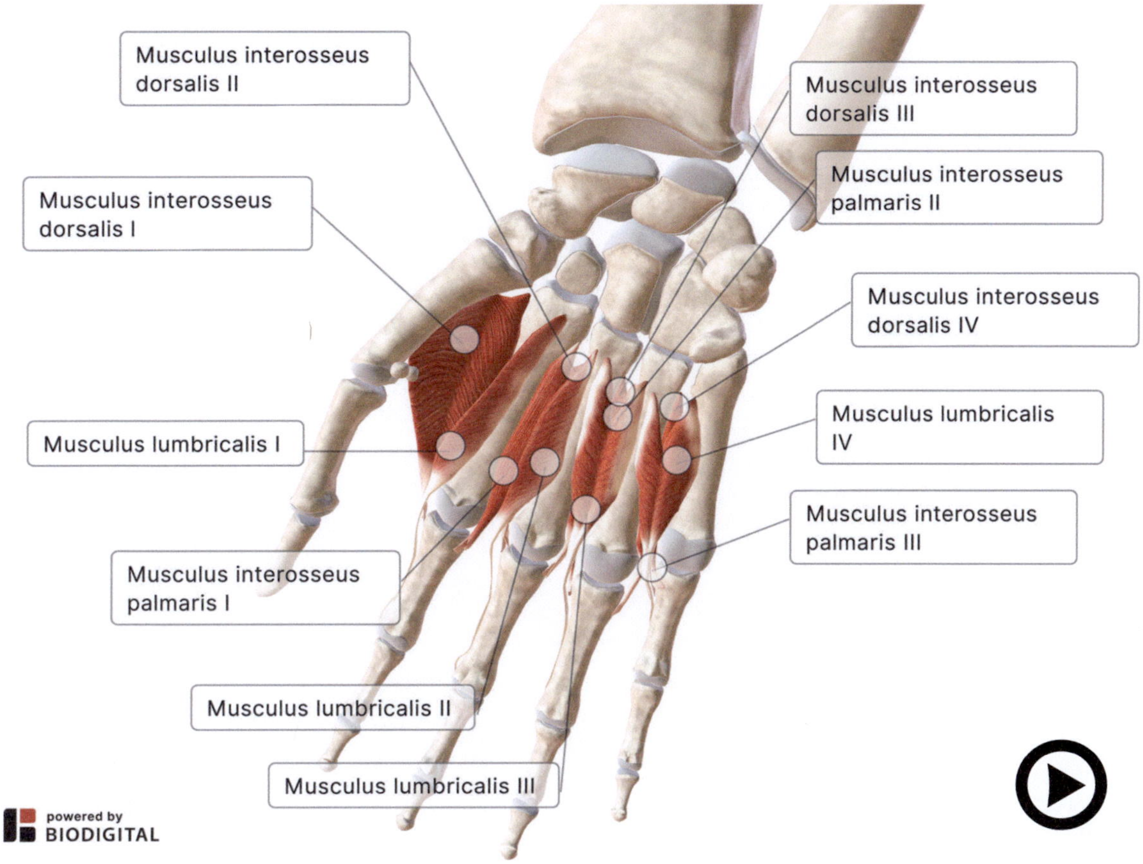

Fig. 5.75 Anatomy and palpation of the middle hand musculature (▶ https://doi.org/10.1007/000-cvn)

nerve from segments C8–Th1. Its main functions include adduction and opposition in the thumb saddle joint and flexion in the thumb metacarpophalangeal joint.

The flexor pollicis brevis muscle, which is located under the abductor pollicis brevis muscle, can be subdivided into a superficial caput, which originates at the distal edge of the retinaculum flexorum and the palmar os trapezium, and a profundal caput with its regions of origin at the os capitatum, the os trapezium and the palmar os trapezoideum. In its distoradial course, it follows the tendon of the flexor pollicis longus and the metacarpal I and inserts with the caput superficiale over the radial sesamoid bone and with the caput profundum over the ulnar sesamoid bone at the base of the proximal phalanx of the thumb. While the superficial portion is innervated by the median nerve from segments C7–Th1, the deep portion receives nerve impulses via the ulnar nerve from segments C8–Th1. Both together perform flexion and opposition in the thumb saddle joint. In the metacarpophalangeal joint of the thumb, both supported flexion as well as the superficial caput supported abduction and the profundal caput supported adduction.

The short and triangular opponens pollicis muscle forms the deepest part of the thenar muscle group and originates at the ossis trapezii tuberculum and palmar at the retinaculum flexorum and partly at the os scaphoideum. It runs distoradially and opens via a rather short tendon at the radial edge of metacarpal I. Functionally, it leads in the thumb tuberculum ossis trapezii. Functionally, it performs an opposition in the thumb saddle joint and also supports adduction and flexion.

The muscles of the ball of the thumb are palpated as a group. The patient is in a supine or sitting position while the therapist seeks contact with the homolateral ball of the thumb. The hand is first placed passively, and the palpating index and middle fingertip are placed flat and centrally in the region of the metacarpal I of palmar. Here the fingers meet directly with the abductor pollicis brevis muscle, which is located superficially. If the patient is asked to move the thumb into abduction around a radioulnar axis, the muscle belly is clearly felt due to the contraction. An opposition movement as well as flexion in the base joint can make palpation even more precise. If the fingertips move a little in the ulnar direction, they hit the space between the I and II metacarpals directly. This is also known as the web. If the therapist pinches the index finger and thumb in this space via the pincer grip and asks the patient to stretch the thumb in the direction of adduction, against his pincer grip, the flat adductor pollicis muscle is clearly felt. Starting from the same grip, the patient is now asked to move the thumb, which is

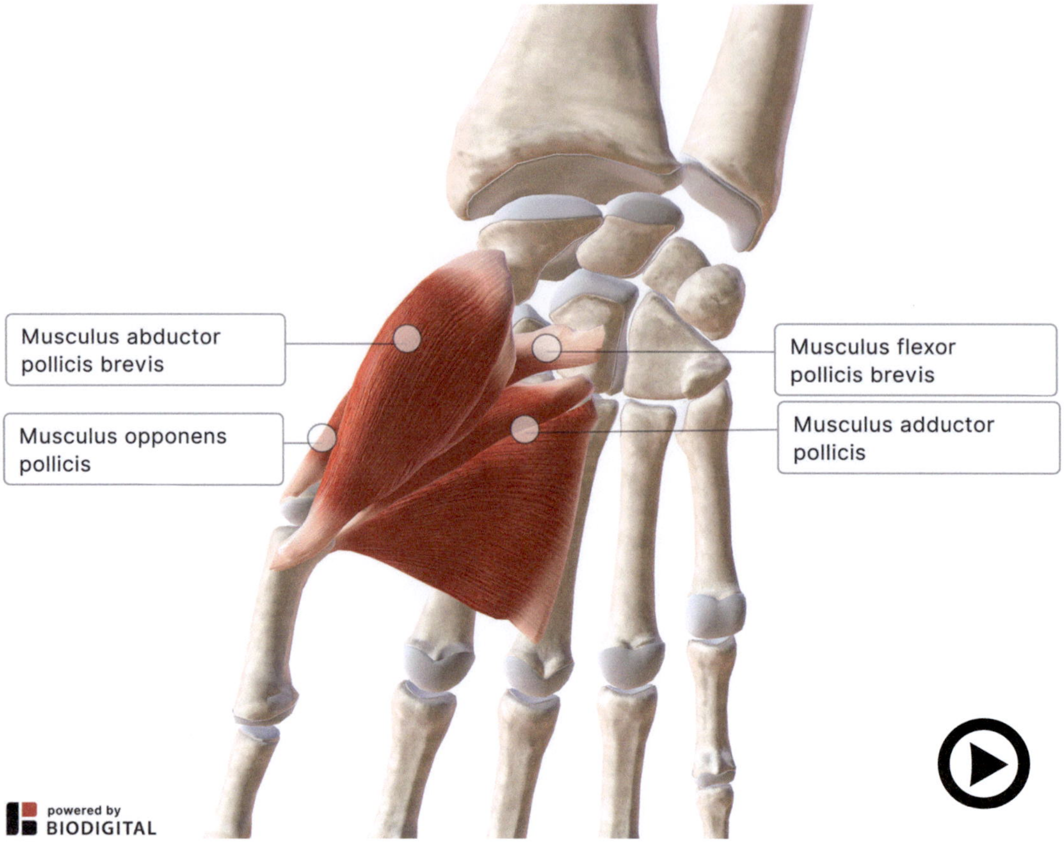

Fig. 5.76 Anatomy and palpation of the thenar group (▶ https://doi.org/10.1007/000-cvp)

passively positioned in opposition, into isolated flexion in the base joint, which clearly leads to palpable contraction of the flexor pollicis brevis muscle in the proximal area of the metacarpals from the palmar side. Palpation of the opponens pollicis muscle can only be achieved by stimulation from the pincer grip. The metacarpal I is grasped from the dorsal side with the index finger and thumb in such a way that they are applied directly to the bony edge from the radial and ulnar sides. Active opposition can then be performed, which can lead to a noticeable contraction at the radial edge if the muscle belly is not overlapped too much by the abductor pollicis brevis muscle.

Implementation Note

In carpal tunnel syndrome, there may be visible and palpable atrophy of the thenar muscle group (Fig. 5.76).

5.10.3 Palpation of the Hypothenar Muscle Group

The muscle group that forms the ball of the little finger in the palmar region consists of the palmaris brevis muscle, the abductor digiti minimi muscle, the flexor digiti minimi brevis muscle and the opponens digiti minimi muscle. The hypothenar muscle group is elementary for grasping, as it essentially moves the little finger in the direction of the thumb, which is essential for both a powerful and precise grip. All four muscles are innervated by the ulnar nerve from segments C8–Th1, and their anatomical location is described below. The overview is followed by instructions for palpation, which covers the entire muscle group. The patient is positioned in the supine or sitting position.

The superficially located m. palmaris brevis stretches as a square muscle from the ulnar edge of the palmar aponeurosis in the region of the art. metacarpophalangealis IV and V in the ulnodistal direction and inserts on the skin of the hypothenar. It tightens the skin in this region as well as the palmar aponeurosis if the palmaris longus muscle (see Sect. 5.9.3) is not present.

The abductor digiti minimi muscle is largely responsible for the shape of the hypothenar. It originates at the os pisiforme and at ligamentous structures of the retinaculum flexorum and the tendon of the m. flexor carpi ulnaris. Its muscle belly, which runs steeply distally along metacarpal V, opens ulnarly at the base of the proximal phalanx of the digitus minimus and in the dorsal aponeurosis. Due to its anatomical position, it performs flexion and abduction in the proximal phalangeal joint, whereas it moves distally following phalanges in extension.

The flexor digiti minimi brevis muscle is located below the abductor digiti minimi muscle and originates from the hamulus ossis hamati and parts of the retinaculum flexorum. Located somewhat radially of the abductor digiti minimi, it follows the same course distally and inserts at the base of the proximal phalanx of the little finger and with some fibres in the dorsal aponeurosis. Functionally, it performs flexion in the joint at the base of the little finger and supports adduction of the digitus quintus.

The rather short and triangular opponens digiti minimi forms the deep ulnar edge of the hypothenar. It has its origin at the hamulus ossis hamati, runs obliquely distoulnar and inserts at the facies lateralis of the metacarpal V in the distal third. The opponens digiti minimi muscle is also called the little finger opposition because it contributes to the curvature of the palm and moves the metacarpal V towards the palmar.

To palpate the ball of the little finger, the therapist uses the pincer grip to encompass the tissue located proximoulnar to metacarpal V with the index finger and thumb. The patient is then asked to move the base of the little finger towards the thumb. The small amount of movement is sufficient to produce a contraction of the hypothenar muscle group. Subsequently, the individual components can be examined separately. If the fingertips move into the palm proximal to the ball of the little finger, a stimulus is applied directly to the palmaris brevis muscle. If the fingertips are applied to the ulnar edge of the metacarpal V, they are directly on the very palpable and relatively large abductor digiti minimi muscle, which plays a decisive role in shaping the shape of the ball. Somewhat radial to the muscle and at the same time on the palmar surface of the metacarpal V is the flexor digiti minimi brevis muscle, which can be stimulated in depth via the steeply positioned fingertips. Slightly ulnar and below the abductor digiti minimi muscle, the opponens digiti minimi muscle can be stimulated in depth via the steeply positioned fingertips.

Implementation Note

In the case of damage to the ulnar nerve, a visible and palpable atrophy of the little finger ball can be recorded (Fig. 5.77).

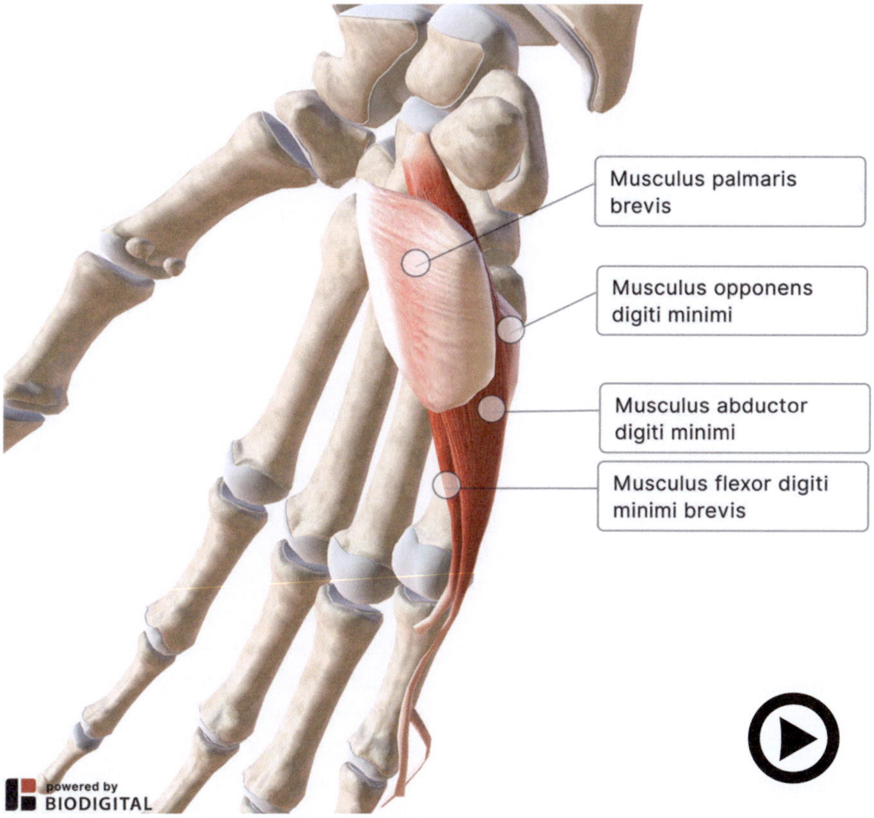

Fig. 5.77 Anatomy and palpation of the hypothenar group (▶ https://doi.org/10.1007/000-cvq)

5.11 Musculature of the Skull

Numerous muscles in the area of the skull ensure that humans can carry out everyday activities such as speaking, chewing and swallowing or communicate non-verbally with the help of facial expressions. These activities, which are essential for survival, are carried out by the musculature, which can be classified into different groups. These include the muscles of the temporomandibular joint; the supra- and infrahyoidal muscles; as well as the mimic muscles of the forehead, eye, nose, mouth, ear and tongue; the platysma; and the external eye muscles. Due to the superficial location, many of the listed structures can be felt without complications.

For palpation, the patient is placed in the supine or sitting position. In the following chapters, the individual representatives of the groups are explained in position and function, and their palpation is described.

5.11.1 Palpation of the Musculature at the Temporomandibular Joint

Chewing is an important process in the processing of food. According to experts, each bite should be chewed thoroughly before swallowing. This promotes hunger-satiety regulation in the body, facilitates nutrient breakdown and thus energy production and leads to better perception of flavours [26]. Numerous muscles are recruited for the process of chewing, and their synergy controls activity. The elementary structures in this context are the temporalis muscle, the masseter muscle and the medial and lateral pterygoid muscles. All four parts are innervated from different branches of the trigeminal nerve, which is the V cranial nerve. Depending on how much or how often a person chews during the day, in the sense of food intake but also in the sense of coping with stress, these muscles are used differently from person to person. In view of the high relevance for daily life, it is important to know the anatomical position of these muscles and to be able to palpate them. For these reasons, this chapter first describes the process in detail and then the palpation of the entire group. The patient is in the supine or sitting position.

An important component for jaw closure is the temporalis muscle [27]. This paired muscle, which is located laterally on the skull, originates extensively at the temporal fossa and the temporal fascia up to the inferior temporal line at the parietal bone and runs obliquely ventrocaudally behind the zygomatic bone. The temporalis muscle is inserted via a bundled tendon on the proc. coronoideus and the crista temporalis on the mandible. In addition to jaw closure, posterior portions of the muscle tend to perform retrusion, while anterior portions tend to initiate protrusion. In addition, it supports unilateral grinding movements. It is innervated via the temporal profundal nerve of the trigeminal nerve (V cranial nerve).

Measured by its size and leverage, the masseter muscle is an important and strong masseter muscle [28]. It is divided into the pars superficialis and the pars profundus and is located on the outside of the temporomandibular joint. The former originates at the anterior two-thirds of the arcus zygomaticus, runs obliquely posterocaudally and inserts over the tuberositas masseterica on the angulus mandibulae. The pars profundus originates at the inferior margo on the posterior third of the zygomatic arc, runs vertically caudally and inserts on the mandibular ramus. In addition to its function of closing the jaw, it supports protrusion and promotes the secretion of the parotid gland by means of the pressure created by contraction. It is innervated by the masseteric nerve of the trigeminal nerve (V cranial nerve).

The medial pterygoid muscle, which is responsible for closing the jaw, arises in the pterygoid fossa at the sphenoid bone and at the lateral lamina of the pterygoid process and runs steeply caudally, becoming somewhat wider. Close to the mandibular angulus, the muscle inserts on the inner pterygoid tuberosity. In addition to closing the jaw, the medial pterygoid muscle forms a muscle loop with the masseter muscle and supports the unilateral protrusion and thus the grinding of the food. It is innervated via the medial pterygoid nerve of the trigeminal nerve (V cranial nerve).

The lateral pterygoid muscle, which belongs to the deep layer, is composed of an inferior caput and a superior caput. While the inferior caput originates on the lateral lamina of the pterygoid process, the superior caput originates on the infratemporal facies and the infratemporal crista on the major ala of the sphenoid bone. Both muscle bellies run horizontally posterolaterally. The caput inferius attaches to the fovea pterygoidea on the proc. condylaris of the mandible. The caput superius inserts on the joint capsule and on the discus articularis of the temporomandibular joint. Functionally, the lateral pterygoid muscle serves protrusion and is the only one of this group to serve abduction (jaw opening). For this purpose, it receives its nerve control through the pterygoid lateral nerve of the same name of the trigeminal nerve (V cranial nerve).

Palpation of the temporomandibular joint muscles begins at the side of the head. The therapist applies his hand directly above the ear on the patient's skull. The patient is then asked to close and clench the jaw. During this activity, the temporalis muscle contracts. This is felt directly under the palm of the hand. During the dynamic jaw opening with subsequent jaw closing, the muscle edges can then be opened with the fingertips.

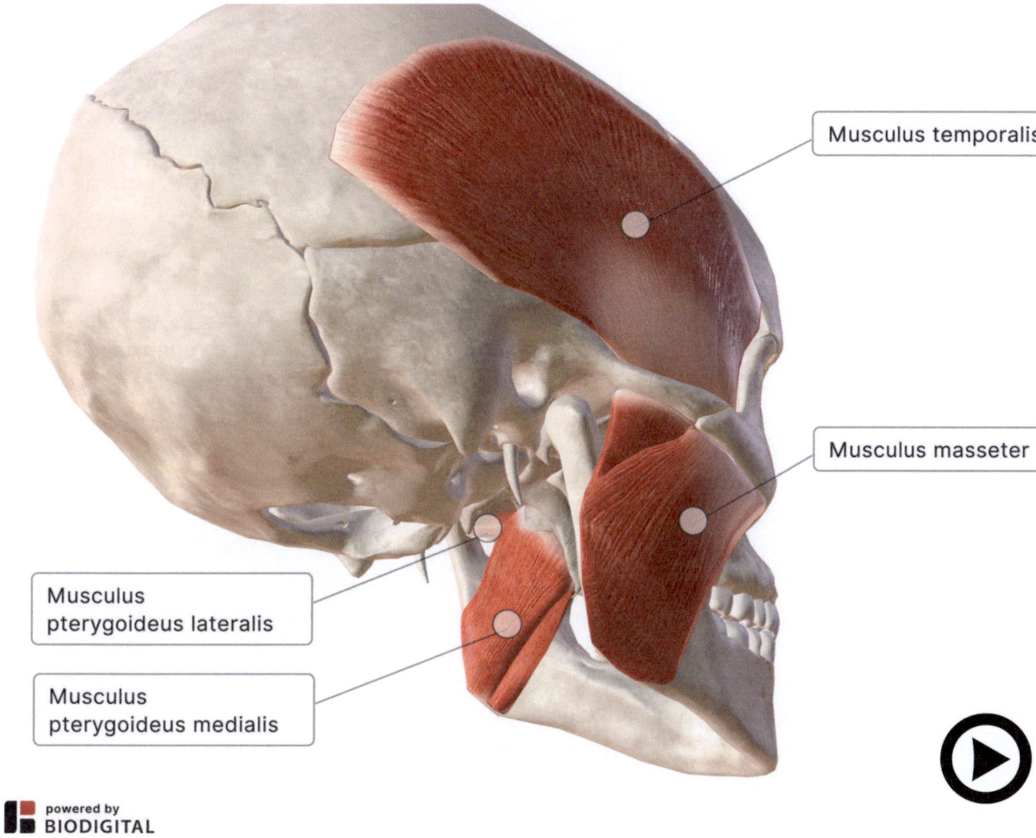

Fig. 5.78 Anatomy and palpation of the musculature of the mandibular joint (▶ https://doi.org/10.1007/000-cvr)

Two finger berries leave the lateral skull in the direction of the ear and move rostrally of the meatus acusticus externus towards the caudal. From about the level of the auditory canal, when the patient clenches again, the masseter muscle can be felt and traced in its expression. It becomes somewhat wider towards the caudal and surrounds the entire mandibular angulus from the outside. In the area below the zygomatic bone, the transverse facial artery can be felt through its pulse wave. This serves as orientation to locate the area of origin of the muscle.

If the finger berries move further around the mandibular angulus, they meet the inner surface of the mandible. When the patient closes the jaw again, a contraction impulse can also be felt in depth here. These muscle fibres are associated with the medial pterygoid muscle, which inserts in this region. Using an oral approach, the muscle belly can also be felt in depth at the posterioinferior inner edge of the mandible.

The lateral pterygoid muscle can only be palpated through the oral cavity. To do this, the patient opens the mouth and moves the lower jaw into laterotrusion to the contralateral side. The therapist uses his index or little finger and applies it between the upper jaw and the cheek of the contralateral side. Then, following the lateral side of the teeth of the upper jaw, the palpating fingertip is progressively shifted occipitally. At the end of this stretch, there is a soft final sensation. This indicates that contact has now been made with the lateral pterygoid muscle.

Implementation Note
If the patient complains of discus clicking during chewing, palpation of the lateral pterygoid muscle may cause severe pain.

In general, the temporomandibular joint musculature can lead to transferred pain to the head or teeth in the case of negative changes caused by bruxism, for example (Fig. 5.78).

5.11.2 Palpation of the Infrahyoid Muscles

The group of infrahyoid muscles is located caudally of the hyoid bone and is elementary for the caudal movement of the hyoid bone, which is essential for the swallowing process but also for phonation. The sternohyoid, sternothyroid, omohyoid, thyrohyoid and levator glandulae thyroideae muscles belong to this group, which can only be activated by stimulation. All parts are innervated via the cervical ansa profunda, from the cervical plexus from segments C1–C3 and are described in the following chapter in their anatomical position and palpation. The patient is in the supine position.

The most superficial sternohyoid muscle runs steeply cranially from the posterior edge of the manubrium and the sternal extremities of the clavicle and inserts at the lower edge of the hyoid bone.

The sternothyroid muscle originates on the dorsal surface of the manubrium and the costa prima, runs steeply cranially behind the sternohyoid muscle and inserts on the thyroid cartilage. Functionally, it moves the thyroid cartilage and thus also the larynx and hyoid bone caudally.

The longest muscle in this group is the omohyoid muscle. It has its origin at the superior margo of the scapula medial to the incisura scapulae, then runs behind the sternocleidomastoid muscle and ends in an intermediate tendon which is connected to the vagina carotica. This intermediate tendon of the inferior portion is followed by the superior portion, which runs steeply cranially and inserts at the lower edge of the os hyoideum. In addition to the functions of swallowing and phonation, the omohyoid muscle keeps the internal jugular vein open. This condition supports harmonious venous return from the head.

As a continuation of the sternothyroid muscle, the thyrohyoid muscle runs cranially from the thyroid cartilage and inserts at the lower edge of the hyoid bone. In addition to the functions already mentioned, it ensures closure of the larynx and trachea during feeding.

As a splitting off the thyrohyoid muscle, the levator glandulae thyroideae muscle runs cranially from the corpus ossis hyoidei and attaches to the isthmus glandulae thyroideae, a small tissue bridge in front of the trachea. It functionally ensures the elevation of the thyroid gland.

Palpation of the infrahyoid muscles is done by stimulation using the fingertips of the branch and middle fingers. The starting point is the os hyoideum in the anterior region of the lower edge. This is the starting point for the palpating fingertips. About one transverse finger to the right and left, they meet directly with the sternohyoid muscle, which they can follow caudally to the sternal manubrium via a stimulus. This stimulus is transmitted directly to the sternothyroid muscle, which is located directly under the first-mentioned muscle belly.

Back at the starting point of the hyoid bone, the fingertips move one transverse finger further in a lateral direction to the contralateral side and meet directly with the insertion of the omohyoideus muscle, which can only be detected by stimulation in this region. One transverse finger further in the dorsolateral direction and thus at the outer edge of the os hyoideum, the fingertips meet the thyrohyoid muscle in depth, which can also only be palpated by indirect stimulation. The levator glandulae thyroideae muscle can only be palpated by direct stimulation from anteriorly via the laryngeal prominence on the Adam's apple. Directly under the palpable tip, the fingers meet the muscle belly of the small muscle.

Implementation Note

All muscles of the infrahyoidal group can only be grasped by stimulation, as they cannot be controlled separately and arbitrarily and thus made to contract. Palpation should also be gentle, as there are numerous nervous and vascular structures in the region of the neck (Fig. 5.79).

5.11.3 Palpation of the Suprahyoid Muscles

The floor of the mouth is formed by the suprahyoid muscles and serves the swallowing process as a whole. It is composed of the digastric muscle, the mylohyoid muscle, the stylohyoid muscle and the geniohyoid muscle. The floor of the mouth thus forms the caudal end and is described below in its anatomical position as well as making the process of palpation transparent in its entirety. The patient is in a supine position with the head underneath, while the therapist stands behind the patient.

The two-bellied digastric muscle runs with its anterior venter from the digastric fossa in the anterior region of the mandible towards the posterior in the direction of the hyoid bone and is fixed to the hyoid bone in this region by an intermediate tendon. This insertion also forms the insertion of the posterior vein, which originates at the incisura mastoidea and runs in an anterioinferior direction to the hyoid bone. While the anterior part of the digastric muscle is innervated by the trigeminal nerve (V cranial nerve), the posterior part receives its nerve impulses via the facial nerve (VII cranial nerve). In addition to its involvement in yawning, speaking and swallowing, the digastric muscle positions the hyoid bone, lifts it with its anterior part and pulls it slightly towards the posterior with its posterior venter.

The mylohyoid muscle forms the basis of the floor of the mouth and arises at the linea mylohyoidea on the facies interna of the mandible in the region of the molars. The rather broad origin runs narrowly towards the posterocaudal and inserts at the corpus of the os hyoideum. At this point, it meets the base of the contralateral muscle belly. Functionally, it moves the hyoid anteriorly, raises it when the mandible is fixed and thus supports the swallowing process as well as speech and breathing, and is synergistically involved in jaw

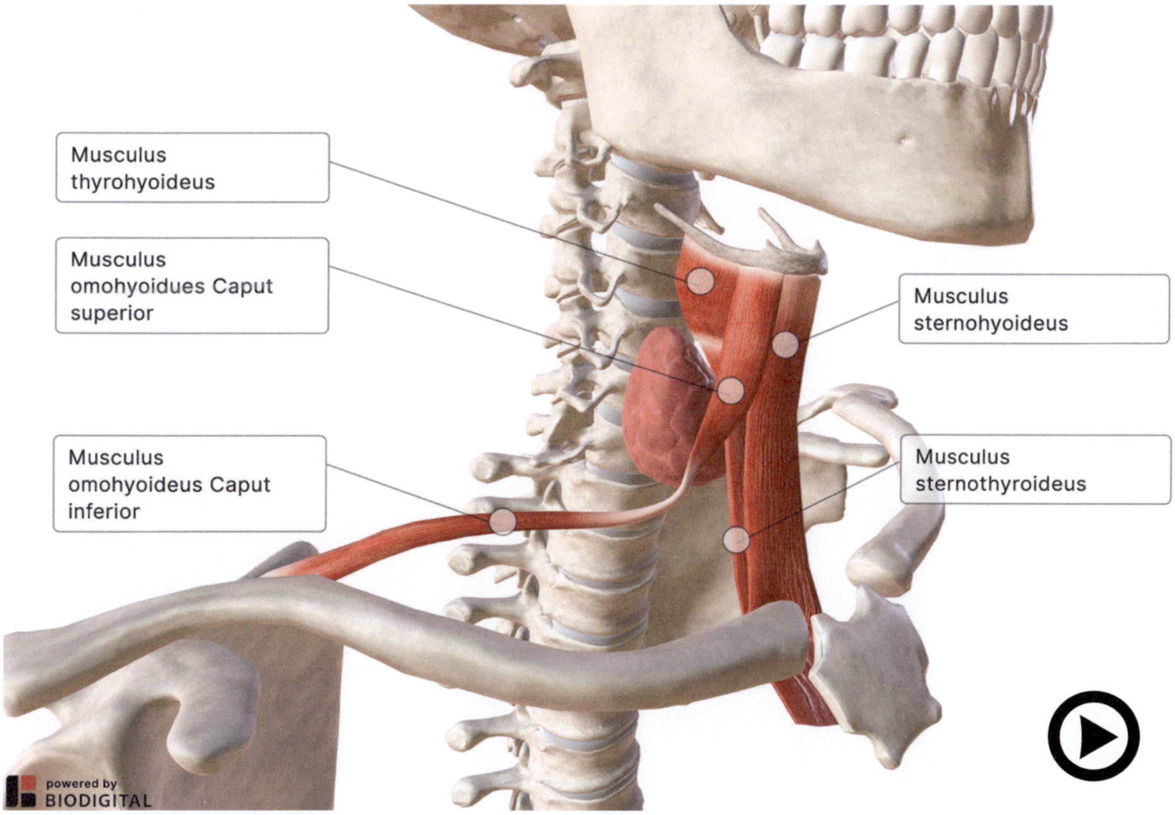

Fig. 5.79 Anatomy and palpation of the infrahyoid musculature (▶ https://doi.org/10.1007/000-cvs)

opening and grinding movements. The mylohyoid muscle receives the innervation for these movements via the trigeminal nerve (V cranial nerve).

The elongated and rather thin stylohyoid muscle originates at the proc. styloideus of the temporal bone, then runs in the anterocaudal direction and inserts at the corpus of the greater cornu and thus at the lateral edge of the hyoid bone. The muscle that serves to tense the floor of the mouth also guides the hyoid bone posterocranially and thus supports the swallowing process as well as the opening of the jaw. These activities can be realised through innervation via the facial nerve (VII cranial nerve).

The geniohyoid muscle, which originates at the spina mentalis and thus anteriorly on the inside of the mandible, runs horizontally in a straight line in the posterioinferior direction and inserts anteriorly on the corpus of the os hyoideum. It moves the hyoid bone in an anterocranial direction and thus supports the swallowing process by conveying the bolus towards the pharynx. In addition, it performs the jaw opening synergistically. The geniohyoid muscle is innervated via the cervical plexus ansa profunda from segments C1–C3.

Palpation of the suprahyoid muscles begins at the patient's chin. The therapist models the steeply positioned fingertips of the II, III and IV fingers of both hands. The therapist models the steeply positioned fingertips of the II, III and IV fingers of both hands coming from the cranial on the anterior lower edge of the mandible and thus directly under the chin. The patient then presses his tongue against the palate, which leads to a noticeable contraction of the muscle group. It should be noted that in the anterior region, a direct stimulus is applied to the anterior part of the digastric muscle as well as the underlying mylohyoid and geniohyoid muscles. Separate palpation is not possible. If the flexed fingers move posteriorly along the inner edge of the mandible, they meet the mylohyoid muscle in the middle third of the mandible, which is not covered by other muscles of this group. The stylohyoid muscle and the posterior part of the digastric muscle are not directly palpable because of their position.

Implementation Note

The area of the floor of the mouth should be gently palpated first, as there are many nerves and vessels in this region. The suprahyoidal muscles may also be sensitive to palpation if swallowing is difficult (Fig. 5.80).

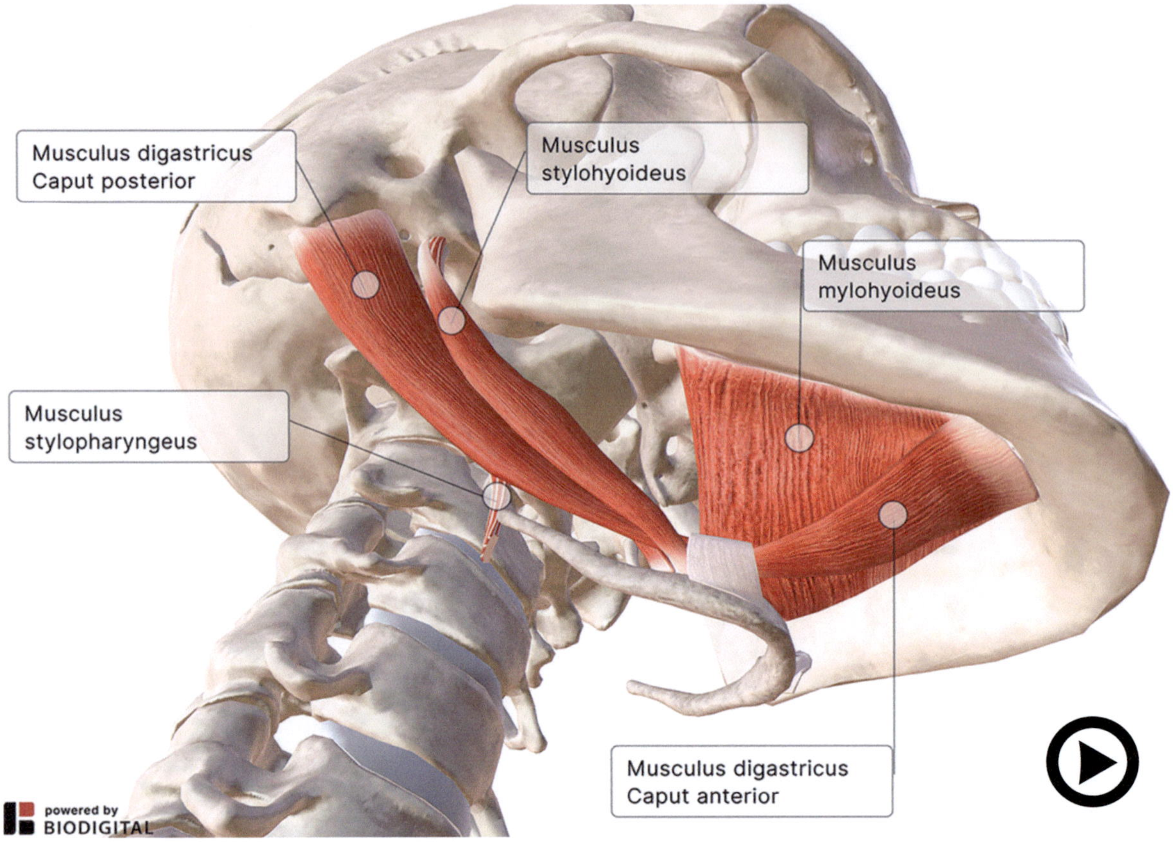

Fig. 5.80 Anatomy and palpation of the suprahyoid musculature (▶ https://doi.org/10.1007/000-cvt)

5.11.4 Palpation of the Facial Mimic Muscles: Forehead

The epicranium is covered by parts of the mimic facial musculature. The occipitofrontalis muscle and the temporoparietalis muscle can be summarised as the epicranius muscle. Both are innervated by the facial nerve (VII cranial nerve) and serve to perform various facial expressions. In the following, they are first described in their anatomical position and then recorded by palpation. The patient is in a lateral or sitting position.

The occipitofrontalis muscle, as its name suggests, is located on the forehead and the back of the head and covers the skull like a bonnet. It is divided into two bellies, the venter frontalis and occipitalis.

The anterior part originates via fascial structures on the margo supraorbitalis at the os frontale and the glabella and is thus also connected to other mimic muscles. The broad muscle belly runs steeply upwards in the cranial direction and also inserts extensively on the galea aponeurotica in the anterior region and thus covers the entire forehead. Functionally, the frontalis muscle performs mimic movements such as frowning, raising the eyebrows and moving the scalp.

The posterior part, which is also known as the occipital muscle, arises at the linea nuchae suprema at the os occipitale and runs in a straight ascending line in the cranial direction. It radiates into the posterior parts of the galea aponeurotica and thus covers the entire back of the head. Due to its position, it functionally tensions the scalp and serves to displace the scalp.

The temporoparietalis muscle is located laterally on the skull and originates with a rather pointed tendon at the fascia of the superior temporalis muscle in the area of the ear. In its superior and slightly rostral course, the muscle fibres diverge so that it inserts into the galea aponeurotica via a broad attachment. Because of these junctions, it can put the scalp under tension and raise the ears.

To palpate the mimic facial muscles in the area of the forehead, the therapist first places the palm of his hand in the centre of the head. The hand is now on the galea aponeurotica, and as soon as the patient begins to raise the eyebrows or move the ears, as far as he is motorically able to do so, a movement of the scalp becomes clearly perceptible. The fingertips then move occipitally and meet directly with the occipitalis muscle. A further orientation aid is provided by the occipital artery, which is located above the muscle and indicates the path to the muscle by its pulse wave. If the fingers, which are placed flat, move in an anterior direction, they meet the frontalis muscle directly in the area between the hairline and the eyebrows and have thus grasped the entire area of the occipitofrontalis muscle. In the region of the forehead, a frown can again improve the sense of touch.

To feel the temporoparietalis muscle, the fingertips make contact with the ear in the superorostral region. If the positioned fingers move from this starting point diagonally to the superorostral area on the scalp, they directly feel the pulsating superficial temporal artery. This artery takes the same course as the temporoparietal muscle, which is located directly under the skin and can thus be subjected to stimulation via the fingers. Moving the ears by the patient increases the sensation of palpation. The muscle ends in the transition to the frontalis muscle in the area of the lateral edge of the forehead.

Implementation Note
Palpation pressure on the temporal artery, to locate the temporoparietalis muscle, may cause headache, so palpation must be started gently at first [29] (Fig. 5.81).

5.11.5 Palpation of the Facial Mimic Muscles: Eye

The eye is an important sensory organ that helps people to orientate themselves in their surroundings. In addition to this function, other movements, such as blinking in the sense of non-verbal communication and closing the eyelids as a protective function of the eye, also play an elementary role. The group of mimic facial muscles in the area of the eye that carry out these activities, among others, is composed of the orbicularis oculi muscle, the corrugator supercilii muscle and the depressor supercilii muscle. All three muscles receive their nervous control via the facial nerve (VII cranial nerve) and are presented below, first individually in their anatomical position and then palpated as a group.

The orbicularis oculi muscle surrounds the eye in a ring and is divided into a pars orbitalis, pars palpebralis and pars lacrimalis. The pars orbitalis, which forms the largest and outer muscular ring, is in bony connection with the proc. frontalis of the maxilla as well as the pars nasalis of the os frontale and encloses the palpebral fissure. The pars palpe-

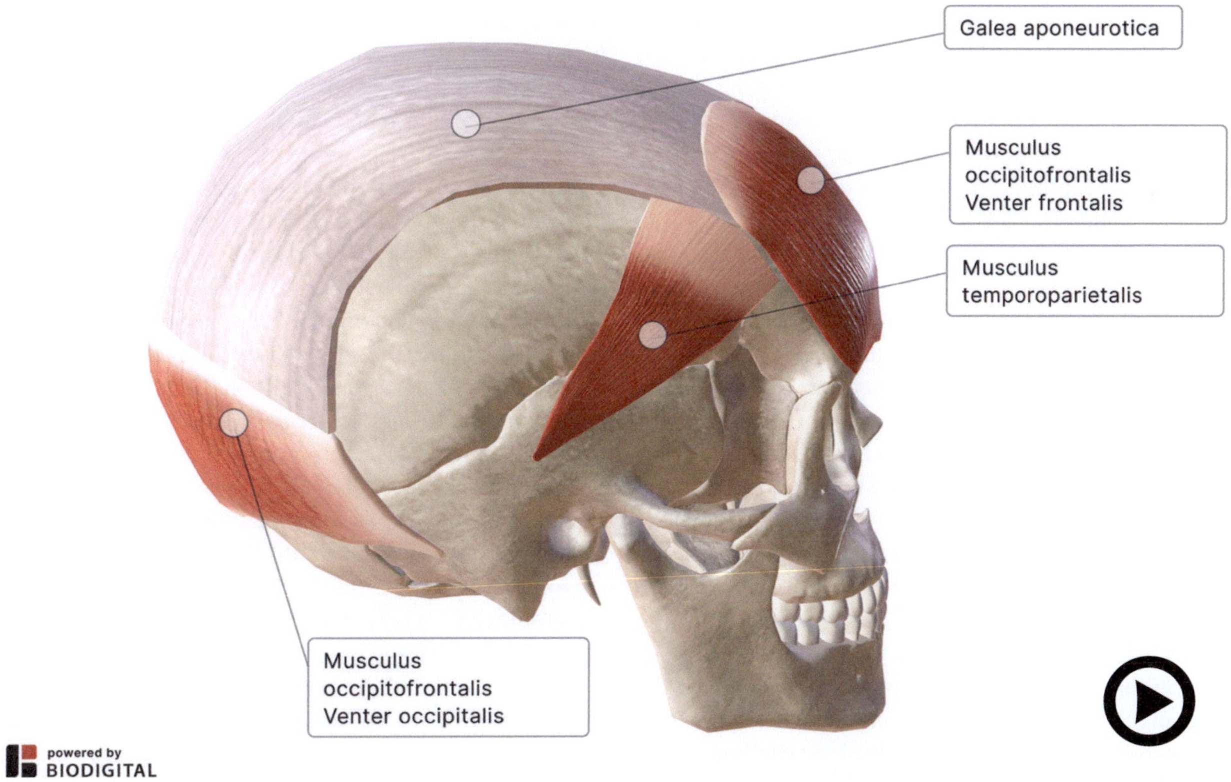

Fig. 5.81 Anatomy and palpation of the mimic facial muscles of the forhead (▶ https://doi.org/10.1007/000-cvv)

bralis is located directly on the eyelid and extends from the medial palpebral ligament at the inner corner of the eyelid to the lateral palpebral raphe. The pars lacrimalis is associated with the pars orbitalis and is connected to the crista lacrimalis posterior and surrounds the saccus lacrimalis medially on the eye. Due to its position, it closes the eyelid, is responsible for the distribution of tear fluid and thus also supports tear drainage. In addition, it can pull the eyebrows caudally and cause the eyelids to close tightly, which is necessary for non-verbal communication.

The corrugator supercilii muscle, which is also named after its function as the eyebrow wrinkler, arises at the pars nasalis of the temporal bone and runs obliquely in the superolateral direction. In its course, it is covered by the frontalis muscle and partially by the orbicularis oculi muscle and then inserts at the galea aponeurotica and in the middle third of the skin of the eyebrow. By being able to functionally pull the eyebrow caudomedially, it provides protection for the eyes by contracting when there is too much light. Due to its course, it causes vertical wrinkles on the forehead when tense, which are also known as frown lines and thus convey a mimic expression in non-verbal communication.

The depressor supercilii muscle has its origin at the arcus superciliaris of the os frontale and at the medial corner of the eye and the proc. frontalis of the maxilla. It runs in a superolateral direction and inserts on the skin in the medial part of the eyebrow. In the region of origin is the angular artery, while in the region of insertion are the supraorbital arteries. Functionally, the depressor supercilii muscle serves to move the eyebrow caudally and thus, as a mimic expression, together with the procerus muscle, can create a horizontal crease on the glabella.

Palpation of the mimic facial musculature in the area of the eye begins with the orbicularis oculi muscle, the parts of which are located directly in the eye socket. The finger berries, which are laid flat, start at the inner corner of the eye, move over the upper eyelid to the eyebrow and move laterally and then to the lower eyelid. They thus outline the muscle in its complete layout and can provide it with a palpatory stimulus. If the patient blinks his eyes or squints them, the palpation sensation can be intensified due to the contraction.

The palpatory starting point for the other two muscles from this group is laterally at the os nasale directly on the pulsating angular artery. Starting from this artery, the rather steeply positioned index finger travels along the bony edge of the eyebrow on the arcus superciliaris in a superolateral direction, thereby applying a direct stimulus to the depressor supercilii muscle. Directly above this muscle runs the corrugator supercilii muscle, which can also be stimulated. Both muscles can be traced to about the medial third of the eyebrow. If the patient is asked to pull the eyebrow in a caudomedial direction and thus show the facial expression of scepticism, both muscles will contract, which in turn facilitates palpation.

Implementation Note

In the area of the eye, palpation should generally be gentle, as sensitive structures such as numerous nerves and vessels are located in this region. In facial nerve palsy, the thematised muscles appear hypotonic and diminished in function. This becomes clear, for example, through a drooping eyelid (Fig. 5.82).

5.11.6 Palpation of the Facial Mimic Muscles: Nose

Millions of olfactory cells are located in the human nose and serve to perceive the environment olfactorily. The human nose is not only used to perceive odours but also for mimic, non-verbal communication. For these special activities, the mimic muscles in the area of the nose are recruited, which move them individually. This group includes the m. levator labii superioris alaeque nasi, the m. procerus, the m. nasalis and the m. depressor septi nasi. All muscles are responsible for mimic movements of the nose and are innervated by the facial nerve (VII cranial nerve). In the following, the individual parts are first described individually in their anatomical position and function and then palpated as a group.

The pyramidal m. procerus, which is also sometimes referred to as the splitting off of the m. frontalis, is located in the area of the glabella and belongs to the mimic facial musculature in the area of the nose. It originates via a narrow tendon on the fascia above the os nasale and in the superior region of the nasal cartilage. In its steep course in the superior direction, the muscle crosses the fibres of the frontalis muscle and radiates broadly into the skin of the glabella and partly into the frontal venter of the occipitofrontalis muscle. Functionally, the procerus muscle pulls the forehead skin and the medial area of the eyebrow caudally. When contracted with the depressor supercilii muscle, it produces a horizontal frown line above the glabella.

Another mimic muscle in the area of the nose is the nasalis muscle, which is composed of a pars transversa and a pars alaris.

The first-mentioned pars transversa originates on the maxilla superolateral to the incisive fossa and the juga alveolaria of the canine or lateral incisor. The superomedial course opens via a thin aponeurosis on the bridge of the nose and via some fibres in the aponeurosis of the procerus muscle.

The pars alaris has its origin in the incisive fossa of the maxilla and the bony area above the second incisor and the juga alveolaria of the canine or lateral incisor. In the course towards the tip of the nose, this part of the nasalis muscle inserts into the cartilago alaris nasi. Due to its anatomical

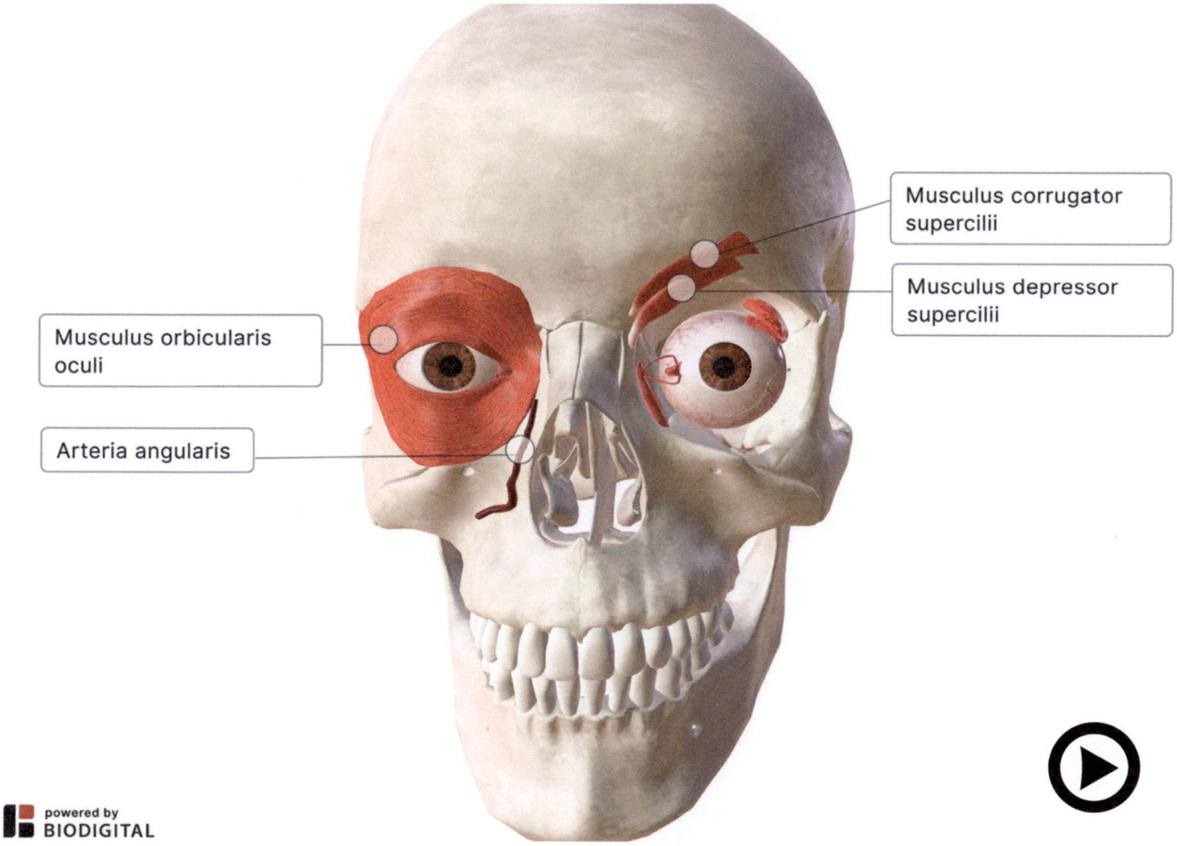

Fig. 5.82 Anatomy and palpation of the mimic facial muscles of the eye (▶ https://doi.org/10.1007/000-cvw)

position, the pars transversa pulls the cartilaginous framework down towards the maxilla and thus narrows the nostril. The pars alaris in turn pulls the nostril laterally and thus serves to widen the nostril and thus facilitate exhalation.

The posterior lateral edges of the nose are marked by the m. levator labii superioris alaeque nasi. It extends caudally on the right and left from the margo infraorbitalis and the facies frontalis and the proc. frontalis of the maxilla and becomes somewhat broader in the area of its attachment to the upper lip and the wings of the nose. In addition, some fibres radiate into the orbicularis muscle and skin areas in this region. Functionally, the levator labii superioris alaeque nasi raises the upper lip and the homolateral nostril and serves to widen the nostril. As it is fused with the skin, it can transmit mimic signs of disgust or disregard.

The depressor septi nasi muscle is located directly under the nose and originates in the incisive fossa of the maxilla, approximately at the level of the anterior maxillary incisors. The superior ascending muscle finds its insertion in the cartilago septi nasi as well as the cartilago alaris nasi. Due to this anatomical position, it pulls the tip of the nose caudally, as well as parts of the nostril, narrowing the nostril.

Palpation from the supine or sitting position begins with the procerus muscle, which is located furthest superiorly. The therapist applies his raised fingertips centrally between the eyebrows and asks the patient to draw his eyebrows together. This creates a transverse crease directly above the procerus muscle, which can be reached by stimulation. If the fingertips move towards the tips of the nose, they cross the nasalis muscle, which can be palpated by stimulation. If the patient moves his nostrils outwards as far as he can, this muscle contracts and becomes more noticeable. Starting from the nostril, palpation is carried out in the direction of the maxilla. Directly at the bony transition and thus the edge of the nose, a stimulus can be applied in depth to the levator labii superioris alaeque nasi muscle on the right and left from the superior beginning of the nose to the nostrils. Directly in the space between the nose and the upper lip, in the anterior middle area, the steeply positioned finger berries meet the depressor septi nasi muscle. Only one stimulation is possible here, as the muscle belly is completely covered by the orbicularis oris muscle.

Implementation Note

With paralysis of the facial nerve, the mimic muscles in the area of the nose can only contract moderately or not at all. As a result, palpation can only be made precise with difficulty or not at all by a change in tone (Fig. 5.83).

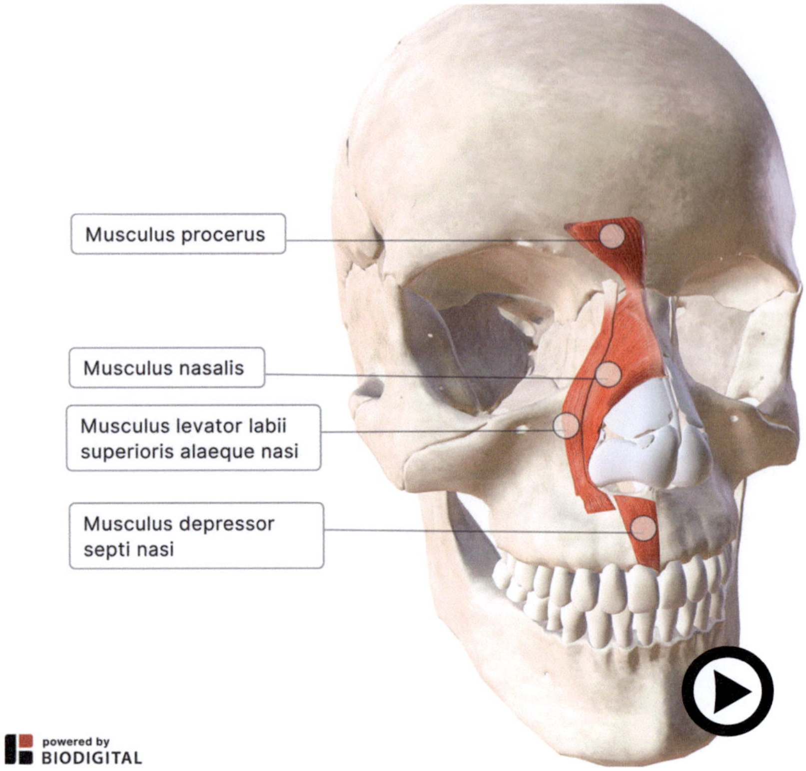

Fig. 5.83 Anatomy and palpation of the mimic facial muscles of the nose (▶ https://doi.org/10.1007/000-cvx)

5.11.7 Palpation of the Facial Mimic Muscles: Mouth

The mouth is assigned numerous everyday functions that are elementary for survival. It is the first instance of food intake and ensures that the food is crushed but also that its texture is examined. The bolus is then prepared in the oral cavity for further swallowing, and the first carbohydrates are broken down. In addition to being the initial source of energy, the mouth also serves the respiratory process and as a resonance body and, via the lips, for voice production. Another task is sucking, which requires a negative pressure inside the mouth. In addition, the mouth is also used for non-verbal mimic communication.

All these functions are controlled by different muscles. A differentiation is made between a superficial and a deep system. The superficial mimic facial musculature in the area of the mouth includes the levator labii superioris, zygomaticus minor, zygomaticus major, risorius, depressor anguli oris, mentalis and orbicularis oris muscles. The deep-lying region is formed by the levator anguli oris muscle, the buccinator muscle and the depressor labii inferioris muscle. All these muscles are innervated via the facial nerve (VII cranial nerve) and are described below in their anatomical course and then discussed as a group in terms of palpation. The recommended starting position is supine or seated. The listed order of the individual structures is chosen according to the order of palpation.

The levator labii superioris muscle is located furthest superior and is divided into a caput angulare, a caput infraorbitale and a caput zygomaticum. It is partially overlapped by the zygomaticus minor muscle along its lateral edge. The caput angulare originates on the proc. frontalis of the maxilla, runs obliquely caudally and inserts on the cartilago alaris major, the skin of the nostril and the lateral part of the upper lip. The infraorbital caput originates from the infraorbital marrow above the infraorbital foramen, converges slightly caudomedially and attaches to the upper lip at the level of the canine, close to the angular caput. The caput zygomaticum originates at the os zygomaticum behind the sutura zygomaticomaxillaris, runs caudomedially and inserts on the upper lip. Throughout, the levator labii superioris muscle serves to raise the lip. This function leads to a mimic expression, which can be associated with disgust.

The zygomaticus minor arises at the os zygomaticum, directly in front of the sutura zygomaticomaxillaris. It runs caudomedially towards the upper lip and then attaches directly to the upper lip and its skin. Functionally, the zygomatic muscle serves to raise the upper lip with a lateral deviation.

The deep-lying levator anguli oris originates in the canine fossa of the maxilla, inferior to the infraorbital foramen, runs caudolaterally towards the homolateral corner of the mouth and is covered in its course by fibres of the levator labii superioris alaeque nasi. In the oral cavity, it is in contact with the maxilla and the oral mucosa. It is inserted at the corner of the mouth, is in contact with the skin and runs together with the zygomaticus major, the depressor anguli oris and the orbicularis oris muscles. In keeping with its name, it serves to raise the corner of the mouth, which together with the risorius muscle is needed for laughter.

The zygomaticus major muscle arises from the proc. temporalis of the os zygomaticum behind the sutura zygomaticotemporalis. It runs caudomedially to the modiolus and inserts on the upper lip and on muscles in the region of the corner of the mouth. It functionally raises the corner of the mouth occipitosuperiorly and thus serves the expression of laughter. This represents a decisive factor for the mimic representation of the current emotional state.

The risorius muscle is called the smile muscle because its course pulls medially from the buccal skin and the fascia of the masseter muscle and the fascia parotidea and inserts directly on the modiolus. It thus pulls the corner of the mouth occipitolaterally and widens the mouth for the purpose of laughing. In addition, it can cause laugh dimples to form on the cheeks.

The deep buccinator muscle, which is localised in the cheek according to its name, has its origin on the external facies of the alveolar processes of the maxilla and mandible at the level of the molars, on the buccinator crest and occipitally on the pterygomandibular raphe. It radiates towards the corner of the mouth and inserts directly on the modiolus and surrounding skin of the lower and upper lip. The muscle belly is perforated by the parotid duct and the parotid gland. Functionally, it shapes the cheeks and pulls them together. Furthermore, the buccinator muscle pushes food pulp between the molars and is important for the sucking process in infants. In the area of facial expression, it supports both laughing and crying.

The triangular depressor anguli oris muscle is in the anterior region of the mandible and arises laterally from the mental tuberosity on the inferior margo of the mandible and is partially fused with the platysma and the depressor labii inferioris muscle. The broad origin tapers in a superior direction and inserts at the corner of the mouth. There, it has contact with the risorius and orbicularis oris muscles. Due to its location, it pulls the corners of the mouth downwards and therefore provides a mimic expression of disappointment or sadness.

In the region of the chin, the depressor labii inferioris muscle is covered regionally by the depressor anguli oris muscle. It originates at the margo inframandibularis in the area of the linea obliqua, between the symphysis mentalis and the mental foramen, and runs ascending in the craniomedial direction. The insertion extends predominantly over the skin of the lower lip, and in part, the fibres intermingle with those of the orbicularis oris muscle. According to its name, it pulls the lower lip downwards when contracted, which corresponds to a mimic expression of sadness and disappointment.

The mentalis muscle is located directly on the surface of the chin and originates anteriorly on the inferior margo of the mandible and the alveolar wall of the second incisor. The superiomedial course opens directly into the skin of the chin, so that it functionally tightens the chin skin and pulls it upwards. The lower lip can also be pushed forward to mimically express displeasure about a situation. This movement can often be observed in small children during pouting.

The orbicularis oris muscle extends annularly around the mouth and thus forms the fleshy basis of the lips. Since it is divided into a pars labialis, which serves more as the basic framework of the lips and runs annularly, and a pars marginalis, which serves as the basic framework of the red of the lips and runs partially perpendicular to the pars labialis, it is not a ring muscle in the classical sense. The facies anterioris of the alveolar processes of the maxilla and mandible serves as the origo. The respective fibres then meet at the corner of the mouth. The orbicularis oris muscle is known by the synonym "kissing muscle" because functionally it performs this activity in addition to closing the mouth and moving the lips when speaking. Furthermore, when contracted, it provides vertical folds on the lips known as tobacco pouch folds.

For palpation of the mimic muscles around the mouth, start superiorly and then palpate across the cheek to the chin and mouth. In most cases, stimulation is only possible via the fingertips. While the patient is in a supine or sitting position, the therapist first applies the index fingertip laterally on the homolateral side of the nose approximately in the middle third with contact to the maxilla. The finger is directly on the levator labii superioris muscle. If the fingers move slightly towards the eye, they meet directly with the origin of the muscle at the lower edge of the orbit. If the patient pulls his lip upwards, a contraction of the muscle is felt. In addition, a pulse wave can be detected because the muscle belly can be located directly above the facial artery.

The fingertip now moves to the lateral edge of the bony orbit in the middle third. In this area, it meets directly with the region of origin of the minor zygomaticus muscle. Starting from this point, a line is mentally drawn in the direction of the homolateral nasal wing on the outer edge, but still on the maxilla. This oblique line describes the course of the muscle so that the finger can apply a stimulus to the structure.

In the region of the insertion of the zygomaticus minor, in the region of the mouth, the fingertips, when they move about one transverse finger in the lateral direction, meet directly with the small levator anguli oris muscle and can provide it with a stimulus.

The finger berries again move further towards the cheek directly to the prominent os zygomaticum. The zygomatic bone has a protrusion that leads directly to the zygomaticus major muscle. If the finger berries are on this point, the patient is asked to pull the homolateral upper lip upwards and outwards. A contraction of the muscle belly can be felt, and the fingertips can palpate the course more precisely.

Starting from this reference point, the finger berries are moved about two transverse fingers in the direction of the mandible and are now directly in the area of the cheek teeth from the outside. They meet the superficial risorius muscle and the underlying buccinator muscle. Note that the risorius muscle extends slightly further occipitally to the level of the mandibular angulus. To make the palpation more precise, the patient is asked to pull the homolateral corner of the mouth straight back. This activity causes the muscle belly to contract, which in turn can be sensed by the fingertips.

To palpate the depressor anguli oris muscle, place the fingertips of the index and middle fingers on the mandible in the region of the canines. The muscle belly is located in this region and can be felt even better if the patient actively moves the homolateral corner of the mouth obliquely caudolaterally.

Starting from this point, the fingertips move one transverse finger anteriorly and meet directly with the m. depressor labii inferioris, which can be reached via stimulation, as it is partly localised under the m. depressor anguli oris. For better orientation, the pulsating A. labialis inferioris can be felt in depth leading to the origin of the muscle.

If the index finger berry is applied laterally to the tip of the chin, it is located directly on the mentalis muscle, which can only be detected by stimulation.

At the end of the palpation journey, palpation of the orbicularis muscle remains, which extends in a ring around the mouth. For an initial overview, the patient is asked to form a kissing mouth, which leads directly to the muscle sought. The orbicularis muscle can then be felt in the regions with steeply placed fingertips. For the upper area on the upper lip, the superior labial artery also serves as a guide for palpation.

Implementation Note

In facial paresis, the muscles cannot be targeted and usually appear hypotonic in this situation (Fig. 5.84).

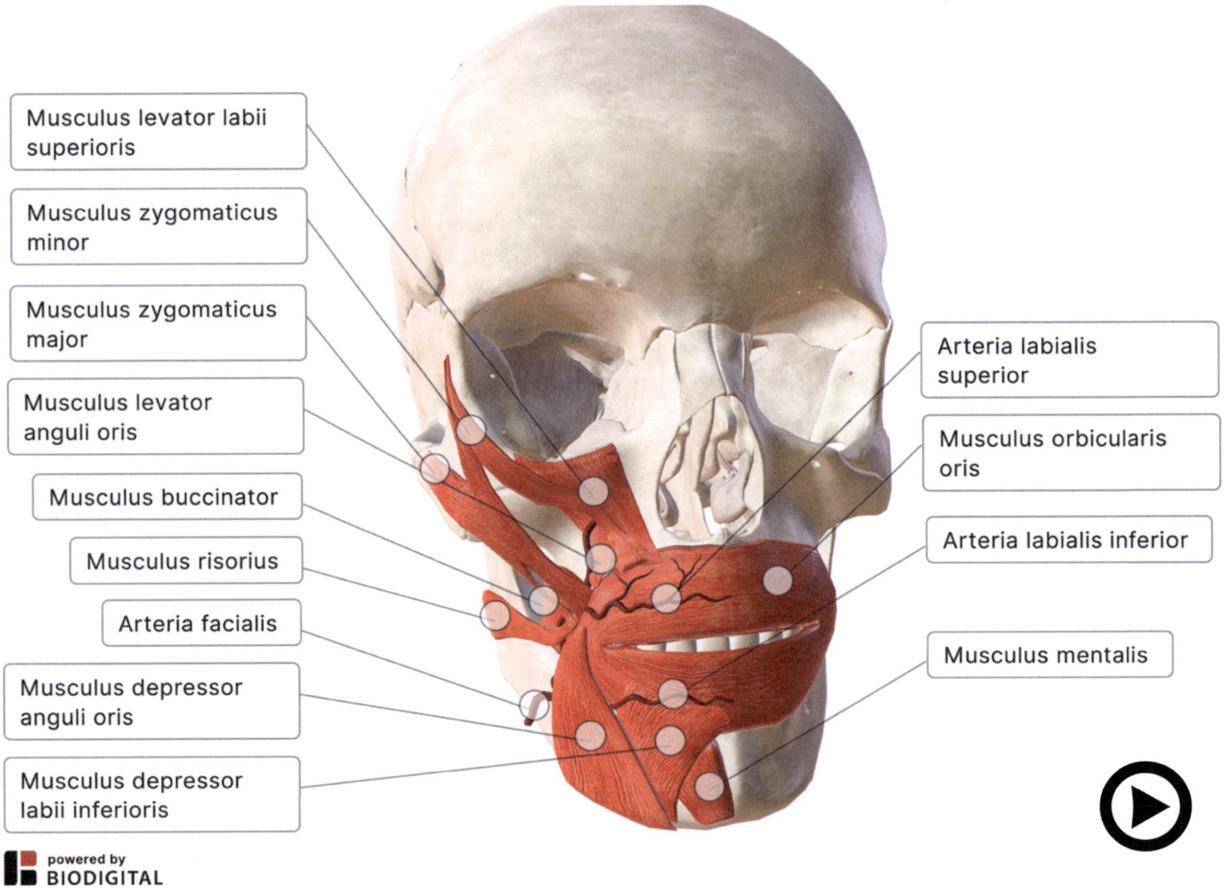

Fig. 5.84 Anatomy and palpation of the mimic facial muscles of the mouth (▶ https://doi.org/10.1007/000-cvy)

5.11.8 Palpation of the Platysma

The Greek word platysma stands for "plate" in German and in the medical context for the cervical fascia, which, similar to a plate, surrounds the neck from anteriorly. This muscular structure is counted as part of the facial mimic musculature and covers the ansa cervicalis superficialis and the vena jugularis externa. The rather thin structure is varied and can be expressed from a massive muscular attachment to connective tissue interruptions. The origo extends from the upper fascia of the pectoralis major and deltoid muscles and the skin of the chest, neck and shoulder. The course of the fibres is individual, depending on the region of origin. Central parts run steeply cranially, and outer parts first run transversely towards the neck and then further craniomedially. In the course, the fibres partly cross those of the contralateral side. In some cases, individual fibres run up to the second rib. The platysma inserts caudally of the linea obliqua on the mandible and the skin and connective tissue of the respective half of the face. Furthermore, it partially radiates into the mentalis muscle, the depressor anguli oris muscle and the orbicularis oris muscle. Due to this anatomical anatomy, the platysma functionally pulls down the lower jaw and the corners of the mouth and tensions connective tissue structures. This tension produces a facial expression of scepticism or fright. The platysma is innervated by the facial nerve (VII cranial nerve).

For palpation of the platysma, the patient is in the supine or sitting position. Before the fingers are placed in the region of the neck, the patient is asked to pull both corners of the mouth downwards in order to tense the cervical fascia. Often, when the tension is intense, a tendinous plate is already visible, which rises up on the neck. The tense structure is then felt with the fingers, as the platysma is not directly palpable in a relaxed state, but can only be palpated by stimulation. This works best in the neck area between the mandible and clavicle. Individual fibres and tendons can often be felt particularly well.

Implementation Note
With age, the skin and connective tissue of the neck increasingly slacken. This can mean that older people sometimes find it difficult to tighten the neck fascia (Fig. 5.85).

5.11.9 Palpation of the Mimic Muscles: Ear

The reception of acoustic signals is realised via the auricle, which in this context is important for communication as well as for orientation in space. It consists mainly of elastic carti-

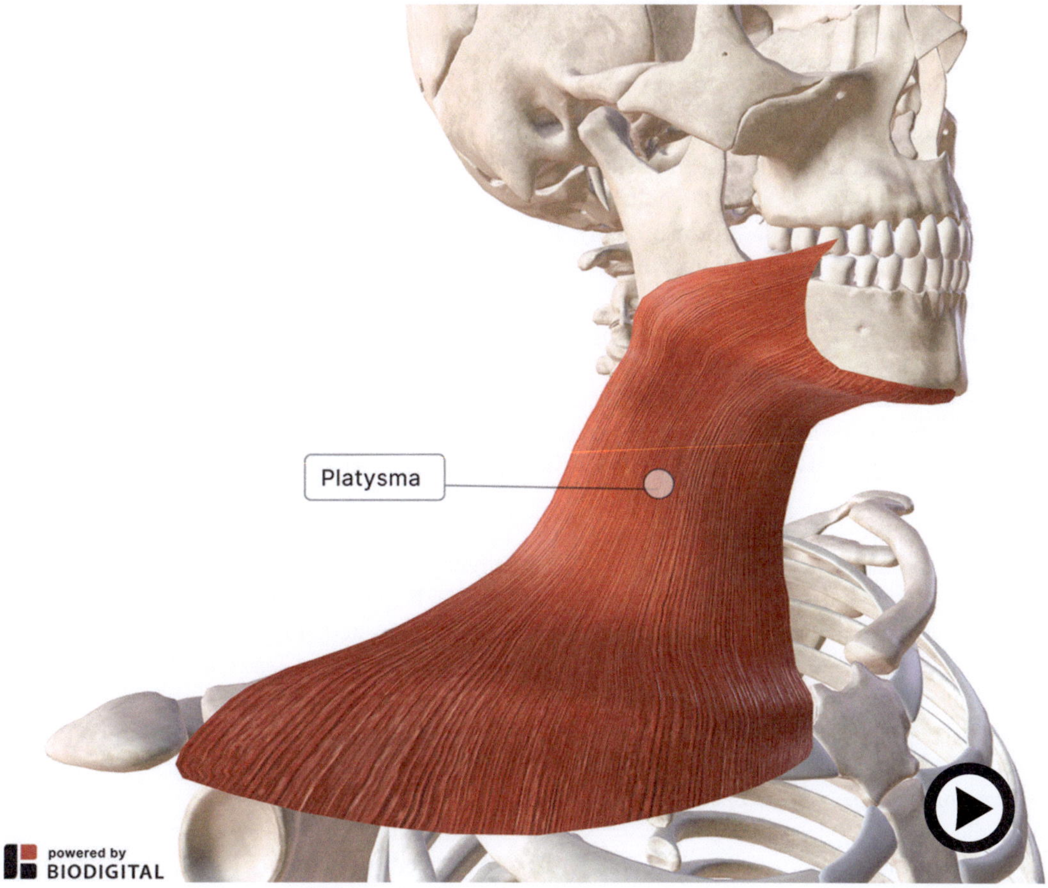

Fig. 5.85 Anatomy and palpation of the platysma (▶ https://doi.org/10.1007/000-cvz)

lage and small muscles that both shape the ear and enable small movements. The ear muscles are mainly recruited for non-verbal communication via mimic signals. There are nine muscles on the human body for this region. These include the anterior auricularis muscle, the posterior auricularis muscle, the superior auricularis muscle and the minor and major helicis muscles, the tragicus and antitragicus muscles, the transversus auriculae muscle and the obliquus auriculae muscle. All of these muscles are innervated by the facial nerve (VII cranial nerve). In this chapter, the anatomical position is first briefly described, and then the palpation journey on the ear is explained. The patient is in a supine or lateral position or in a sitting position.

The anterior auricular muscle is located on the side of the head above the temporal bone. It arises at the lateral edge of the galea aponeurotica, runs obliquely to the occipitocaudal and inserts at the facies anterior to the helix as well as at the auricle auris. Functionally, the anterior ear muscle can move the auricle anteriorly.

The superior auricular muscle lies directly above the ear and has its origin at the lateral edge of the galea aponeurotica. Its tapered course in the inferior direction ends at the upper part of the auricle. Because of this attachment, it can move the ear in the superior direction.

The posterior auricular muscle is located behind the ear and originates at the mastoid muscle of the temporal bone and runs in two to three thin strands, slightly obliquely anterosuperiorly. The muscle belly covers the retroauricular lymph nodes and inserts on the posterior wall of the ear cartilage. When contracted, it can move the ear occipitally.

The small, intrinsic minor helicis muscle arises at the base of the helical crus and the anterior margin of the helix and runs obliquely to the insertion at the front of the helical crus above the tragus and the auricular cartilage. Functionally, it is only structurally involved in the adaptation of the anterior margin of the auricular cartilage.

The greater helicis muscle runs like a ligament along the anterior superior border of the ear. It originates at the anterior edge of the helix, pulls anteroinferiorly and inserts at the spina helicis as well as the tragus and partly at the anterior edge of the helix. Functionally, it serves to structurally adjust the anterior edge of the auricle.

The tragicus muscle is located in the anterior region of the ear, directly in front of the meatus acusticus externus. This small muscle originates at the lamina tragi, runs steeply superiorly and inserts at the incisura intertragica. Like all intrinsic ear muscles, it serves to shape the auricle.

The antitragicus muscle is located in the lower part of the ear and has its origin at the antitragicus. It runs obliquely occipitosuperiorly and inserts at the helix and the antitragohelic fissure. Functionally, it serves to open the auditory canal and to shape the ear.

The obliquus auriculae muscle is located in the upper part of the back of the ear. It runs over the helix and the eminentia fossae triangularis to the eminentia conchae at the back of the ear cartilage and functionally pulls the antihelix slightly inwards.

The transversus auricular muscle is located at the back of the ear in the posterior region. Its transverse course extends from the eminentia conchae to the eminentia of the scapha to its insertion at the back of the ear cartilage. When contracted, it pulls the helix downwards and forms the ear.

Palpation of the mimic musculature in the area of the ear is oriented towards the associated picture as well as the following sequence and begins at the os temporale. It should be noted that only stimulation of the structures is possible. Only if the patient is able to move his ears actively can a contraction under the fingertip be recorded under certain circumstances. The palpation journey begins with the auricularis anterior muscle. The steeply erect finger berries are located at the upper outer edge of the homolateral orbit and move occipitally towards the temple. In doing so, they meet the muscle belly directly after the bony structure. During this, the superficial temporal artery is also felt pulsatingly in the anterior region. The fingertips are moved further occipitally until they meet an imaginary line which, starting from the meatus acusticus externus, projects steeply superiorly. Directly two transverse fingers after this line, the steeply erect fingertips meet the superior auricularis muscle. In the upper region of this muscle, the pulsating superficial temporal artery is also palpable in the posterior region. If an imaginary horizontal line is drawn, starting from the cartilaginous part which lies directly superior to the auditory canal on the helix, the posterior auricularis muscle is located adjacent to the auricle towards the occipital on the skull. The steeply positioned fingertips can thus apply a stimulus to the structure.

The palpation journey of the mimic musculature, which is located directly at the auricle, starts from the meatus acusticus externus, which again serves as a reference point. The steeply positioned index finger berry travels directly superiorly and encounters a cartilaginous protrusion. A stimulus is applied to the minor helicis muscle. In the anterosuperior direction, along the ear, the anterior edge of the auricle is felt. At the level of the arch, when the ear extends occipitally, the helicis major muscle is located along the cartilage and can be grasped by applying a stimulus with the index finger. Directly in front of the auditory canal, a cartilaginous projection can be palpated, at the superior end of which the tragicus muscle is located. Targeted palpation with the steeply positioned index finger leads to an irritation. If the fingertip moves to the earlobe, it encounters the antitragicus muscle in the posterior region, which can also be grasped with a forceps grip. If the patient actively moves the ear, a movement in this area can be perceived.

The obliquus auriculae and transversus auriculae muscles are located on the back of the auricle in the upper area. Starting from a vertical line projecting superiorly through the

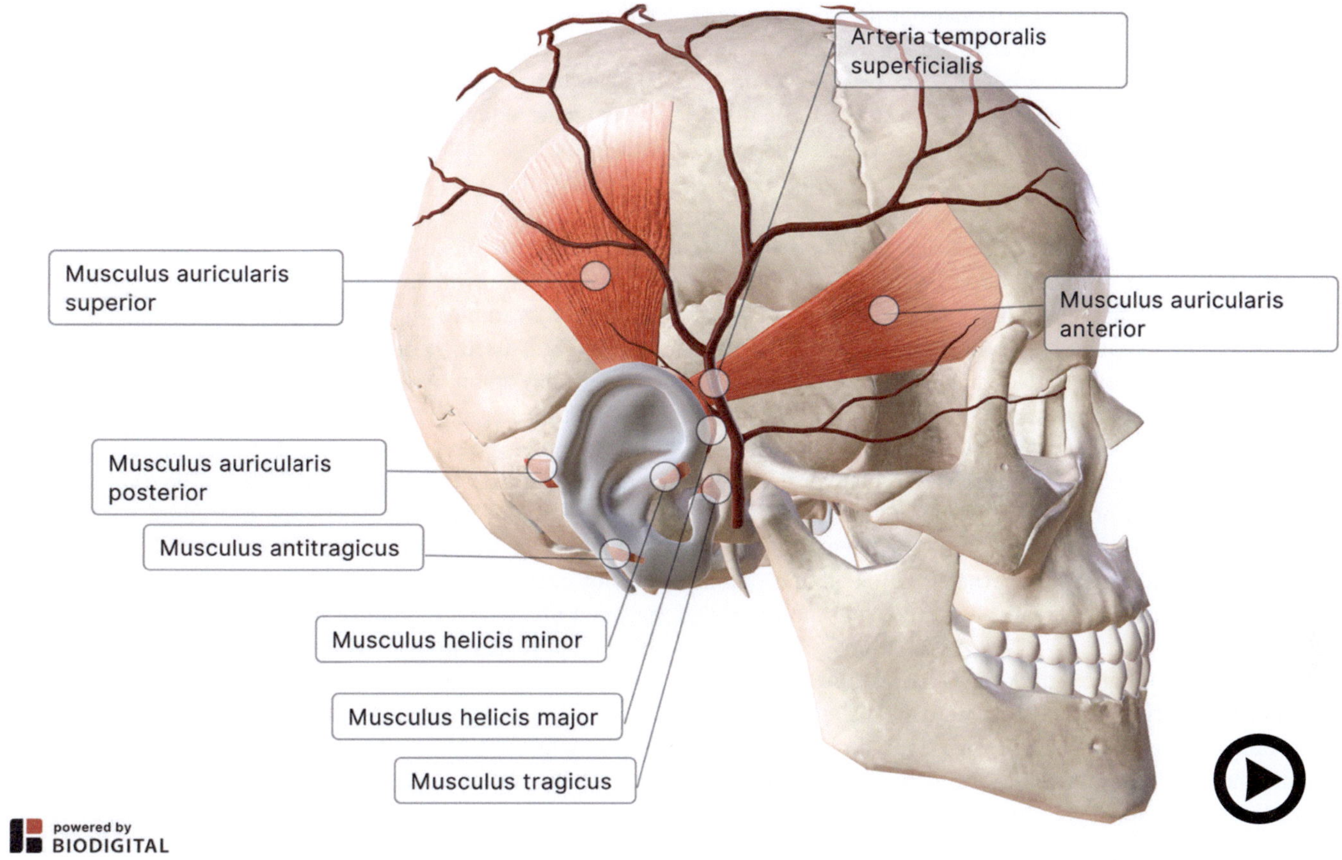

Fig. 5.86 Anatomy and palpation of the mimic facial muscles of the ear (▶ https://doi.org/10.1007/000-cw0)

auditory canal, the pincer grip is applied in the upper area of the auricle. About two transverse fingers of the line occipitally is the region of the obliquus auriculae muscle, while about three transverse fingers of the transversus auriculae muscle is adjacent.

Implementation Note
As the muscles of the ear are extremely delicate structures, it is essential that palpation is carried out gently and superficially (Fig. 5.86).

5.11.10 Palpation of the External Eye Muscles

The sense of sight is elementary for humans to orientate themselves in their environment and to communicate non-verbally. The eye must be controlled individually in order to meet these requirements. The muscles responsible for this must be active almost constantly during the day to fulfil their function. The external eye muscles include the m. rectus superior, the m. rectus inferior as well as the m. rectus medialis and the m. rectus lateralis, the m. obliquus superior and the m. obliquus inferior. The anatomical position of these six muscles is described below, followed by a discussion of palpatory stimulation. The patient is positioned in the sitting or supine position.

The superior rectus muscle originates at the common tendon and then runs in a straight line anterolaterally, crosses the tendon of the superior oblique muscle, continues towards the base of the sclera and inserts at the ocular bulb, anterior to the bulbous equator. Functionally, the superior rectus muscle performs elevation of the eyeball and slight internal rotation and adduction of the eye. It is innervated by the oculomotor nerve (III cranial nerve).

The inferior rectus muscle originates at the common tendon and then runs slightly obliquely anteriolaterally, merging with the sclera at the lower edge of the eye and inserting into the lower surface of the ocular bulb slightly anterior to the bulbous equator. Functionally, it is responsible for the depression of the eyeball. It also performs adduction and external rotation of the eye. It is innervated by the oculomotor nerve (III cranial nerve).

The strongest muscle in the group of external eye muscles is the rectus medialis muscle. It originates at the annulus tendineus communis and runs along the orbital wall straight anteriorly, attaching to the medial surface of the bulbus oculi slightly anterior to the equator bulbi. Contraction of the muscle assists elevation during strong upward gaze and depression during downward gaze. In addition, it performs adduction of the eyeball. It receives the innervation for these activities via the oculomotor nerve (III cranial nerve).

The lateral rectus muscle originates at the common tendon and then runs horizontally anteriorly in a slightly arched shape. It is inserted from the lateral side over the sclera on the lateral bulb of the eye, more anteriorly to the equator bulb. When the muscle is contracted, the eye is moved in the direction of abduction. In addition, it supports a slight elevation when looking upwards and a slight depression when looking downwards. This activity occurs via innervation by the abducens nerve (VI cranial nerve).

The inferior oblique muscle arises from the anterior lacrimal crest on the maxilla next to the entrance of the nasolacrimal duct. Its horizontal attachment runs occipitolaterally around the eyeball, undercrosses the inferior rectus muscle in its course and merges into a fan-like terminal tendon which inserts at the inferior border of the orbit over the sclera at the posterior inferior temporal portion of the bulbus oculi. Functionally, it performs elevation of the eyeball and supports abduction as well as external rotation of the bulbus oculi. The nerve control is realised via the oculomotor nerve (III cranial nerve).

The superior oblique muscle is located at the upper edge of the eye and originates in the corpus of the sphenoid, the periorbita and the dural sheath of the optic nerve. In its particular course, it passes over the rectus medialis muscle in a rostral direction through the connective tissue trochlea, which serves as a hypomochleon or pulley. Continuing, it extends more posterolaterally after the deflection and then attaches to the superior temporal quadrant of the eyeball posterior to the equatorial line via the sclera. Functionally, it rotates the eye backwards (depression), supports abduction and rotates the upper half of the globe inwards. In addition, it can act as a depressor in an adducted position. It is innervated by the trochlear nerve (IV cranial nerve).

The palpation of the external eye muscles can only be achieved by stimulation. For this purpose, the fingertip of the little finger is used, which is placed steeply and with the fingernail pointing outwards, as described below.

Palpation begins superiorly at the eye by palpating the little finger directly in the space between the eye and the upper orbital rim. This applies a stimulus to the superior rectus and oblique muscles. The same procedure is then performed on the inferior rim of the eye, thereby palpating the inferior rectus and obliquus muscles. Medial to the eye, between the bony structure of the skull and the eye itself, is the medial rectus and lateral rectus. Both are again grasped via the same procedure.

Implementation Note

When palpating the eye, it is imperative to be gentle as the muscular structures can be very sensitive (Fig. 5.87).

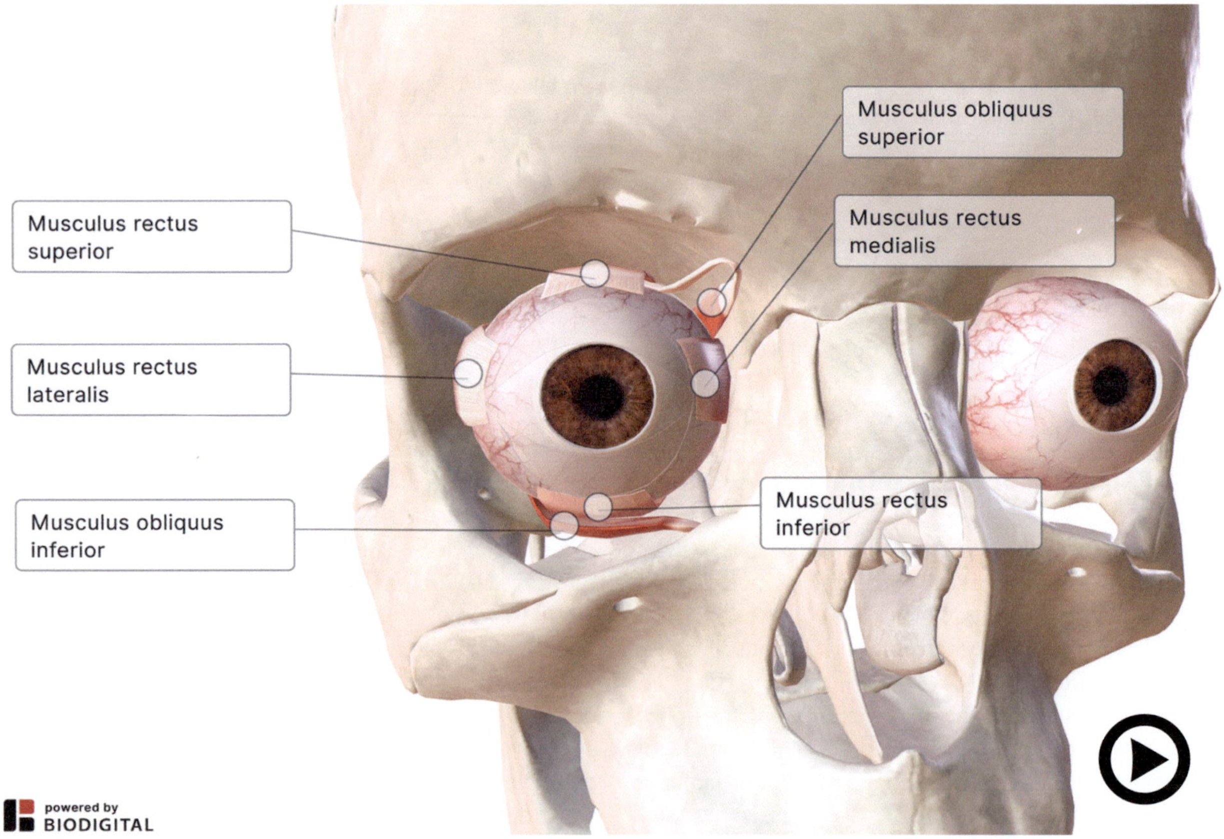

Fig. 5.87 Anatomy and palpation of the outer eye musculature (▶ https://doi.org/10.1007/000-cw1)

References

1. Ohlendieck, K. (2013). Proteomics research and the molecular mechanisms of muscle adaptations and muscular disorders. *Nervenheilkunde, 32*(06), 389–394. https://doi.org/10.1055/s-0038-1628512
2. Fürst, D., & Gautel, M. (1995). The anatomy of a molecular giant: How the sarcomere cytoskeleton is assembled from immunoglobulin superfamily molecules. *Journal of Molecular and Cellular Cardiology, 27*(4), 951–959. https://doi.org/10.1016/0022-2828(95)90064-0
3. Liu, Y., & Palmer, J. (2012). Iliacus tender points in young adults: a pilot study. *The Journal of the American Osteopathic Association, 112*(5), 285–289.
4. Dragieva, P., Zaharieva, M., Kozhuharov, Y., Markov, K., & Stoyanov, G. (2018). Psoas minor muscle: A cadaveric morphometric study. *Cureus., 10*(4), e2447. https://doi.org/10.7759/cureus.2447
5. Kirschner, J., Foye, P., & Cole, J. (2009). Piriformis syndrome, diagnosis and treatment. *Muscle & Nerve, 40*(1), 10–18. https://doi.org/10.1002/mus.21318
6. Kassarjian, A., Tomas, X., Cerezal, L., Canga, A., & Llopis, E. (2011). MRI of the quadratus femoris muscle: anatomic considerations and pathologic lesions. *AJR. American Journal of Roentgenology, 197*(1), 170–174. https://doi.org/10.2214/AJR.10.5898
7. Schneider, O., Scharf, H.-P., Stein, T., Knapstein, S., Hermann, C., & Flechtenmacher, J. (2016). Incidence of knee injuries: Numbers for outpatient and inpatient care in Germany. *Orthopade, 45*(12), 1015–1026. https://doi.org/10.1007/s00132-016-3301-6
8. Roger, J., Bertani, A., Vigouroux, F., Mottier, F., Gaillard, R., Have, L., & Rongièras, F. (2020). ACL reconstruction using a quadruple semitendinosus graft with cortical fixations gives suitable isokinetic and clinical outcomes after 2 years. *Knee Surgery, Sports Traumatology, Arthroscopy, 28*(8), 2468–2477. https://doi.org/10.1007/s00167-020-06121-2
9. Niemitz, C. (2010). The evolution of the upright posture and gait—a review and a new synthesis. *Die Naturwissenschaften, 97*(3), 241–263. https://doi.org/10.1007/s00114-009-0637-3
10. Rossetto, M. (2006). Wie viel Bewegung ist gesund? *FIT for LIFE, 1/2-06*, 52–55.
11. Joshi, S., Joshi, S., & Athavale, S. (2006). Morphology of peroneus tertius muscle. *Clinical Anatomy, 19*(7), 611–614. https://doi.org/10.1002/ca.20243
12. Vlaic, J., Josipovic, M., Bohacek, I., & Jelic, M. (2019). The plantaris muscle: too important to be forgotten. A review of evolution, anatomy, clinical implications and biomechanical properties. *The Journal of Sports Medicine and Physical Fitness, 59*(5), 839–845. https://doi.org/10.23736/S0022-4707.18.08816-3
13. Gabel, J. (2015). Funktionsanalyse des Fußes. *Trauma und Berufskrankheit, 17*, 4–9. https://doi.org/10.1007/s10039-013-1991-0
14. Sasaki, H., & Polus, B. (2012). Can neck muscle spindle afferents activate fusimotor neurons of the lower limb? *Muscle & Nerve, 45*(3), 376–384. https://doi.org/10.1002/mus.22300
15. Rarreck, T. (2011). Thoracic-Outlet-Syndrom (TOS). *Deutsche Heilpraktiker-Zeitschrift, 6*(1), 20–23. https://doi.org/10.1055/s-0030-1270406
16. Natsis, K., Piagkou, M., Repousi, E., Apostolidis, S., Kotsiomitis, E., Apostolou, K., & Skandalakis, P. (2016). Morphometric variability of pyramidalis muscle and its clinical significance. *Surgical and Radiologic Anatomy, 38*(3), 285–292. https://doi.org/10.1007/s00276-015-1550-4
17. Harper, C., Shahgholi, L., Cieslak, K., Hellyer, N., Strommen, J., & Boon, A. (2013). Variability in diaphragm motion during normal breathing, assessed with B-mode ultrasound. *The Journal of Orthopaedic and Sports Physical Therapy, 43*(12), 927–931. https://doi.org/10.2519/jospt.2013.4931
18. Kocjan, J., Adamek, M., Gzik-Zroska, B., Czyżewski, D., & Rydel, M. (2017). Network of breathing. Multifunctional role of the diaphragm: A review. *Advances in Respiratory Medicine, 85*(4), 224–232. https://doi.org/10.5603/ARM.2017.0037
19. Reinold, M., Macrina, L., Wilk, K., Fleisig, G., Dun, S., Barrentine, S., Ellerbusch, M. T., & Andrews, J. (October-December 2007). Electromyographic analysis of the supraspinatus and deltoid muscles during 3 common rehabilitation exercises. *Journal of Athletic Training, 42*(4), 464–469.
20. El-Naggar, M. (2001). A study on the morphology of the coracobrachialis muscle and its relationship with the musculocutaneous nerve. *Folia Morphologica, 60*(3), 217–224.
21. Ferner, H. (1938). Der Nervus musculocutaneus, seine Verlaufsvarietäten am Oberarm und deren Beziehung zur Entwicklung eines Caput tertium musculi bicipitis. *Zeitschrift für Anatomie und Entwicklungsgeschichte, 108*, 567–586. https://doi.org/10.1007/BF02118846
22. Sturzenegger, M., Béguin, D., Grünig, B., & Jakob, R. (1986). Muscular strength after rupture of the long head of the biceps. *Archives of Orthopaedic and Trauma Surgery, 105*, 18–23. https://doi.org/10.1007/BF00625654
23. Thompson, N., Mockford, B., & Cran, G. (2001). Absence of the palmaris longus muscle: a population study. *The Ulster Medical Journal, 70*(1), 22–24.
24. Amin, N., Kumar, N., & Schickendantz, M. (2015). Medial epicondylitis: evaluation and management. *The Journal of the American Academy of Orthopaedic Surgeons, 23*(6), 348–355. https://doi.org/10.5435/JAAOS-D-14-00145
25. Zancolli, E., Zancolli, E., & Perrotto, C. (2012). New mini-invasive decompression for pronator teres syndrome. *The Journal of Hand Surgery, 37*(8), 1706–1710. https://doi.org/10.1016/j.jhsa.2012.05.033
26. Miquel-Kergoat, S., Azais-Braesco, V., Burton-Freeman, B., & Hetherington, M. (2015). Effects of chewing on appetite, food intake and gut hormones: A systematic review and meta-analysis. *Physiology & Behavior, 151*, 88–96. https://doi.org/10.1016/j.physbeh.2015.07.017
27. Arnaud-Brachet, M., Foletti, J., Graillon, N., Chaumoître, K., Chossegros, C., & Guyot, L. (2020). Could mastication modify the shape of the orbit? A scannographic study in humans. *Surgical and Radiologic Anatomy, 42*(1), 63–67. https://doi.org/10.1007/s00276-019-02315-7
28. Peyron, M., Lassauzay, C., & Woda, A. (2002). Effects of increased hardness on jaw movement and muscle activity during chewing of visco-elastic model foods. *Experimental Brain Research, 142*(1), 41–51. https://doi.org/10.1007/s00221-001-0916-5
29. Katano, H., Nishikawa, Y., Yamada, H., Shibata, T., Miyachi, S., & Mase, M. (2019). Association of superficial temporal artery dilatation with headache after revascularization in adult moyamoya disease. *World Neurosurgery, 129*, e594–e606. https://doi.org/10.1016/j.wneu.2019.05.228

Palpation of the Nerves

6

Contents

Supplementary Information The online version contains supplementary material available at https://doi.org/10.1007/978-3-662-69186-1_6. The videos can be accessed individually by clicking the DOI link in the accompanying figure caption or by scanning this link with the SN More Media App.

R. Bauer, S. Wolfram, *Atlas of Palpation*, https://doi.org/10.1007/978-3-662-69186-1_6

6.1 Basics of Palpation of Nerves

The control centre of the human body is the central nervous system, consisting of the brain and the spinal cord. To fulfil this function, a connection between the periphery and the central nervous system is needed. The perfect link is provided by the peripheral nervous system. This ensures harmonious communication via efferents and afferents. This construct can also be called the sensorimotor system. The word nerve comes from the ancient Greek and when translated into German means "cord" or "thread". If all these "threads" are strung together in the body, the result is a distance of about 5.8 million kilometres, which could be laid 145 times around the earth's equator [1]. This enormous network must function properly, and the axoplasm must flow so that the electrical impulses arrive in the target cell and functions can be triggered. The system can be compared to a light switch that, when pressed, transports the current via the wires to the lamp and makes it light up. If there is a problem with this transmission, the lamp will not emit light. Transmitted to the body, various information can be disturbed in its transmission in the case of bottlenecks or other damage.

For this reason, it is important to know the anatomical position and function of the most important nerves in the human body. In addition, they can be located through targeted palpation. In the following chapters, the exact course and palpation of the palpable nerves will therefore be discussed. It is regionally subdivided into pelvis, lower extremity, abdomen, upper extremity and head. Similar to vessels, the nerves are palpated with the fingertips. The feeling of palpation is comparable to the side of a guitar. Some nerves are localised in depth, which only allows stimulation at various reference points. The exact procedure is described in the following chapters. The client is to be positioned in a relaxed starting position. If a nerve is compressed by pressure, the axoplasmic flow is temporarily reduced. This can cause discomfort.

6.2 Pelvis/Lower Extremity

Precise control via the peripheral nervous system is elementary for optimal functionality of the musculature and other structures of the lower extremity. Nerves from the lumbosacral plexus provide the nervous supply to the tissues. In addition to motor information, these nerves also receive and connect sensitive stimuli. In the following chapters, the most important nerves are described in terms of their position and function as well as palpation via specific reference points. These include the femoral nerve, the genitofemoral nerve, the obturator nerve, the ilioinguinal nerve, the lateral cutaneus femoris nerve and the superior and inferior gluteus nerve. The pudendal nerve, saphenous nerve, sciatic nerve, common fibular nerve, superficial and deep fibular nerve, sural nerve, tibial nerve, lateral and medial plantar nerve and lateral, intermediate and medial dorsal cutaneous nerve are also palpable. Depending on the region, direct palpation or only stimulation of the structure can be realised.

6.2.1 Palpation of the Femoral Nerve

The powerful nerve that innervates the front of the thigh arises from segments L1–L4 and runs between the quadratus lumborum muscle and the psoas major muscle at its lateral edge deep into the iliac fossa and then over the iliac muscle towards the groin. Together with the parts of the iliopsoas muscle, it passes through the lacuna musculorum lateral to the arcus iliopectineus and directly lateral to the femoral artery in a distal direction. Immediately after the lacuna musculorum and the ramus superior ossis pubis, it gives off branches that extend over the thigh to innervate it motorically and sensitively. One of the main branches is the saphenous nerve, which is explained in more detail in Sect. 6.2.8. The psoas major, quadriceps femoris, sartorius, iliacus and pectineus are supplied by the femoral nerve itself.

The region of passage through the lacuna musculorum is suitable for palpation of the femoral nerve. The patient is positioned supine while the therapist feels the pulse of the femoral artery in the groin with the fingertips (see Sect. 7.1.1.2). Directly one transverse finger of the client lateral to the artery, the fingertips meet the femoral nerve, which is perceived as a firm elastic round structure and can be followed somewhat distally [2].

Implementation Note

The nerve runs directly on the iliopsoas muscle, which comes up via active hip flexion and can be used for better orientation in the groin (Fig. 6.1).

6.2.2 Palpation of the Genitofemoral Nerve

The genitofemoral nerve arises from the segments L1–L2, which in its steep distal course perforates the psoas major muscle in the upper third [3]. It follows the same course as the muscle up to the inguinal ligament, then bends slightly medially and runs together with the femoral artery through the lacuna vasorum as the ramus femoralis. It moves distally directly above the artery and then dips down into the depths. The second branch runs into the pelvis as the ramus genitalis. While the ramus femoralis supplies sensation to the inner side of the thigh, the ramus genitalis innervates the cremaster muscle as well as the skin of the scrotum in men and the labia majoris in women.

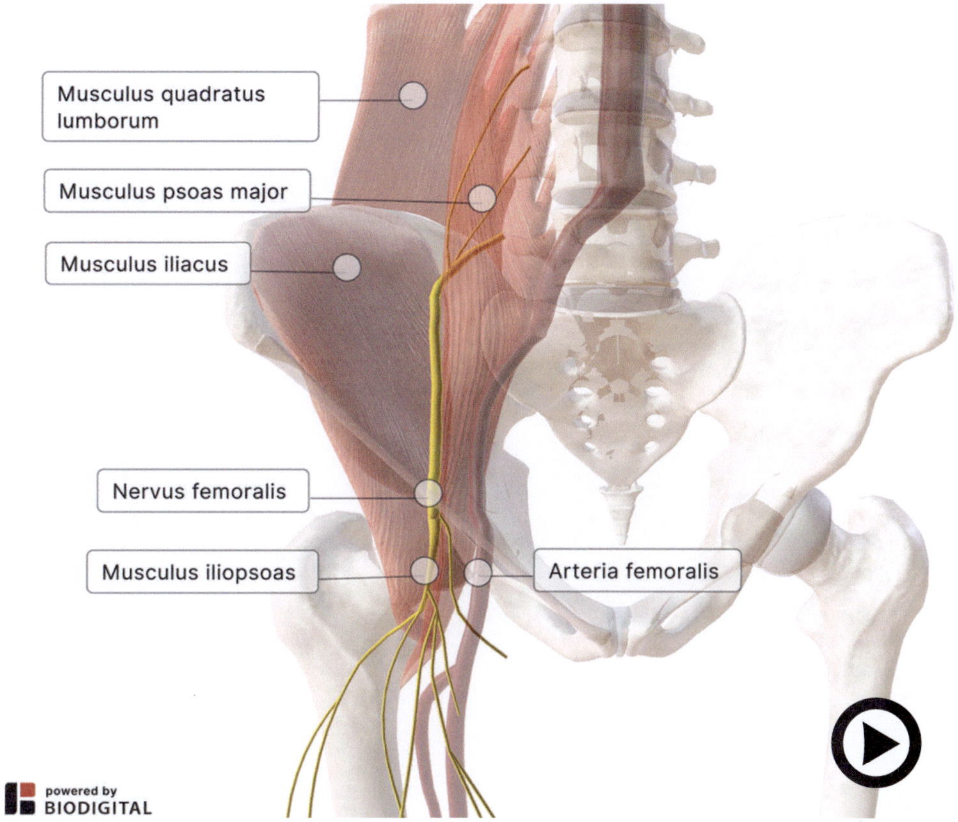

Fig. 6.1 Anatomy and palpation of the N. femoralis (▶ https://doi.org/10.1007/000-cx1)

Palpation of the ramus femoralis is done from the supine position. The therapist stands sideways and orients himself to the homolateral femoral artery with his index and middle fingers placed flat on the surface. Directly distal to the inguinal ligament, a stimulus can be applied to the nerve by applying pressure to the artery.

The ramus genitalis can only be detected by a direct stimulus from the cranial side with steeply positioned fingertips on the ramus superior ossis pubis. It should be noted that the ilioinguinal nerve follows the same course and is also detected by compression.

Implementation Note
Palpation is only possible via stimulation, which also detects other structures. An improved topographical orientation can be implemented via a contraction in hip flexion as well as the pulse wave of the femoral artery (Fig. 6.2).

6.2.3 Palpation of the Obturator Nerve

The obturator nerve, which originates from segments L2–L4, carries both somatosensory and somatomotor fibres and supplies part of the adductor muscles (adductor longus and brevis, gracilis and pectineus) and the skin area medial to the thigh via the anterior ramus. The external obturator muscle as well as the adductor magnus muscle and sensitive areas around the knee joint are controlled via the posterior ramus. After leaving the segments, it runs distally with the greater psoas muscle, which it partially perforates. In the region of the iliac fossa, it moves anteriorly towards the obturator foramen, which it crosses in the upper region, directly under the superior osseous ramus. In the area of the foramen, it divides into a posterior ramus, which pierces the external obturator muscle and runs distally, and an anterior ramus, which runs distally posterior to the pectineus muscle. Both then follow the adductor brevis muscle in depth from posterior and anterior, respectively, in the medial area of the thigh to the distal.

For palpation, the patient is positioned in a supine position with the legs in a straight line, while the therapist stands laterally at the level of the pelvis. As the obturator nerve is located in the upper third behind the aorta in depth, stimulation is only possible in the middle third via a pelvic approach and in the distal third on the inner side of the thigh. Here, the practitioner's approach is based on that of the m. obturatorius externus (see Sect. 5.2.13). The therapist contacts the proximal inner side of the thigh with the index and middle

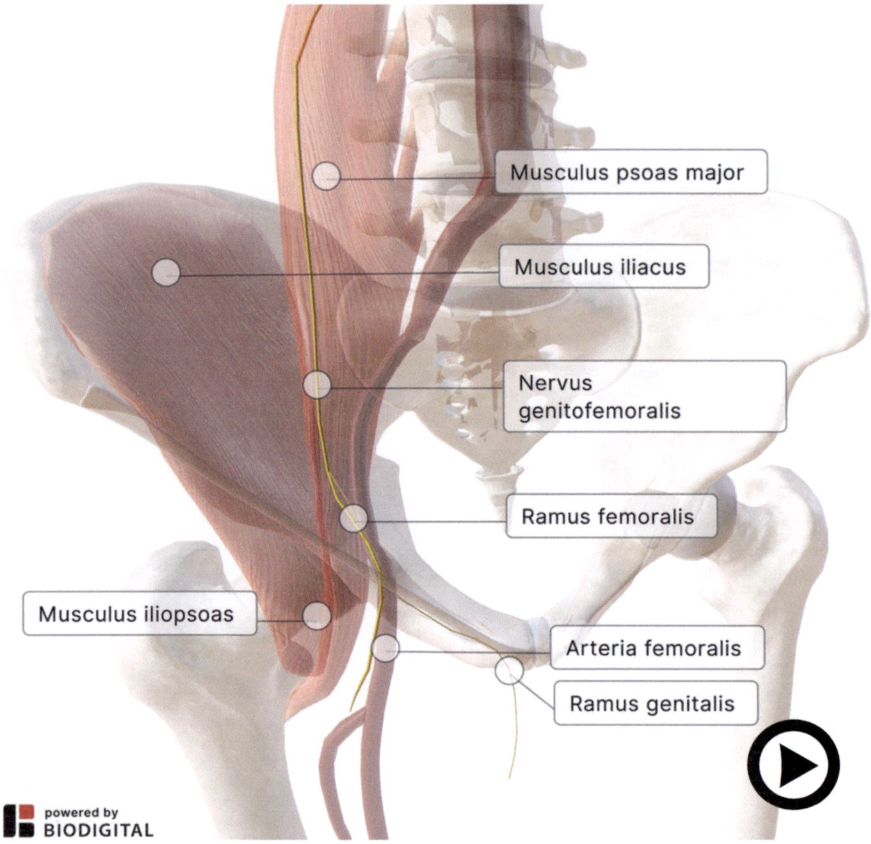

Fig. 6.2 Anatomy and palpation of the N. genitofemoralis (▶ https://doi.org/10.1007/000-cw3)

fingertips steeply raised and palpates in the direction of the pelvis. In the area of the origin of the adductor longus muscle, the femoral artery and directly under the ramus superior ossis pubis, the fingers meet the obturator foramen, in whose superior area a stimulus can be applied to the nerve. As the fingers pass through numerous structures, direct palpation is not possible. A second access can be made on the inner thigh via the adductor longus muscle (see Sect. 5.2.8). Directly at its anterior edge, pressure can be applied from medial to lateral on the ramus anterior via the steeply positioned finger berries and on the posterior edge of the muscle belly on the ramus posterior.

Implementation Note
As only a stimulus is applied, the direct round structure of the nerve cannot be recorded or can only be recorded with difficulty (Fig. 6.3).

6.2.4 Palpation of the Ilioinguinal Nerve

Emerging from the lumbar plexus, the ilioinguinal nerve first runs from segment L1 below the iliohypogastric nerve.

As the name of the nerve already suggests, it finds its way posterior to the kidney and laterally to the iliac crest, passing through the psoas major muscle and then running on the quadratus lumborum muscle.

Starting from there, along the lateral abdominal wall, piercing the transversus abdominis muscle or not, depending on the individual, it reaches the inguinal ligament.

At the level of the latter, running between the obliquus abdominis and transversum abdominis muscles, its path is determined by the medial canalis inguinalis to the periphery.

Here, the possible further course differs according to gender.

In the male, the sensitive fibres, together with the funiculus spermaticus, are found at the scrotum. This occurs via the course through the inguinal canal further through the superficial annulus inguinalis. The scrotal anterior nerves from the ilioinguinal nerve are present at this point.

The course is determined differently in the female sex, where the fibres, together with the lig. teres, lead through the inguinal canal and the external inguinal ring (annulus inguinalis superficialis) to the labia majora. The labial anterior nerves are then found there.

The ilioinguinal nerve is both motor and sensitive, supplying the periphery. It therefore innervates the transversus abdominis muscle (caudal parts), the obliquus internus abdominis muscle (main branch of the ilioinguinal nerve) as well as the skin of the base of the penis and cranial parts of

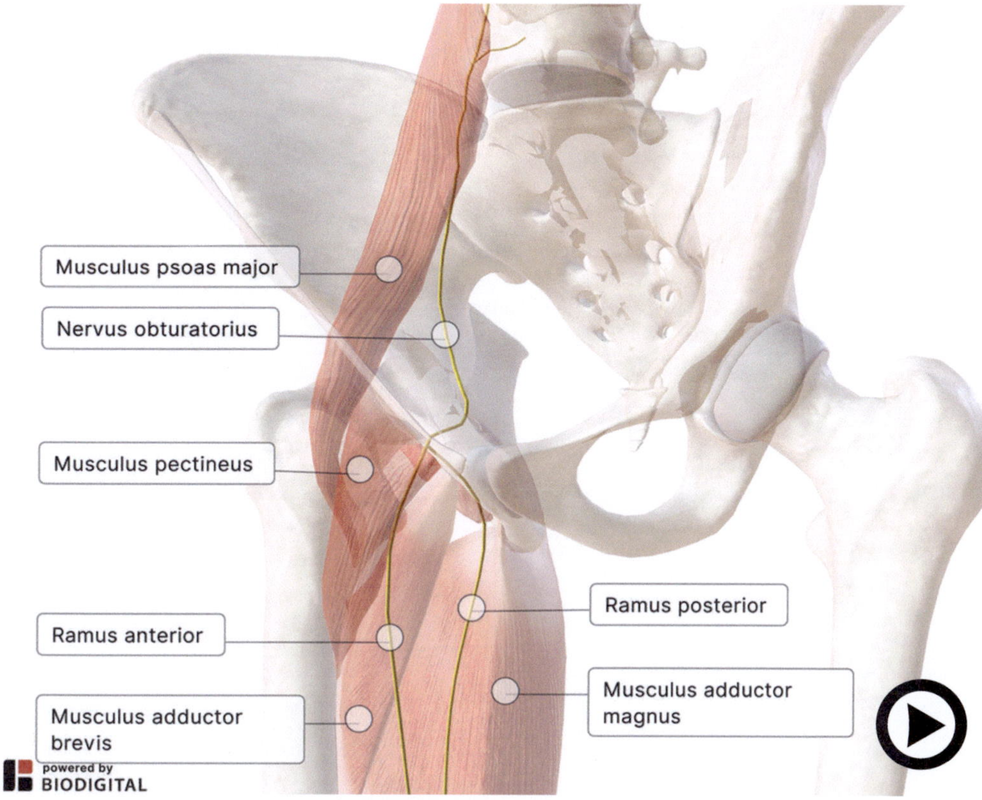

Fig. 6.3 Anatomy and palpation of the N. obturatorius (▶ https://doi.org/10.1007/000-cw4)

the scrotum (scrotal anterior nerves). In women, it sensitively supplies the mons pubis and the labia majora via the labial anterior nerves [4].

Palpation is performed by stimulating the area of the iliac crest. The patient is positioned in the supine position while the therapist, standing laterally, contacts the middle third of the iliac crest, coming from the side, with the fingertips of the index, middle and ring fingers. The patient is positioned in the supine position while the therapist, standing laterally, contacts the middle third of the iliac crest, coming from the side, with the fingertips of the index, middle and ring fingers. The stimulus is applied directly via pressure on the inside of the homolateral iliac crest. The palpation is then continued via the pecten ossis pubis and the ramus superior ossis pubis.

Implementation Note

Numerous structures overlap the nerve in its course, which makes it difficult to feel the roundish structure directly (Fig. 6.4).

6.2.5 Palpation of the Lateral Cutaneous Femoris Nerve

The nerve, which is located laterally in the surface of the thigh, arises from the segments L2–L3 and runs dorsally of the psoas major muscle distolaterally into the iliac fossa. Continuing anteriorly towards the SIAS, it passes through

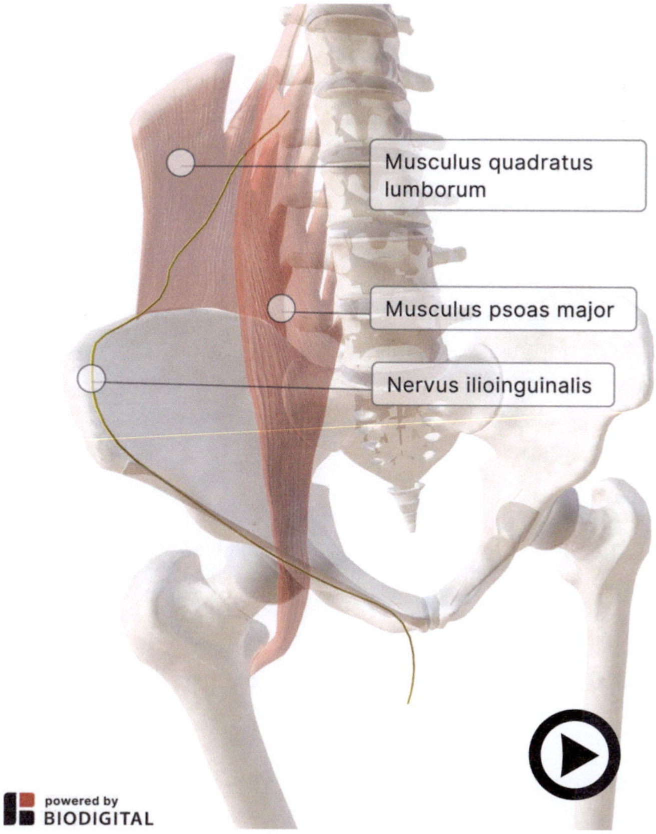

Fig. 6.4 Anatomy and palpation of the N. ilioinguinalis (▶ https://doi.org/10.1007/000-cw5)

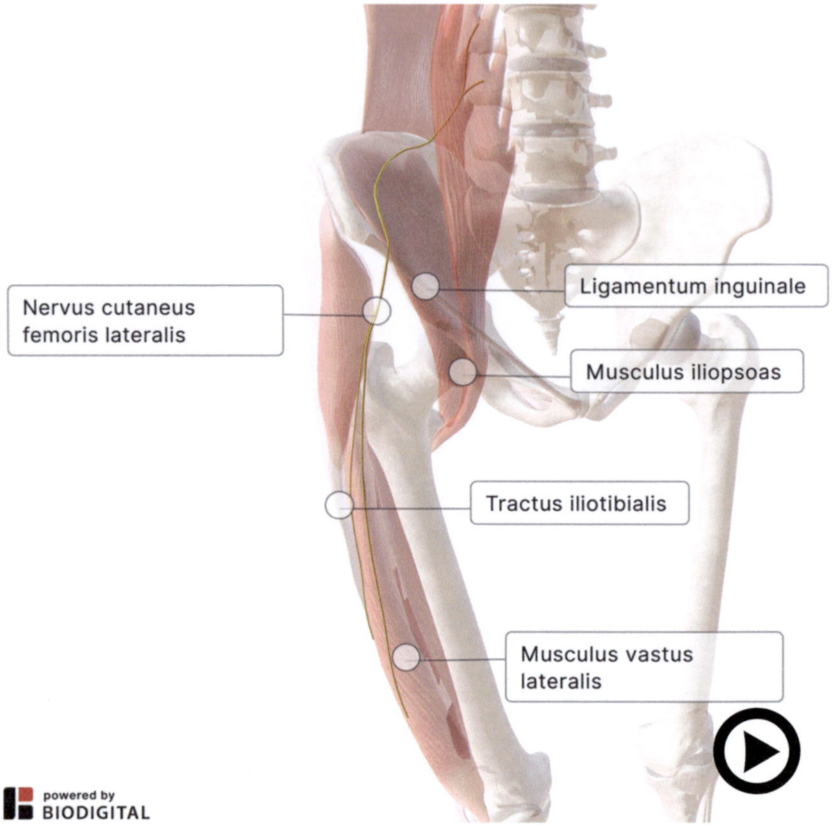

Fig. 6.5 Anatomy and palpation of the N. cutaneus femoris lateralis (▶ https://doi.org/10.1007/000-cw6)

the lacuna musculorum and bends laterally over the sartorius muscle. In a similar course to the rectus femoris muscle, the lateral cutaneous femoral nerve, true to its name, runs laterally and ends at the level of the distal third of the vastus lateralis muscle. As it is a somatosensitive nerve, it supplies the skin of the lateral thigh [5].

Palpation of the nerve is done from the supine position. The therapist stands sideways and makes contact with the origin of the homolateral sartorius muscle via the SIAS. The finger berries, which are placed flat, then move about two transverse fingers distally along the muscle and meet the crossing lateral cutaneous femoris nerve. Depending on the anatomical condition, this can be felt or merely provided with a stimulus.

Implementation Note
As the nerve then splits into finer branches, it is difficult to follow it as it progresses (Fig. 6.5).

6.2.6 Palpation of the Superior and Inferior Gluteal Nerve

Both nerves originate from the sacral plexus, with the superior part originating from segments L4–S1 and the inferior part from segments L5–S2. Both initially descend into the lesser pelvis before extending laterally through the foramen ischiadicum majus. The superior gluteal nerve passes through the suprapiriform foramen and the inferior gluteal nerve through the infrapiriform foramen. Both then differentiate into small branches and innervate the gluteus medius and minimus and tensor fasciae latae muscles superiorly and the gluteus maximus and hip joint capsule inferiorly.

For the stimulation of the respective nerves, the starting position should be in the prone position with the therapist standing sideways at the level of the buttocks. The fingertips first grasp the piriformis muscle (see Sect. 5.2.6) and then move in the direction of the sacrum. Shortly before the muscle origin at the facies pelvica, the steeply positioned fingers will apply pressure deep into the tissue at the superior and inferior edges of the muscle, respectively. This will apply a stimulus to the superior and inferior gluteal nerve.

Implementation Note
Direct sensing of the roundish structures is not possible (Fig. 6.6).

6.2.7 Palpation of the Pudendal Nerve

The pubic nerve originating from segments S2–S4 first runs laterally through the infrapiriform foramen and then

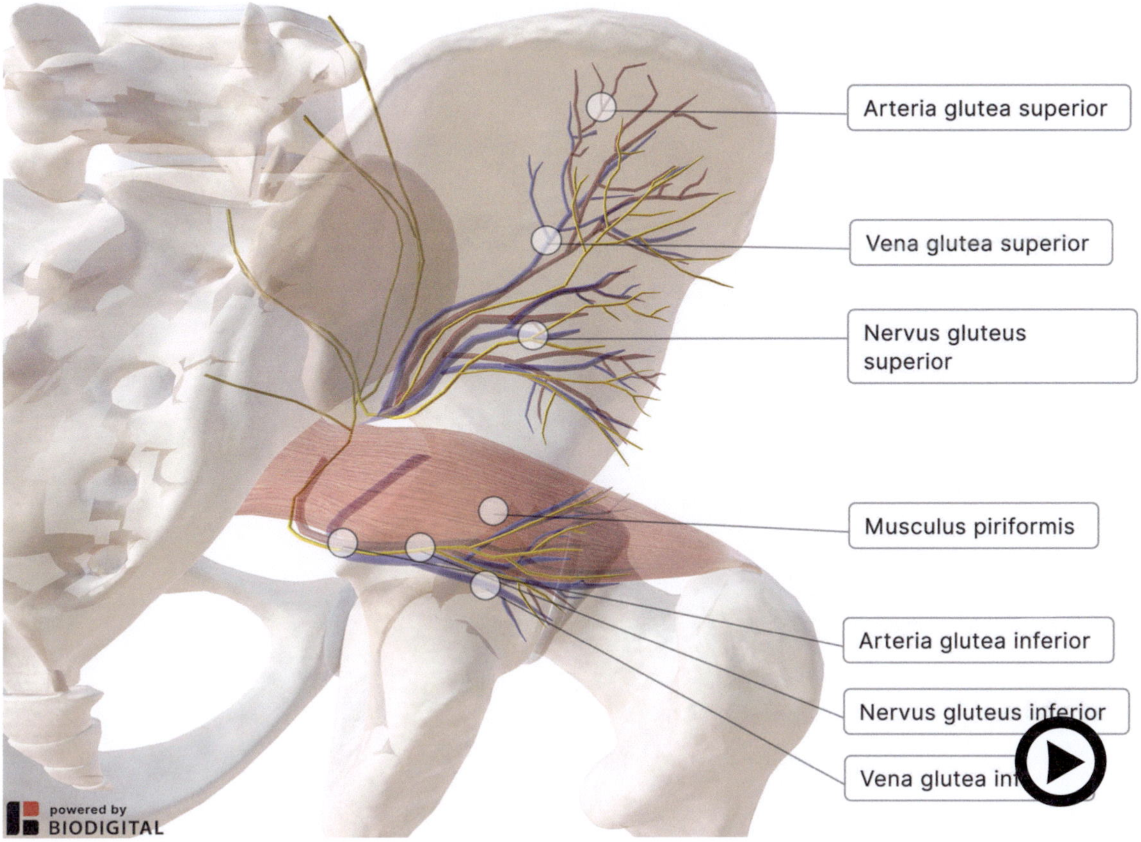

Fig. 6.6 Anatomy and palpation of the N. gluteus superior et inferior (▶ https://doi.org/10.1007/000-cw7)

steeply distally through the foramen ischiadicum minus into the pelvis. It is completely covered by the gluteus maximus muscle and limited medially by the sacrotuberal ligament. In the pelvis, it takes an anterocaudal course, passes through Alcock's canal and then splits into its branches. The terminal branches (inferior rectal nerve, perineal nerve, dorsal penile nerve and dorsal clitoral nerve) provide somatomotor control of various sphincter and pelvic floor muscles as well as somatosensory innervation of the skin in this region.

Palpation takes the form of stimulation of the nerve. The client is positioned supine while the therapist first contacts the sacrotuberal ligament (see Sect. 4.2.1.3) via the steeply positioned fingertips. Starting from this structure, the fingers move slightly medially so that they slide into a depression at the lateral edge of the ligament. Directly in this region, they meet the pudendal nerve.

Performance

Prolonged palpation and prolonged pressure may cause paresthesia in the genital region. This abnormality can often be observed when cycling [6] (Fig. 6.7).

6.2.8 Palpation of the Saphenous Nerve

As a splitting off the femoral nerve, the saphenous nerve, shortly after passing through the lacuna musculorum, runs steeply distomedially with the femoral artery and vein. It initially runs deep until it then emerges within the adductor canal towards the surface, between the adductor longus muscle, the gracilis muscle and the sartorius muscle. Medially on the knee, it then emerges between the tendon of the sartorius muscle and that of the gracilis muscle in the area of the superficial pes anserinus and then moves steeply distally, where it runs directly superficial to the medial edge of the tibial crest. Finally, it bends towards the foot directly at the level of the medial malleolus and ends in the dorsum of the foot. In its course, the saphenous nerve gives off numerous sensory branches that provide sensation to the skin medially at the knee joint as well as the lower leg.

Palpation of the nerve is first done by stimulating the adductor canal (see Sect. 7.1.1.8). To do this, the client should be positioned in the supine position with the knee joints underneath. Then the client can be grasped distally with the fingertips of the index and middle fingers applied

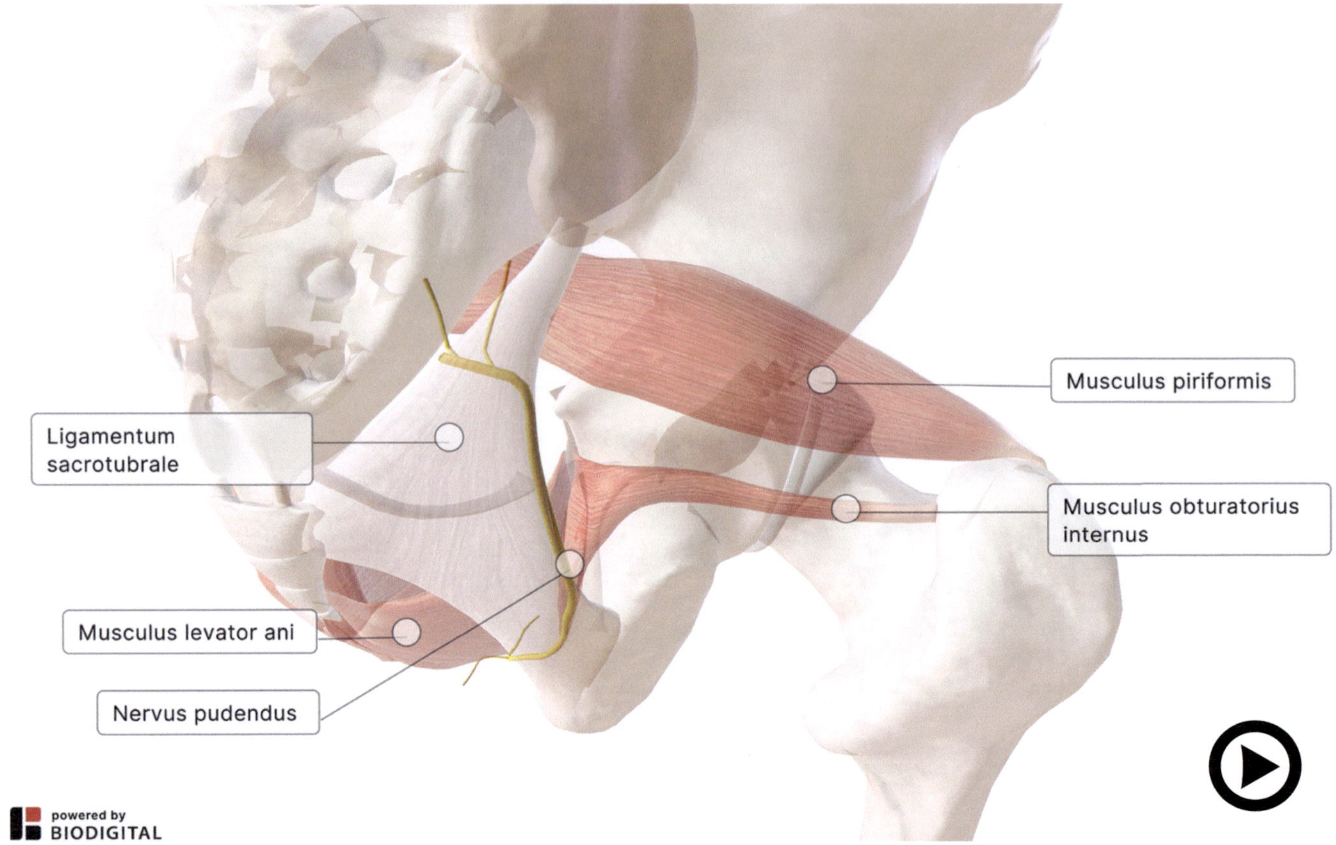

Fig. 6.7 Anatomy and palpation of the N. pudendus (▶ https://doi.org/10.1007/000-cw8)

over a wide area both medially on the knee and, even better, on the facies medialis of the tibia. It is advisable to move the tissue transversely to the bone to delineate the round structure. Depending on the anatomical conditions, the quality of palpation may vary.

Execution Advice
To avoid discomfort in the sensitive area of the saphenous nerve, a gentle approach is advised (Fig. 6.8).

6.2.9 Palpation of the Sciatic Nerve

The colossal nerve arises from the segments L4–S3 of the sacral plexus and supplies large parts of the leg both motor and sensory via its numerous branches. It is about as strong as one's own little finger and experiences a high clinical significance due to its far-reaching influence on the lower extremity.

Emerging from the sacral plexus in a lateral direction, it bends in the middle third of the piriformis muscle below it and runs steeply distally. It also partially pierces the muscle, which is important in terms of clinical hypothesis formation in the sense of a possible constriction. After crossing the pelvitrochanteric muscles, the sciatic nerve runs between the biceps femoris and semitendinosus muscles in depth towards the popliteal fossa. It is bounded anteriorly by the adductor

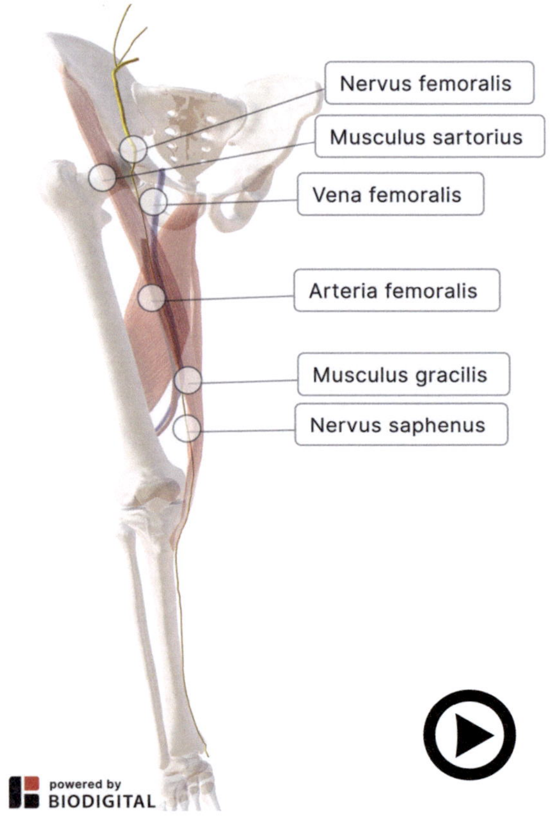

Fig. 6.8 Anatomy and palpation of the N. saphenus (▶ https://doi.org/10.1007/000-cw9)

magnus muscle. Shortly before it enters the popliteal fossa, the enormous nerve divides into the tibial nerve, which runs posteriorly, and the common fibular nerve, which runs anteriorly along the lower leg. This division point is variable in height [7]. Subsequently, these branches supply the lower leg. Due to its complexity, only the sciatic nerve as such up to its entry into the popliteal fossa will be discussed in this chapter, while the branches will be dealt with in separate chapters. Strictly speaking, both parts run as separate nerves from the beginning, but are combined as the sciatic nerve due to the common sheath. The main motor supply areas of the nerve in the area of the thigh include the ischiocrural muscles (except for the caput breve of the biceps femoris muscle) and the adductor magnus muscle via the tibial fibres. The fibular fibres exert a motor influence on the caput breve of the biceps femoris muscle and, further distally, a somatosensory influence on the lower leg and foot.

The stimulation of the sciatic nerve is done in the prone position. The therapist has a choice of two approaches. Proximal palpation takes place via the piriformis muscle, which must first be located. Around the middle third, the steeply positioned fingertips move downwards along the inferior edge of the muscle and meet the nervous structure. Since the gluteus maximus muscle is superficial, the fingers must first glide through the muscular structure and into depth. The distal approach is also made with the fingertips steeply positioned directly between the muscle bellies of the biceps femoris and semitendinosus muscles. The therapist orientates himself on a groove that separates the two muscles and feels his way deeper. At this point, a direct stimulus can be applied to the nerve. It should be noted that the nerve usually splits about a hand's width proximal to the knee joint space. Thus, the stimulus can be applied approximately to the beginning of the femoral condyles.

Implementation Note
Depending on the anatomical situation, the division point of the sciatic nerve can also be located further proximally (Fig. 6.9).

6.2.10 Palpation of the Common Fibular Nerve

As a splitting branch of the sciatic nerve, the common fibular nerve follows the distolateral tendon of the biceps femoris muscle to its insertion at the caput fibulae, where it branches into the superficial and profundal fibular nerve. Thus, the nerve has a rather short and superficial course. Directly after splitting off from the sciatic nerve, the common fibular nerve gives off the sural nerve, which projects steeply distally (see Sect. 6.2.13).

The somatomotor fibres innervate the caput breve of the biceps femoris muscle, while the somatosensory fibres, which run further, supply the skin in the lateral region of the lower leg.

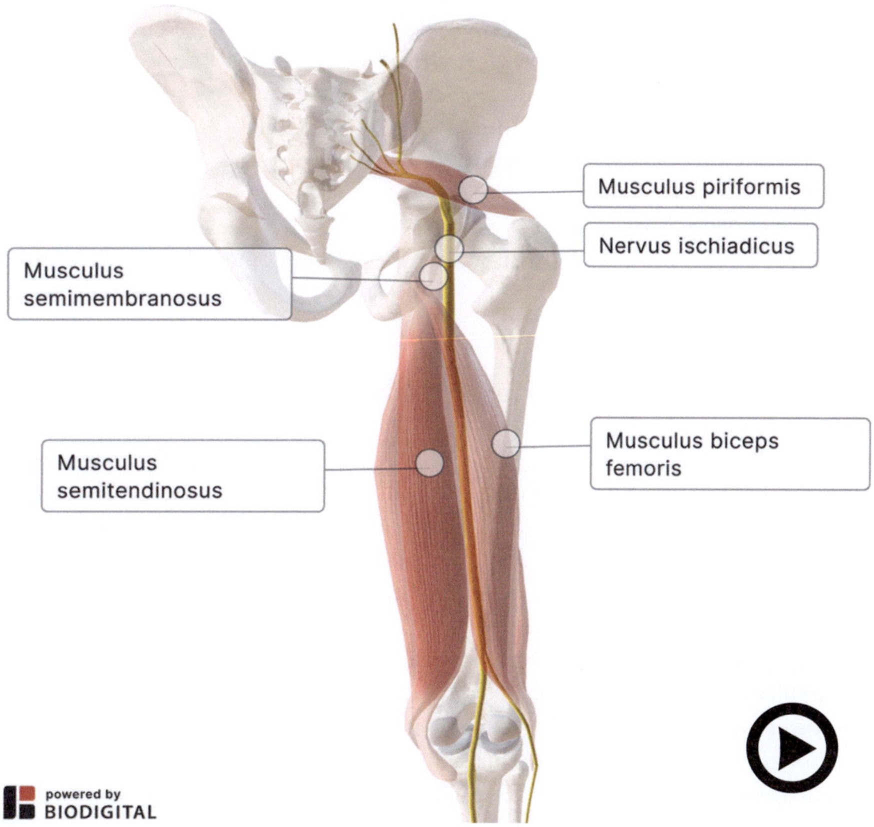

Fig. 6.9 Anatomy and palpation of the N. ischiadicus (▶ https://doi.org/10.1007/000-cwa)

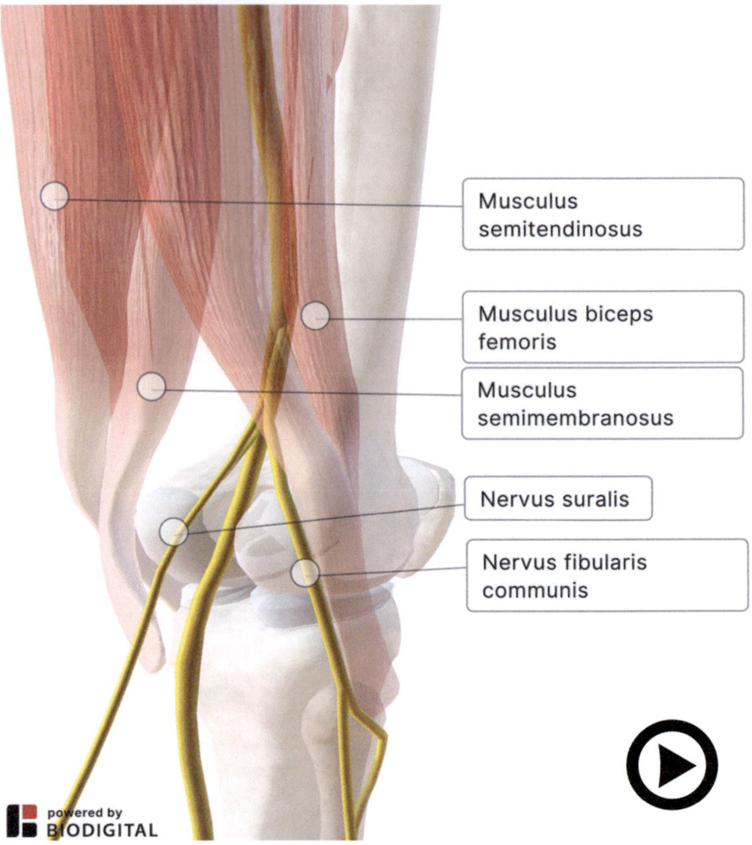

Fig. 6.10 Anatomy and palpation of the N. fibularis communis (▶ https://doi.org/10.1007/000-cwb)

For palpation, the client is positioned in the supine position while the therapist orientates himself with the flatly placed fingertips on the attachment tendon of the biceps femoris muscle (see Sect. 5.3.7). From there, they move slightly in the posterior direction and, after the muscle edge, meet directly with the nerve, which can be grasped in depth by direct stimulation. In some cases, the fingertips must be flexed under the distal phalanges in order to feel the round, firm, nerve structure.

Implementation Note
The caput fibulae provides optimal guidance for finding the common fibular nerve (Fig. 6.10).

6.2.11 Palpation of the Superficial Fibular Nerve

Directly posterioproximal to the caput fibulae, the superficial fibular nerve arises as a division of the common fibular nerve. Between the muscle origins of the fibularis longus muscle and the soleus muscle, the nerve moves in a distoanterior direction and then runs under the fibularis longus muscle and laterally of the extensor digitorum longus muscle to the lateral malleolus. It emerges in the distal third of the tibia or at the lower edge of the fibularis longus muscle belly. At the anterior edge of the lateral malleolus, it divides into the dorsal cutaneous pedal nerves (see Sect. 6.2.16), which provide sensory supply to the dorsum of the foot through further branches. The somatomotor innervation of the superficial fibular nerve is provided by the fibularis longus muscle and the fibularis brevis muscle.

Two regions are considered for palpation of the nerve, with the client positioned in the supine position. The therapist stands sideways and contacts the homolateral caput fibulae with the fingertips of the index and middle fingers. If the fingertips move posteriorly in the proximal area, they meet directly with the bifurcation of the common fibular nerve and its posterior branch, the superficial fibular nerve. For better orientation, the attachment tendon of the biceps femoris muscle can serve as a guide, which is located anterior to the nerve.

The second palpation area is located in the anteriodistal third of the tibia between the extensor digitorum longus and the fibularis longus or brevis muscles. The fingertips move flatly on the facies anterior to the fibula in the distal third transversely to the course of the nerve and, depending on the anatomical condition, can grasp the nerve in its course distally.

The splits on the dorsum of the foot can be optimally grasped with a final inversion of the foot. In this case, parts often emerge whose palpation is reminiscent of that of a thin guitar side.

Implementation Note
In the foot region, the lateral malleolus serves as an osseous landmark for locating the superficial fibular nerve (Fig. 6.11).

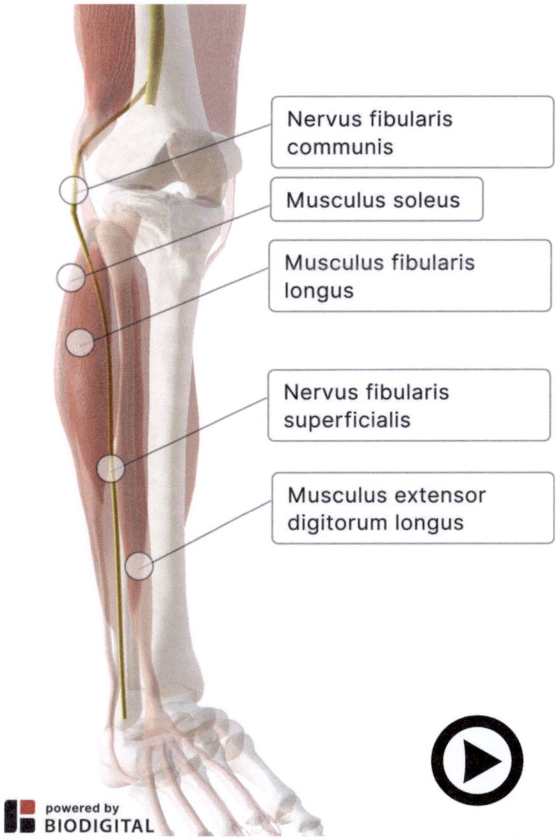

Fig. 6.11 Anatomy and palpation of the N. fibularis superficialis (▶ https://doi.org/10.1007/000-cwc)

6.2.12 Palpation of the Profundal Fibular Nerve

Posterioproximal to the caput fibulae, the profundal fibular nerve arises as a branch of the common fibular nerve. In contrast to its superficial equivalent, the deep nerve runs directly anteriorly and, after the tendon of origin of the fibularis longus muscle, dives under the extensor digitorum muscle and the tibialis anterior muscle in the direction of the medial tibial margo. It then runs distally with the tibial artery along the anterior edge of the tibia to the talus. From there, the fibular profundus nerve radiates medially of the extensor hallucis brevis muscle distally to the distal third of the metatarsal I. It also follows the further course of the medial tibial artery. It also follows the course of the anterior tibial artery, which splits into the dorsal pedal artery and then the dorsal metatarsal artery. The mixed nerve supplies the skin somatosensitively in the area between the big toe and the second toe as well as the tibialis anterior, extensor hallucis longus, extensor digitorum longus, extensor hallucis brevis, extensor digitorum brevis and fibularis tertius muscles somatomotorically.

For palpation of the profundal fibular nerve, which is performed from the supine position, two areas are available to the therapist. For the first palpation area, the fingertips are applied directly proximal to the caput fibulae to be able to hit the nerve branch proximal to the tendon of the fibularis longus muscle. As there are also fascial extensions of the tractus iliotibialis in this area, depending on the anatomical situation, only one stimulus can be generated in some cases.

The second palpation area is distal to the tibia. The fingertips are first placed on the tendon of the extensor digitorum longus muscle (see Sect. 5.4.3). From there, they move in a lateral direction and, after the pulsating anterior tibial artery, meet the profundal fibular nerve, which can then be grasped as far as the middle of the metatarsal I.

Implementation Note
With prolonged pressure on the nerve, paraesthesia may occur in the area between the big toe and the second toe. This may briefly serve for more precise differentiation during palpation (Fig. 6.12).

6.2.13 Palpation of the Sural Nerve

Immediately after the common fibular nerve splits off from the sciatic nerve, it gives off the sural nerve in the popliteal fossa as a branch, which then rises steeply distally, previously picking up fibres from the medial cutaneous surae nerve from the tibial nerve proximally. It then runs distolaterally between the two gastrocnemius heads, perforates the Achilles tendon in the distal third and extends distally of the lateral malleolus on the lateral edge of the foot to the fifth toe. The predominantly somatosensitive nerve supplies the heel as well as the lateral edge of the foot and posteriolateral parts of the lower leg.

The superficially located nerve can be grasped via the steeply placed fingertips transverse to its course. The client is positioned in the prone position while the therapist makes contact between the two heads of the gastrocnemius. Depending on the anatomical condition, the sural nerve can be felt or merely palpated by applying a stimulus. In the area of the foot, the fingers move to the lateral edge of the Achilles tendon in order to palpate the nerve in depth. Distal to the lateral malleolus, the nerve is more superficial, which allows direct palpation with the fingertips laid flat, perpendicular to its course.

Implementation Note
The gastrocnemius muscle can be seen as a guide muscle for the sural nerve and thus serves as a guide (Fig. 6.13).

6.2.14 Palpation of the Tibial Nerve

From the beginning, the sciatic nerve leads the common fibular and tibial nerves in a sheath. Only in the proximal area of the popliteal fossa does it divide, so that the tibial part then continues steeply distally. While it is still located quite superficially in the region of the popliteal fossa, it dives into the

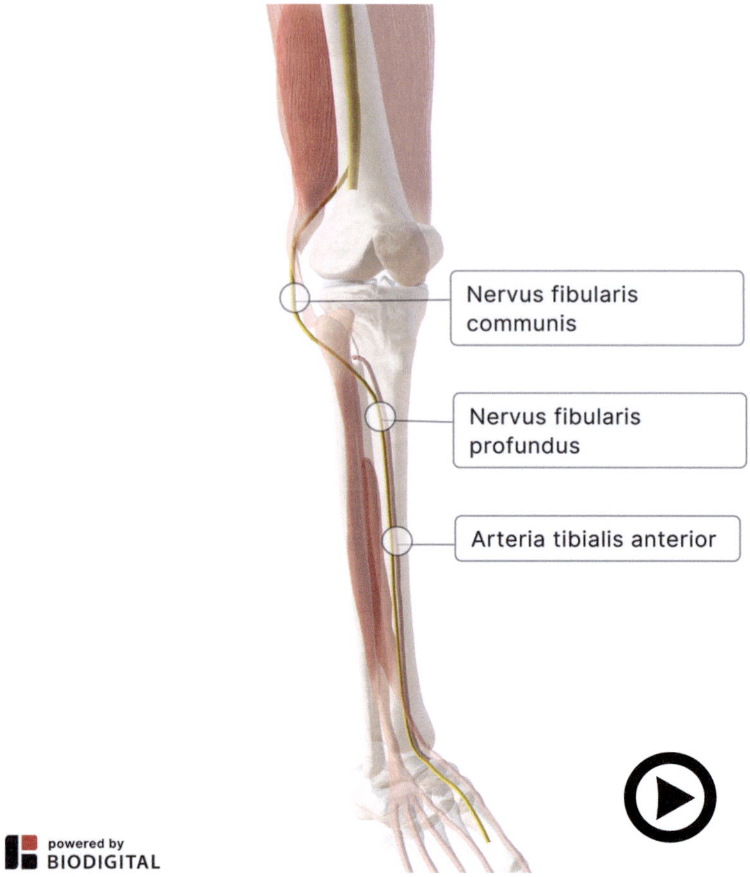

Fig. 6.12 Anatomy and palpation of the N. fibularis profundus (▶ https://doi.org/10.1007/000-cwd)

depths of the calf muscles between the gastrocnemius heads to follow the posterior tibial artery and vein. Only in the distal part does the posterior tibial nerve of the medial malleolus and medial Achilles tendon come to the surface again. It is bordered anteriorly by the tendon of the posterior tibialis muscle and the tendons of the flexor digitorum and hallucis longus muscles. Following the pulsating posterior tibial artery, the tibial nerve enters the sole of the foot in the malleolar canal distal to the talus sustentaculum to split into the medial and lateral plantar nerves. Via numerous branches that the nerve gives off in its course, it supplies, among other things, the posterior skin surface of the lower leg as well as those of the dorsum and sole of the foot in a somatosensitive manner. With its somatomotor nerve fibres, it also innervates almost all plantar muscles of the foot, all dorsal muscles of the lower leg as well as the popliteus muscle, the biceps femoris muscle (caput longum) and the semitendinosus and semimembranosus muscles. It therefore has a great influence on the functionality of the lower extremity and can be palpated as follows.

The client is positioned in the prone position so that two regions on the homolateral side are available for the therapist to palpate. For the first region, the steeply placed fingertips of the index and middle fingers are placed directly in the popliteal fossa between the origins of the gastrocnemius muscle. They can sense the pulse of the tibial artery and, when they move laterally, reach the tibial nerve. In the distal area of the Achilles tendon, the fingertips palpate in a medial direction and, following the tendinous border and somewhat in depth, encounter the rather firm, roundish, nerve structure. The nerve can then still be provided with a palpatory stimulus, running directly next to the artery, until it enters the sole of the foot.

Implementation Note
After a medial tarsal tunnel syndrome and nerve damage, there may be discomfort in the sensitive catchment area of the tibial nerve [8] (Fig. 6.14).

6.2.15 Palpation of the Lateral and Medial Plantar Nerves

Plantar, slightly anterior to the sustentaculum tali, the rather short lateral and medial plantar nerves arise from the tibial nerve. These two nerves branch out towards the sole of the foot, each producing a portion which extends medially and laterally distally, respectively.

The medial plantar nerve first runs distally under the abductor hallucis muscle until it appears plantarly at the level of the medial cuneiform bone. It then radiates with the tendon of the flexor hallucis longus muscle into the distal phalanx of the hallux. On this path, the nerve is additionally accompanied by the plantar artery on the big toe.

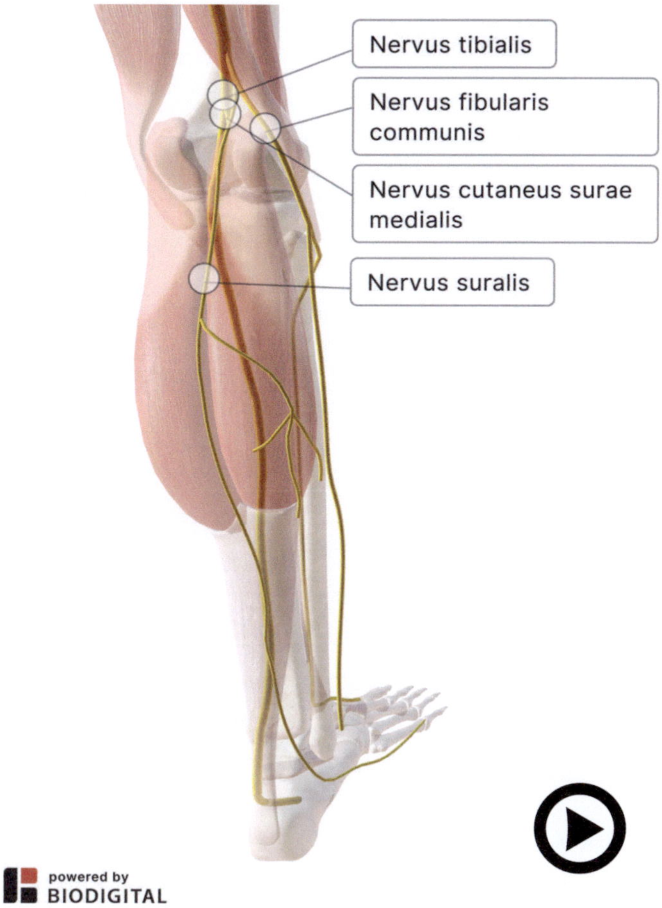

Fig. 6.13 Anatomy and palpation of the N. suralis (▶ https://doi.org/10.1007/000-cwe)

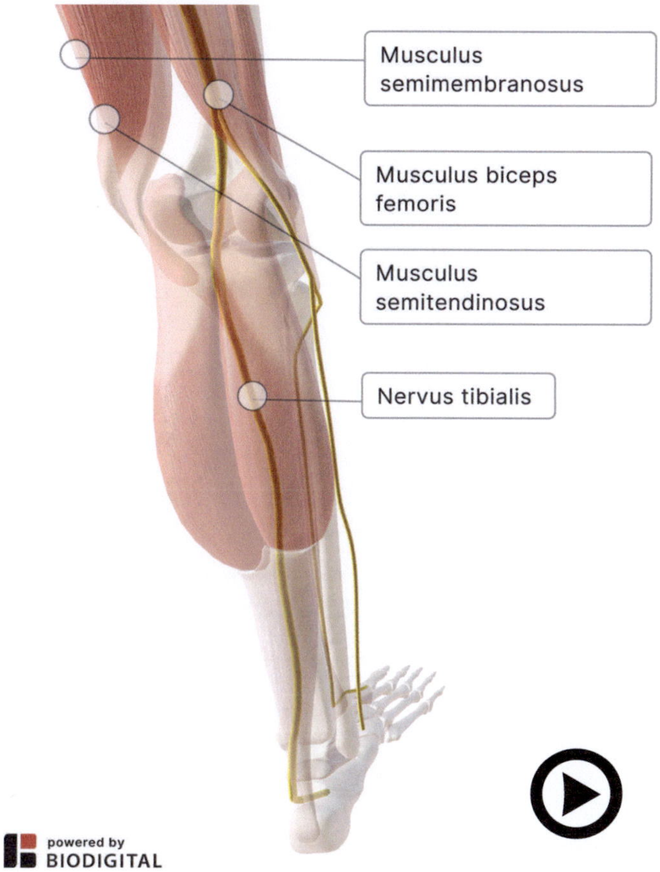

Fig. 6.14 Anatomy and palpation of the N. tibialis (▶ https://doi.org/10.1007/000-cwf)

The lateral plantar nerve runs obliquely laterodistally under the tarsal bones and emerges at the level of the metatarsal V tuberosity between the abductor digiti minimi and flexor digitorum brevis muscles. It then continues distally along the side of the little toe and is also accompanied by laterally running arteries of the metatarsus and the phalanx.

The lateral and medial plantar nerve is palpated from the prone position with the knee joint flexed. The therapist applies a stimulus from the medial and lateral sides of the metatarsals I and V with the steeply positioned fingertips, thus stimulating the nerve. The muscles mentioned serve as orientation.

Implementation Note
Due to the strong expression of surrounding soft tissue, it is usually only possible to stimulate the medial and lateral plantar nerve (Fig. 6.15).

6.2.16 Palpation of the Cutaneous Dorsal Pedal Nerve

The superficial cutaneous nerves that sensitively innervate the dorsum of the foot can be grouped into different groups. These include the medial dorsal cutaneous nerve and the intermediate dorsal cutaneous nerve from the superficial fibular nerve, as well as the lateral dorsal cutaneous nerve as a division of the sural nerve. Both the medial and intermedial parts are located anterior to the lateral malleolus, while the lateral dorsal cutaneous nerve runs distal to the process. In their course distally, they split several times so that they unfold their network over the entire dorsum of the foot.

From the supine position, the individual nerves can be grasped by stimulating the dorsum of the foot with the fingertips. Due to the decreasing number of branches and the anatomical position, it is hardly possible to palpate individual nerve cords in isolation. An exception is the cutaneous dorsalis pedis intermedius nerve, which is partially exposed proximolaterally on the dorsum of the foot with maximum inversion of the foot. The nerve can then be moved and felt with the steeply placed index fingertip, similar to the side of a guitar.

Implementation Note
The nn. cutanei dorsales pedis are extremely delicate in their structure and can therefore only be subjected to gentle stimulation (Fig. 6.16).

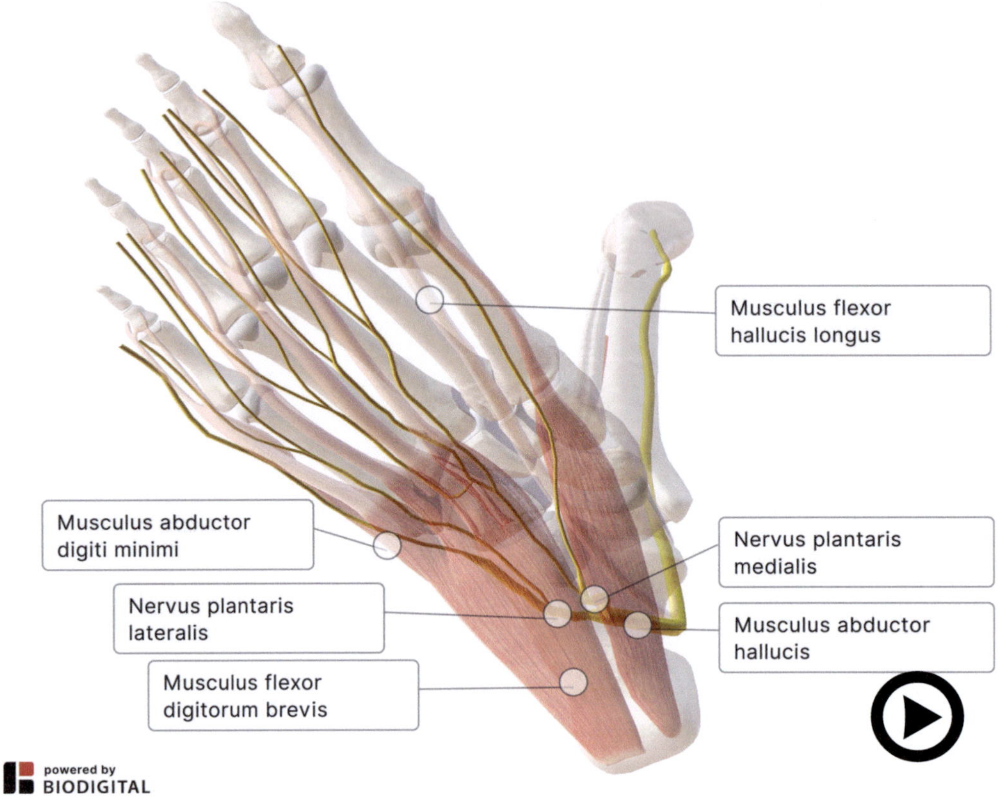

Fig. 6.15 Anatomy and palpation of the N. plantaris medialis et lateralis (▶ https://doi.org/10.1007/000-cwg)

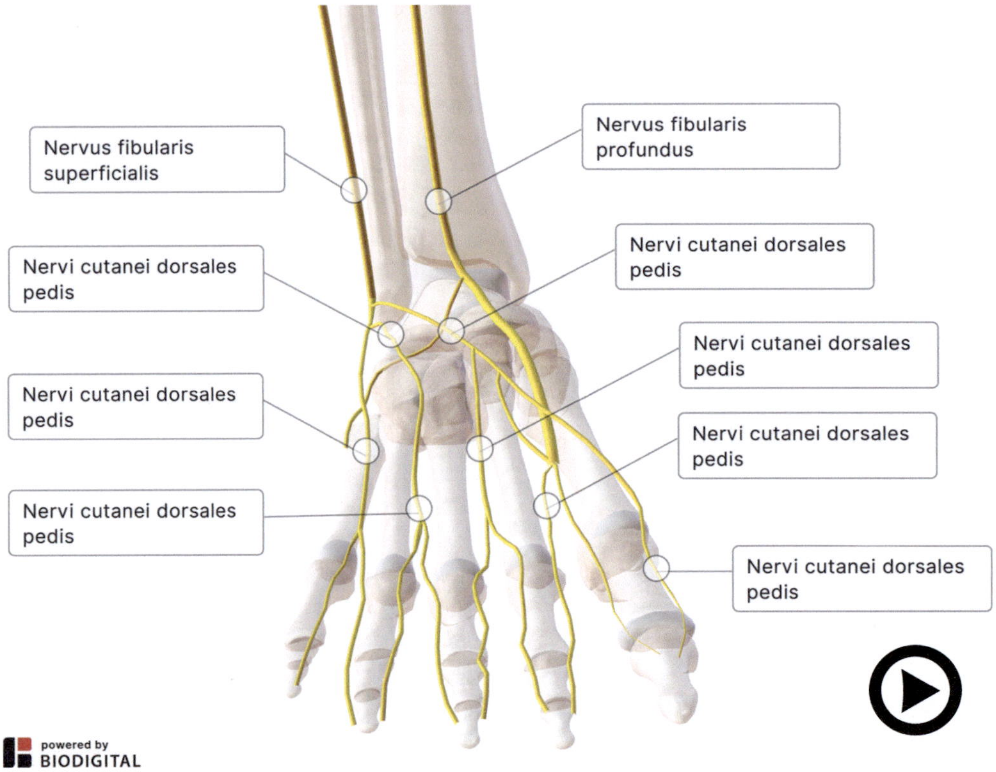

Fig. 6.16 Anatomy and palpation of the Nn. cutanei dorsales pedis (▶ https://doi.org/10.1007/000-cwh)

6.3 Nerves in the Area of the Abdomen and Trunk

There are numerous nerves in the abdominal region that innervate the abdominal cavity both motorically and sensitively. In addition, organs with their receptors ensure the reception and transmission of various information that is of great importance for the homeostasis of the organism. Vital organs are protected by the thorax, which also provides a large area for nerve courses. Since there are numerous soft tissues in the abdomen and trunk, only the intercostal nerves and the iliohypogastric nerve can be palpated by stimulation. The anatomical knowledge of the location is relevant in order to be able to locate the nerve courses. For this reason, the following chapters first describe the anatomy and then the palpation with the client in the supine position.

6.3.1 Palpation of the Intercostal Nerves

The intercostal nerves arise directly from the 12 paired thoracic nerves from the rami anteriores and run ventrally in the intercostal spaces on the thorax. Eleven paired intercostal nerves are completed caudally of the 12th rib by the two subcostal nerves, so that all 12 thoracic nerves have ventral branches. In the thoracic region, the intercostal nerves 1–6 innervate the intercostal muscles motorically and the thoracic skin sensitively. The intercostal nerves 7–11 and the subcostal nerves also provide motor supply to parts of the abdominal muscles and sensitive supply to large parts of the skin in the abdominal region. In some cases, the nerves can become constricted as they perforate various fasciae in their course. This can lead to unpleasant sensations.

To stimulate the intercostal nerves, the client can be positioned individually according to the region to be palpated so that the therapist can reach the intercostal spaces with the fingertips. The fingers are positioned steeply in the region of a rib so that they can then move cranially or caudally into the intercostal space. Once in the intercostal space, the fingertips can palpate from dorsal to ventral to the junction with the sternum to achieve stimulation in the nerve course of the intercostal nerves. The nerve cords run directly along the edges of the ribs and, depending on the region, are overlaid by the abdomen or chest muscle culture, which makes direct palpation impossible.

Implementation Note

The ribs serve as an osseous orientation aid in order to be able to provide the intercostal nerves with a targeted stimulus (Fig. 6.17).

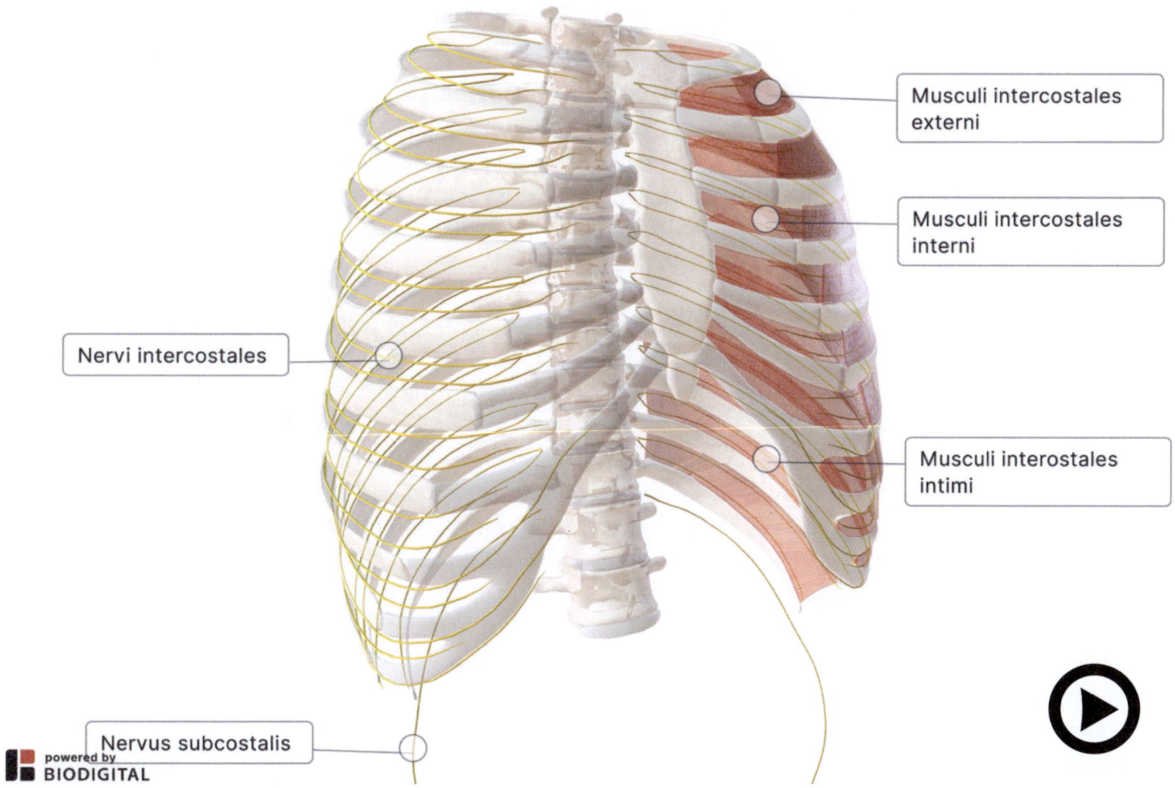

Fig. 6.17 Anatomy and palpation of the Nn. intercostales (▶ https://doi.org/10.1007/000-cwj)

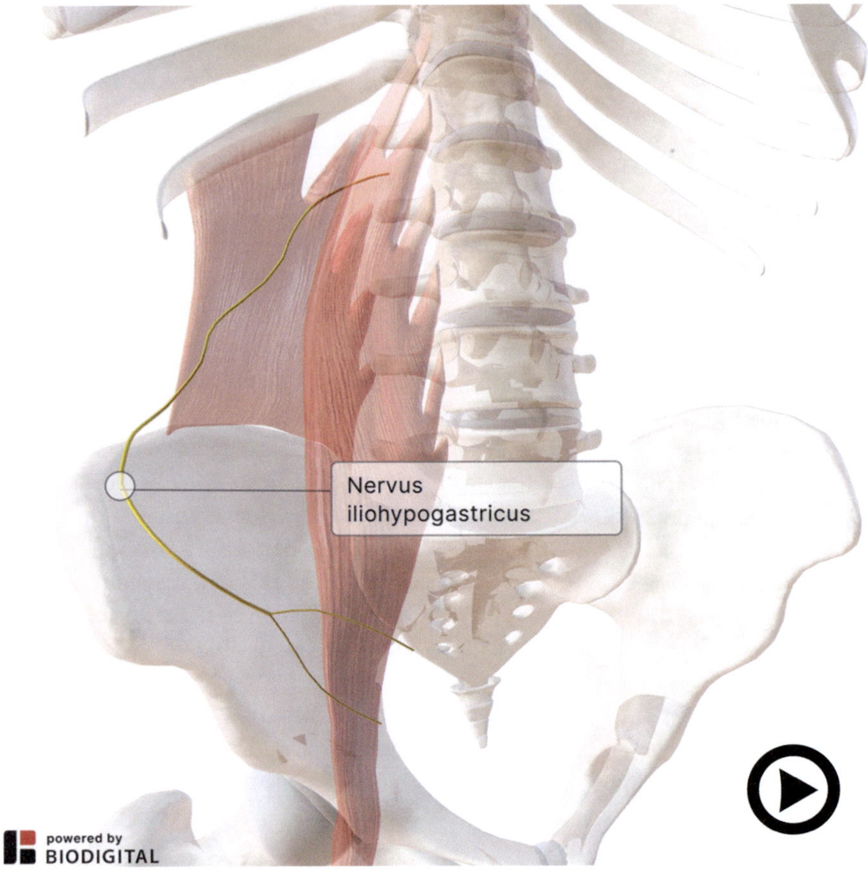

Fig. 6.18 Anatomy and palpation of the N. iliohypogastricus (▶ https://doi.org/10.1007/000-cwk)

6.3.2 Palpation of the Iliohypogastric Nerve

From the lumbar plexus, the iliohypogastric nerve arises dorsally of the kidney from the associated segments Th12 and L1. It then runs laterally between the psoas major and quadratus lumborum muscles. Continuing towards the iliac crest, the nerve perforates the transversus abdominis muscle and radiates cranially along the iliac crest ventrally between the transversus abdominis muscle and the obliquus internus abdominis muscle. After leaving the bony iliac crest at the level of the SIAS, the branching nerve continues to follow the inguinal ligament medially. The mixed iliohypogastric nerve supplies the transversus abdominis and the obliquus internus somatomotorly and proportionately. Somatosensitively, it supplies the skin region cranial to the inguinal ligament and lateral to the hip joint.

As the nerve is covered by numerous soft tissues in its course near the crista iliaca, only one stimulation is possible. The client is to be positioned in a supine position. The therapist first makes contact with the homolateral crista iliaca in the anterior area of the posterior third with steeply positioned fingertips. If the fingertips move about one to two transverse fingers in the direction of the cranial part of the iliac crest, they meet the iliohypogastric nerve, which can be followed ventrally at this height parallel to the iliac crest.

Implementation Note
The ilioinguinal nerve is located directly on the iliac crest, which is why palpation of the iliohypogastric nerve should be performed one to two transverse fingers cranial to the iliac crest to avoid confusion (Fig. 6.18).

6.4 Nerves in the Upper Limb

The somatosensory as well as somatomotor supply to the upper extremity is provided by the cervicobrachial plexus, which is composed of the spinal nerves C1–Th1. The nerve plexus then moves laterally across the shoulder girdle and divides into individual peripheral nerves that innervate the skin and muscles of the upper limb as well as the head. Of these nerves, those that can be subjected to palpatory stimulation are described in the following chapters. These include the thoracic long nerve, the suprascapular nerve, the supraclavicular nerve, the thoracodorsal nerve and the dorsal scapular nerve, the medial and lateral pectoral nerve, the axillary nerve, the musculocutaneous nerve, the median nerve, the radial nerve and the ulnar nerve. Depending on the anatomical position, the optimal starting position of the client is adopted for palpation so that the nerve can be subjected to stimulation. In the following chapters, the anatomical position is discussed before palpation takes place.

6.4.1 Palpation of the Thoracic Longus Nerve

The somatomotor long thoracic nerve receives its fibres from the supraclavicular portion of the brachial plexus. It runs laterally from segments C5 to C7, perforates the scalenus medius muscle and then passes under the clavicle and over the costa prima to the caudolateral. Still under the axillary artery, it passes together with the lateral thoracic artery over the serrated insertions of the anterior serratus muscle to about the level of the middle of the trunk. The thoracic long nerve is responsible for the innervation of the serratus anterior muscle and can thus favour the scapula alata when irritated [9].

The palpation is carried out by stimulating the area of the neck and the torso. It is recommended to start with the head in a passive position in order to relax the neck muscles. The steeply positioned fingertips orientate themselves on the scalenus medius muscle (see Sect. 5.6.3) between the dorsal edge of the sternocleidomastoid muscle and the ventral edge of the trapezius pars descendens muscle and apply a horizontally directed pressure in the lateral cervical region in the direction of the spine. In doing so, they apply a stimulus to an area in which, in addition to the thoracic long nerve, the dorsal scapular nerve and the supraclavicular nerve as well as parts of the brachial plexus are located. Direct palpation in this region is therefore not possible.

To stimulate the caudal part of the nerve, the fingertips orientate themselves to the intersection between the caudal edge of the pectoralis major muscle and the insertions of the serratus anterior muscle. There, the fingers, which are initially placed flat, meet the lateral thoracic artery. The nerve is located directly dorsal to the artery, which can be grasped by stimulation and followed caudally.

Implementation

The thoracic long nerve is susceptible to injury due to its superficial location. A gentle approach is therefore advisable (Fig. 6.19).

6.4.2 Palpation of the Suprascapular Nerve

Originating from segments C5 to C6, the suprascapular nerve is part of the brachial plexus and supplies the supra- and infraspinatus and somatosensory dorsal parts of the shoulder joint capsule. The suprascapular nerve tapers out of the brachial

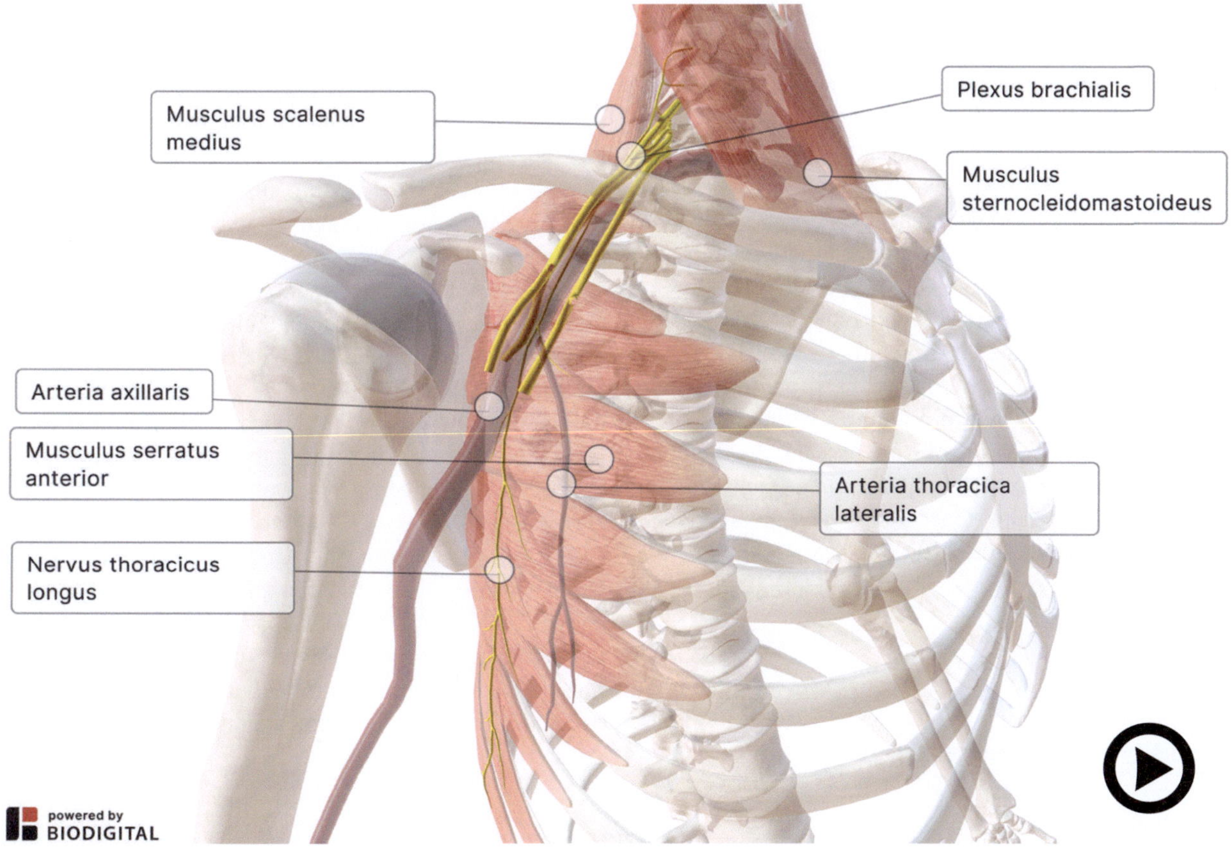

Fig. 6.19 Anatomy and palpation of the N. thoracicus longus (▶ https://doi.org/10.1007/000-cwm)

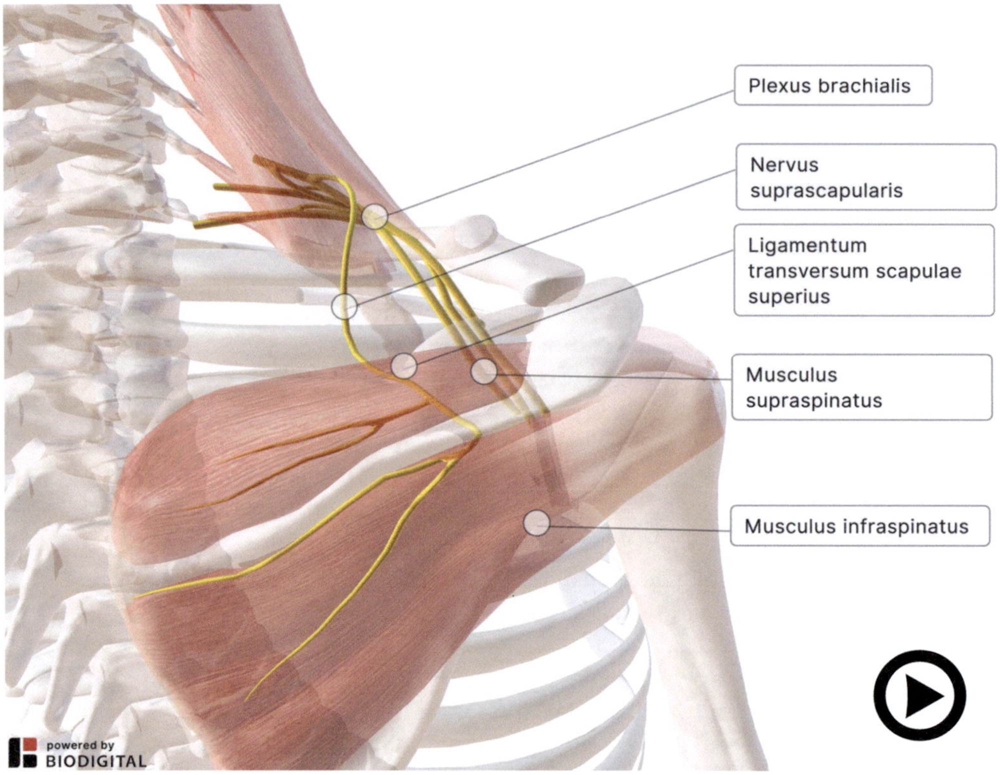

Fig. 6.20 Anatomy and palpation of the N. suprascapularis (▶ https://doi.org/10.1007/000-cwn)

plexus through the posterior scalenus gap between the scalenus anterior and medius muscles and then passes dorsolaterally under the omohyoideus pars inferior towards the scapula. In this region, the nerve is covered by the trapezius pars descendens muscle until it arrives through the incisura scapulae in the suprascapular fossa below the muscle of the same name. After giving off some branches, the suprascapular nerve runs laterally of the spina scapulae through the incisura spinoglenoidalis and finally ends broadly cross-linked in the infraspinous fossa. In this part, it is covered by the deltoideus pars spinalis muscle and the infraspinatus muscle.

The nerve is overlapped by numerous structures, which makes palpation difficult and only allows stimulation. The client is positioned in the prone position so that the therapist can make contact with the homolateral spina scapulae with his steeply placed fingertips. Once there, the fingers move in a caudal direction so that they can apply a stimulus to the nerve directly at the lower edge of the scapular bone.

Implementation Note

The suprascapular nerve passes through several potential constrictions along its course, which may compress it if there are structurally negative changes (Fig. 6.20).

6.4.3 Palpation of the Supraclavicular Nerves

The naming of these nerves describes their local proximity to the clavicle. They originate from segments C3 to C4 and are thus part of the cervical plexus. The supraclavicular nerves can be divided into medial, intermedial and lateral components and supply the skin in the area of the lower neck, shoulder and upper chest somatosensitively.

After leaving the cervical plexus, the parts of the supraclavicular nerves run caudolaterally between the sternocleidomastoid muscle and the scalenus anterior or medius muscle in the cranial region. They wrap around the external jugular vein before the individual parts continue their way medially, intermedially and laterally to the clavicle. Their entire course is covered by the platysma, which they partially perforate.

For the stimulation, the patient is placed in a supine or sitting position while the therapist contacts the homolateral clavicle. The fingertips are positioned steeply in the acromion and begin to move on the superior margo in the direction of the sternal extremities. During this, they repeatedly encounter parts of the supraclavicular nerves, which can be registered by stimulation.

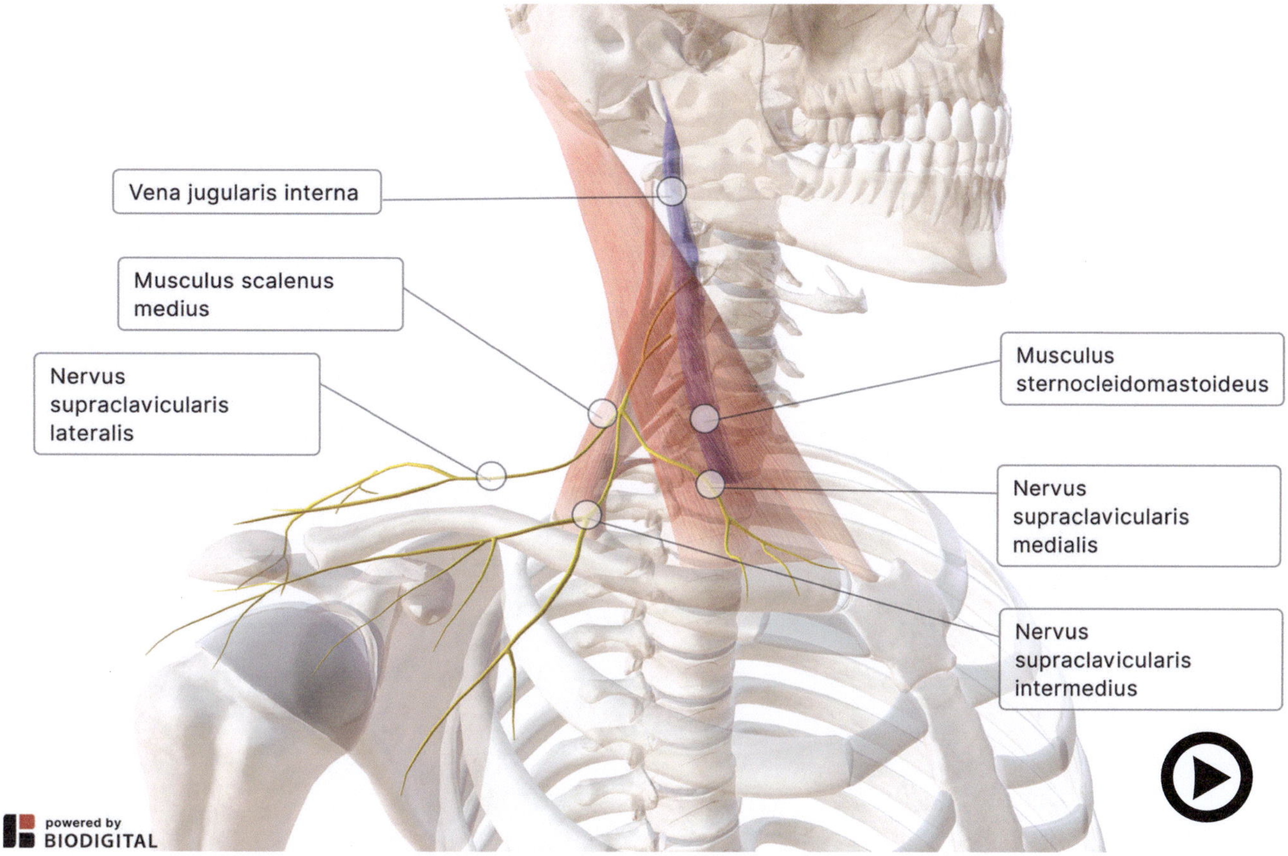

Fig. 6.21 Anatomy and palpation of the N. supraclavicularis (▶ https://doi.org/10.1007/000-cwp)

Instructions for Use
Due to the anatomical conditions, direct palpation of the supraclavicular nerve is not possible (Fig. 6.21).

6.4.4 Palpation of the Thoracodorsal Nerve

The thoracodorsal nerve extends under the scapula and originates as a motor nerve from the brachial plexus. In the area of the axilla, the nerve runs caudally between the serratus anterior muscle and the subscapularis muscle and is accompanied by the thoracodorsal artery and vein on its way in the distal third. In its course, it gives off further branches which are responsible for the innervation of the teres major muscle and the latissimus dorsi muscle.

For palpation, the client should be in a prone or sitting position. The therapist stands at the level of the scapula and orients his or her finger berries on the inferior angulus of the scapula. As the finger berries travel along the margo lateralis towards the axilla, they cross the thoracodorsal nerve, as a rounded and solid structure about midway. It is important that the finger berries are not directly on the bony scapula, but just before it, on the serratus anterior muscle and between the teres major muscle and the latissimus dorsi muscle.

Implementation Note
During palpation, there may be sensory disturbances which are expressed in the direction of the latissimus dorsi muscle (Fig. 6.22).

6.4.5 Palpation of the Dorsal Scapular Nerve

The dorsal scapular nerve arises from the brachial plexus, especially from segment C5, and then passes caudolaterally between the medius and posterior scalenus muscles. After passing through, the nerve is oriented towards the superior angulus of the scapula and divides into a portion that runs dorsally towards the supraspinous fossa and a second portion that runs ventrally of the levator scapulae towards the medial margo of the scapula. The second portion then follows the scapula along the medial edge to the inferior angulus and is covered by the rhomboid and levator scapulae muscles. Before the division, the somatomotor nerve, which innervates the levator scapulae and the rhomboid muscles, is extensively overlapped by the descending and transverse trapezius muscles.

For the stimulation, the client is positioned in a prone or seated position so that the therapist has optimal access from

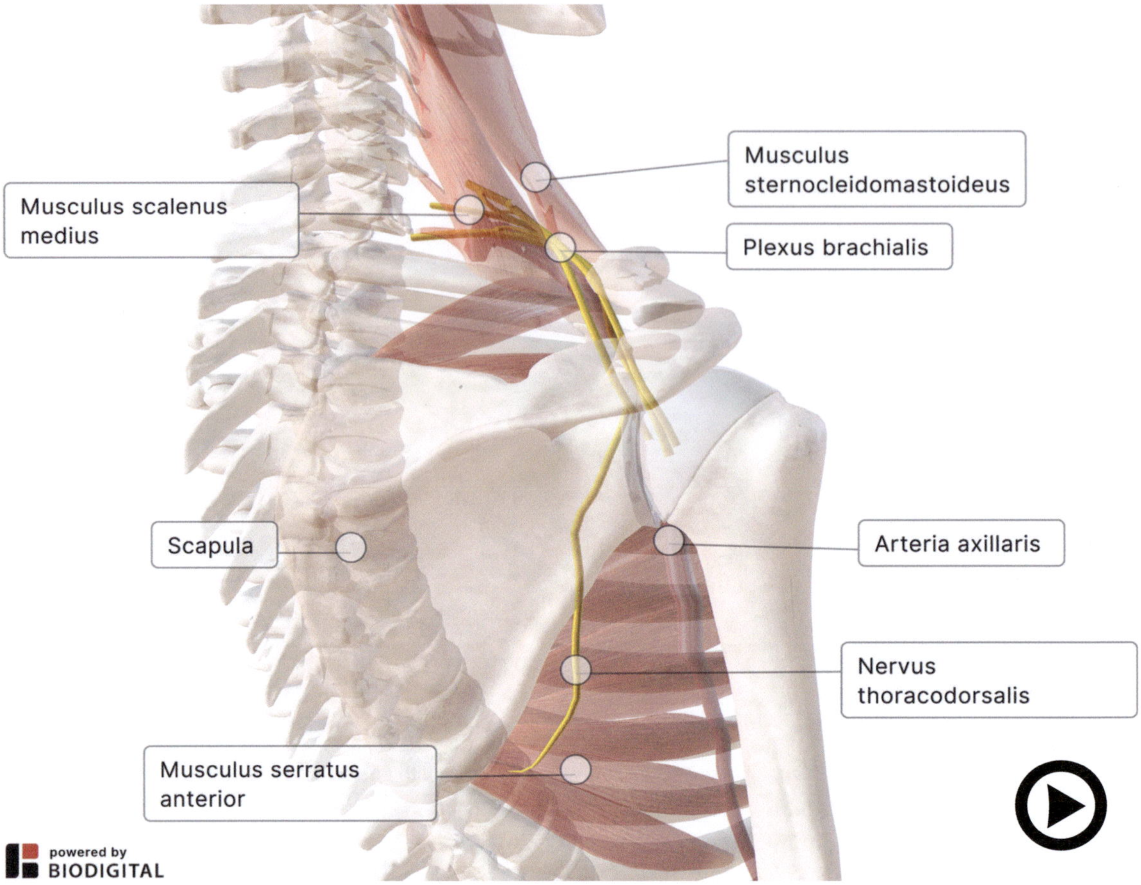

Fig. 6.22 Anatomy and palpation of the N. thoracodorsalis (▶ https://doi.org/10.1007/000-cwq)

the dorsal side. The fingertips are positioned steeply at the superior angulus of the scapula, where they meet the tendon of the levator scapulae muscle (see Sect. 5.7.1). From there, they move to the lateral edge and meet the dorsalis scapulae nerve in the depression, which can be reached by stimulation.

In addition, palpation impulses can be given in the region of the margo medialis scapulae by moving the fingertips slightly medial to the bony edge from cranial to caudal and applying a stimulus in depth. At the same time, the artery and vein of the same name are palpated.

Implementation Note
As the fingers must first palpate through various muscles, an explicit recording of the dorsalis scapulae nerve is not possible (Fig. 6.23).

6.4.6 Palpation of the Pectoral Nerves

The pectoral medial and lateral nerves arise from the brachial plexus and supply the thoracic region. It should be noted that the name medial derives only from the medial division and that the nerve is located more laterally on the thorax. This contrasts with the lateral portion which originates laterally but then passes caudally of the clavicle to the medial. Both nerves are separated by the axillary artery and vein, respectively, with the lateral pectoral nerve running anteriorly and the medial pectoral nerve posteriorly to the vessels. The former runs directly under the pectoralis major pars clavicularis towards the extremitas sternalis, while the pectoralis medialis nerve takes the same course as the pectoralis minor, which it perforates at times. Both nerves supply the pectoralis major and minor somatomotor nerves.

For the stimulation of the nerves, the patient is positioned in a supine or sitting position while the therapist orientates himself on the proc. coracoideus with the fingertips placed flat. From there, the fingertips move horizontally towards the sternum to apply a stimulus to the lateral pectoral nerve caudal to the clavicle. If the steeply positioned finger berries move in a caudomedial direction and follow the pectoralis minor muscle, they apply a stimulus to the pectoralis medial nerve.

Implementation Note
Due to the superimposition of the chest muscles, direct sensation of the pectoral nerves is not possible (Fig. 6.24).

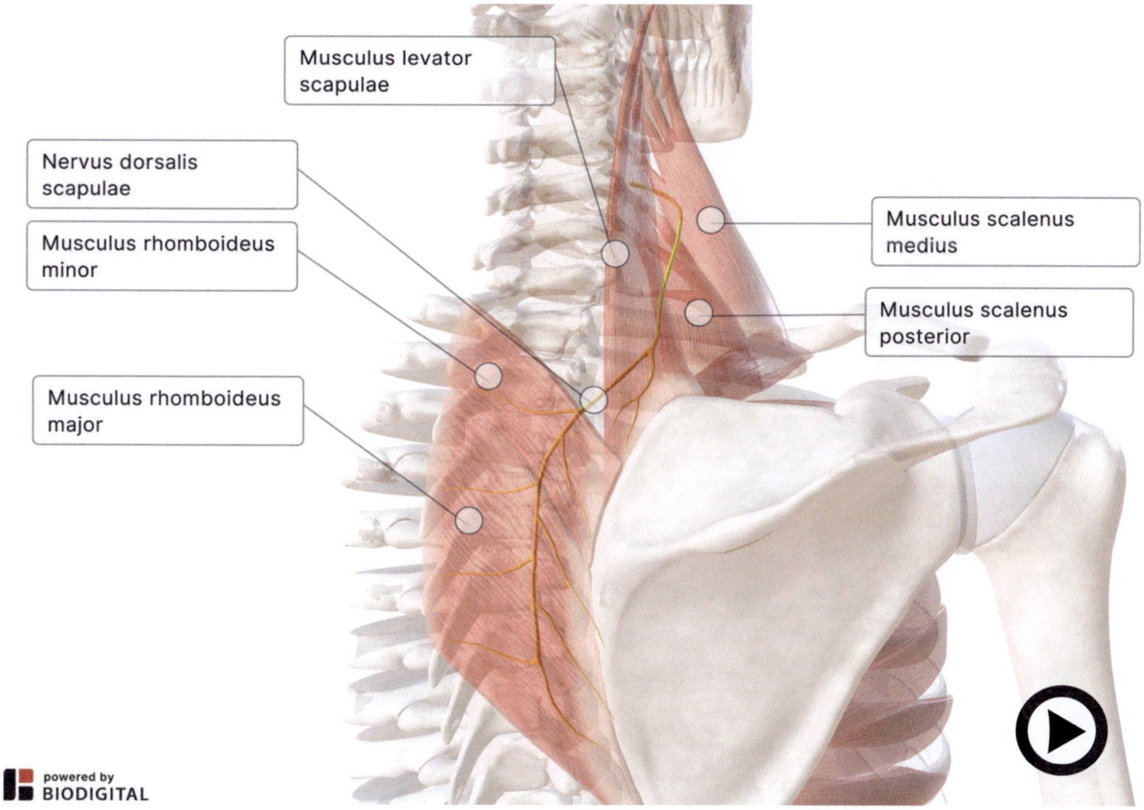

Fig. 6.23 Anatomy and palpation of the N. dorsalis scapulae (▶ https://doi.org/10.1007/000-cwr)

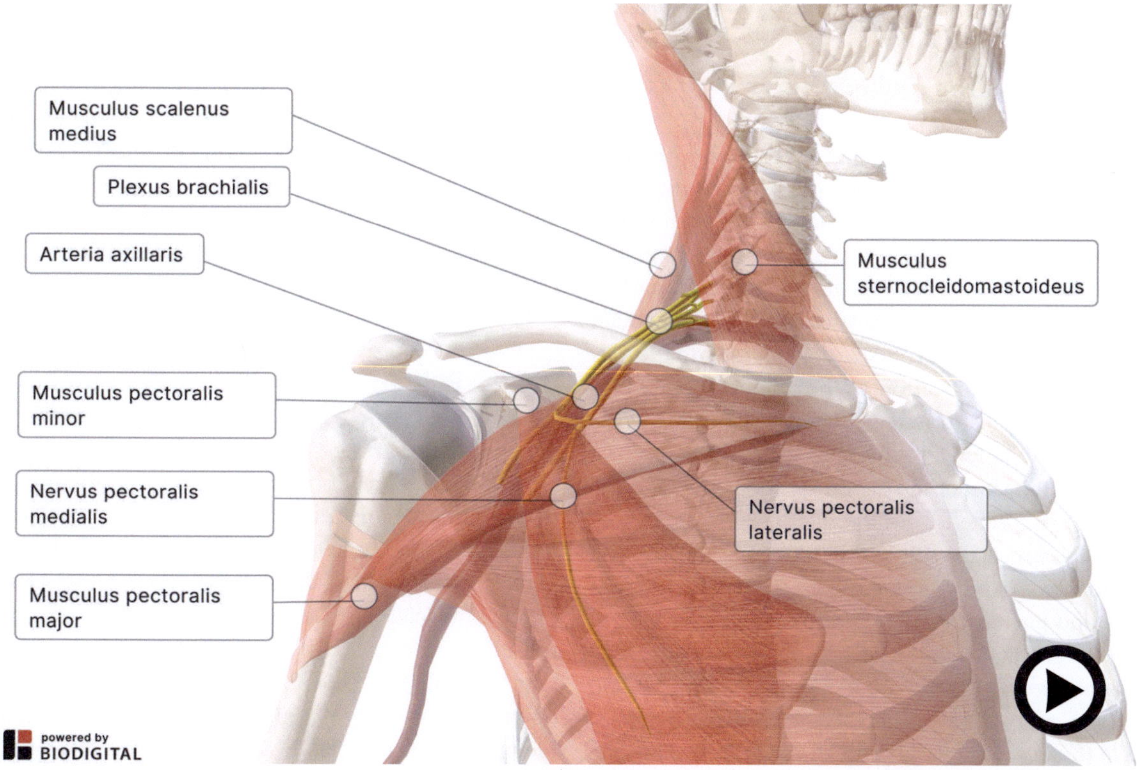

Fig. 6.24 Anatomy and palpation of the N. pectoralis medialis et lateralis (▶ https://doi.org/10.1007/000-cws)

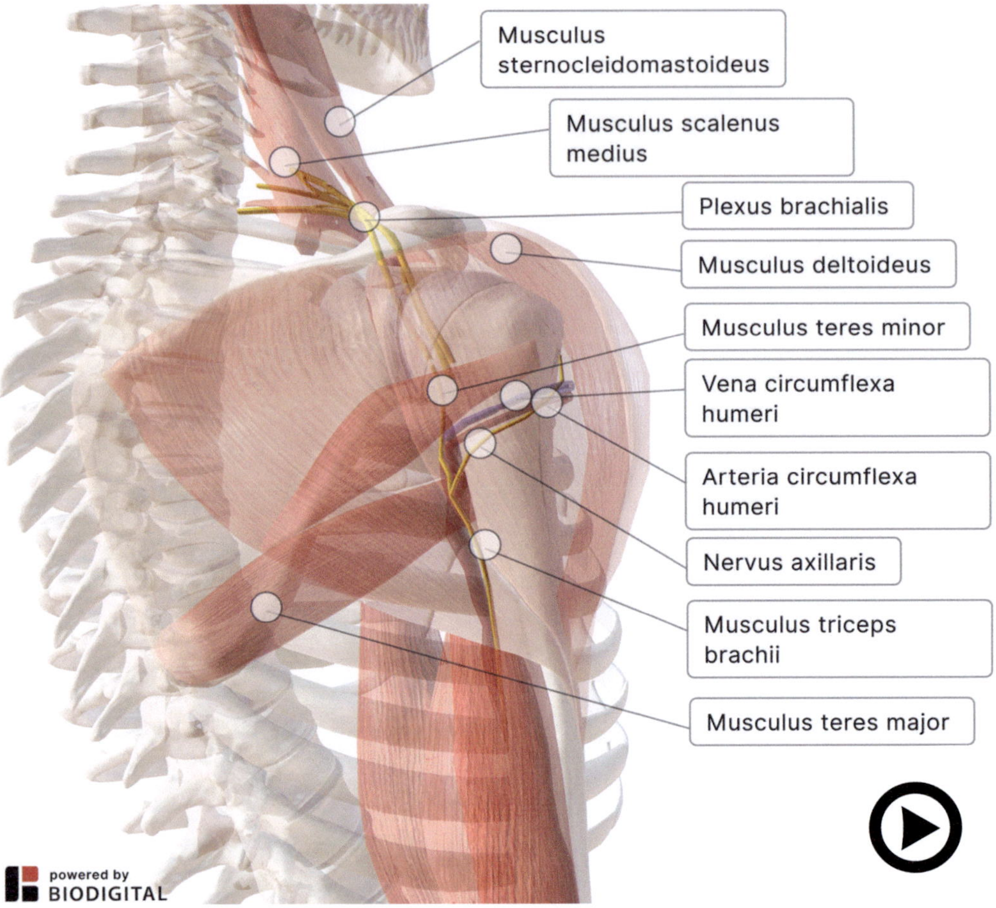

Fig. 6.25 Anatomy and palpation of the N. axillaris (▶ https://doi.org/10.1007/000-cwt)

6.4.7 Palpation of the Axillary Nerve

In the axilla, the axillary nerve arises from the brachial plexus. It then runs distodorsally, passing directly between the muscle belly of the teres minor and teres major muscles. It then runs anteriorly with one branch around the proximal portion of the humerus together with the humeral circumflex artery and vein, while the other branch runs distally between the heads of the triceps brachii muscle and laterally to the deltoid muscle. The interconnection of the axillary nerve covers a large area, so that it provides motor innervation to the deltoid muscle and the teres minor muscle. Somatosensitive parts also supply the skin of the lateral shoulder region.

The nerve is stimulated from the lateral position so that the therapist has access to the overlying arm. It should be noted that the nerve is predominantly covered by the deltoid pars spinalis and pars acromialis muscles and therefore cannot be directly grasped. Finger berries make contact under the deltoid muscle with the proximal part of the humerus and the teres minor and major muscles. Exactly at the intersection of these three structures, a deep stimulus is applied via the steeply positioned finger berries. In addition, a stimulus can be applied to the axillary nerve between the caput longum and caput laterale of the triceps brachii muscle and at the distal edge of the deltoid muscle, but this is so overlaid by the surrounding tissue that direct detection is not possible.

Implementation Note
The intensity of the stimulation of the axillary nerve depends on the individual constitution of the client (Fig. 6.25).

6.4.8 Palpation of the Musculocutaneous Nerve

Dorsal to the coracobrachialis muscle, in the proximal third of the humerus, the musculocutaneous nerve arises from the brachial plexus. It is thus covered in its area of origin by the pectoralis major muscle and the caput breve of the biceps brachii muscle. The nerve then traces the coracobrachialis muscle, pulling distolaterally on its upper edge. Approximately in the medial third of the humerus, the musculocutaneous nerve continues between the brachialis and biceps brachii muscles towards the lateral humeral epicondyle. Perforating the biceps brachii muscle, it sends the lateral cutaneous antebrachii nerve into the crook of the elbow

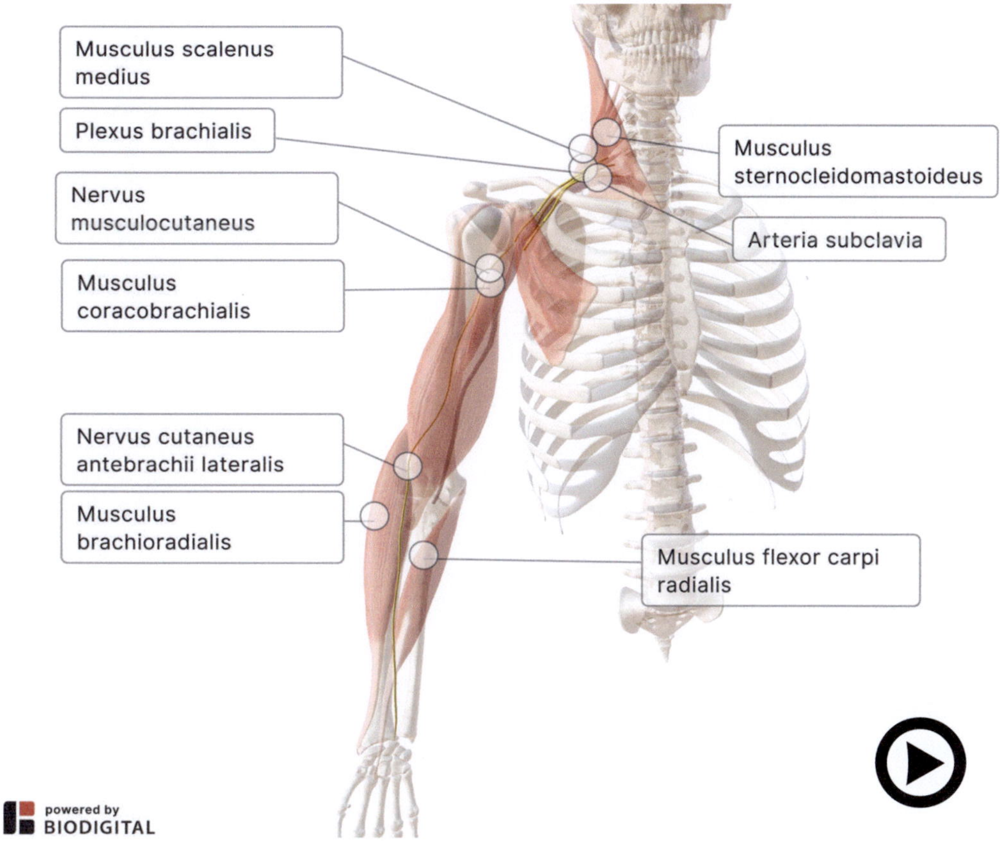

Fig. 6.26 Anatomy and palpation of the N. musculocutaneous (▶ https://doi.org/10.1007/000-cwv)

near the radial nerve and the radial artery as a continuing branch located between the brachioradialis and flexor carpi radialis muscles in the ventral forearm. A second branch of the musculocutaneous nerve, the cutaneous antebrachii medialis, splits off already in the middle third of the humerus and follows the medial side of the upper arm as well as the ulnar side of the forearm into the distal third in the region of the ulna.

Due to its mixed fibre content, the nerve somatomotorically innervates the coracobrachialis, brachialis, and biceps brachii muscles, while somatosensitively it supplies the elbow joint capsule and radial and ventral skin areas of the forearm.

Two areas are suitable for stimulating the musculocutaneous nerve with the client in the supine position. The therapist stands sideways and first makes contact with the biceps brachii muscle anteriorly in the middle of the humerus. The fingertips, placed flat, trace the muscle in a proximal direction, following the caput breve. In the area where the two heads split, the fingertips slide down to meet the coracobrachialis muscle and thus also the musculocutaneous nerve.

The second approach is made in the crook of the elbow. For this, the finger berries, which are placed flat, are oriented at the intersection of the lateral edge of the biceps brachii muscle and the medial edge of the brachioradialis muscle. Directly in the depression, the finger berries meet both the musculocutaneous nerve and the radial nerve. If they follow the medial edge of the brachioradialis muscle, the lateral cutaneous antebrachii nerve, which is a splitting branch, is palpated.

Implementation Note

Depending on the anatomical anatomy, the musculocutaneous nerve can pierce the coracobrachialis muscle [10] (Fig. 6.26).

6.4.9 Palpation of the Median Nerve

The nerve originating from the brachial plexus runs in the medial region of the anterior upper and lower arm, as its name suggests. Directly in the axilla between the tendon of the latissimus dorsi muscle and the coracobrachialis muscle, the nerve runs together with the axillary artery and then the brachial artery distolaterally under the biceps brachii muscle towards the crook of the elbow. Directly in the cubital fossa, the median nerve briefly comes to the surface medial to the brachial artery and then enters the depths of the forearm under the pronator teres muscle. In the area of the deep forearm muscles, the nerve runs between the flexor pollicis longus muscle and the flexor digitorum profundus muscle distally towards the hand. Arriving palmar and centrally on the hand, it passes between the tendons of the m. flexor digitorum superficialis and the m. flexor carpi radialis under the retinaculum flexorum into the palm and divides into individual branches that continue into the fingers. The somatomotor parts of the nerve supply almost all forearm flexors except for the flexor carpi ulnaris muscle and, in the hand, the abductor pollicis brevis muscle, the opponens pollicis muscle, the superficial caput of the flexor pollicis brevis muscle and the lumbrical I and II muscles. In addition, somatosensory fibres innervate the skin areas above the ball of the thumb and the radial half of the palm. Furthermore, it supplies the skin of the pollex, the index and the digitus medius, as well as the radial half of the digitus anularis. On the dorsal side, the nerve sensitively innervates the distal ends of digits I–III from half of the medial phalanx, as well as the radial half of the distal phalanx at digit IV.

If the nerve is stimulated by the steeply positioned fingertips, it is recommended to position the client in a supine position with the arm in a passive position. The therapist stands laterally at the level of the upper arm and applies the fingertips directly in the sulcus bicipitalis medialis, which is bordered by the caput breve of the m. biceps brachii and the m. triceps brachii as well as the septum intermusculare mediale. Starting from this reference point medially on the upper arm, the fingers follow the groove distally and meet the pulsating brachial artery in the crook of the elbow (see Sect. 7.1.3.3), which can be found in the cubital fossa medial to the biceps brachii muscle (see Sect. 5.8.4). Directly medial to the artery, the finger berries move gently into the depths and also meet the median nerve.

A second region suitable for palpation is palmar at the level of the joint space of the art. radiocarpalis. Here, the nerve is located between the tendons of the palmaris longus muscle and the common tendon sheath of the flexor pollicis longus and flexor carpi radialis muscles. A stimulus can be produced in this region by applying pressure in depth.

Implementation Note
Depending on the anatomical anatomy, the median nerve can pierce the pronator teres [11] (Fig. 6.27).

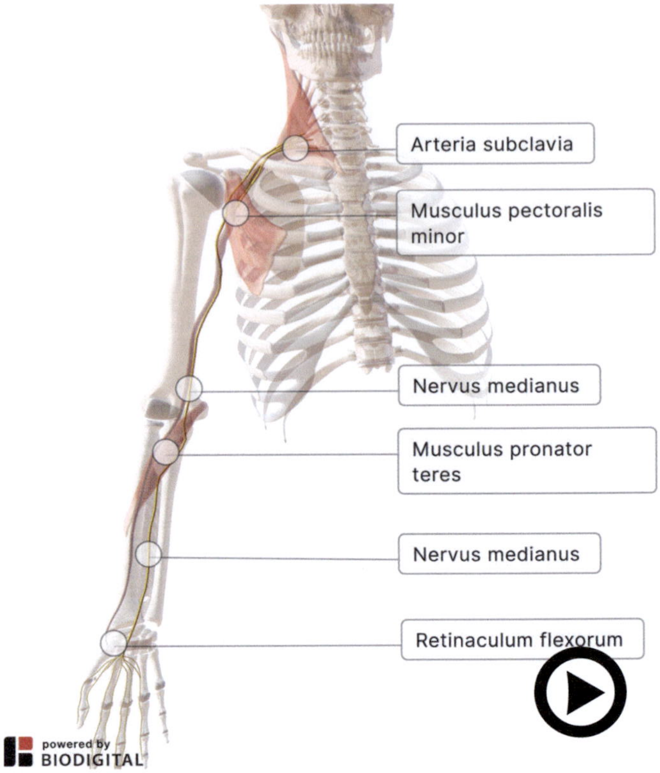

Fig. 6.27 Anatomy and palpation of the N. medianus (▶ https://doi.org/10.1007/000-cww)

6.4.10 Palpation of the Radial Nerve

In the axilla, the radial nerve arises from the brachial plexus and begins its long course distolateral to the humerus. Posteriorly in the proximal region on the humerus, it takes a similar course to the profunda brachii artery and loops laterally around the humerus in about the middle third. Directly between the muscle bellies of the lateral caput of the triceps brachii muscle and the brachialis muscle, the radial nerve then rises and runs along the anterior edge of the brachioradialis muscle and the lateral edge of the long caput of the biceps brachii muscle to the anterior of the lateral humeral epicondyle into the cubital fossa.

There, it dives into the depths together with the radial artery and runs distally as the superficial ramus directly under the brachioradialis muscle along the radius. After passing under the pronator teres muscle in the middle third of the radius around the tendon of attachment, it wraps around the radius to reach the distal part of the forearm in a dorsal direction. There, it crosses several extensors until it divides into further branches under the retinaculum extensorum, which continue to the thumb, index finger and middle finger.

The pars profunda of the radial nerve, which extends further into the depths at the level of the circumferentia radii, runs dorsally under the supinator muscle, wrapping around the radius in the proximal third. On the forearm, the nerve branch is oriented dorsally on the membrana interossea antebrachii and ends in the distal area of the radius.

Due to its length, the nerve has a great motor influence and innervates, among others, the triceps brachii muscle as well as the anconeus muscle and almost all muscles of the dorsal forearm muscle group. Somatosensitively, it is responsible for the supply of the skin areas in the lateral and dorsal areas of the arm, the thumb, and the index and middle fingers.

Two regions are suitable for palpation, with the patient in a sitting position with the arm in a passive position. The first access to the nerve is laterally on the upper arm between the

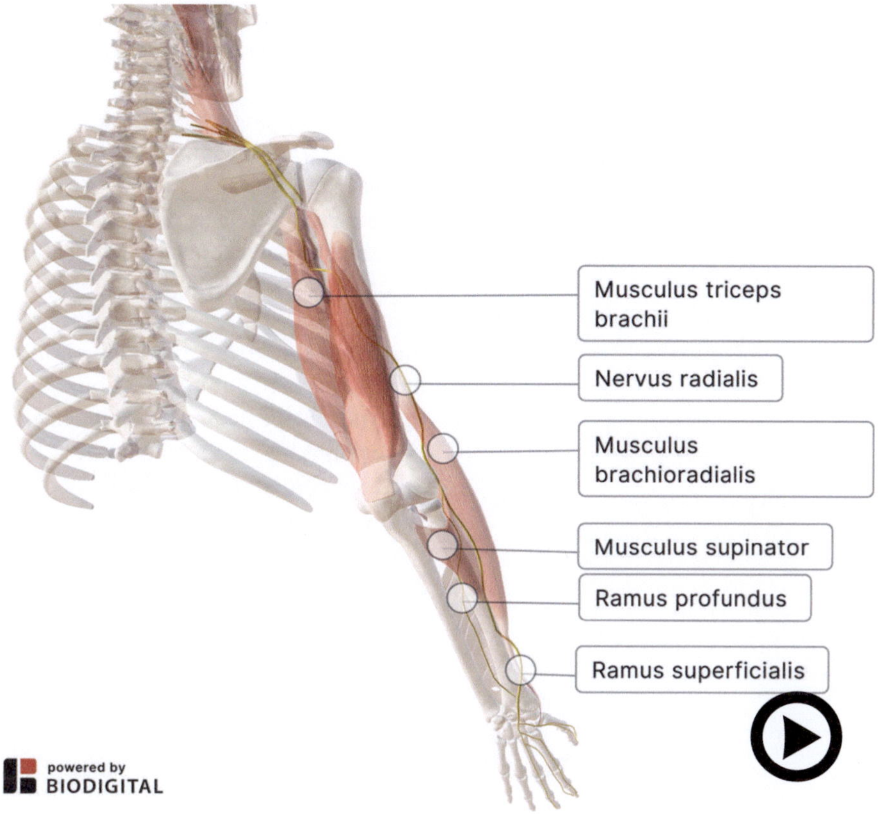

Fig. 6.28 Anatomy and palpation of the N. radialis (▶ https://doi.org/10.1007/000-cwx)

lateral edge of the caput breve of the biceps brachii muscle and the medial edge of the brachioradialis muscle. The fingertips are placed flat in the described region and begin to palpate directly at the anterior border of the brachioradialis muscle in depth. They then move distally until they reach the anterior region of the lateral humeral epicondyle. Also in this region is the profunda brachialis artery, which accompanies the nerve in this section.

The second approach is to the distal part of the radius. The fingertips grasp the radial pulse as proximally as possible and meet the radial artery between the brachioradialis and flexor carpi radialis muscles, as well as the superficial part of the nerve of the same name. Then, with moderate pressure, the fingers applied flatly follow the sinuous course to the dorsum of the hand ulnar to the dorsal tuberosity on the radius in order to provide the radial nerve with a stimulus.

Implementation Note
Depending on the anatomical anatomy, the radial nerve can pierce the supinator muscle [12] (Fig. 6.28).

6.4.11 Palpation of the Ulnar Nerve

In the axilla, the ulnar nerve arises from the brachial plexus and then travels medially on the upper arm together with the axillary artery and the median nerve in a distal direction. It passes medially on the humerus through the medial bicipital sulcus, which is bordered by the caput breve of the biceps brachii muscle and the triceps brachii muscle and the medial intermuscular septum. Arriving dorsomedially at the elbow, the ulnar nerve passes distally between the epicondylus medialis humeri and the olecranon through the sulcus nervi ulnaris, along the ulna. It is covered in this section by the flexor carpi ulnaris muscle. At about the middle third of the forearm, it loops into the surface between the flexor digitorum superficialis and flexor carpi ulnaris muscles and pulls distally with the ulnar artery towards the hand. Ulnar to the hand, the ulnar nerve passes through the Loge de Guyon, which is bounded by the retinaculum flexorum, the lig. carpi palmare as well as the hamulus ossis hamati, the os pisiforme and the lig. pisohamatum. The nerve then divides into further branches, which mainly run to the little and ring fingers. While the somatosensitive wiring of the nerve is limited to the skin in the area of the ball of the little finger from the palmar and dorsal sides as well as the ulnar side of the ring finger, it has a greater influence somatomotorly. Motorically, it supplies the flexor carpi ulnaris and flexor digitorum profundus muscles as well as large parts of the hand muscles in the hypothenar, metacarpal and thenar regions.

Several reference points are suitable for palpating the nerve with the client in the supine position, as it is largely

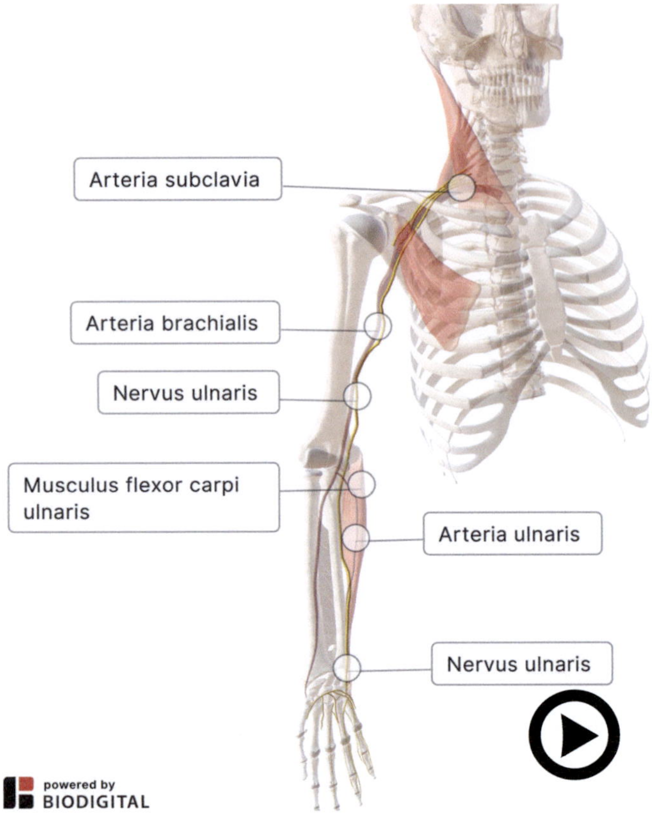

Fig. 6.29 Anatomy and palpation of the N. ulnaris (▶ https://doi.org/10.1007/000-cwy)

on the surface. The therapist stands laterally at the level of the upper arm and applies the steeply positioned fingertips directly in the medial bicipital sulcus, which is bordered by the caput breve of the biceps brachii muscle and the triceps brachii muscle as well as the medial intermuscular septum. In addition to the ulnar nerve, it also meets the median nerve, which runs through the same groove. Following the medial border of the triceps brachii muscle, the finger berries then move distally until they reach the ulnar nerve sulcus dorsomedially of the medial humeral epicondyle. Directly in this depression, the nerve can be felt across its course.

Another approach is made at the beginning of the distal forearm. The steeply placed fingertips meet the ulnar nerve directly between the flexor digitorum superficialis and flexor carpi ulnaris. The pulsating ulnar artery is indicative of this, as it is located in the immediate vicinity of the nerve. If the fingertips move distally, the nerve can be palpated in the remaining course.

Implementation Note

Especially in the ulnar nerve sulcus, the ulnar nerve is susceptible to injury due to its superficial location [13]. Palpation should therefore be carried out carefully (Fig. 6.29).

6.5 Palpation of the Nerves in the Area of the Head/Neck

People communicate with each other even if they do not exchange a word. This happens mainly through non-verbal signals such as facial expressions and gestures. Communication takes place specifically with the eyes, nose, mouth or throat by controlling the muscles in such a way that an emotion such as joy, affection, dislike, fear or anger is expressed. Direct eye contact during conversation is also an important clue to the exchange of information. In addition to these aspects of communication, other elementary functions must take place in the area of the head, such as speaking, eating or blinking, to name but a few. This requires nerves that send specific signals to the respective effectors or that can receive and transmit stimuli from them. Numerous nerves in the area of the head and neck perform this task. In the following chapters, only selected nerves are discussed which can be palpated by means of stimulation. Since the anatomical position must be clarified in advance, the course of the nerve is described in the first part before the palpation instructions follow. The nerves described in this section of the book include the facial nerve, the trigeminal nerve, the greater and lesser occipital nerves and the phrenic nerve.

6.5.1 Palpation of the Facial Nerve

The VII cranial nerve leaves the brain in the angulus pontocerebellaris between the truncus cerebri and the cerebellum in the direction of the parotid gland. In the area of the parotid gland, it divides further into a pars temporofacialis and a pars cervicofacialis, which continue to supply the head and face with sensory, motor and parasympathetic information. There are numerous nerve branches which split off in the further course. In addition to the sensory innervation of the taste buds, the sensitive innervation of the skin of the external meatus acusticus and the tympanic membrane, the mixed nerve fibres also supply numerous motor muscles. These include, for example, the mimic muscles in the entire area of the face as well as parts of the suprahyoidal musculature up to the stapedius muscle in the ear itself.

In facial nerve palsy, a person can be observed communicating without facial expressions, as it is precisely these muscles that are controlled.

The palpatory stimulation of the facial nerve can be carried out from any starting position and refers only to the region just before it splits into its two larger terminal branches. The fingertips are placed flat and with only moderate pressure in the anterior region of the earlobe, caudal to the temporomandibular joint. They also meet the pulsating external carotid artery and the superficial temporal vein. If gentle pressure is now applied in depth, the facial nerve is

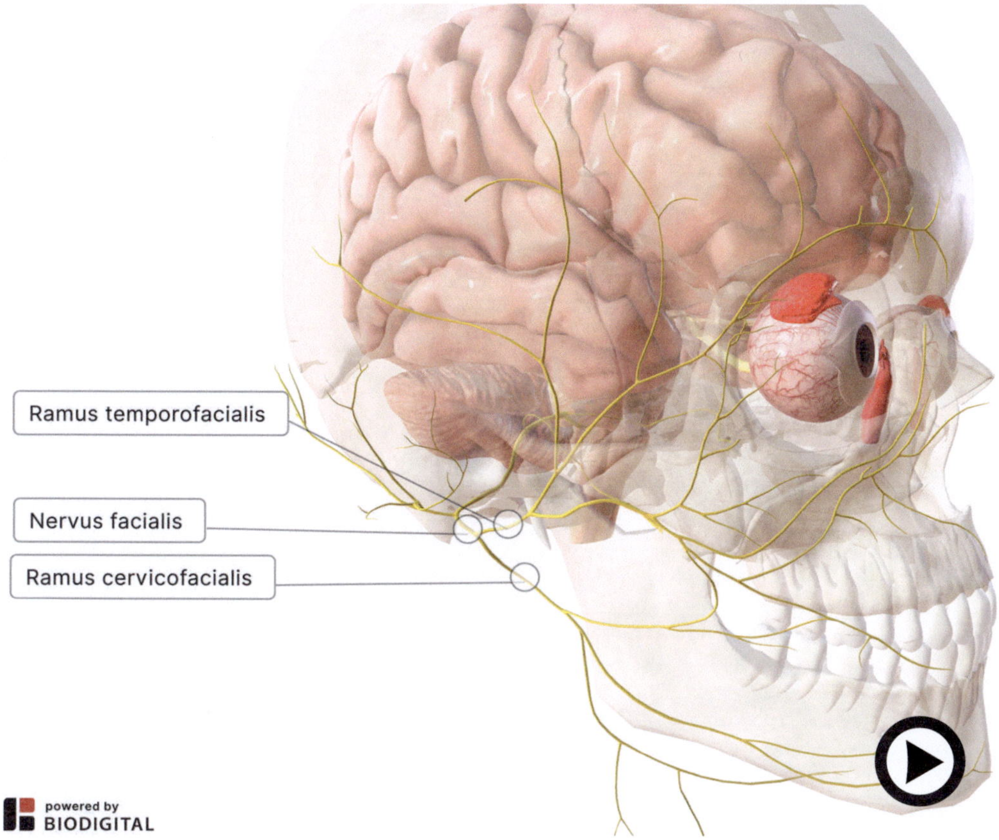

Fig. 6.30 Anatomy and palpation of the N. facialis (▶ https://doi.org/10.1007/000-cwz)

also reached via a stimulus. The terminal branches can be influenced by applying pressure over a wide area with the fingers.

Another branch of the facial nerve is the posterior auricular nerve, which, true to its name, is located behind the ear. A stimulus can be produced on the muscle via the finger berries placed flat in this region, by moving the fingers transversely to the course of the nerve in a superior and inferior direction.

Implementation Note

The stimulation takes place through the parotid gland and should therefore be gentle (Fig. 6.30).

6.5.2 Palpation of the Trigeminal Nerve

The trigeminal nerve is also called the fifth cranial nerve and carries both specific visceromotor and general somatosensory nerve fibres. The nerve originates in the outer area of the pons and travels to the pars petrosa ossis temporalis to pass through the dura mater. During its rostral course, the trigeminal nerve expands to the trigeminal ganglion and then subdivides into its terminal branches, the ophthalmic nerve, the maxillary nerve and the mandibular nerve. The names of the three branches directly indicate their location on the skull, so that the V_1 is located at the eye, the V_2 at the upper jaw and the V_3 at the lower jaw. Furthermore, the V cranial nerve gives off numerous branches that extend over further branches on the face and innervate musculature as well as skin areas, teeth and other structures. At this point, it should be mentioned that this chapter only describes the branches that can be subjected to direct palpatory stimulation.

For palpation, the client is positioned in a supine or seated position.

The V_1 is located as the frontal nerve at the supraorbital foramen, which can be felt at the eyebrow (see Sect. 2.12.1.1). The fingertip is placed medially on the eyebrow and begins to follow it laterally. In the course, small bony depressions become palpable, in which the branches of the frontal nerve are located. This area is referred to as the supratrochlear nerve, which in turn is a branch of the frontal nerve.

The V_2 is stimulated below the eye in the area of the infraorbital foramen (see Sect. 2.12.2.3). In this area, the infraorbital nerve exists as a splitting off the maxillary nerve. Another division that can be stimulated obliquely laterocaudal to the eye, at the os zygomaticum, is the zygomaticofacial nerve. Also, as a splitting off of the maxillary nerve, it comes to the surface through the zygomatico-orbital foramen (see Sect. 2.12.2.1). This bony depression can be grasped laterocaudally of the eye.

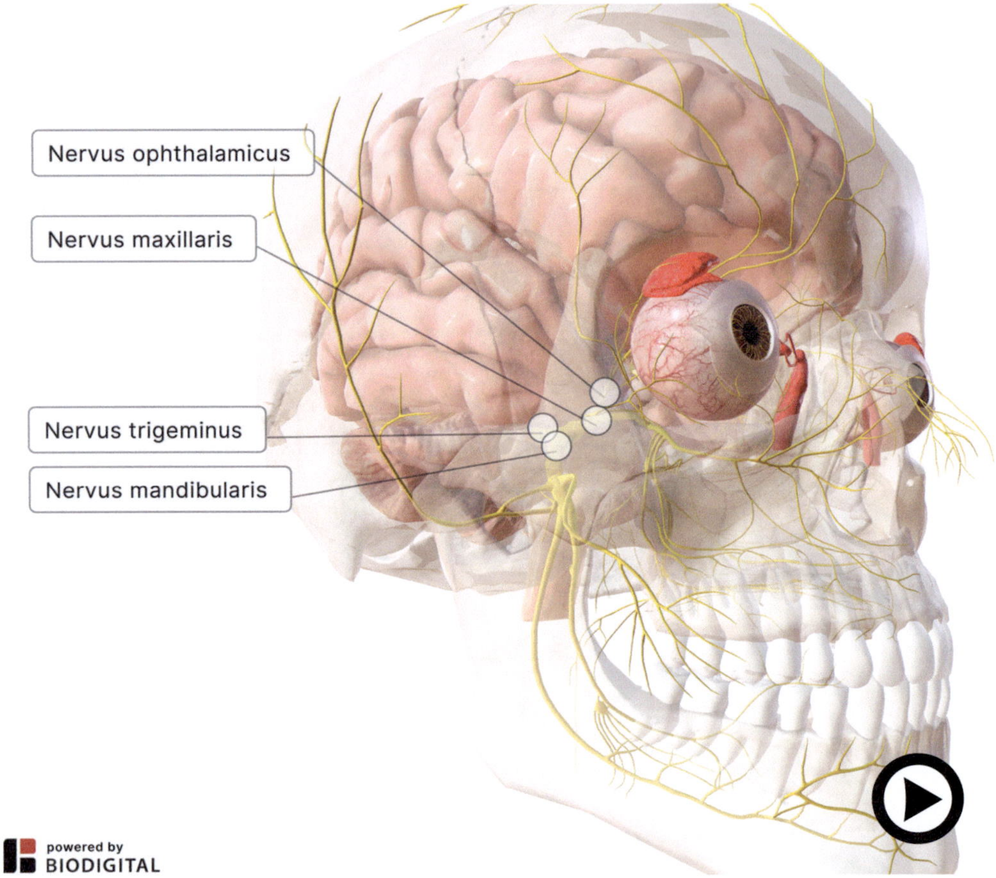

Fig. 6.31 Anatomy and palpation of the N. trigeminus (▶ https://doi.org/10.1007/000-cx0)

The V_3 is stimulated in the anterior region of the mandible by applying pressure to the mental foramen with the fingertip (see Sect. 2.12.2.4). The inferior alveolar nerve is palpated as the terminal branch, which leaves the mental foramen with the mental artery.

Implementation Note
Palpation of the trigeminal nerve should be done gently to avoid discomfort (Fig. 6.31).

6.5.3 Palpation of the Greater and Lesser Occipital Nerves

The greater occipital nerve and the lesser occipital nerve arise from the originating segments C2 and C3. Both originate from the cervical plexus, and while the greater occipital nerve also generates somatomotor innervation, the lesser part consists only of somatosensitive fibres. After their exit, both nerves run in a dorsolateral direction to the os occipitale. From there, both run across the occiput in a cranial direction, with the greater occipital nerve extending more medially and the lesser occipital nerve laterally. In this course, the lesser occipital nerve passes between the splenius capitis and sternocleidomastoid muscles, while the greater occipital nerve, together with the occipital artery, passes along the bone, perforating the splenius capitis and parts of the erector spinae.

To stimulate the nerve, a starting position should be chosen in which good access to the back of the head can be achieved. The lateral or sitting position is recommended. The therapist orientates himself bony at the lower edge of the os occipitale and can grasp the pulsating A. occipitalis with the fingertips (see Sect. 7.1.4.11). Directly in this region, palpation also produces a stimulus on the occipital nerve, which can be followed even further occipitally. At the outer edge of the erector spinae muscle, a palpation stimulus can be applied to the nerve at the back of the head.

For the lesser occipital nerve, the fingertips are oriented towards the posterior border of the sternocleidomastoid mus-

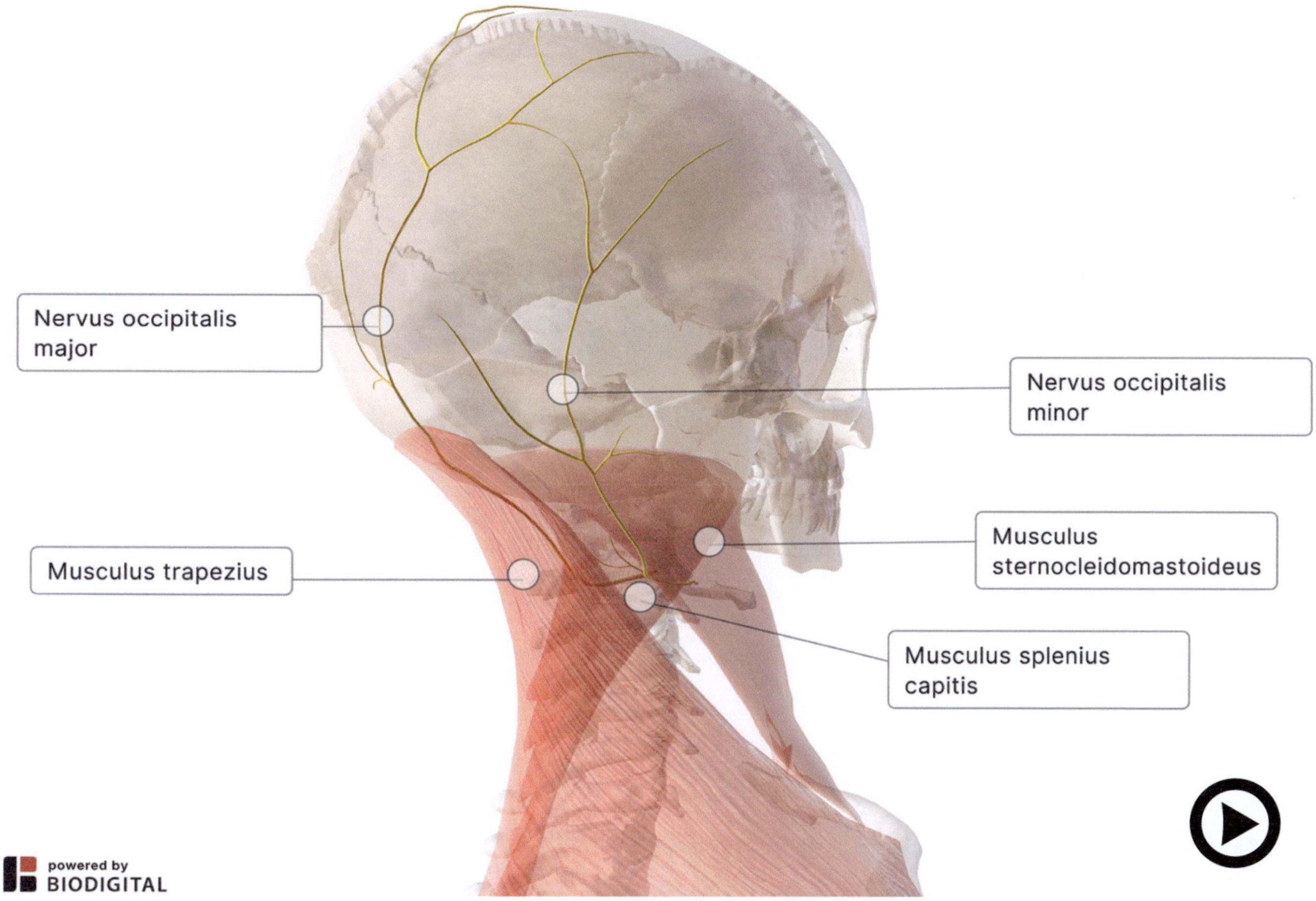

Fig. 6.32 Anatomy and palpation of the N. occipitalis major et minor (▶ https://doi.org/10.1007/000-cw2)

cle, in the proximal quarter of which the nerve comes to the surface. A flat stimulus can be given globally via the applied fingertips.

Execution Advice
Palpation of the greater and lesser occipital nerves should be performed gently to avoid any sensory disturbance (Fig. 6.32).

6.5.4 Palpation of the Phrenic Nerve

The deep phrenic nerve arises from segments C3 to C5 and innervates the diaphragm motorically. After its exit from the cervical plexus, the anterior scalene nerve runs caudally between the subclavian artery and vein towards the lungs and diaphragm. On this path, it sends numerous branches which also take over the somatosensitive innervation of the pleura parietalis, the pericardium as well as the peritoneum in the area of the cardia, the hepar and the vesica biliaris.

Direct palpation of the phrenic nerve is not possible, but a stimulus can be produced with the help of the steeply placed fingertips of the index and middle fingers. The client is in a supine position so that the head is in a passive position and contact can be made with the scalenus anterior muscle (see Sect. 5.6.3). In this region, approximately at the level of the sixth cervical vertebra, pressure is created in the direction of the spine so that a stimulus can be applied to the phrenic nerve at depth.

Implementation Note
Due to the nerve- and vessel-rich region, palpation should be done gently (Fig. 6.33).

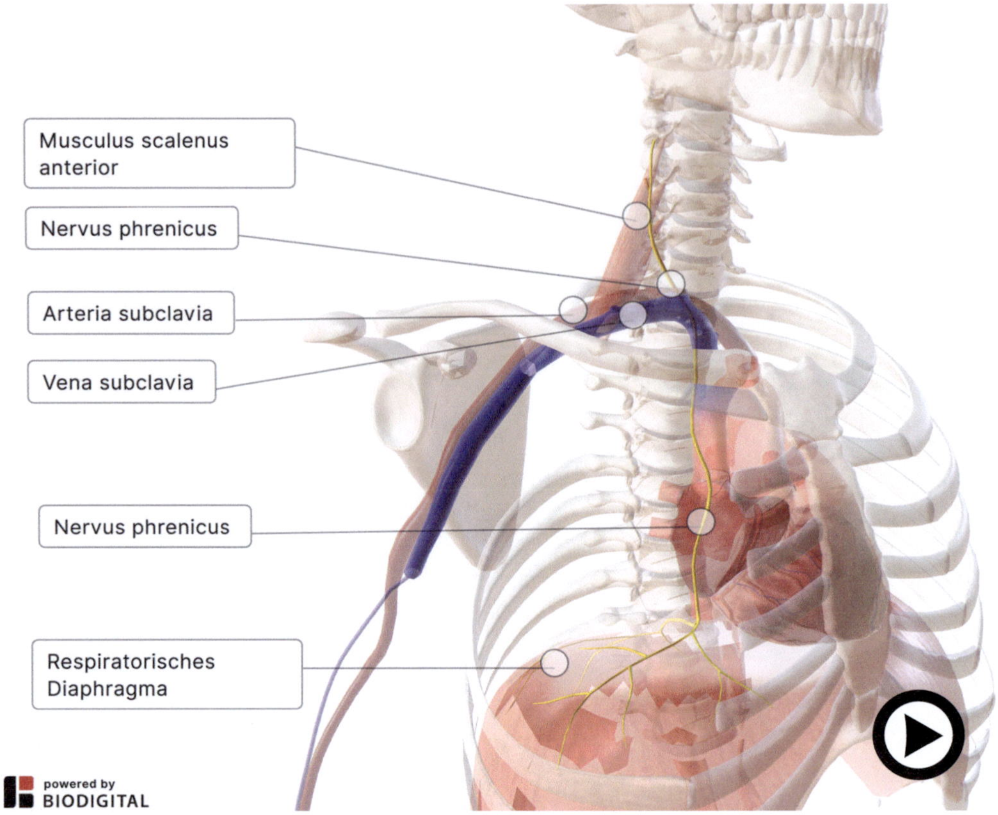

Fig. 6.33 Anatomy and palpation of the N. phrenicus (▶ https://doi.org/10.1007/000-cx2)

References

1. Markert, B., Fraenzle, S., & Tieben, C. (2009). Information und Informationsverarbeitung. *Umweltwissenschaften und Schadstoff-Forschung, 21*, 483–486. https://doi.org/10.1007/s12302-009-0088-7
2. Fingleton, C., Dempsey, L., Smart, K., & Doody, C. (2014). Intraexaminer and interexaminer reliability of manual palpation and pressure algometry of the lower limb nerves in asymptomatic subjects. *Journal of Manipulative and Physiological Therapeutics, 37*(2), 97–104. https://doi.org/10.1016/j.jmpt.2013.12.006
3. Iwanaga, J., Simonds, E., Schumacher, M., Kikuta, S., Watanabe, K., & Tubbs, R. (2019). Revisiting the genital and femoral branches of the genitofemoral nerve: Suggestion for a more accurate terminology. *Clinical Anatomy, 32*(3), 458–463. https://doi.org/10.1002/ca.23327
4. ter Meulen, B., Peters, E., Wijsmuller, A., Kropman, R., Mosch, A., & Tavy, D. (2007). Acute scrotal pain from idiopathic ilioinguinal neuropathy: Diagnosis and treatment with EMG-guided nerve block. *Clinical Neurology and Neurosurgery, 109*(6), 535–537. https://doi.org/10.1016/j.clineuro.2007.03.011
5. Carai, A., Fenu, G., Sechi, E., Crotti, F., & Montella, A. (2009). Anatomical variability of the lateral femoral cutaneous nerve: Findings from a surgical series. *Clinical Anatomy, 22*(3), 365–370. https://doi.org/10.1002/ca.20766
6. Chiaramonte, R., Pavone, P., & Vecchio, M. (2021). Diagnosis, rehabilitation and preventive strategies for pudendal neuropathy in cyclists, a systematic review. *Journal of Functional Morphology and Kinesiology, 6*(2), 42. https://doi.org/10.3390/jfmk6020042
7. Akasaka, N., Sasakawa, T., Onodera, Y., Otomo, S., & Iwasaki, H. (2015). The distance between the sciatic nerve bifurcation and popliteal fossa in Japanese. *Masui, 64*(2), 205–207.
8. Ahmad, M., Tsang, K., Mackenney, P., & Adedapo, A. (2012). Tarsal tunnel syndrome: A literature review. *Foot and Ankle Surgery, 18*(3), 149–152. https://doi.org/10.1016/j.fas.2011.10.007
9. Nguyen, C., Guérini, H., Roren, A., Zauderer, J., Vuillemin, V., Seror, P., & Lefèvre-Colau, M.-M. (2015). Neuromuscular dynamic scapular winging: Clinical, electromyographic and magnetic resonance imaging diagnosis. *Presse Médicale, 44*(12 Pt 1), 1256–1265. https://doi.org/10.1016/j.lpm.2015.08.006
10. Pećina, M., & Bojanić, I. (1993). Musculocutaneous nerve entrapment in the upper arm. *International Orthopaedics, 17*(4), 232–234. https://doi.org/10.1007/BF00194185
11. Soubeyrand, M., Melhem, R., Protais, M., Artuso, M., & Crézé, M. (2020). Anatomy of the median nerve and its clinical applications. *Hand Surgery and Rehabilitation, 39*(1), 2–18. https://doi.org/10.1016/j.hansur.2019.10.197
12. Gilan, İ., Gilan, V., & Öztürk, A. (2020). Evaluation of the supinator muscle and deep branch of the radial nerve: Impact on nerve compression. *Surgical and Radiologic Anatomy, 42*(8), 927–933. https://doi.org/10.1007/s00276-020-02480-0
13. Assmus, H., Antoniadis, G., Bischoff, C., Hoffmann, R., Martini, A.-K., Preissler, P., & Wüstner-Hofmann, M. (2011). Cubital tunnel syndrome: A review and management guidelines. *Central European Neurosurgery, 72*(2), 90–98. https://doi.org/10.1055/s-0031-1271800

Palpation of the Vessels

7

Contents

7.1 Palpation of the Arteries

The three-layer vessels are characterised by the fact that they carry blood away from the heart. This is oxygen-rich in the systemic circulation and oxygen-poor in the pulmonary circulation. In this way, they organise the oxygen supply and the associated metabolism in the entire body. The heart is the central motor that makes the blood flow through the arteries. Kinetic energy is converted into potential energy by the wind kettle function of the arteries close to the heart. The resulting pulse wave is considered the most important identification criterion when palpating arterial vessels.

The following chapters deal with the arteries that are palpable on the human body. Anatomical knowledge is indispensable, which is why the individual vessels are first described in their position before the palpation procedure is described. The client is to be placed in a relaxed starting position while the therapist gently palpates from the surface to the depth with the flatly placed fingertips of the index and middle fingers. This basic approach is important so as not to push off the pulse wave in advance. Arteries are often felt in different areas of the body, as they repeatedly come to the surface during the examination. Therefore, those structures are predominantly recorded selectively. With small arteries, the detection of the pulse wave is more challenging. It is therefore generally recommended to close the eyes during palpation in order to focus on the essentials.

7.1.1 Arteries in the Area of the Pelvis and Lower Extremity

In order to ensure locomotion, which is largely ensured by the lower extremity, the supply of oxygen- and energy-rich blood is elementary. The superior gluteal artery, the femoral artery, the popliteal artery, the anterior and posterior tibial arteries, the dorsal pedal artery and the dorsal metatarsal arteries are suitable for palpation and stimulation in the pelvic region and the lower extremity. All of the above structures can be individually recorded or stimulated. The methodology of palpation is presented in the individual chapters after a brief description of the location.

7.1.1.1 Palpation of the Superior Gluteal Artery

The superior gluteal artery forms the largest branch of the iliac artery and supplies the tensor fasciae latae muscle,

Supplementary Information The online version contains supplementary material available at https://doi.org/10.1007/978-3-662-69186-1_7. The videos can be accessed individually by clicking the DOI link in the accompanying figure caption or by scanning this link with the SN More Media App.

R. Bauer, S. Wolfram, *Atlas of Palpation*, https://doi.org/10.1007/978-3-662-69186-1_7

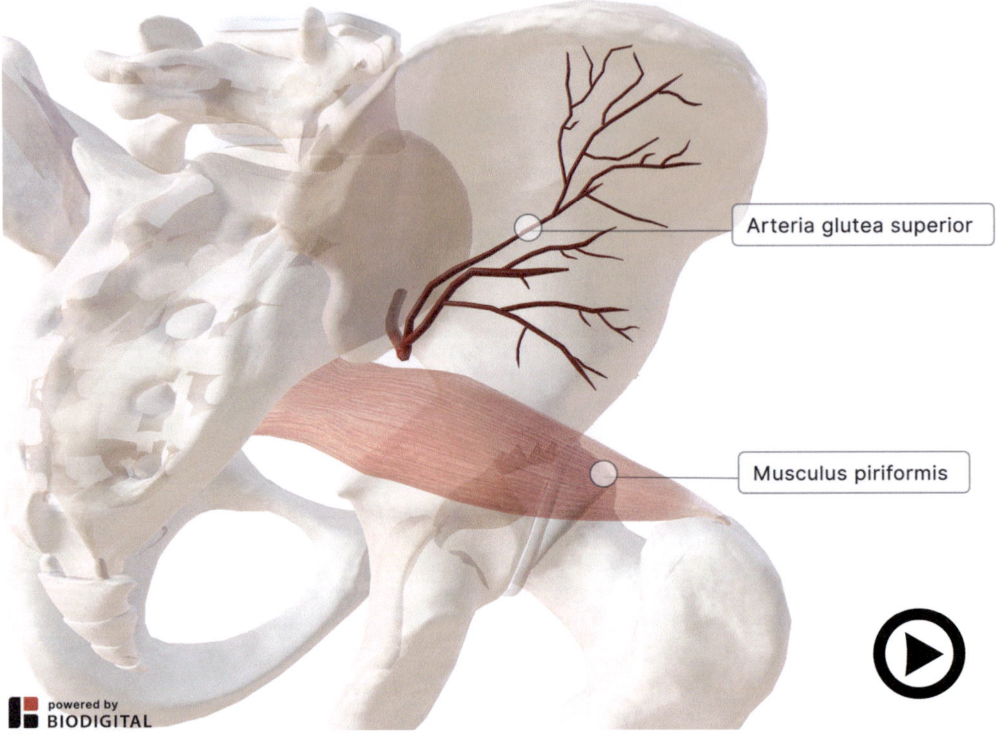

Fig. 7.1 Anatomy and palpation of the A. gluteasuperior (▶ https://doi.org/10.1007/000-cyg)

the gluteal muscles, the piriformis muscle and some areas of skin in the gluteal region. It runs ventrally between the lumbosacral trunk and the upper sacral nerves dorsolaterally through the incisura ischiadica majus, inferior to the SIPI, craniolaterally. Its entire course is covered by the gluteus maximus and minimus muscles. It runs directly above the piriformis muscle, which is used as orientation for palpation.

While the patient is in the prone position and the therapist has felt the homolateral piriformis muscle (see Sect. 5.2.6), the steeply positioned fingertips are placed on the upper muscle edge of the medial third. Depending on the muscular characteristics, a stimulus can be applied in depth to the superior gluteal artery.

Implementation Note
The piriformis muscle can irritate the superior gluteal artery when overloaded. This can lead to an undersupply of the muscles fed by it, which can result in an increase in tone of the target structures (Fig. 7.1).

7.1.1.2 Palpation of the Femoral Artery

The femoral artery is a direct branch of the external iliac artery and arises in the area of the inguinal ligament, close to the lacuna vasorum. It provides arterial blood flow for the entire leg. Numerous branches in its course are responsible for feeding the thigh muscles. The profunda femoris artery, which splits off in the proximal third from the femoral artery in the direction of the femur, plays a significant role.

After passing through the lacuna vasorum, the femoral artery runs anterolaterally and then steeply distally. In the upper third, it is still superficial until it then moves into the depths under the sartorius and vastus medialis muscles. In its course, along the sartorius muscle, it remains anterior to the adductor longus muscle and forms the hiatus adductorius with the femoral vein (see Sect. 7.1.1.8). After the adductor canal, the artery runs distoposteromedially in the direction of the popliteal fossa, passes through both attachments of the adductor magnus muscle and merges with the popliteal artery.

There are two access points for palpation with the client in the supine position with the knee joints underneath. First, the therapist contacts the medial area of the groin with the fingertips laid flat. Here, the fingertips point in the direction of the inguinal ligament. The index and middle fingers move gently into the depths until they perceive a pulsating structure [1]. You are now directly on the artery you are looking for. For the second reference point, the steeply positioned fingertips probe downwards in the area of the adductor canal, between the sartorius or vastus medialis muscle and the adductor longus muscle in the distal third of the anteromedial thigh. They are now directly on the femoral artery in the distal part of the thigh.

Implementation Note
In the region of the lacuna musculorum, the femoral artery can be directly perceived superficially. In the region of the adductor canal, palpation in depth is necessary [2] (Fig. 7.2).

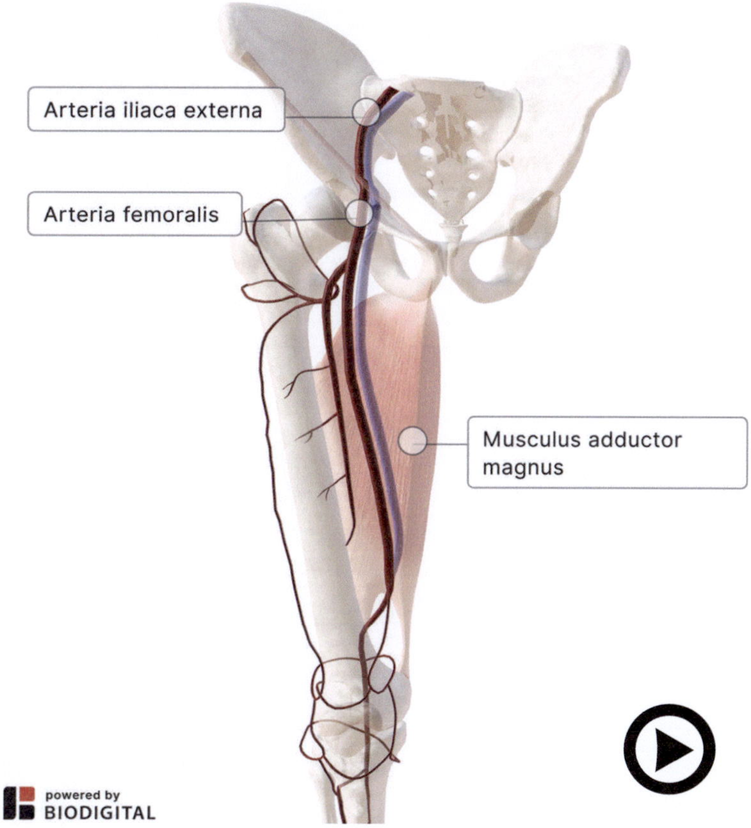

Fig. 7.2 Anatomy and palpation of the A. femoralis (▶ https://doi.org/10.1007/000-cx4)

7.1.1.3 Palpation of the Popliteal Artery

The popliteal artery arises from the femoral artery; then runs posteriorly between the semimembranosus, semitendinosus and biceps femoris muscles distally; and merges with the posterior tibial artery between the two heads of the gastrocnemius in the upper third of the lower leg. With the help of its outgoing branches, it contributes to the supply of the structures surrounding the knee joint.

During palpation, the patient is in prone position. The therapist stands sideways and passively flexes the homolateral leg at the knee joint. Then the steeply positioned fingertips, coming from posterior, are placed centrally on the knee joint gap. They feel their way anteriorly between the attachments of the ischiocrural muscles and the heads of the gastrocnemius and meet the pulsating popliteal artery at depth.

Implementation Note

The tibial nerve is in direct positional relation to the popliteal artery. A gentle approach should avoid irritation of the neural structure. Muscular hypertrophy can lead to narrowing of the popliteal artery [3] (Fig. 7.3).

7.1.1.4 Palpation of the Anterior Tibial Artery

In the distal area of the popliteal artery, the anterior tibial artery splits off, which then runs horizontally to the side and perforates the posterior tibial muscle and the interosseous membrane in the proximal area. For this purpose, there is an opening in the membrana interossea cruris, directly medial to the caput fibulae. In this area, the artery is covered by numerous structures such as the soleus muscle, the fibularis longus muscle or the extensor digitorum longus muscle. It then runs steeply distally anterior to the anterior edge of the tibia and posterior to the tibialis anterior muscle. In this course, it is completely covered by the tibialis anterior muscle and accompanied by the vein of the same name and the profundal fibular nerve. Only in the distal area of the lower leg does the anterior tibial artery appear as soon as the muscle belly of the foot lifter merges with the tendon of attachment. After passing under the extensor hallucis longus muscle, it merges with the dorsalis pedis artery in the region of the talus. Throughout its course, the artery has numerous branches that supply the structures of the lower leg with blood.

For palpation, the patient is placed in a supine position while the therapist contacts the homolateral lower leg in the distoanterior third with the fingertips. The patient is then asked to actively move the big toe in extension. This leads to a noticeable contraction of the extensor hallucis longus muscle (see Sect. 5.4.2). Directly in the area of the tendon, the fingertips are placed steeply and then palpated in depth. In a muscularly relaxed state, the pulsating anterior tibial artery can now be perceived.

Implementation Note

Due to the close anatomical positional relationship, the anterior tibialis muscle can have a direct influence on the anterior tibial artery (Fig. 7.4).

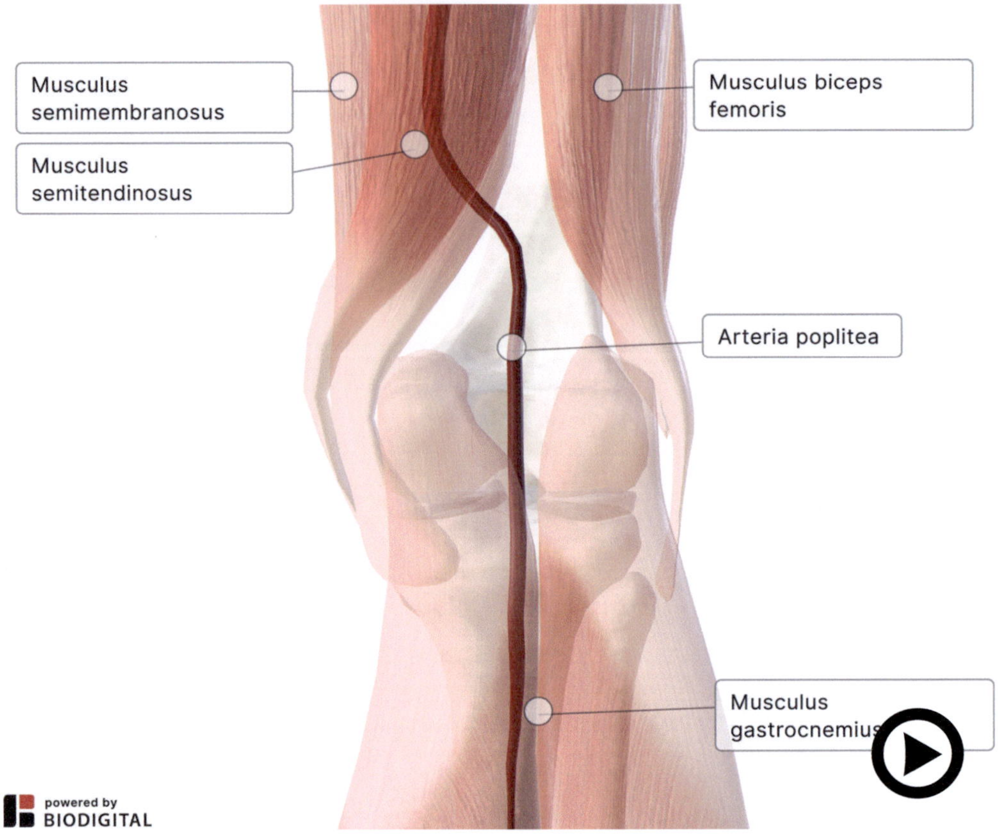

Fig. 7.3 Anatomy and palpation of the A. popliteal (▶ https://doi.org/10.1007/000-cx5)

Fig. 7.4 Anatomy and palpation of the A. tibialis anterior (▶ https://doi.org/10.1007/000-cx6)

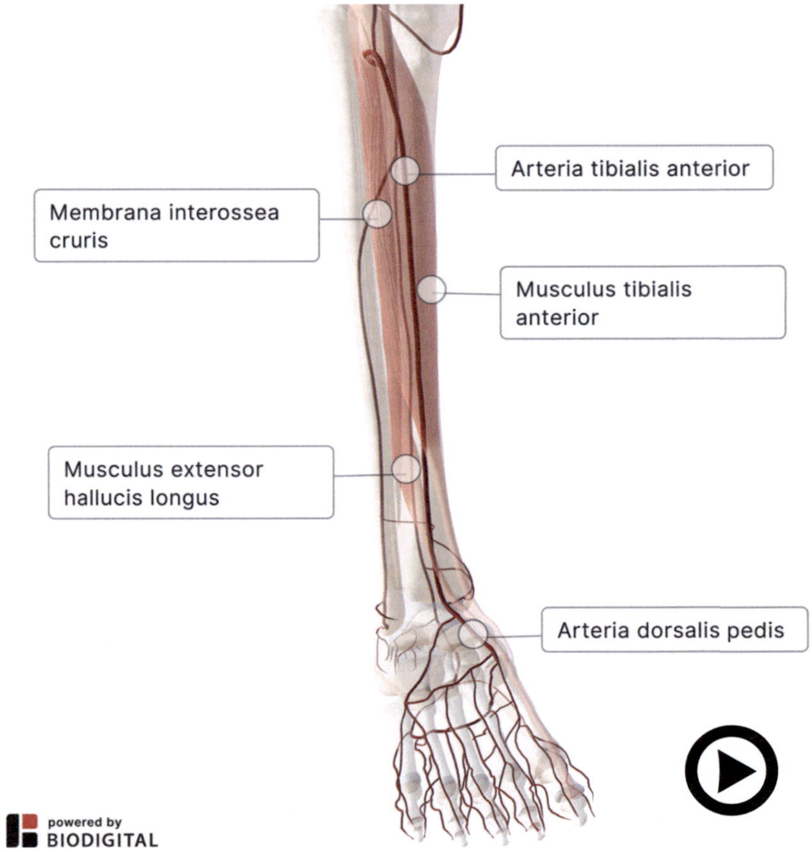

7.1.1.5 Palpation of the Posterior Tibial Artery

As a continuation of the popliteal artery, the posterior tibial artery runs steeply from the popliteal fossa along the tibia distally. Together with the posterior tibial vein and the tibial nerve, it is covered by the gastrocnemius and soleus muscles. Only in the distal third of the lower leg does the artery emerge between the tendon of the flexor digitorum longus and the tendon of the flexor hallucis longus posterior to the medial malleolus of the tibia. Distal to the medial malleolus, the posterior tibial artery bends towards the foot and runs distal to the talus sustentaculum towards the sole of the foot. It is accompanied by the flexor digitorum longus tendon. At the level of the talus or the os naviculare, the artery is covered again by the abductor hallucis muscle before it then flows into the plantar artery, which splits into a medial and lateral branch. It thus ensures the forwarding of blood to the foot and additionally supplies structures on the posterior lower leg via splits in its course.

As the artery is largely covered by muscles, pulse palpation is only possible in the vicinity of the medial malleolus. Palpation can be performed in all starting positions. The therapist applies the fingertips of the index and middle fingers over a large area, posterior to the medial malleolus. In this region, the pulse wave can be felt directly, and the course of the artery can be recorded.

Implementation Note

In peripheral arterial disease, the posterior tibial artery is often affected by stenosis [4] (Fig. 7.5).

7.1.1.6 Palpation of the Dorsalis Pedis Artery

As a continuation of the anterior tibial artery, the anterior dorsal pedal artery runs along the talus in a distomedial direction along the extensor hallucis longus muscle on the lateral side to the transition from the medial cuneiform bone to the first metatarsal. This rather small section of a vessel is located superficially and serves to convey blood to the arterial branches which supply structures of the foot further on.

For palpation of the dorsalis pedis artery, the supine position is recommended, although due to the anatomy, other starting positions also lead to an acceptable palpation sensation. The therapist contacts the ankle joint from anteriorly with the finger berries placed flat and asks the patient to actively extend the big toe. This allows tension to be felt in

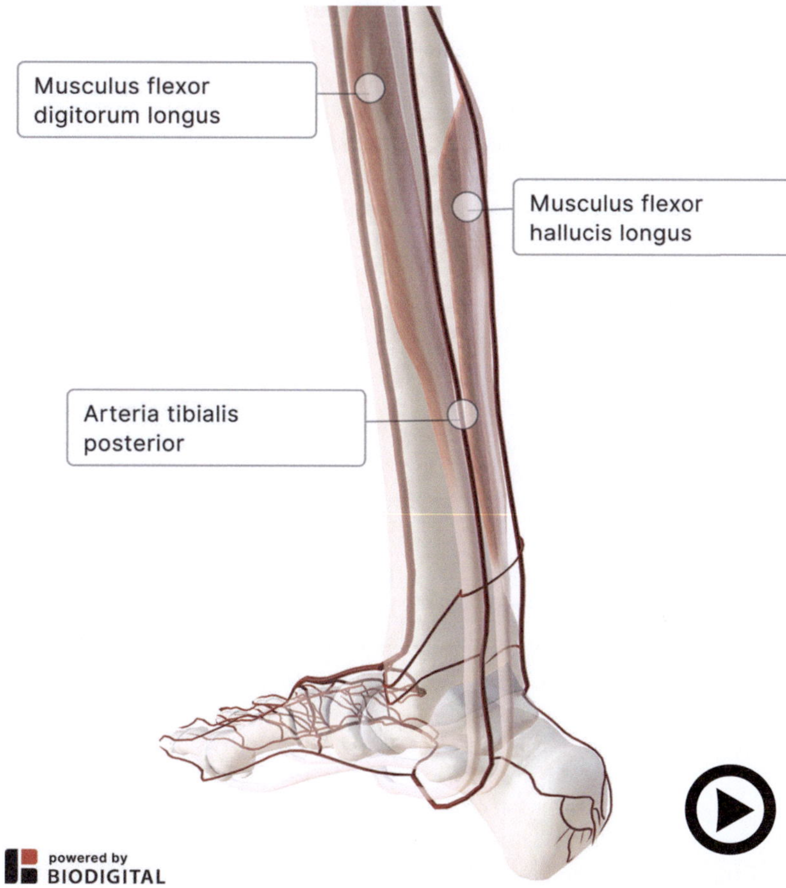

Fig. 7.5 Anatomy and palpation of the A. tibialis posterior (▶ https://doi.org/10.1007/000-cx7)

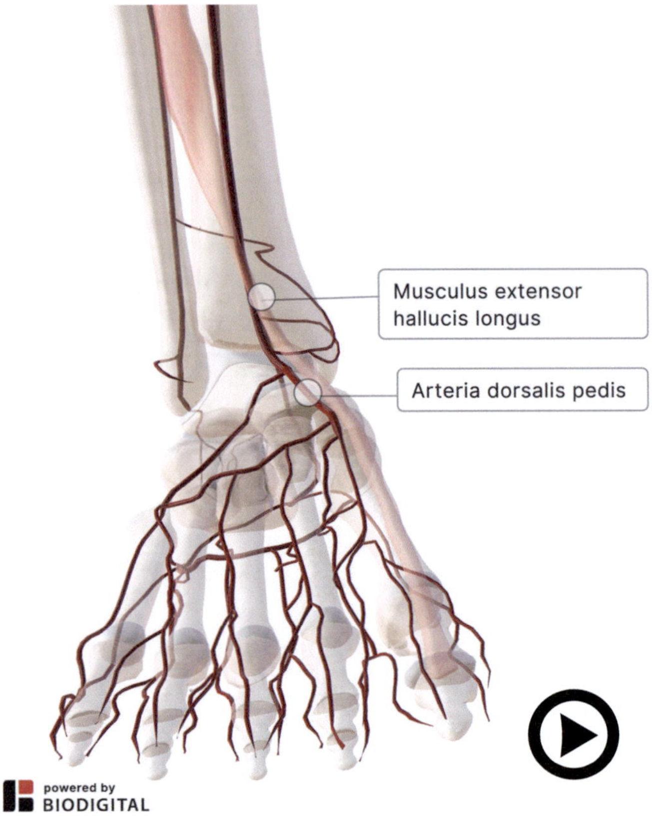

Fig. 7.6 Anatomy and palpation of the A. dorsalis pedis (▶ https://doi.org/10.1007/000-cx8)

the tendon of the extensor hallucis longus, which guides the fingers directly to the artery. The finger berries move directly lateral to the tendon distally towards the metatarsal I and will record a pulse wave over the os naviculare as well as the os cuneiforme mediale.

Implementation Note
The dorsalis pedis artery is used to analyse the vascular status because the pulse can be felt very well if there are no stenoses in the proximal area.

Different variants of the system exist [5] (Fig. 7.6).

7.1.1.7 Palpation of the Dorsal Metatarsal Arteries

The dorsal arteries arise from the dorsalis pedis artery and the arcuate pedis artery, each of which extends distally along a metatarsal. With their branches, they supply the structures in the area of the foot and flow into the digital dorsal arteries of the individual toes.

As various soft tissue structures are located above the arteries, palpation depends on the anatomical variation of the foot. For palpation with the client in the supine position, the fingertips are applied steeply from the lateral side at the base of each metatarsal. After a pulse wave is felt, the arteries are located distally along the metatarsal.

Implementation Note
Precise palpation from the surface to the depth is necessary to feel the pulse and not to push it off directly at the beginning (Fig. 7.7).

7.1.1.8 Palpation of the Adductor Canal

The adductor canal is an important region in relation to the nervous but also the arterial and venous supply to the knee joint and should be considered during palpation. It is revealed on palpation of the medial edge of the vastus medialis muscle at the junction with the adductor magnus muscle. The longitudinal groove between the two muscles is lined by an aponeurosis and carries the saphenous nerve from the femoral nerve as well as the femoral artery and vein and the descending genal artery.

Due to the important supply function of this region, it is indispensable to be able to feel the state of tension with the fingertips. For this purpose, the person to be palpated is positioned in a supine position with the knee joints underneath. The therapist stands sideways and contacts the medial edge of the homolateral vastus medialis muscle in its distal third via the fingertips. Directly in the transition to the adductor magnus muscle, a furrow is clearly noticeable, which allows the fingertips to slide into the depths. Directly in this region is the adductor canal, which can only be subjected to stimulation on the membrana vastoadductoria in the distal area. A more precise differentiation can be produced by an active movement in knee joint extension, as this causes the vastus medialis muscle to contract.

Implementation Note
The membrana vastoadductoria can cause pain when irritated as it carries numerous nerves and vascular pathways. A cautious approach is therefore required (Fig. 7.8).

7.1.2 Arteries in the Trunk and Abdomen Area

In the area of the trunk, there are numerous arteries that supply the organs. As they are protected under the strong muscular sheath of the trunk muscles and the bony thorax, only the aorta and the superficial epigastric artery can be palpated in selected regions. For this purpose, the client is positioned in the supine position. Precise anatomical knowledge of the position as well as the characteristic feeling of the pulse wave helps in tracing. In the following chapters, the vessels mentioned are described anatomically, and the palpation procedure is described.

7.1.2.1 Palpation of the Aorta

The largest artery in the human body originates directly at the ventriculus sinister, receives oxygen-rich blood during

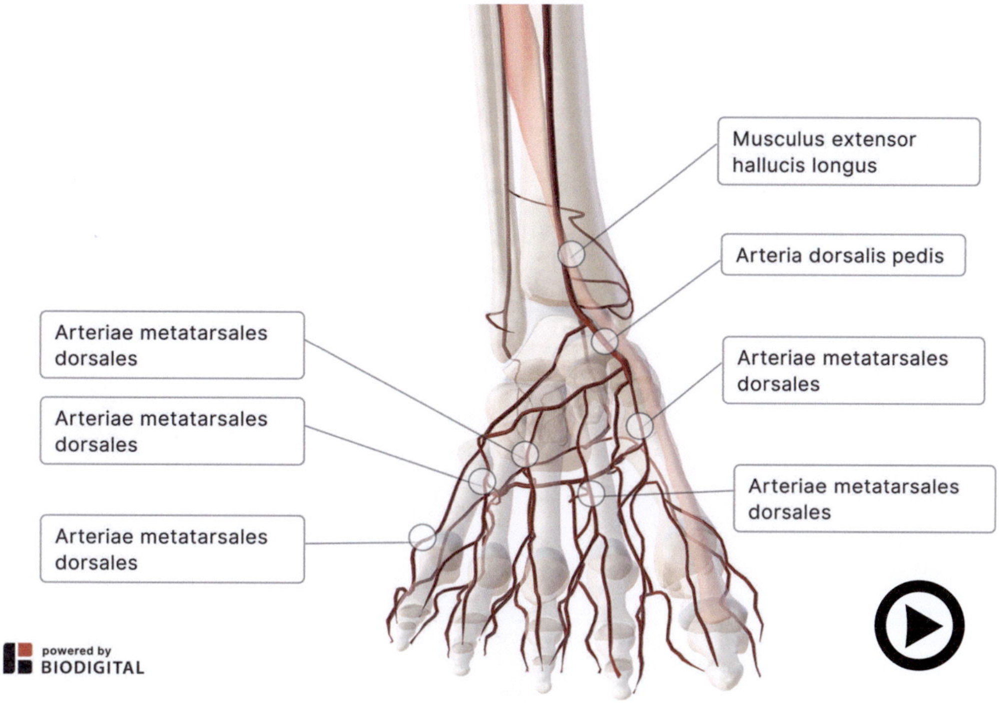

Fig. 7.7 Anatomy and palpation of the A. metatarsales dorsales (▶ https://doi.org/10.1007/000-cx9)

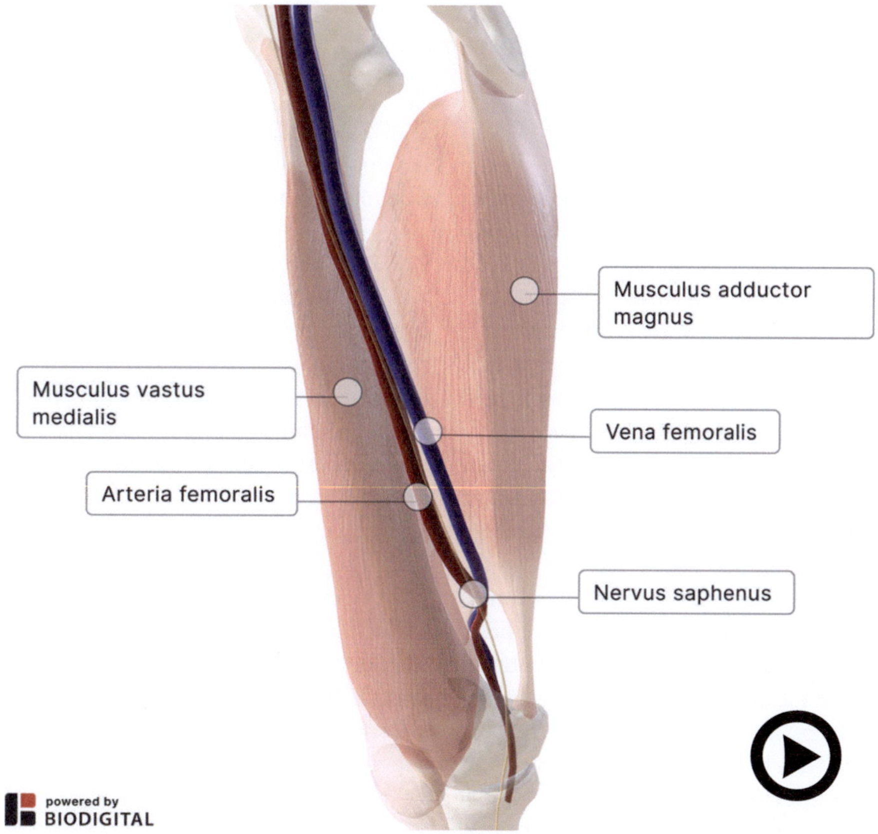

Fig. 7.8 Anatomy and palpation of the adductor canal (▶ https://doi.org/10.1007/000-cxa)

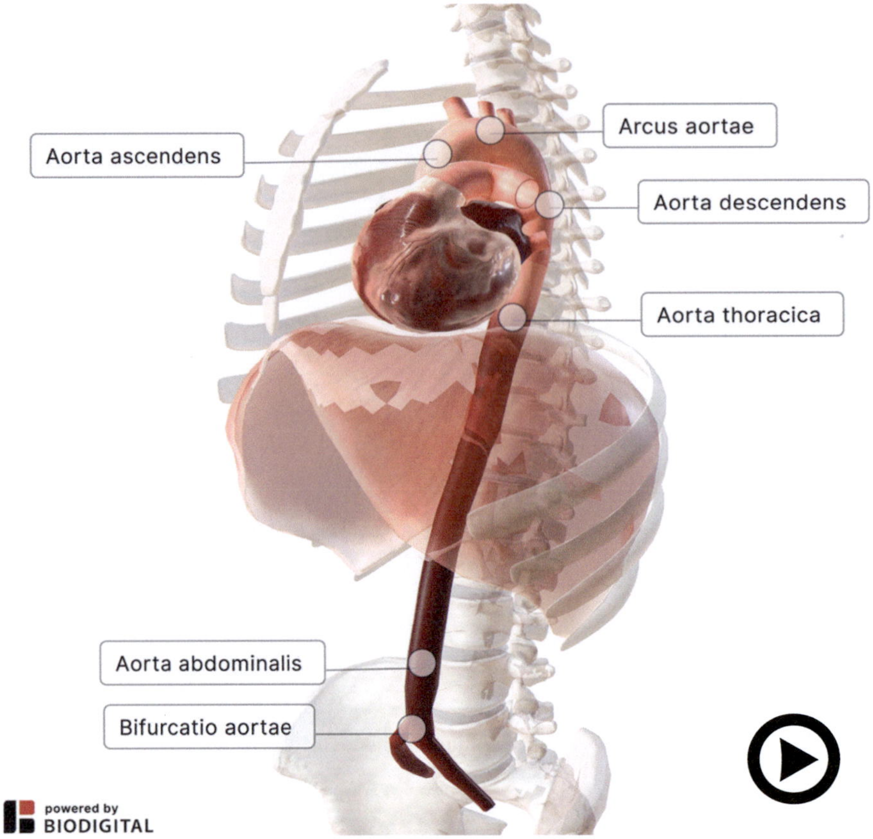

Fig. 7.9 Anatomy and palpation of the aorta (▶ https://doi.org/10.1007/000-cxb)

the expulsion phase of the heart through the valva aortae and distributes the "elixir of life" throughout the body with the help of the "Windkessel" function. Directly at the heart, it first runs upwards in the direction of the cranial. The aorta then merges into the arcus aortae, which supplies the head and the upper extremities with the help of numerous branches. After the arch, the pulsating vessel runs slightly to the left of the centre of the body, descending steeply towards the caudal. This approximately 2.5–3.5 cm thick and 30–40 cm long pars descendens first perforates the respiratory diaphragm and gives off numerous secretions, for example to the kidney, adrenal gland, liver or sex organs. Subsequently, at about the level of the umbilicus, the large body artery divides via the bifurcatio aortae into the two aa. iliacae communes, which then run into the lower extremity.

For palpation, the client is positioned in the supine position with the knee joints underneath. The therapist stands on the left side at the level of the navel and places the steeply placed fingertips of the index, middle and ring fingers on the left side of the umbilicus. They then slide slowly dorsomedially into the depths in the direction of the spine. The typical pulse wave can now be felt in the abdominal part of the aorta.

Implementation Note

An abdominal aortic aneurysm is an absolute contraindication to palpation [6] (Fig. 7.9).

7.1.2.2 Palpation of the Superficial Epigastric Artery

Immediately after the femoral artery leaves the lacuna vasorum, the superficial epigastric artery splits off, which then rises steeply craniomedially. In the region of the navel, it splits into numerous small branches which supply structures in the lower region of the abdomen and the groin with oxygenated blood.

For palpation, the patient is positioned in the supine position. The therapist places the fingertips of the index and middle fingers flat in the area of the lacuna vasorum on the femoral artery so that they point in the craniomedial direction, about three to four transverse fingers next to the navel. On this imaginary line, the stimulation is now applied to the superficial epigastric artery, which is located directly superficially.

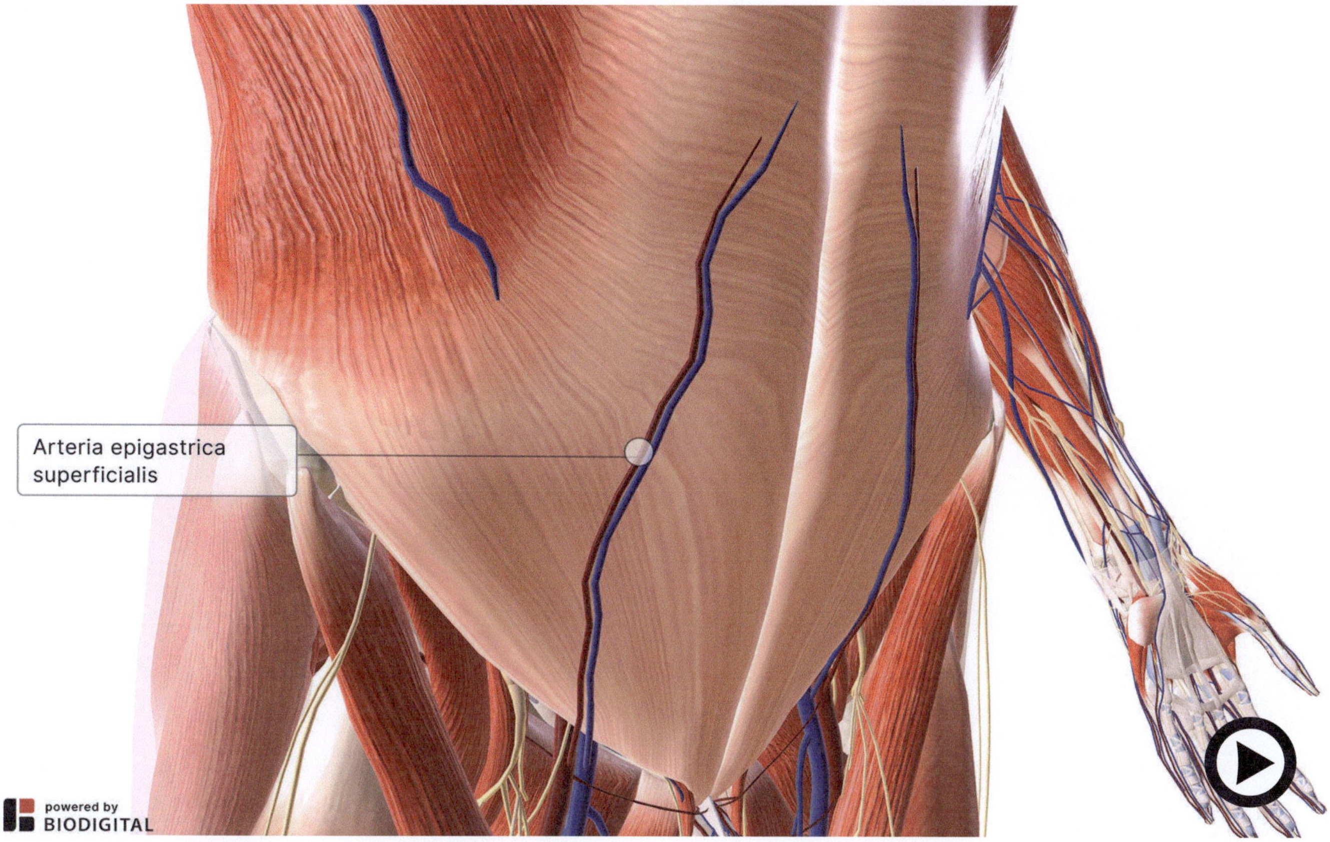

Fig. 7.10 Anatomy and palpation of the A. epigastrica superficialis (▶ https://doi.org/10.1007/000-cxc)

Implementation Note
Palpation must be gentle as the artery is superficial and therefore the pulse can be quickly squeezed off during palpation (Fig. 7.10).

7.1.3 Arteries in the Area of the Upper Extremity

An arterial supply to the skeletal muscles is indispensable for the functionality of the shoulder girdle, shoulder joint, elbow joint and hand. The entire upper extremity is supplied by the continuing vessels of the subclavian artery, which originates in the area of the shoulder girdle. The subclavian artery is followed distally by the axillary artery, then the brachial artery and finally the ulnar and radial arteries. In the area of the hand, the arteries converge into the Aa. digitales palmares propriae. All the vessels mentioned are presented in the following chapters, first in their anatomical position and then in their palpation. The recommended starting position is supine or sitting.

7.1.3.1 Palpation of the Subclavian Artery

The subclavian artery arises on the right side of the body from the brachiocephalic trunk and on the left side of the body directly from the aortic arch, as this is already on the left side and therefore no transition is needed. Both then first run in the direction of the craniolateral, passing dorsally of the art. sternoclavicularis and beyond the clavicle. They then each pass through the posterior (middle, depending on the literature) scalenus gap between the scalenus anterior and scalenus medius muscles, continue laterally and join the axillary artery behind the clavicle at the lateral end of the medial third. The subclavian artery is covered by the platysma and the sternocleidomastoid muscle. In the medial area, the sternohyoideus and sternothyroidus muscles are also located anterior to the subclavian artery. The vessel serves to conduct blood into the axillary artery and supplies the region of the shoulder girdle, parts of the thorax and abdominal wall as well as the neck via numerous branches. A large branch of the subclavian artery is the vertebral artery, which runs along the cervical spine and supplies the head from the occipital region as an equivalent to the common carotid arteries.

During palpation, the client is positioned in the supine position with the head underneath or in the sitting position with the arm in a passive position. The therapist stands laterally at the level of the shoulder girdle and makes contact with the homolateral clavicle in the medial third coming from the cranial. Starting from this reference point, the fingertips of

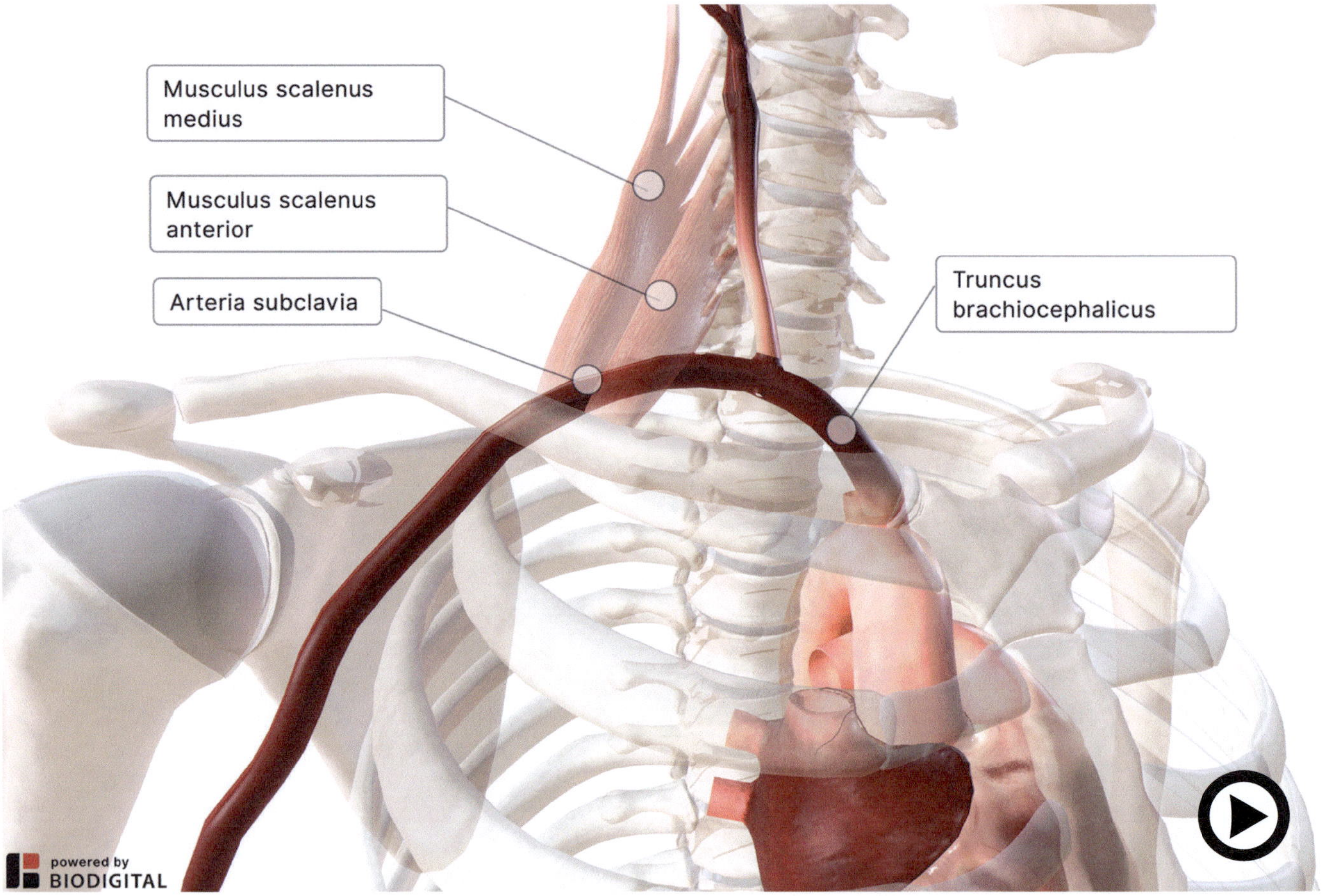

Fig. 7.11 Anatomy and palpation of the A. subclavia (▶ https://doi.org/10.1007/000-cxd)

the index and middle fingers move dorsally and slide directly into a depression in which the pulsating subclavian artery can be perceived. The palpation site is called the lateral cervical region. This is located between the descending trapezius muscle and the sternocleidomastoid muscle.

Implementation Note
Palpation should be gentle as the subclavian vein and brachial plexus are also located in the region described (Fig. 7.11).

7.1.3.2 Palpation of the Axillary Artery

The axillary artery arises from the subclavian artery dorsal to the middle third of the clavicle and lateral to the costa prima. It then runs distolaterally to the end of the proximal third of the humerus and merges with the brachial artery. It is thus tangential to the axilla, which gives it its appropriate name. In its course, it is accompanied by the brachial plexus and the axillary vein. Its numerous branches serve to supply the shoulder, axillary and thoracic regions, while the axillary artery itself ensures that the blood is passed on to the adjoining brachial artery.

For palpation, position the patient supine or seated while the therapist contacts the homolateral caput breve of the biceps brachii muscle on the inner side of the upper arm with the fingertips of the index and middle fingers. The fingers follow the muscle proximally directly into the axilla between the pectoralis major and subscapularis muscles. Directly in the axilla, they then meet the pulsating brachial artery.

Implementation Note
Due to the anatomical proximity to the brachial plexus as well as to the axillary lymph nodes, a gentle approach is advisable (Fig. 7.12).

7.1.3.3 Palpation of the Brachial Artery

The brachial artery runs directly in the sulcus bicipitalis medialis between the caput breve of the m. biceps brachii and the caput longum of the m. triceps brachii on the inner side of the upper arm. It is the direct continuation of the axillary artery and runs distally to be partially covered by the biceps brachii muscle. In the region of the crook of the elbow, it divides directly at the level of the pronator teres muscle into the ulnar and radial arteries. The brachial artery itself

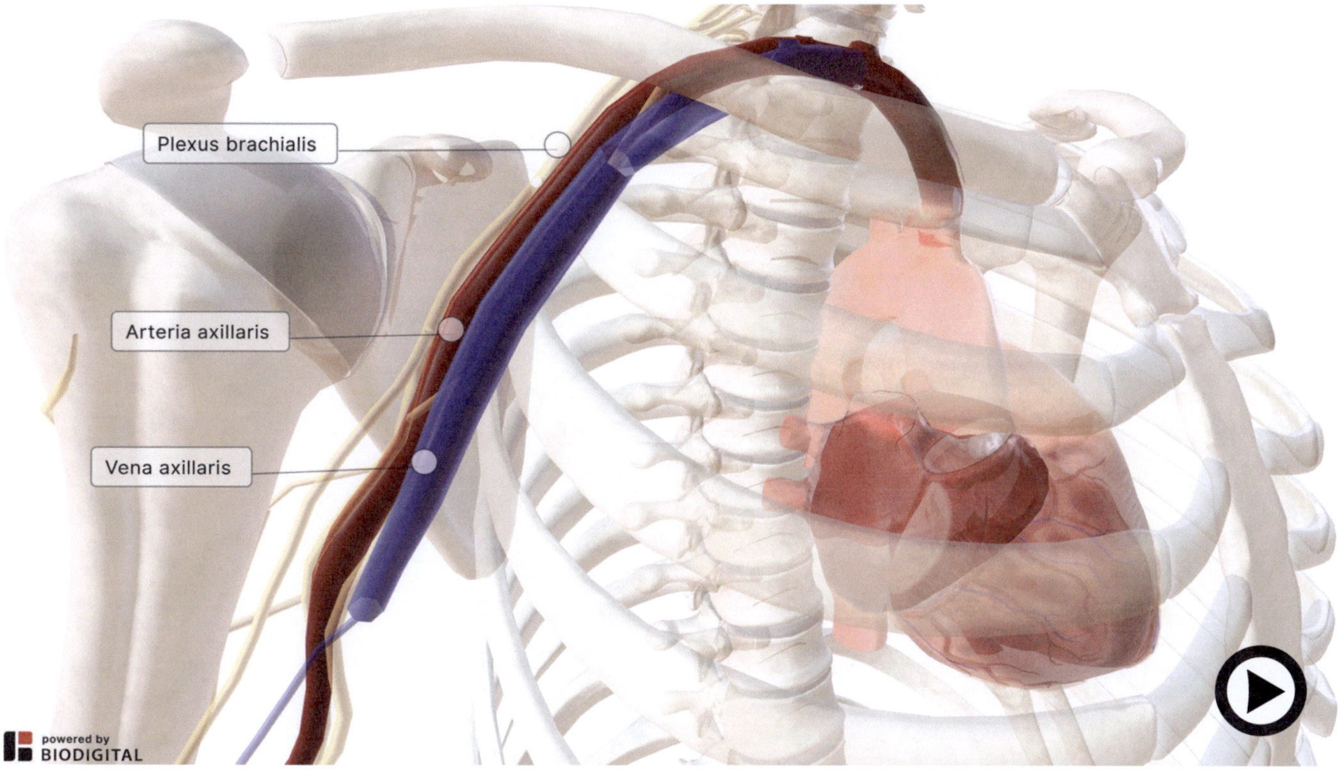

Fig. 7.12 Anatomy and palpation of the A. axillaris (▶ https://doi.org/10.1007/000-cxe)

serves to convey blood to the forearm, whereas the numerous branches in its course serve to supply the muscles of the upper arm.

The starting position for palpation is the supine or sitting position. The therapist stands sideways at the level of the upper arm and palpates from anteriorly on the biceps brachii muscle in the middle third medially. The steeply positioned fingertips meet a depression on the inner side of the upper arm, where the pulsating brachial artery can be perceived. The fingers are now between the biceps brachii and triceps brachii muscles and distal to the tendon of the latissimus dorsi muscle on the vessel. Another palpation of the brachial artery can be done in the crook of the elbow. For this purpose, the therapist orients himself at the transition to the attachment tendon of the biceps brachii muscle at the ulnar muscle edge. Directly in the depression on the medial side, the branch of the artery can be grasped via the steeply positioned fingertips.

Implementation Note
Muscular structures can irritate the brachial artery in rare cases. This can lead to an undersupply of the muscles fed by it [7] (Fig. 7.13).

7.1.3.4 Palpation of the Radial Artery

The radial artery arises from the bifurcation of the brachial artery in the bend of the elbow medial to the tendon of the biceps brachii muscle and then runs distoradially along the medial edge of the brachioradialis muscle. Thus, it passes through the radial antebrachial sulcus along the forearm into the hand, runs radially of the scaphoid bone dorsally and passes under the abductor pollicis longus muscle and the extensor pollicis brevis and longus muscles. On the dorsum of the hand, the radial artery then divides at the level of the trapezium into the dorsal metacarpal arteries and the dorsal carpal and metacarpal ramus and radial palmar arteries. It thus serves to convey the oxygenated blood into the hand and supplies parts of the elbow, radial side of the forearm, parts of the carpus and the thenar as well as other fingers via outgoing branches.

Since palpation of the radial artery serves as a prime example of pulse palpation, this artery is the most suitable for starting vascular palpation. The pulse can be palpated from any position, whereby the starting position of the client is supine or sitting. The therapist stands sideways and contacts the radial palmar surface of the distal radius with the index and middle fingertips placed flat. The radial pulse can

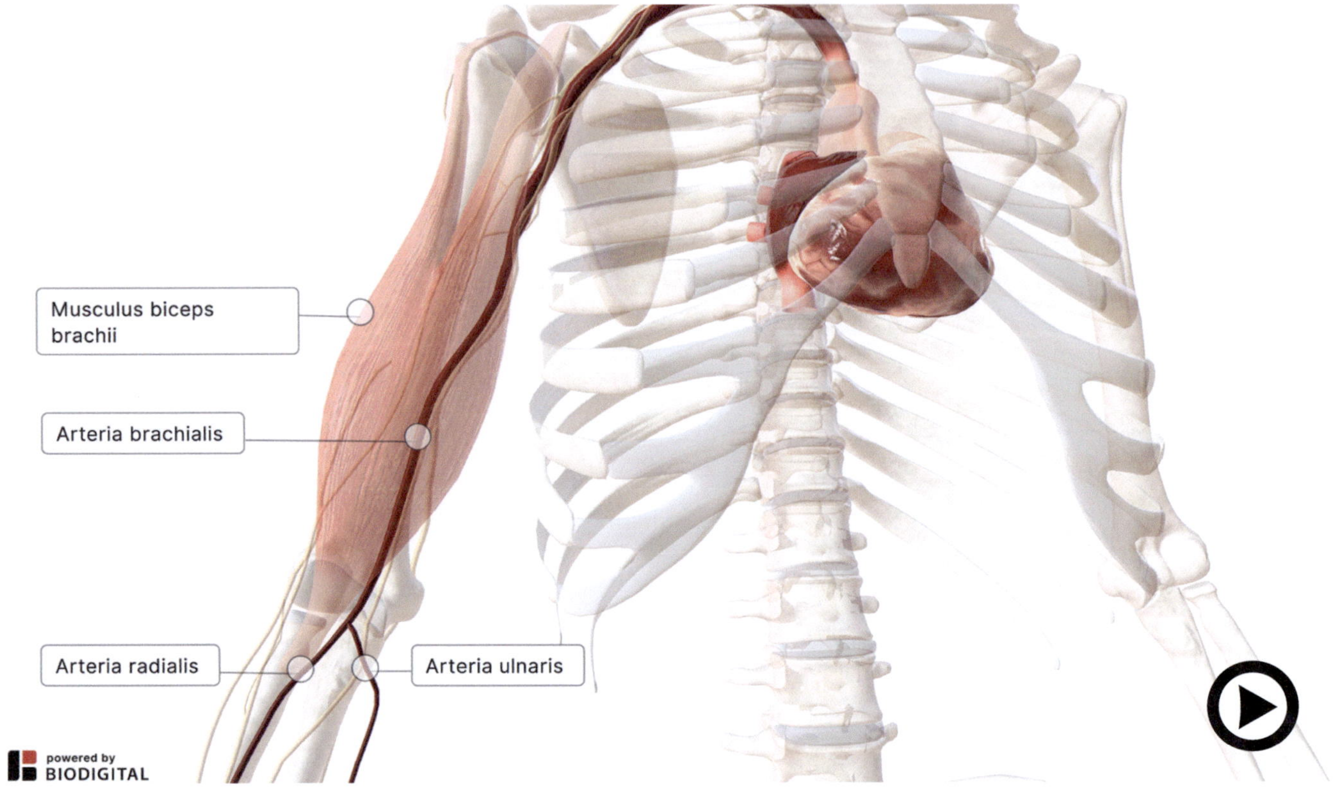

Fig. 7.13 Anatomy and palpation of the A. brachialis (▶ https://doi.org/10.1007/000-cxf)

be felt directly radial to the flexor tendons in the soft tissue-lined depression. Depending on the anatomy of the arm and the strength of the pulse, the artery can then be traced further proximally by palpation. The steeply positioned fingertips always orient themselves radially to the flexor tendons.

Implementation Note
The pressure over the fingertips should be gentle at the beginning so as not to squeeze the radial artery (Fig. 7.14).

7.1.3.5 Palpation of the Ulnar Artery

The ulnar artery arises from the bifurcation of the brachial artery in the bend of the elbow medial to the tendon of the biceps brachii muscle and then runs distoulnar over the pronator teres muscle and under the flexor carpi radialis and flexor digitorum superficialis muscles. At the ulnar edge of the forearm, it runs steeply distally, taking the same course as the palmaris longus muscle between the flexor carpi ulnaris muscle and the flexor digitorum profundus muscle. In the distal area of the ulnar or in the transition to the carpus, the ulnar artery is located directly ulnar to the flexor tendons of the fingers and palmar to the tendon of the flexor carpi ulnaris muscle. In the region of the carpus, it is often also called the superficial ulnar artery, which passes through the Loge de Guyon with the ulnar nerve [8]. At about the level of the os pisiforme, the ulnar artery then merges into the arcus palmaris superficialis, which extends on the palm side and transports the blood further into the fingers. The ulnar artery, with its branches in its course, is thus responsible for supplying the regions at the elbow, on the ulnar side of the forearm, as well as parts of the carpus and the hypothenar and the other fingers.

For palpation of the ulnar artery, the patient is positioned supine or seated with the forearm in a passive position. The therapist stands to the side and applies the finger berries of the index and middle finger, laid flat, directly radial to the os pisiforme. In this region, the fingertips move with moderate pressure further and further into the depths until they meet the rather weakly pulsating vessel. The ulnar artery can then be felt proximally by orienting the fingertips along the ulnar edge of the flexor tendons.

Implementation Note
The ulnar artery is often rather weak in its pulsation, so that sensitive palpation is required (Fig. 7.15).

7.1.3.6 Palpation of the Aa. Digitales Palmares Propriae and Digitales Dorsales Manus

The fingers are supplied by arteries located radially and ulnarly, both palmar and dorsal. They are called digital pal-

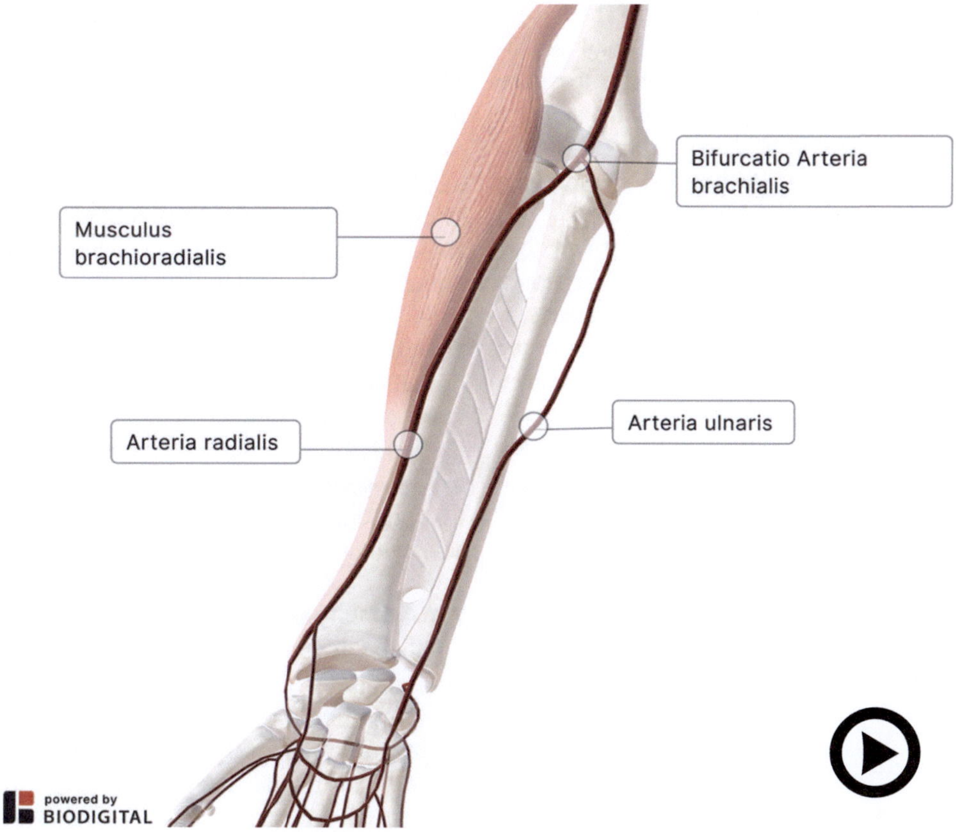

Fig. 7.14 Anatomy and palpation of the A. radialis (▶ https://doi.org/10.1007/000-cxg)

Fig. 7.15 Anatomy and palpation of the A. ulnaris (▶ https://doi.org/10.1007/000-cxh)

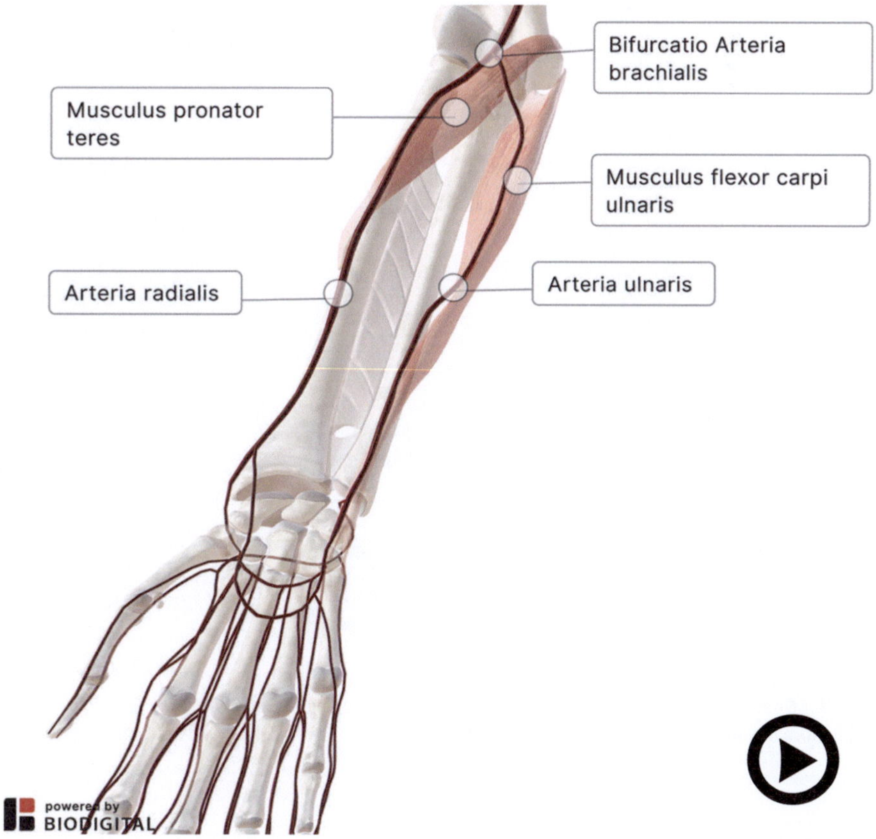

mares propriae and digital dorsal manus arteries. The former arise from the Aa. digitales palmares communes and the latter from the Aa. metacarpales dorsales. In addition, there are splits from the radial artery, which supply the thumb and part of the index finger, and splits from the ulnar artery, which supply the little finger with blood. Altogether, they provide the blood supply of oxygenated blood to the fingers.

To feel the pulse of the digital palmares propriae and digital dorsal manus, the client is positioned supine or seated with the arm in a passive position. The therapist stands in front of the patient and contacts the proximal phalanx of the index finger from the ulnar side. If the fingertip is moved slightly dorsally and palmar at the proximal phalanx, the pulsating digital arteries can be recorded. Subsequently, the entire index finger can be palpated from radial and ulnar and the other fingers using the same procedure.

Implementation Note

The pressure should be gentle at the beginning; otherwise, the arteries can quickly be squeezed, which means that the pulse wave can no longer be felt (Fig. 7.16).

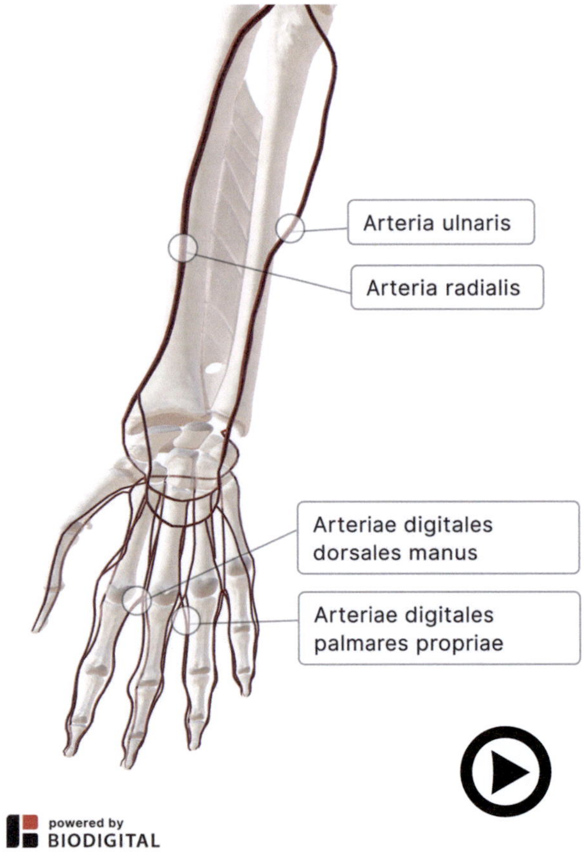

Fig. 7.16 Anatomy and palpation of the Aa. digitales propriae et digitales dorsales manus (▶ https://doi.org/10.1007/000-cxj)

7.1.4 Arteries in the Area of the Head

The skull is supplied by two separate arterial accesses: on the one hand, the A. carotis communis dexter and sinister lead oxygen-rich blood to the head from anterior, and on the other hand, the A. vertebralis dexter and sinister from posterior. These arteries originate from the arcus aortae or, on the right side, from the truncus brachiocephalicus. Numerous branches of these two supply areas radiate over the entire head. The palpable arterial vessels include the common carotid artery, the superficial temporal artery, the zygomatico-orbital artery, the facial artery, the angular artery, the dorsal nasal artery, the supratrochlear artery, the supraorbital artery, the posterior auricular artery and the occipital artery. In the following chapters, the anatomical location of the vessels is first presented, and then the palpation process is developed. The patient is in the supine or sitting position.

7.1.4.1 Palpation of the Common Carotid Artery

On the right side, the carotid artery arises from the aortic arch via the brachiocephalic trunk, while the left common carotid artery arises directly from the aortic arch. Both run to the anteriolateral side of the neck and then rise steeply towards the cranial. They run directly under the sternocleidomastoid muscle and the overlying platysma. Posteriocaudally, approximately in the region of the angulus mandibulae, it divides into the external carotid artery, which runs laterally along the skull, and the internal carotid artery, which dips into the skull. The vessel, which is about 6.5 mm thick in males and 6.1 mm thick in females, runs together with the internal jugular vein and the vagus nerve in the vagina carotica up to the division point described. There are interindividual differences regarding the diameter [9].

Palpation of the common carotid artery is performed from the sitting or supine position. The therapist stands sideways to the client and orients himself to the arcus mandibulae on the contralateral side. The flatly placed fingertips of the index and middle fingers move about two transverse fingers from the mandibular arch distally and meet the pulsating carotid artery anterior to the sternocleidomastoid muscle. It can then be grasped in the course cranially in front of or below the sternocleidomastoid muscle.

Implementation Note

Due to the carotid sinus reflex, palpation should always be gentle and one-sided (Fig. 7.17).

7.1.4.2 Palpation of the External Carotid Artery

The external carotid artery arises as a branch of the common carotid artery occipital to the mandibular angulus. It

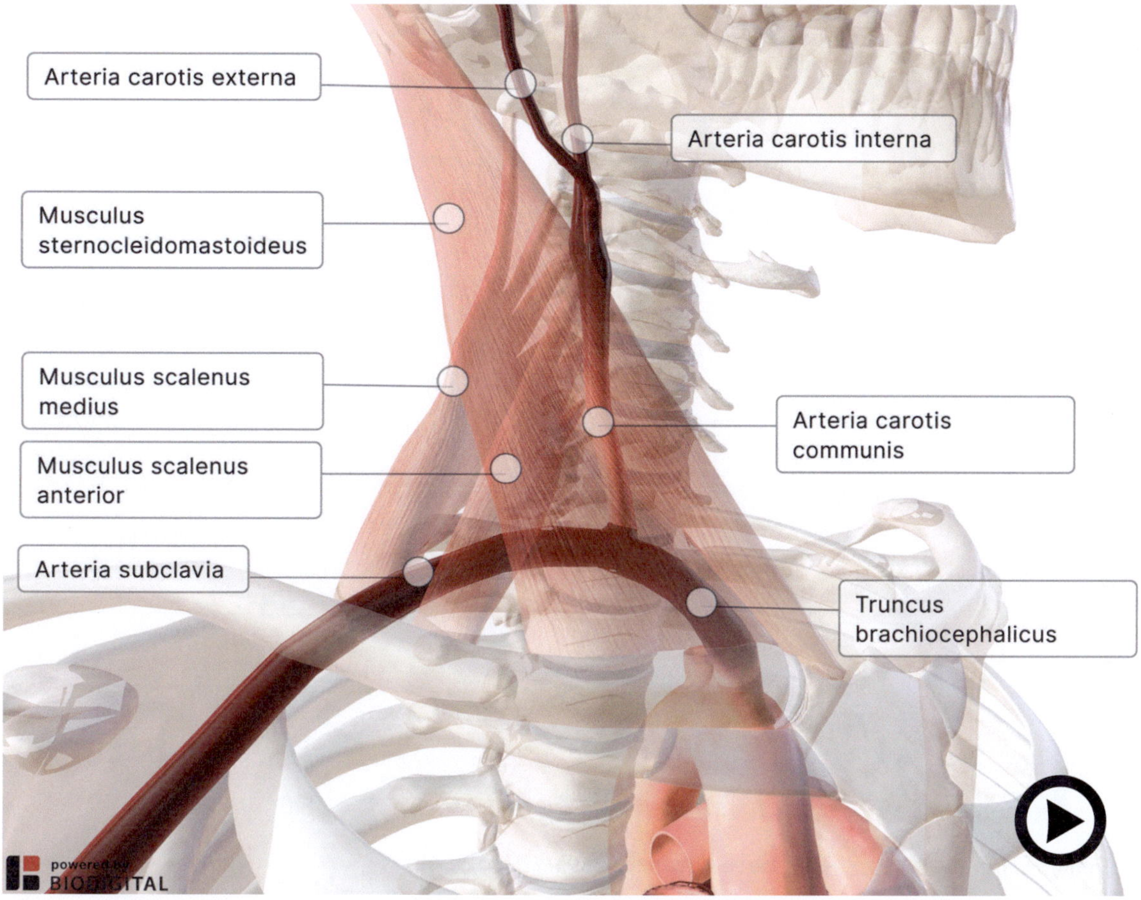

Fig. 7.17 Anatomy and palpation of the A. carotis communis (▶ https://doi.org/10.1007/000-cxk)

then rises steeply and runs anterior to the ear parallel to the ramus mandibulae. At about the level of the external acoustic meatus, it merges with the superficial temporal artery. In its course, the external carotid artery forms numerous branches such as the facial artery, the maxillary artery, the zygomatico-orbital artery, the posterior auricular artery and the occipital artery. Based on these numerous branches, it is clear that the vessel supplies large parts of the head and neck. In addition, it ensures the arterial blood supply to the dura mater.

For palpation, which is done in the supine or sitting position, the therapist stands sideways in front of the client and makes contact with the homonymous ramus mandibulae. For this purpose, the fingertips of the index and middle fingers are placed on the occipital surface of the lower jaw and anterior to the earlobe. With gentle deep pressure, the pulsating external carotid artery can be perceived.

Implementation Note

Palpation should be gentle, as the artery can be irritated with even a little pressure, resulting in a reduced pulse response (Fig. 7.18).

7.1.4.3 Palpation of the Superficial Temporal Artery

The superficial temporal artery arises from the external carotid artery and spreads over the lateral surface of the skull. Its origin is anterior to the external meatus acusticus. In its ascending course towards the superior, the superficial temporal artery has numerous branches that supply areas of the jaw and ear as well as structures of the face and lateral skull. It finally runs out into a frontal ramus and a parietal ramus.

The temporal pulse is felt in the supine or sitting position. The therapist applies the fingertips of the index and middle fingers anterior to the auditory canal so that one finger is located on the ramus zygomaticus and one finger above it. With little pressure, the pulsatile superficial temporal artery can be palpated. In addition, the fingertips can trace the vessel further towards the cranial vault.

Implementation Note

Palpation should be gentle, as the artery can be compressed with little pressure, so that the pulse is no longer palpable. If the superficial temporal artery is already well defined, giant cell arteritis may be the cause [10] (Fig. 7.19).

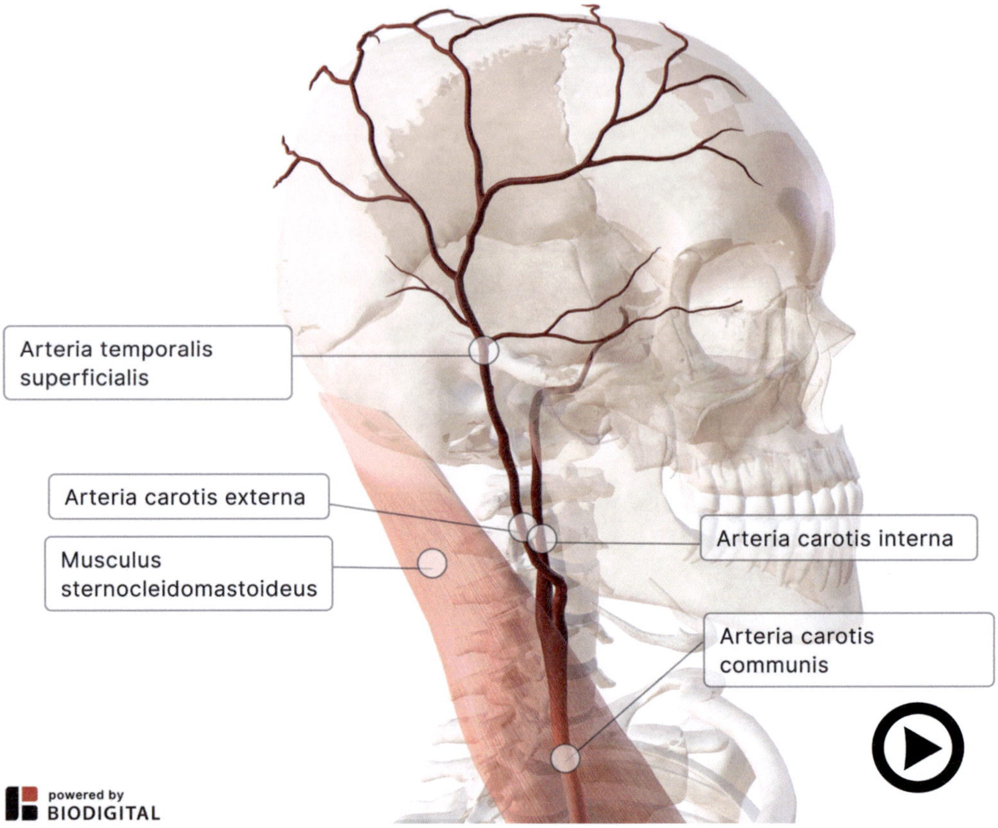

Fig. 7.18 Anatomy and palpation of the A. carotis externa (▶ https://doi.org/10.1007/000-cxm)

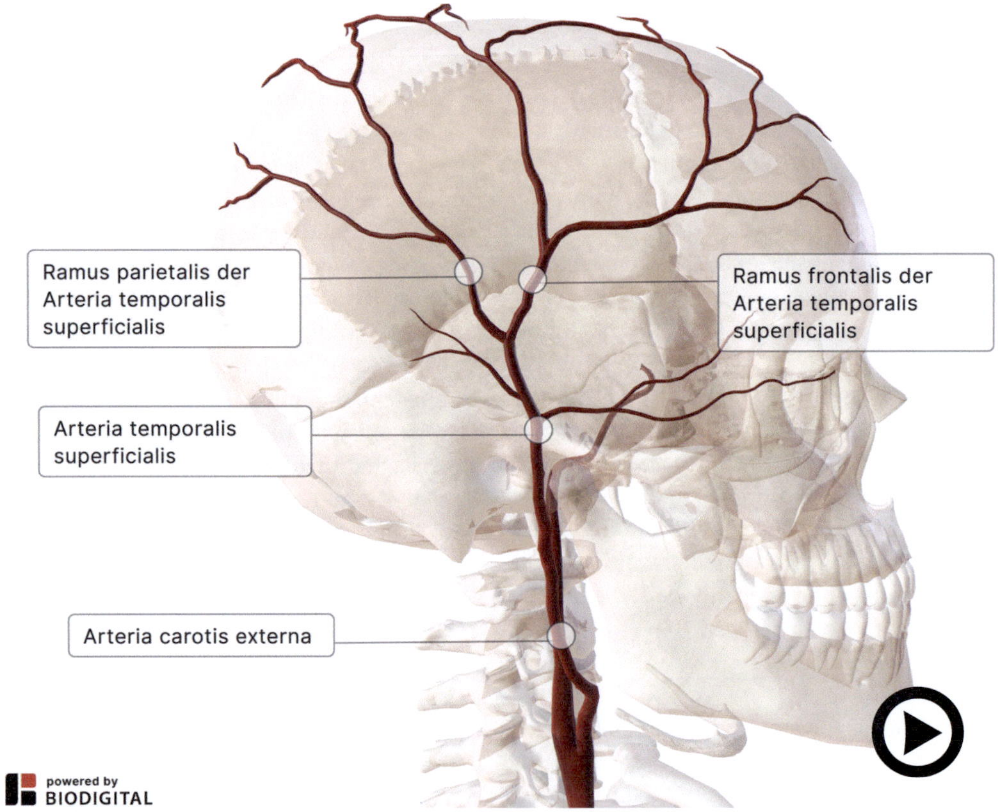

Fig. 7.19 Anatomy and palpation of the A. temporalis superficialis (▶ https://doi.org/10.1007/000-cxn)

7.1.4.4 Palpation of the Zygomatico-Orbital Artery

The rather inconstant zygomatico-orbital artery owes its name entirely to its location. As a branch of the superficial temporal artery or, in rare cases, of the median temporal artery, it runs above the proc. zygomaticus ossis temporalis towards the eye. It lies directly superficial to the temporalis muscle and supplies structures in the region of the eyes, such as the eyelids.

For palpation, with the patient in the supine or sitting position, the therapist applies the fingertips of the index, middle and ring fingers above the proc. zygomaticus ossis temporalis with the fingertips facing superiorly. As soon as the patient clenches, a clear contraction can be felt. In a relaxed jaw position, if the artery is present, a gentle pulse wave can be perceived through the fingers.

Implementation Note

Palpation must be gentle from the surface to the depth; otherwise, the zygomatico-orbital artery may be squeezed (Fig. 7.20).

7.1.4.5 Palpation of the Facial Artery

The facial artery, occipitocaudal to the mandibular angulus, arises from the external carotid artery and then runs first along the mandible to its centre. As it continues, it rises from the cheeks over the teeth towards the nose. It has numerous branches that supply all the structures in the area of the face with arterial blood. In the area lateral to the nostrils, the facial artery merges with the angular artery.

Palpation of the artery is done in a sitting or supine position and can only be done directly at two points, as it is covered by numerous muscles. For the first reference point, the therapist places the fingertips of the index and middle fingers, pointing towards the nose, flat on the mandible at about the level of the corner of the mouth or the second molar. With the application of gentle pressure in depth, the pulsating artery can be detected. The second reference point exists lateral to the nostril. To detect this pulse wave, a mental line is drawn from the pupil caudally, intersecting a horizontal line that runs along the lower edge of the nostril. At this intersection, the index finger berry gently searches for the pulsating facial artery, which then merges with the angular artery in this area.

Implementation Note

The pressure should be applied gently from the surface to the depth, as some structures cover the artery (Fig. 7.21).

7.1.4.6 Palpation of the Angular Artery

As a branch of the facial artery, the ophthalmic artery runs ascending along the nose. Its region of origin is directly

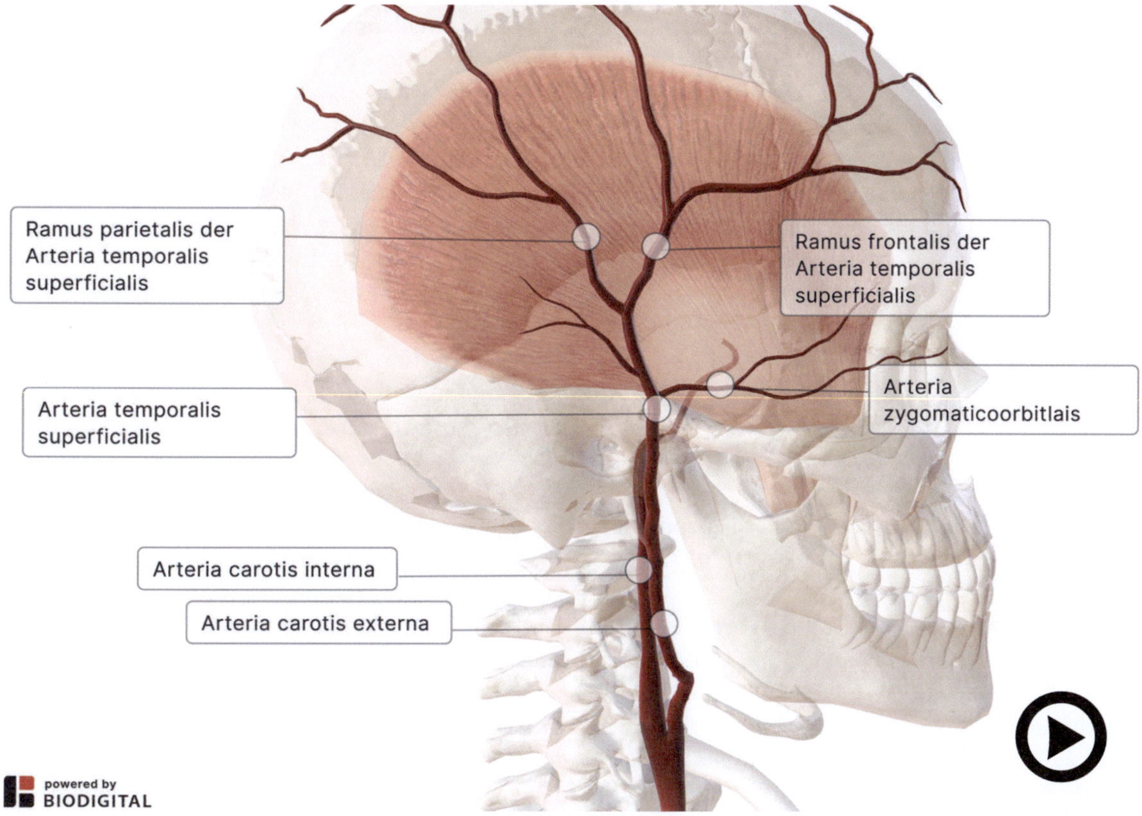

Fig. 7.20 Anatomy and palpation of the A. zygomaticoorbitalis (▶ https://doi.org/10.1007/000-cxp)

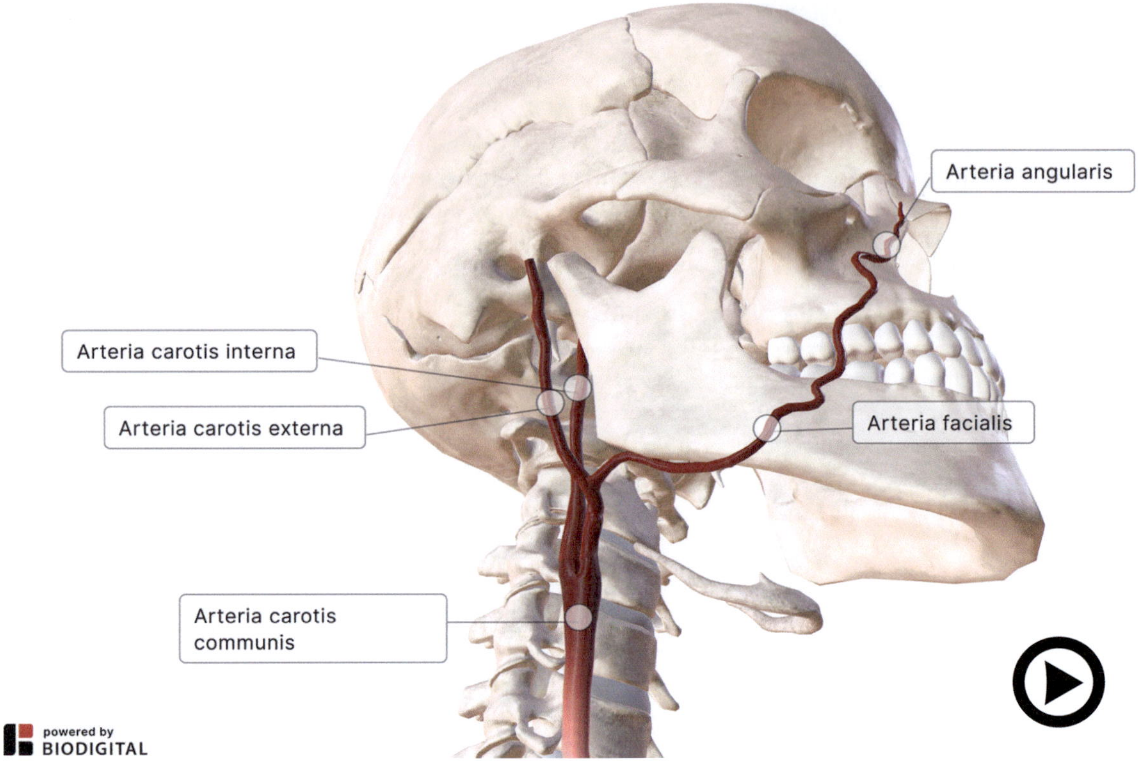

Fig. 7.21 Anatomy and palpation of the A. facialis (▶ https://doi.org/10.1007/000-cxq)

under the levator labii superioris muscle at about the intersection of the vertical line of extension of the pupil and the horizontal line of extension of the lower edge of the nostril. From there, it ascends to the transition of the cartilago nasi lateralis to the os nasale. In this region, the angular artery merges with the nasal artery. Numerous small branches supply the skin in the region of the mouth and below the eye and also the saccus lacrimalis and the orbicularis oculi muscle.

Palpation of the artery takes place in the lateral area of the nose. The client is positioned in the sitting or supine position while the therapist places the fingertip of the index and middle fingers flat next to the nostril. It is important to palpate slowly in depth below the os nasale until the pulsating angular artery is felt.

Implementation Note
Palpation must be gentle from the surface to the depth; otherwise, the angular artery may be compressed (Fig. 7.22).

7.1.4.7 Palpation of the Dorsal Nasal Artery

Originating from the ophthalmic artery, the dorsal nasal artery runs from the superiomedial edge of the orbit towards the nose, which it supplies with oxygenated blood. Lateral to the nostrils, at the transition of the os nasale to the cartilago nasi lateralis, the artery anastomoses with the angular artery. On the bridge of the nose, there is another connection with the artery of the same name on the contralateral side. Thus, the blood circulations are in close contact and can react compensatorily in case of stenosis. In its area of origin, the artery is covered by the orbicularis oculi muscle and the depressor supercilii muscle.

The nasal artery is palpated from the supine or sitting position. The therapist places the index fingertip from the lateral side on the os nasale of the contralateral side and slowly begins to feel from the surface into the depth. The pulsating wave of the vessel can be detected.

Implementation Note
Palpation must be gentle from the surface to the depth; otherwise, the nasal dorsal artery may be squeezed (Fig. 7.23).

7.1.4.8 Palpation of the Supratrochlear Artery

As an ascending branch of the ophthalmic artery, the supratrochlear artery originates at the superiomedial edge of the orbit and then moves into the medial region of the forehead. In its region of origin, it is covered by the orbicularis oculi muscle and the depressor and corrugator supercilii muscles and partly by the procerus muscle. In its further course, it pulls superficial to the frontalis muscle on the forehead and anastomoses with the artery of the same name on the contralateral side as well as with the homolateral supraorbital artery. This extensive anastomosis allows the supratrochlear

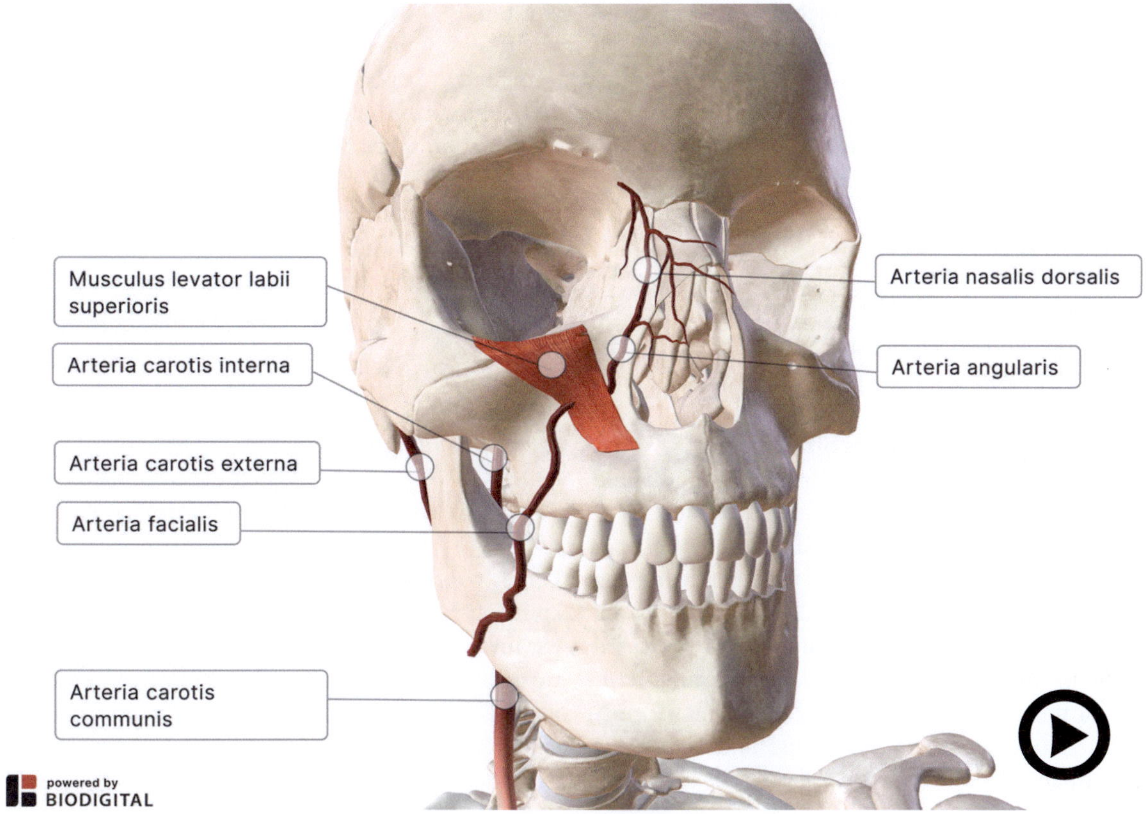

Fig. 7.22 Anatomy and palpation of the A. angularis (▶ https://doi.org/10.1007/000-cxr)

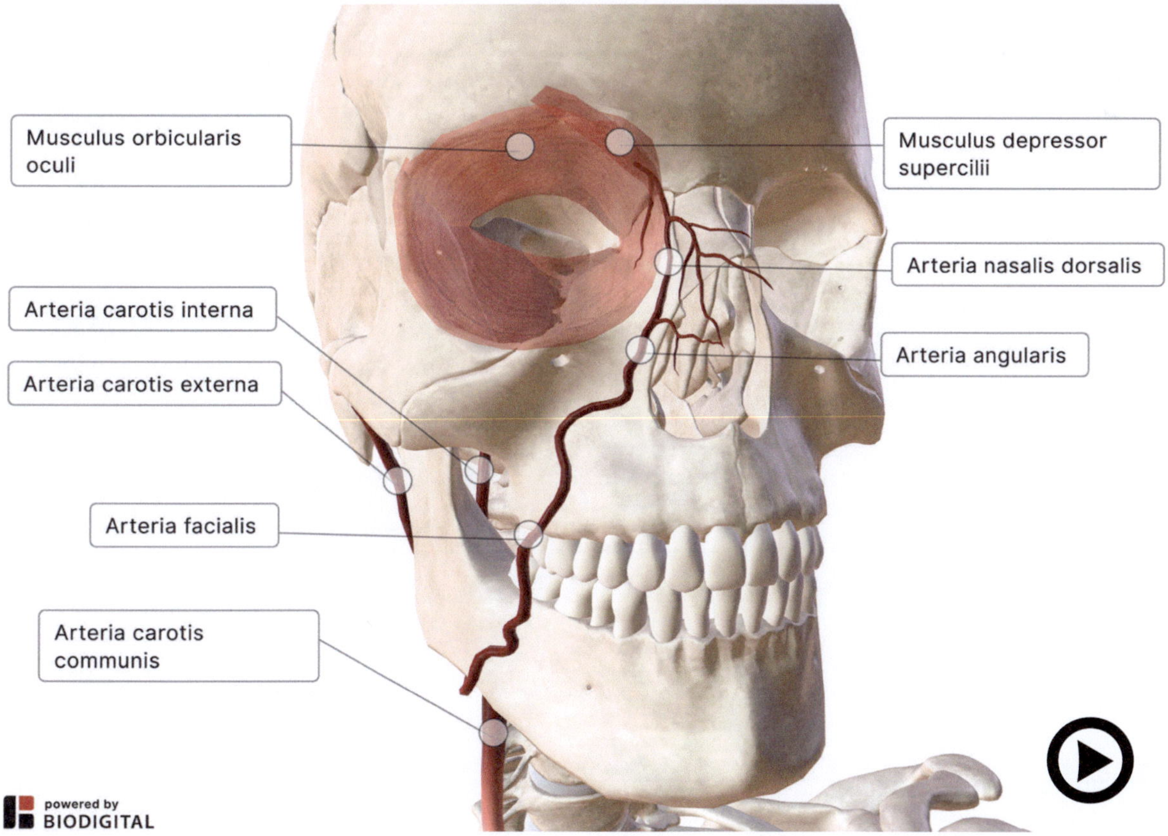

Fig. 7.23 Anatomy and palpation of the A. nasalis dorsalis (▶ https://doi.org/10.1007/000-cxs)

artery to supply blood to structures such as the skin, bone and mimic muscles in the region of the forehead.

Palpation of the artery is done in the supine or sitting position. The therapist places the index fingertip on the upper inner edge of the orbit with the forehead facing flat and begins to gently palpate the depth. The weak pulse wave can be detected by the overlying muscles. The fingertips are located at the medial end of the eyebrow.

Implementation Note

Palpation must be gentle from the surface to the depth; otherwise, the supratrochlear artery may be squeezed (Fig. 7.24).

7.1.4.9 Palpation of the Supraorbital Artery

The superior ophthalmic artery arises from the ophthalmic artery at about the beginning of the medial third of the superior orbit. As a split-off, it first emerges slightly anteriosuperiorly from the orbit and then runs together with the supraorbital nerve and the supraorbital vein through the supraorbital foramen superiorly to the forehead. It is covered by the orbicularis oculi muscle and the depressor and corrugator supercilii muscles. In the region of the frontalis muscle, it divides into a superficial and a profundal part and supplies the structures in the region of the forehead. It also anastomoses with the supratrochlear and superficial temporal arteries. In its region of origin, it ensures the blood supply to the rectus superior muscle and the levator palpebrae muscle within the orbit.

Palpation takes place over the supraorbital foramen (see Sect. 2.12.1.1), which can be easily found as a bony reference point at the beginning of the middle third of the eyebrow. The client is in a supine or seated position while the therapist applies the index fingertip to the foramen. With gentle pressure, the pulse wave can be detected.

Implementation Note

Palpation must be gentle from the surface to the depth; otherwise, the supraorbital artery may be compressed (Fig. 7.25).

7.1.4.10 Palpation of the Posterior Auricular Artery

Directly below the earlobe, the posterior auricular artery splits off from the external carotid artery, first runs under the ear towards the occipital and then rises proportionally superiorly behind the ear or continues towards the occiput. Due to its location, it supplies numerous structures in the area of the ear, including the eardrum, as well as the scalp in the region behind the ear with oxygenated blood.

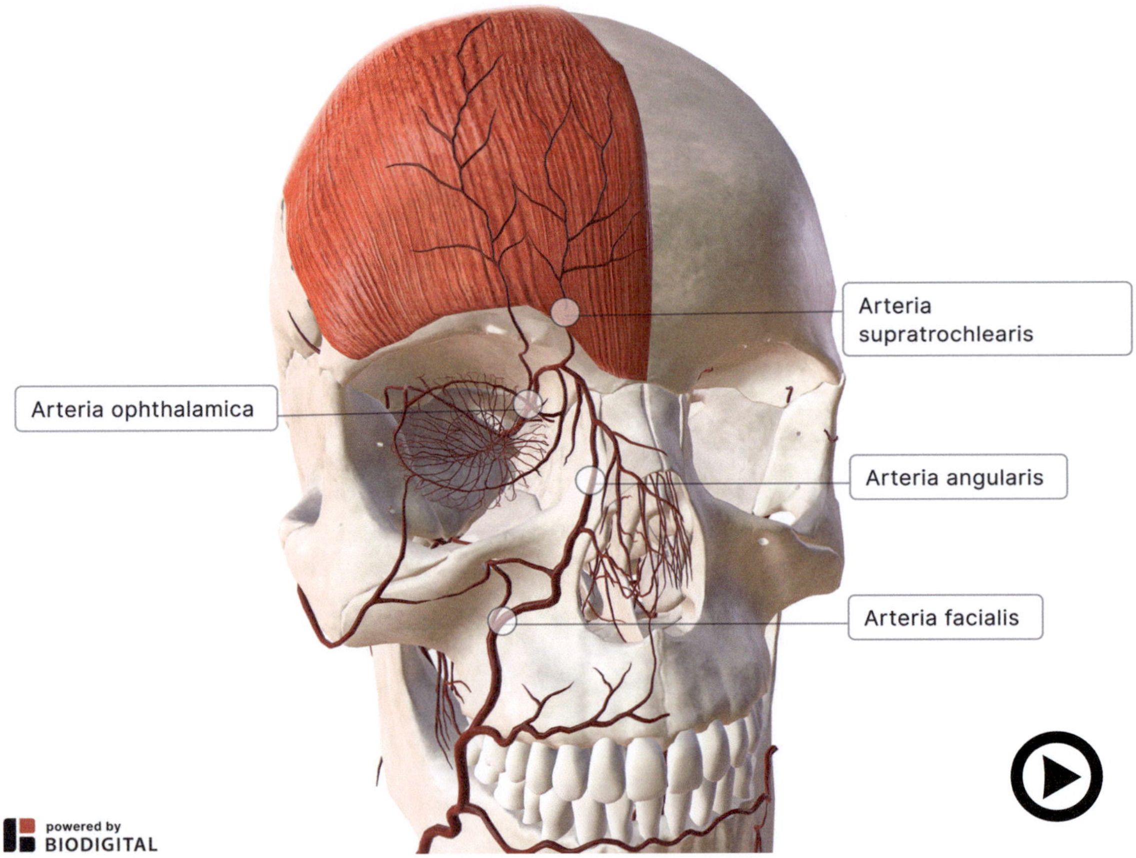

Fig. 7.24 Anatomy and palpation of the A. supratrochlearis (▶ https://doi.org/10.1007/000-cxt)

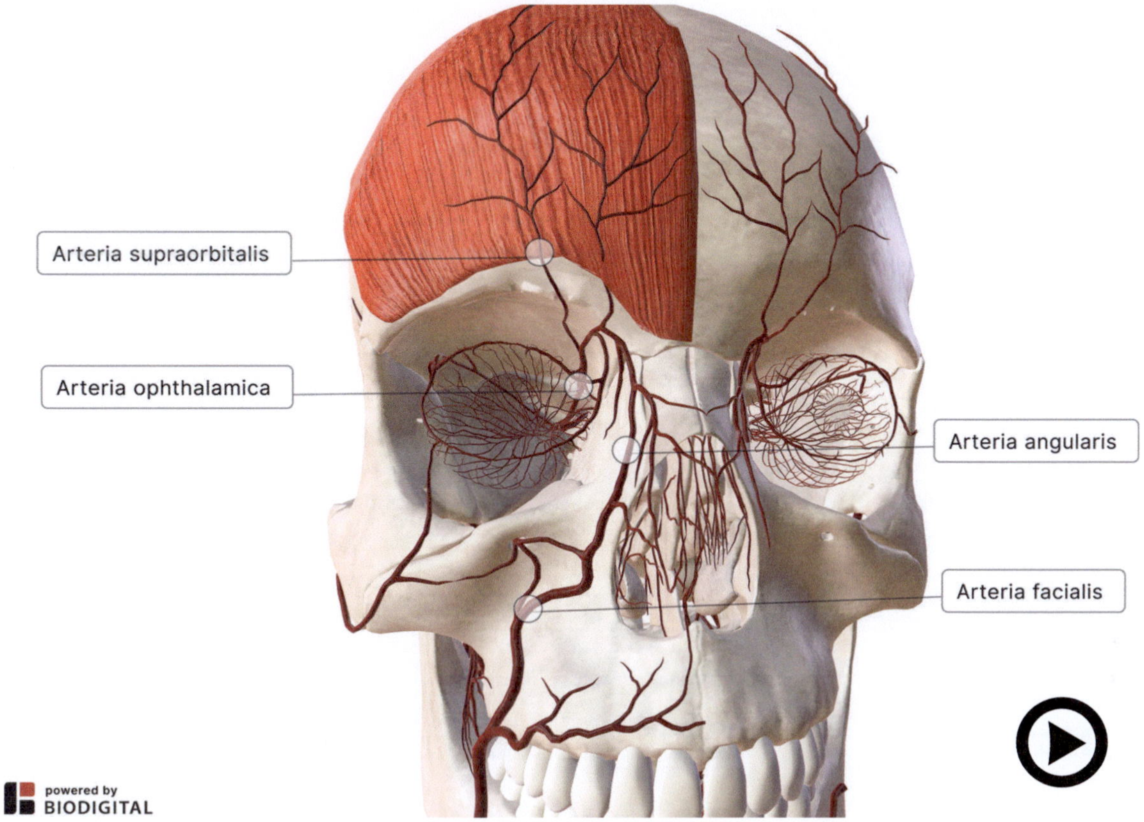

Fig. 7.25 Anatomy and palpation of the A. supraorbitalis (▶ https://doi.org/10.1007/000-cxv)

The posterior auricular artery is very easy to palpate because there are hardly any other structures above it in this region. The client is in a supine or sitting position, and the therapist places the index and middle fingertips flat on the skin below the auricle. The pulse wave can be felt, and the artery can be palpated in its further course without pressure in the depth.

Implementation Note
Palpation must be gentle from the surface to the depth; otherwise, the posterior auricular artery may be squeezed (Fig. 7.26).

7.1.4.11 Palpation of the Occipital Artery

The occipital artery arises laterally on the neck at the level of the mandibular angulus from the external carotid artery. It then ascends to the mastoid muscle, which it runs behind, and then moves occipitally in the occipital artery sulcus at the lower edge of the temporal bone and the occipital bone. On its way, it is directly accompanied by the hypoglossal nerve and the greater occipital nerve. In the area of the trapezius pars descendens, the occipital artery rises and radiates over the entire back of the head. Numerous secondary branches of the artery provide blood supply to the structures in the posterior cervical region as well as the occipital region. In addition, it transports blood to the region of the auricle and to the dura mater and anastomoses with the posterior auricular and superficial temporal arteries. In its course, the occipital artery is covered by the sternocleidomastoid muscle, the splenius capitis muscle and the longissimus capitis muscle.

For palpation of the artery, it is important that the client's head is in a passive position to relax the muscles in this region. Therefore, the supine position is most suitable. The therapist first grasps the proc. mastoideus and palpates its depth directly occipital with steeply placed fingertips. The pulse wave of the occipital artery can be clearly palpated. The fingertips then move further occipitally along the bony lower edge of the occiput and can feel the vessel in some places. In the area of the occiput, it is advisable to first lay the fingers flat to be able to detect the pulse wave. Afterwards, precise palpation is carried out via the fingertip.

Implementation
Due to the direct proximity to the occipital nerves and other nerves in the region of the artery, it is recommended that the pressure on the artery is not too intense in order to avoid excessive compression of both blood flow and nervous structures (Fig. 7.27).

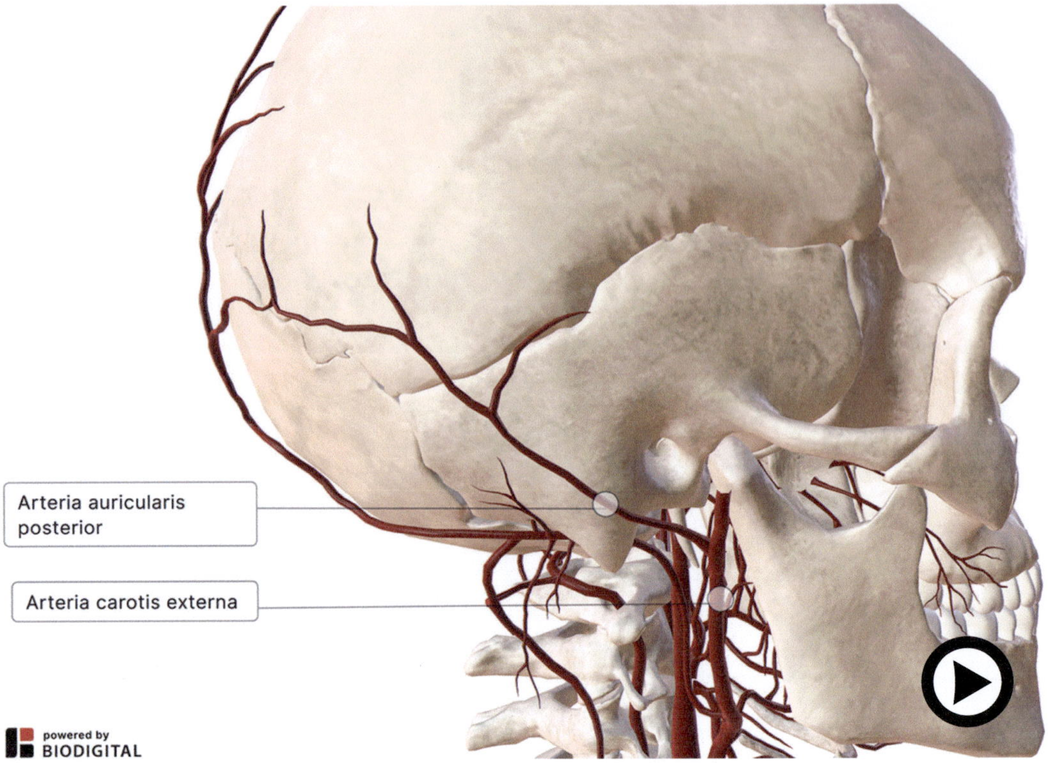

Fig. 7.26 Anatomy and palpation of the A. auricularis posterior (▶ https://doi.org/10.1007/000-cxw)

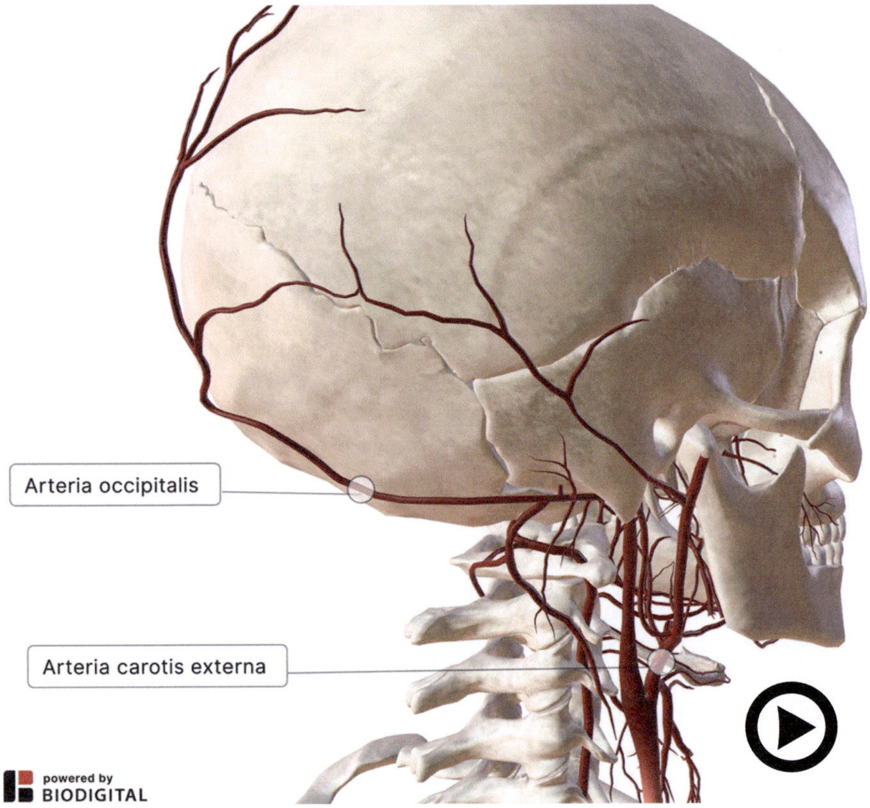

Fig. 7.27 Anatomy and palpation of the A. occipitalis (▶ https://doi.org/10.1007/000-cxx)

7.2 Palpation of the Veins

Like the arteries, the veins are made up of three layers of walls. The difference is that they have a larger lumen and only a thin muscular layer. In addition, they have venous valves, which arise from the tunica intima and serve as a return flow mechanism. They carry oxygen-poor blood in the systemic circulation and oxygen-rich blood in the pulmonary circulation towards the heart. Veins therefore serve to dispose of carbon dioxide, which is a by-product of metabolism, and to supply oxygen, which is transported by respiration from the capillary region of the lungs to the heart. Thus, the venous valves exist only in the systemic circulation. Other return mechanisms that support the venous vessels are the muscle pump [11], the suction effect of the heart and lungs and the local proximity to the arteries and its pulse wave, also known as arteriovenous coupling in the area of the haemodynamic functional unit. If veins are altered in their normal anatomical structure or if the client suffers from diseases that cause congestion in the veins, they may appear as prominent structures up to a manifestation as varicose veins. Already in the visual findings, veins can appear in well-trained patients whose body fat content is very low, and the muscle percentage is very high at the same time.

Due to their proximity to arteries, some veins are palpable or can be provided with a palpatory stimulus. In the following chapters, the palpable veins are first described in their anatomical position, and then instructions are given for precise palpation. In addition to knowledge of the position, a relaxed starting position of the client is of great importance. In contrast to arteries, veins do not have a pulse wave and can therefore be felt as a round, soft and elastic structure that can be easily distinguished from the surrounding tissue. Superficial veins are often somewhat bluish and can therefore already be visually perceived. Palpation is performed with the index or middle fingertip placed on the surface. If the vessel is compressed in advance, there is often a congestion of blood, which makes the vein enlarged and thus facilitates palpation. In addition, there may be a livid colouration of the skin distal to the pressure point. Furthermore, the difficulty of feeling the venous structures can be made easier by closing the eyes and thus removing the visual stimulus. The following chapters describe palpation of the veins in the pelvis, lower extremity, abdomen, upper extremity and head.

7.2.1 Veins in the Area of the Pelvis and Lower Extremity

The lower extremity, which carries people through life every day, is equipped with numerous muscles that require a lot of energy. Metabolism produces numerous metabolic waste products that have to be excreted from the body in various ways. Carbon dioxide, for example, is transported through the veins from the periphery towards the heart and then into the lungs to be replaced with oxygen in the gas exchange. Some of these veins can be palpated or stimulated in the lower extremity. For better orientation, the arteries of the same name often help, as they are usually located in local proximity to the veins.

The venous vessels that can be reached via the fingers are part of the following chapters. The anatomical position of the superior gluteal vein, the femoral vein, the popliteal vein, the anterior tibial vein, the great and parietal saphenous veins and the dorsal venous pedicle are described.

In the presentation, it should be noted that the veins run from the periphery in the proximal or centripetal direction and thus allow the blood to flow in the opposite direction to the arteries. Therefore, the sequence will extend from the smaller to the larger vessels.

The client is in a relaxed starting position in order to avoid tissue tension as far as possible and thus strengthen the feeling of palpation. The supine, prone or side position is recommended.

7.2.1.1 Palpation of the Superior Gluteal Vein

From the gluteal facies at the iliac artery, the strongly branched superior gluteal vein runs together with the superior gluteal artery and the superior gluteal nerve in a caudomedial direction under the SIPI. It is covered by the gluteus maximus muscle. Above the piriformis muscle, it passes through the suprapiriform foramen and the foramen ischiadicum majus and continues into the pelvis, where it opens into the internal iliac vein on the homolateral side.

As it follows a similar course to its namesake artery, the therapist will use the pulse wave of the superior gluteal artery as well as the SIPI as a guide for palpation with the client in the prone position. The fingertips are placed on the SIPI in a steep position. They move slightly caudally and meet the nerve and vascular cord directly in the first depression above the piriformis muscle. Palpation of the vein is by stimulation only.

Implementation Note

If the volume of the gluteal muscles is large, the pulse wave of the superior gluteal artery cannot be used as a guide (Fig. 7.28).

7.2.1.2 Palpation of the Femoral Vein

The popliteal vein joins the femoral vein medioposteriorly in the area of the distal third of the femur. The transition occurs near the hiatus adductorius, the opening between the tendons of the adductor magnus muscle. It then runs in the adductor

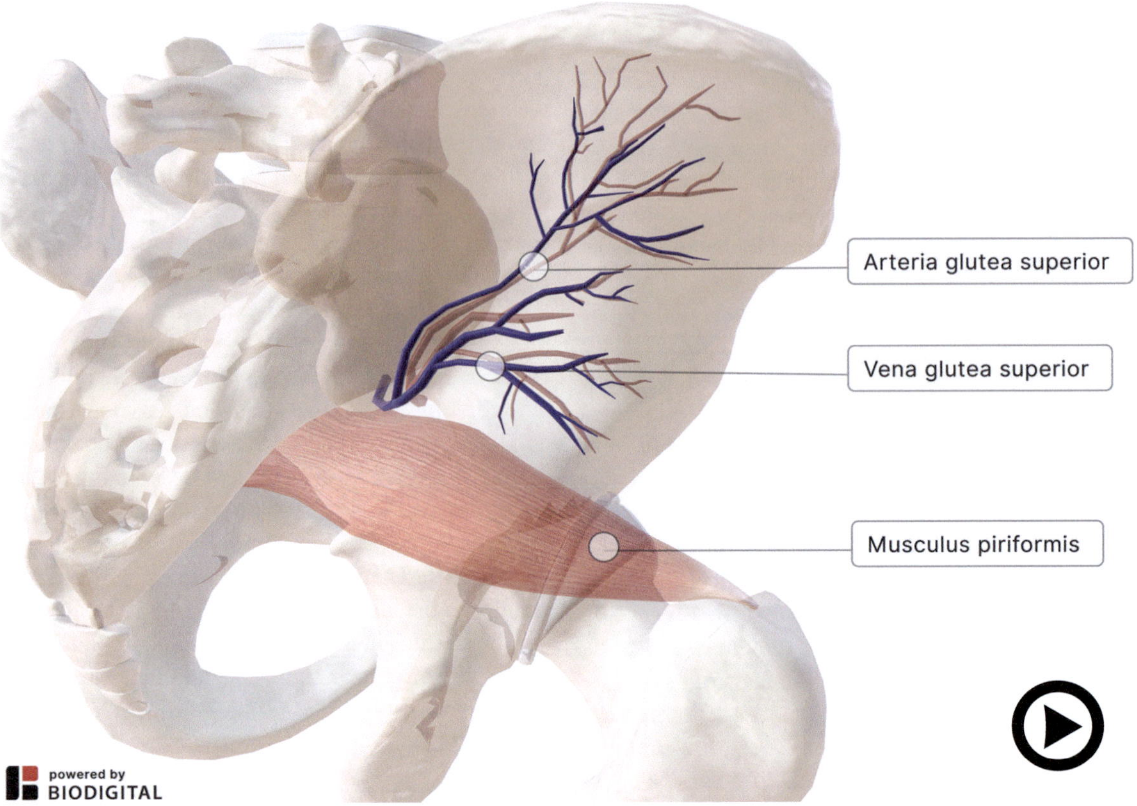

Fig. 7.28 Anatomy and palpation of the V. glutea superior (▶ https://doi.org/10.1007/000-cxy)

canal, receives tributaries from other veins and rises steeply proximally in the medial region of the thigh. In this course, it is in close connection with the femoral artery and the saphenous nerve. Below the inguinal ligament, the venous vessel opens in the lacuna vasorum into the external iliac vein on the homolateral side.

The groin is a suitable approach for palpation. For this purpose, the patient is positioned in the supine position. The therapist first searches for the pulsating femoral artery (see Sect. 7.1.1.2) with the fingertips placed flat. If the middle finger is on the artery, the finger that follows medially lies directly on the femoral artery. The vessel can be palpated with the steeply placed fingertips of the index and middle fingers. In the adductor canal (see Sect. 7.1.1.8), a further stimulus can be applied to the femoral vein.

Implementation Note
Access to the vein is only possible via the groin region, which is covered by thigh muscles such as the sartorius muscle and distally by the vastus medialis muscle (Fig. 7.29).

7.2.1.3 Palpation of the Popliteal Vein

The popliteal vein originates posteriorly at the level of the knee joint space from the anterior and posterior tibial veins and the saphenous vein and runs upwards in a proximal direction. At its origin, it is accompanied by the plantar muscle (see Sect. 5.4.10). Above the femoral condyles, it runs proximomedially and flows into the femoral vein in the hiatus adductorius. In its course, it takes up numerous veins from the region of the knee joint and is accompanied by the popliteal artery and directly in the popliteal fossa by the tibial nerve.

The client is in a prone position with the ankle joints underneath and is oriented towards the femoral artery in the area of the back of the knee during palpation. As soon as the fingertips of the index and middle fingers are flat on the pulsating vessel, a stimulus is also applied to the popliteal vein, which is located slightly in front of the artery. The soft-elastic, round and non-pulsating venous vessel can then be located via the steeply positioned fingertips.

Implementation Note
Palpation of the popliteal vein should be gentle at first because of its proximity to the tibial nerve (Fig. 7.30).

7.2.1.4 Palpation of the Anterior Tibial Vein

The deep anterior tibial vein arises posteriorly in the medial region of the talus or the os naviculare from the dorsalis pedis vein and then runs steeply upwards to the proximolateral. It is accompanied by the anterior tibial artery and the fibular nerve

Fig. 7.29 Anatomy and palpation of the V. femoralis (▶ https://doi.org/10.1007/000-cxz)

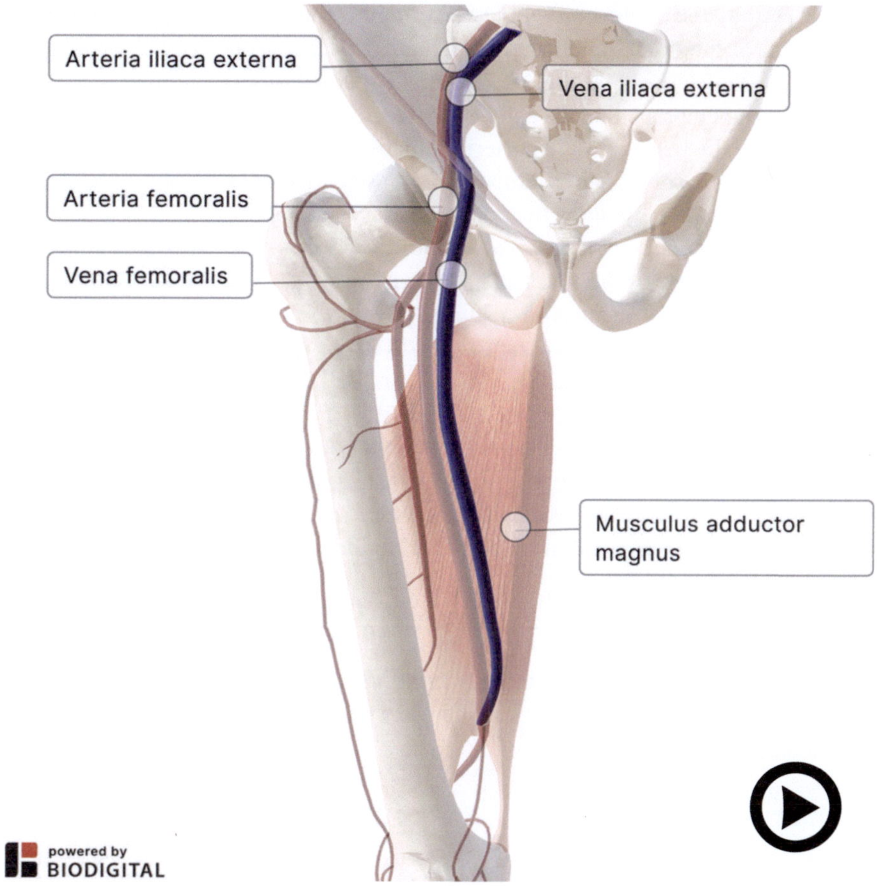

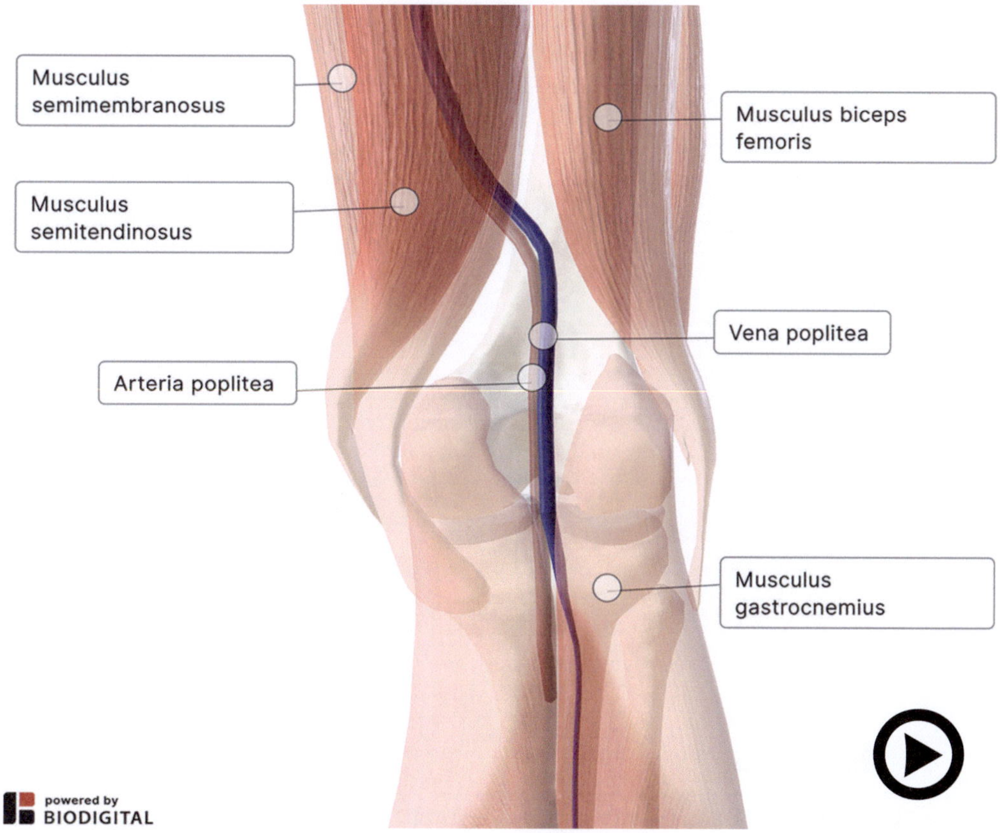

Fig. 7.30 Anatomy and palpation of the V. poplitea (▶ https://doi.org/10.1007/000-cy0)

and covered by the anterior tibial muscle from the end of the distal third of the tibia. Together with the artery of the same name, it runs posteriorly through the proximal opening of the interosseous membrane directly inferior to the proximal tibial artery. It partially perforates the posterior tibialis muscle, then ascends under the soleus and gastrocnemius muscles and over the popliteus muscle and joins the popliteal artery in the popliteal fossa. In its course, it receives venous blood from the lower leg via numerous branches and passes it on.

For palpation, the client is in a supine position with the knee joints underneath. The therapist stands at the level of the feet and first feels the tendon of the extensor hallucis longus and the tibialis anterior muscle (see Sects. 5.4.2 and 5.4.1). The anterior tibial vein is located directly between the two tendons and anterior to the distal tibia. The round, venous and easily movable vessel is then grasped in a relaxed state with the fingertips of the index and middle fingers placed flat on the surface.

Implementation Note

The anterior tibial vein is often confused with the great saphenous vein, which, however, runs directly over the anterior tibial tendon (Fig. 7.31).

7.2.1.5 Palpation of the Great Saphenous Vein

Numerous superficial veins in the lower leg exist under the umbrella term saphenous vein. They are represented both anteriorly and posteriorly and are named according to their, partly individual, localisation. As soon as these veins are pathologically changed in their structure, they can be discovered as so-called varices or better known as varicose veins on the legs already in the visual findings. The largest superficial vein in this group is the great saphenous vein, which arises dorsomedially in the area of the base of the metatarsal bone I from the arcus venosus dorsalis pedis. It then runs directly laterally next to the tendon of the tibialis anterior muscle in the direction of the ankle joint and then rises with it proximally. In the medial third of the tibia, the venous vessel takes a change of direction to the medial region at the knee joint, where it then subsequently passes over the thigh in the anteromedial region to the groin and opens into the femoral vein. Throughout its course, it takes in numerous branches such as those of the saphenous vein medialis and lateralis, the arcuate vein anterior and posterior and the epigastric vein superficialis and forms anastomoses to the deep leg veins via perforating veins. It is conspicuous because of its high number of venous valves [12].

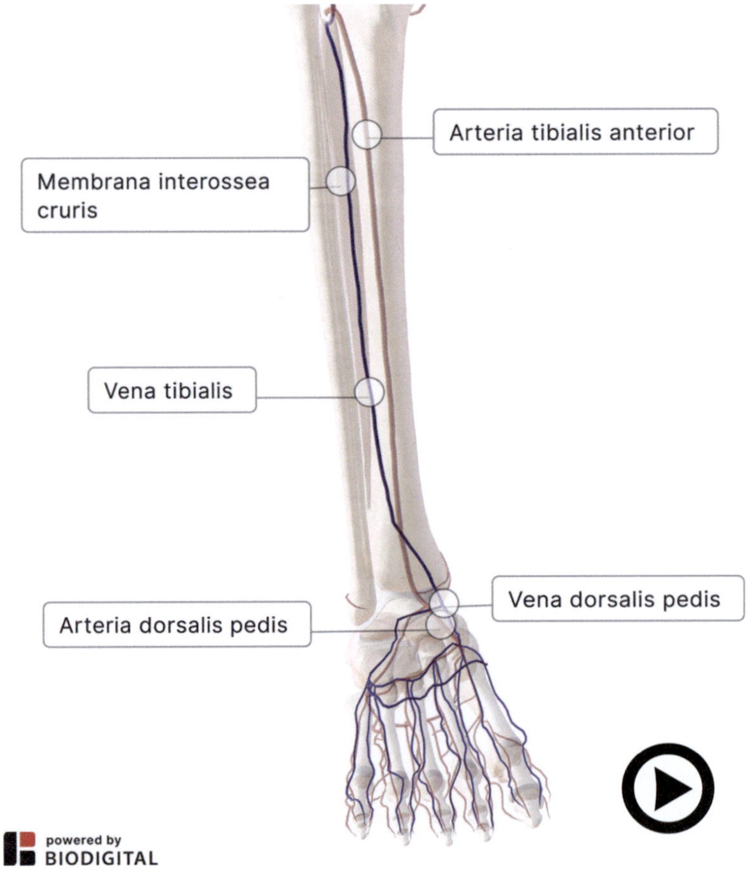

Fig. 7.31 Anatomy and palpation of the V. tibialis anterior (▶ https://doi.org/10.1007/000-cy1)

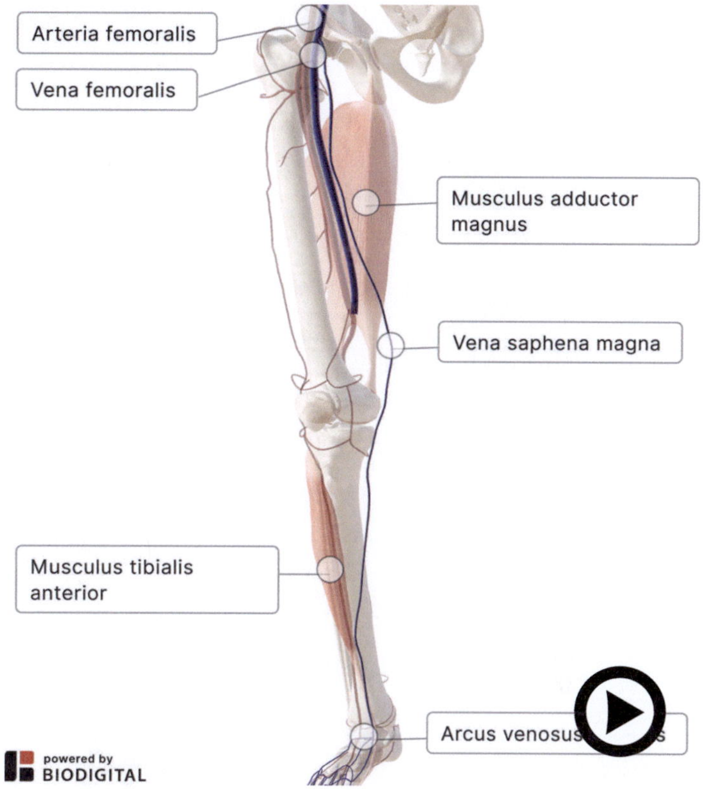

Fig. 7.32 Anatomy and palpation of the V. saphena magna (▶ https://doi.org/10.1007/000-cy2)

Due to the size of the great saphenous vein, it can be easily palpated in the supine position. Depending on the anatomical condition of the client, the venous vessel can already be visually detected in the area of the medial dorsum of the foot or the distal third of the lower leg. First, the medial malleolus is located. The finger berries, laid flat, then move slightly laterally and then meet the roundish, elastic and easily displaced often bluish great saphenous vein. This can then be followed proximally. Small branches can often be felt or seen in the medial area above the malleolus, which are in contact with the posterior tibial vein as perforating veins.

Implementation Note
Other branches of the great saphenous vein should only be palpated if the anatomical conditions allow this (Fig. 7.32).

7.2.1.6 Palpation of the Saphenous Vein

The superficial V. saphena parva rete venosum dorsale pedis arises as a tapering branch of the V. poplitea in the area of the base of the metatarsal V. It then runs in the direction of the ankle joint, where it can appear visually for the first time behind the lateral malleolus. It then rises steeply proximally above the Achilles tendon and between the two heads of the gastrocnemius and joins the popliteal vein in the region of the popliteal fossa under the plantar muscle. In its course, it takes in further venous branches and forms anastomoses to the deep leg veins by means of perforating veins.

The palpation is done from the sitting or supine position. The sitting position is therefore well suited because more blood is in the distal area of the lower leg due to gravity and thus the vein is more “bulging” with blood. The palpatory approach is perceived behind the lateral malleolus. Directly in this posterior setting, the fingertips are placed flat and the V. saphena parva is detected as a round, blue, elastic and easily movable structure.

Implementation Note
Depending on the anatomical condition, the vein can be felt further along its course proximally (Fig. 7.33).

7.2.1.7 Palpation of the Rete Venosum Dorsale Pedis

The dorsal veins are grouped together as a complex and form a venous network that originates from the tributaries of the dorsal metatarsal veins. They then form a venous network on the dorsum of the foot and ultimately flow medially into the great saphenous vein and laterally on the foot into the saphenous vein. Often, the numerous branches can already be seen as roundish and bluish vascular cords. If they are well filled and the anatomical conditions permit, the rete venosum dorsale pedis even lifts up under the skin and thus becomes even more accessible to palpation.

The patient is positioned supine or seated for palpation while the therapist stands sideways at the level of the feet.

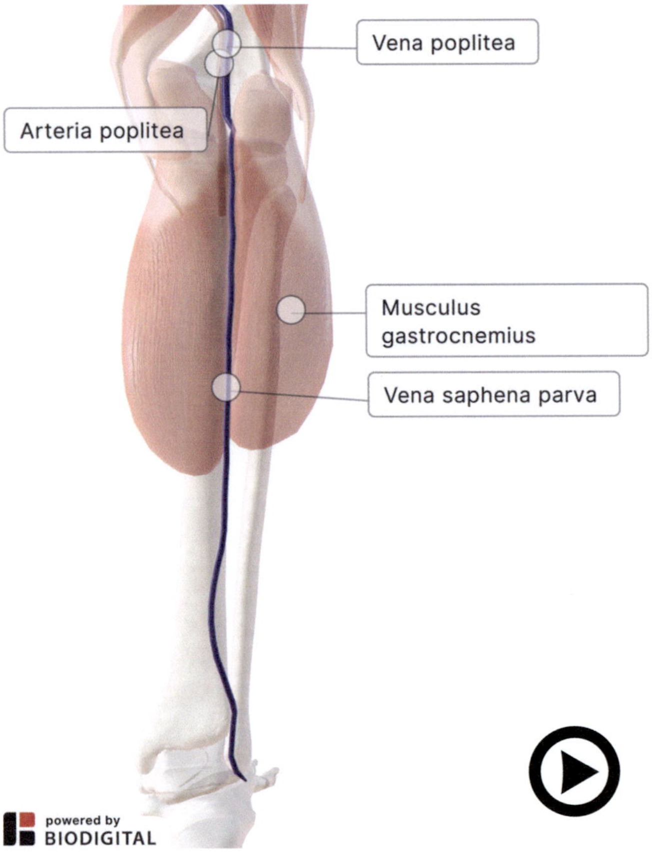

Fig. 7.33 Anatomy and palpation of the V. saphena parva (▶ https://doi.org/10.1007/000-cy3)

The fingertips are placed flat on the dorsum of the foot and begin to palpate transversely from medial to lateral. During this movement across the dorsum of the foot, structures repeatedly appear under the fingers that are roundish, soft elastic on palpation and easily movable in relation to the surrounding tissue. These isolated strands are those of the rete venosum dorsale pedis.

Implementation Note
If the lower leg is pressed down a little in advance in a circular fashion, the blood is dammed up in the veins, which often makes them even more visible (Fig. 7.34).

7.2.2 Veins in the Trunk and Abdomen Area

Numerous veins exist in the abdominal region, which carry the deoxygenated blood from the organs to the heart. The blood is collected in the inferior vena cava, where it meets the venous blood from the extremities via the superior vena cava and is then transported via the dexter atrium through the valva tricuspidalis into the dexter ventriculus. From there, it is pumped through the valva trunci pulmonalis into the truncus pulmonalis and finally reaches the pulmonary circulation. There, it is re-oxygenated and then passes via the atrium sinister through the valva bicuspidalis into the ventriculus sinister and via the valva aortae into the aorta and thus into the systemic circulation. This mechanism is an elementary

Fig. 7.34 Anatomy and palpation of the Rete venosum dorsale pedis (▶ https://doi.org/10.1007/000-cy4)

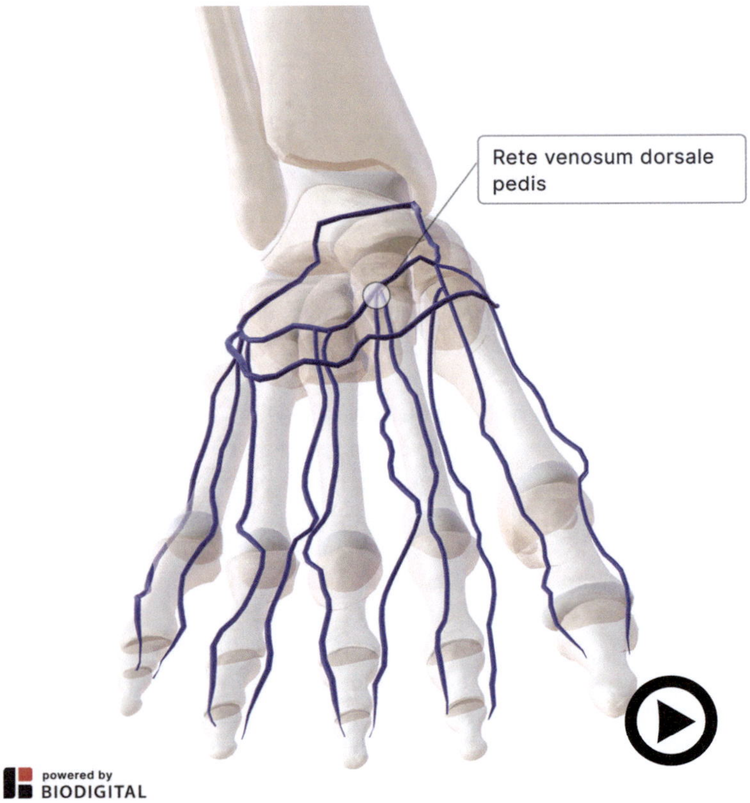

basis for understanding the position of the vena cavae in the human body. The inferior vena cava is also the only vein that can be reached by palpatory stimulation. It is therefore briefly described in the following chapter in its anatomical position before the palpation instructions follow.

7.2.2.1 Palpation of the Inferior Vena Cava

In the previous chapter, the function of the vena cava was already described in the overall complex, which is why this chapter will go into more detail about its anatomical location and the stimulation via the finger berries. The vena cava is divided into an inferior and a superior part, both of which flow into the atrium dexter. The inferior vena cava arises approximately at the level of the 4th–5th lumbar vertebrae from the junction of the right and left iliac veins. It then rises steeply in front of the vertebral bodies and runs to the right of the aorta. Before entering the chest cavity, it perforates the respiratory diaphragm. Arriving on the right side of the heart, it opens within the pericardium into the sinus venarum cavarum of the dexter atrium. On its way, it receives the deoxygenated blood from the abdominal cavity as well as the lower extremity.

The superior vena cava arises dorsally of the manubrium from the tributaries of the right and left brachiocephalic veins. It thus transports the deoxygenated blood from the upper extremity and the head or neck region in a caudal direction via the sinus venarum cavarum into the atrium dexter.

Only the inferior vena cava is suitable for palpation, which is performed in the supine position. For this, the knee joints are placed underneath so that the abdominal wall can be palpated in a relaxed position. The therapist, standing on the left side, first feels the aorta by applying deep pressure in the abdomen with the steeply positioned fingertips. If the fingertips move from the left to the right side of the body, they leave the aorta and immediately meet the inferior vena cava and can stimulate it.

Implementation Note

Palpation should be gentle as it is done through the abdominal wall and organs and may be felt as uncomfortable in depth (Fig. 7.35).

7.2.3 Veins in the Area of the Upper Extremity

The upper limb is disposed of by veins that carry deoxygenated blood from the periphery to the heart so that it can then

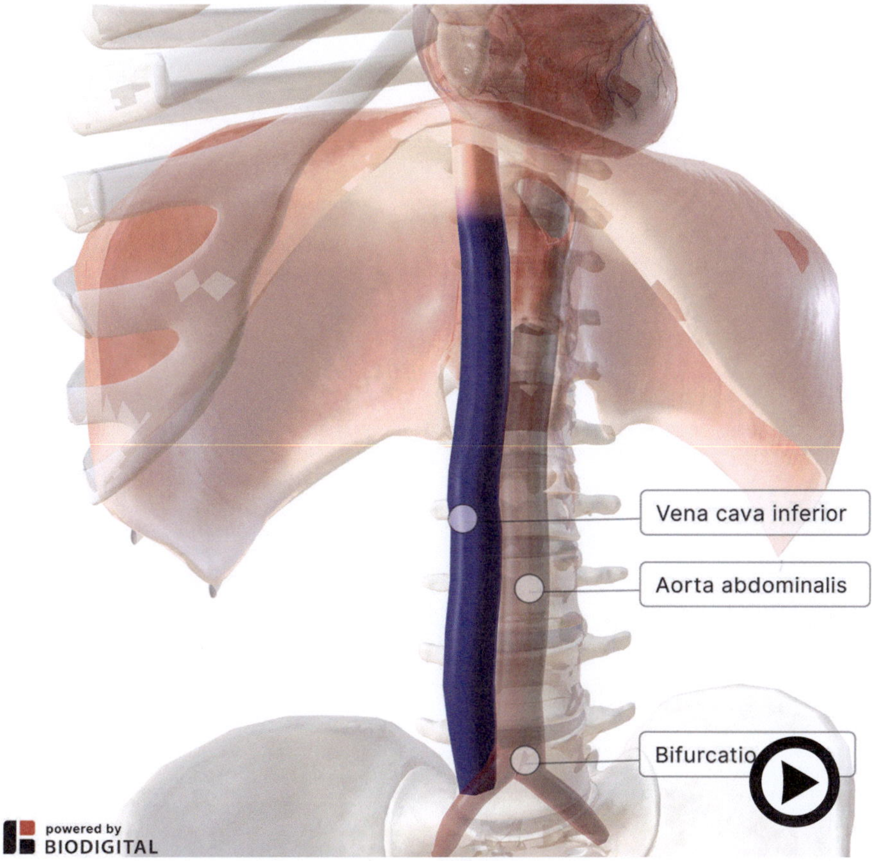

Fig. 7.35 Anatomy and palpation of the V. cava inferior (▶ https://doi.org/10.1007/000-cy5)

be re-oxygenated via the pulmonary circulation and run back to the periphery in the arteries. There are numerous veins that transport blood from the fingers to the homolateral subclavian vein. In the following chapters, the veins that can be reached by palpation are listed thematically. These include the subclavian vein, the axillary vein, the basilic and cephalic veins and the median cubital vein, the superficial veins of the forearm and the dorsal venous rete of the manus. In the presentation, it should be noted that the veins run from the periphery in a proximal or centripetal direction and thus allow blood to flow in the opposite direction to the arteries. Therefore, the sequence will extend from the smaller to the larger vessels.

The client is in a relaxed starting position so that tissue tension is largely avoided to facilitate the palpation sensation. The supine position is recommended.

7.2.3.1 Palpation of the Subclavian Vein

The subclavian vein originates from the axillary vein about two transverse fingers medial to the coracoid muscle and runs dorsal to the clavicle together with the subclavian artery towards the neck. Both vessels are separated by the scalenus anterior muscle, so that the vein anterior to it continues to flow in the direction of the middle of the body in the anterior scalenus gap. In its course, the venous vessel has a direct attachment to the periosteum of the clavicle via the fascia clavipectoralis. In its centripedal course, the subclavian vein joins the internal jugular vein to form the brachiocephalic vein, which then gives rise to the right and left venous angles. The right angulus venosus receives an inflow via the ductus lymphaticus dexter, whereas the left venous angle is fed with lymphatic fluid from the ductus thoracicus. Through numerous inflows, the subclavian vein drains deoxygenated blood from the arm, as well as the homolateral neck and head region, and at the same time forms a potential access for a central venous catheter [13].

The vein is palpated by stimulating the lateral cervical region with the client in the supine position. The therapist, standing on the homolateral side, applies his fingertips, which are initially placed flat, so that the clavicle is located caudally, the sternocleidomastoid muscle medially and the trapezius pars descendens laterally. In this lateral part of the neck, the fingertips are gradually placed more steeply in order to palpate in depth. They meet the pulsating subclavian artery, which is located dorsal to the subclavian vein. Thus, they are applied ventrally to the artery to provide a direct stimulus to the accompanying venous vessel.

Implementation Note

The palpation should be done carefully at the beginning, as there are also nervous structures of the brachial plexus in this region (Fig. 7.36).

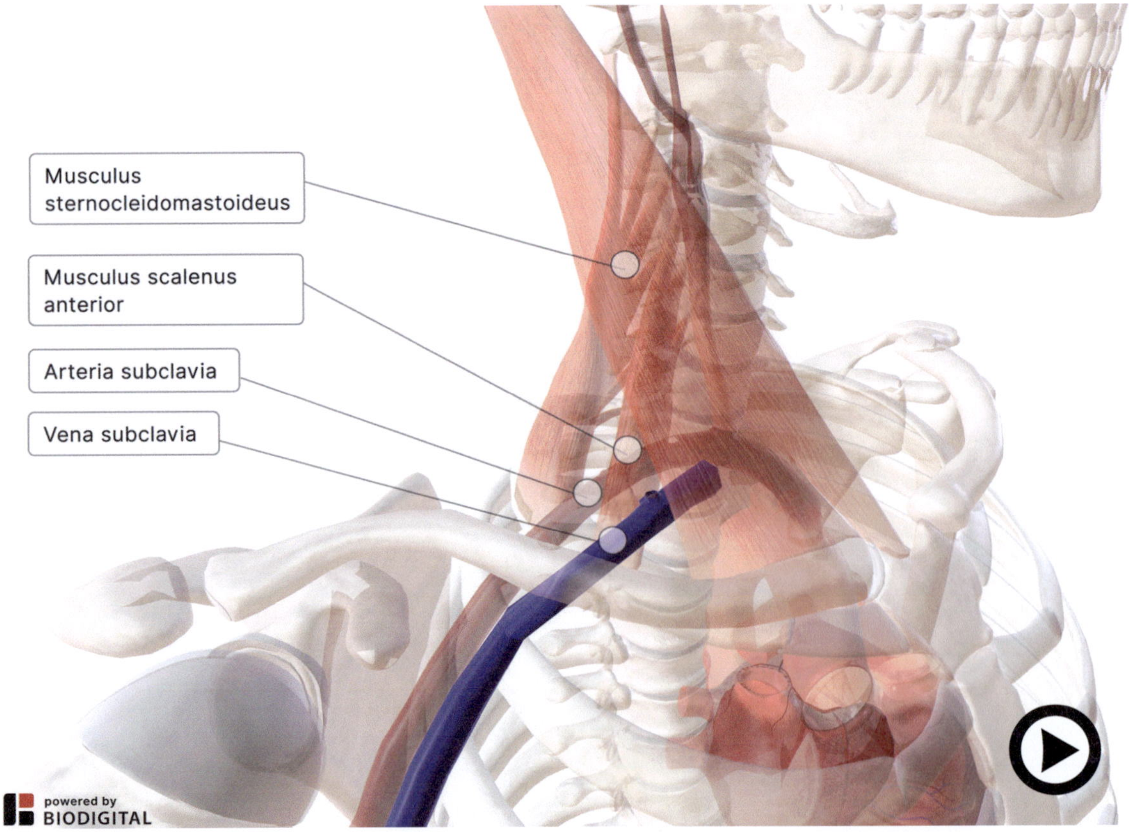

Fig. 7.36 Anatomy and palpation of the V. subclavia (▶ https://doi.org/10.1007/000-cy6)

7.2.3.2 Palpation of the Axillary Vein

The axillary vein, as its name suggests, is located in the axilla and connects the brachial vein and the basilic vein with the subclavian vein. It arises in the proximal third of the humerus from the junction of the first two veins and runs along the medial edge of the upper arm in a proximomedial direction until it joins the subclavian vein. In its course, it receives numerous branches from the shoulder region and thus drains deoxygenated blood from the arm and shoulder region as well as the lateral thoracic wall towards the heart.

For palpation, the patient is positioned supine, and the arm is passively positioned in slight abduction in the shoulder joint. The therapist applies the index and middle fingertips at the intersection between the lower edge of the pectoralis major muscle and the caput breve of the biceps brachii muscle in the medial region of the upper arm. These cross in the axillary region and lead directly to the axillary vein. The venous vessel lies directly in front of its accompanying artery, so that the pulse wave of the axillary artery can also be used for better orientation during palpation. The fingertips are positioned steeply in the area described and begin to generate pressure proximolaterally in the direction of the axilla. In doing so, they meet the round, elastic and flexible axillary vein directly.

Implementation Note

The palpation should be started gently at first, as the ulnar nerve is located directly near the vein, which can cause discomfort in the arm during palpation (Fig. 7.37).

7.2.3.3 Palpation of the Basilic Vein

The basilar vein originates ulnarly from the rete venosum dorsale manus and runs anteroulnar proximally to the cubital fossa. From the crook of the elbow, it extends medially along the arm together with the brachial artery and the ulnar and median nerves proximally along the upper arm. It perforates the basilic hiatus in the middle third of the humerus until it passes medially of the coracobrachialis muscle or the caput breve of the biceps brachii muscle and anteriorly of the teres major muscle and the latissimus dorsi muscle, together with the brachial vein, into the axillary vein.

For palpation, the client is positioned supine or seated with the arm in a passive position. The therapist stands laterally at the level of the bend of the elbow and first feels the pulse of the brachial artery with the fingertips, which is located slightly ulnar to the centre. Starting from this pulsating vessel, the fingertips move proximoulnar along the medial edge of the biceps brachii muscle and meet the roundish basilic vein, which is easily movable in relation to the surrounding tissue. Often this can already be found in the visual findings as it lies superficial in the crook of the elbow and receives the converging branch of the transverse median cubital artery. If the upper arm is compressed proximally, congestion occurs in the vein, which can make palpation more precise. This procedure is also performed for intravenous access in medicine, where the basilic vein can also be used. Depending on the anatomical condition, the vein can then be grasped in its further course proximally and distally. However, as it is overlaid by other structures, palpation in other regions is challenging.

Implementation Note

The further course of the basilic vein can only be recorded by palpation if the anatomical conditions allow this (Fig. 7.38).

7.2.3.4 Palpation of the Cephalic Vein

The large-lumen cephalic vein, which is often used for venous access in the crook of the elbow due to its anatomical features, arises radiodorsally from the rete venosum dorsale manus in the region of the thumb [14]. Its proximal course, along the radius, takes a small turn at the proximal end of the distal third of the forearm in the direction of the palmar or anterior and then pulls steeply along the medial edge of the brachioradialis muscle into the crook of the elbow. There, it often comes to the fore centrally until it then dips over the lateral edge of the caput longum of the biceps brachii muscle into the deltoideopectoral sulcus. From the anterior border of the deltoid pars clavicularis muscle, it passes medially towards the clavicle through the infraclavicular region and enters the axillary vein. In its course, the vein is accompanied by the radial nerve and the musculocutaneous nerve. The cephalic vein drains deoxygenated blood from the entire arm in the direction of the axilla due to numerous feeder branches and anastomoses in the elbow region.

The vein is palpated from the supine or sitting position. The therapist first orientates himself visually directly in the centre of the bend of the elbow. Here, the roundish and bluish cephalic vein is often already clearly visible. For clarification, the arm can be moved to maximum extension or the backflow of blood in the upper arm can be reduced by circular compression, which leads to a clearly visible congestion of blood in the vein. The venous vessel can then be grasped with the fingertips and examined. The elastic vein is easily movable and can be palpated in its further course depending on the anatomical condition.

Implementation Note

Depending on body fat content and training status, it can be recorded throughout the course (Fig. 7.39).

7.2.3.5 Palpation of the Median Cubital Vein

The median cubital vein is a transverse venous vessel found in the cubital fossa, and its proximomedial course connects the radial cephalic vein with the ulnar basilic vein. The vessel, which is rather short in relation to other venous structures, is located superficially and can usually already be

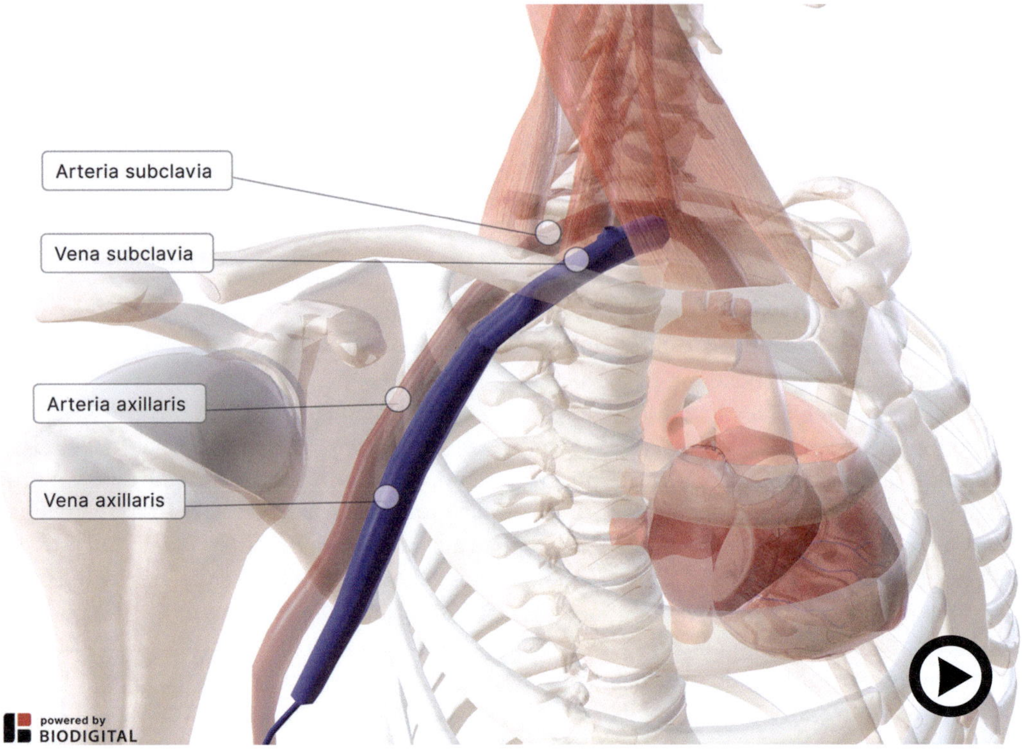

Fig. 7.37 Anatomy and palpation of the V. axillaris (▶ https://doi.org/10.1007/000-cy7)

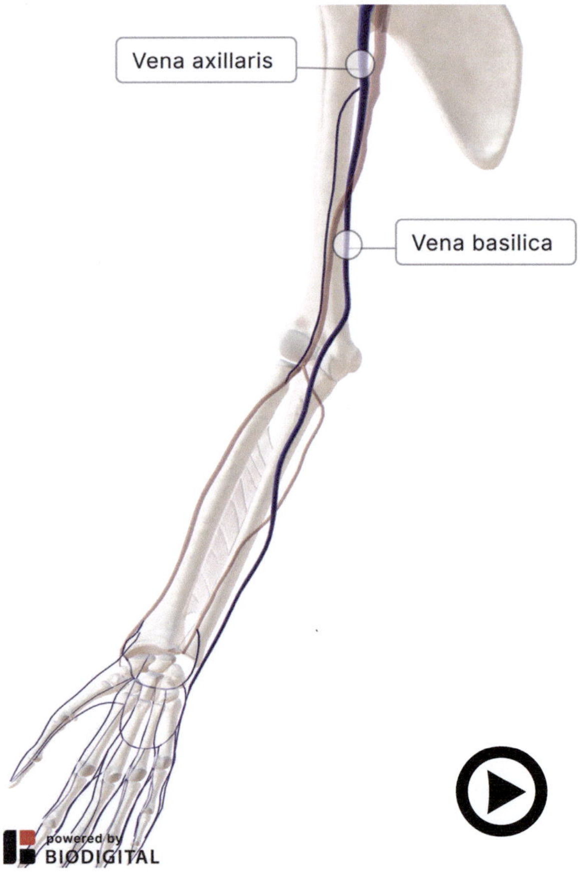

Fig. 7.38 Anatomy and palpation of the V. basilica (▶ https://doi.org/10.1007/000-cy8)

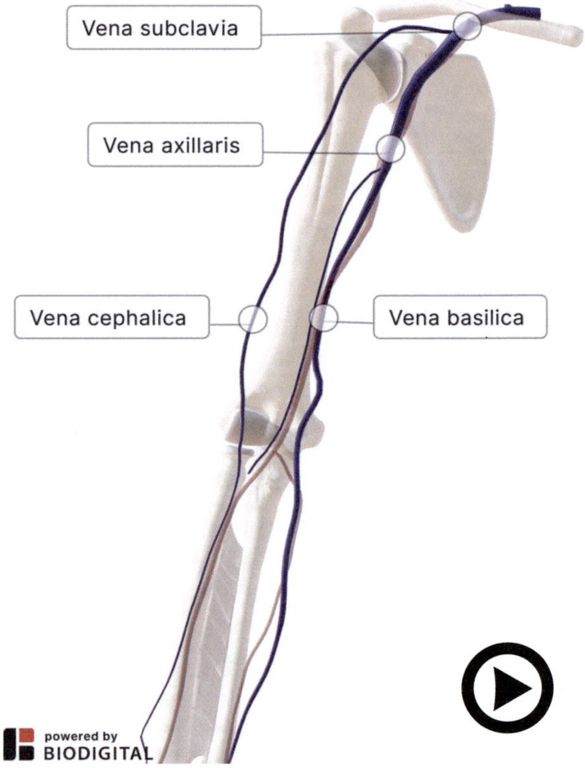

Fig. 7.39 Anatomy and palpation of the V. cephalica (▶ https://doi.org/10.1007/000-cy9)

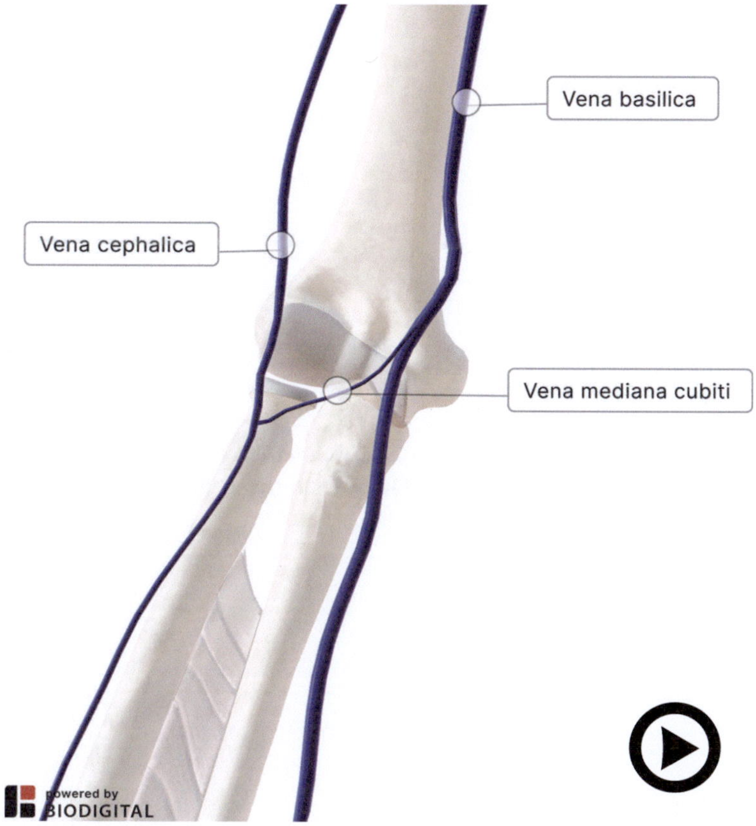

Fig. 7.40 Anatomy and palpation of the V. mediana cubiti (▶ https://doi.org/10.1007/000-cya)

identified as an oblique vein in the visual findings. Due to its location and size, it is suitable for venous access and blood sampling in the crook of the elbow.

For palpation, it is recommended to position the client in a supine or sitting position. The therapist stands sideways and orients himself to the transverse vessel in the bend of the elbow. For reinforcement, the arm can be stretched, or the blood flow can be reduced via a tourniquet on the upper arm so that the vein is better revealed. The bluish, roundish and slightly displaceable vessel is then grasped with the fingertips.

Implementation Note

For better orientation, the pronator teres muscle (see Sect. 5.9.3), which follows the same course, is used and the median cubital vein is located on its proximal edge (Fig. 7.40).

7.2.3.6 Superficial Veins on the Forearm

The entire forearm is covered by superficial veins that carry deoxygenated blood from the hand and forearm proximally into the main veins. There are numerous vessels on the palmar or anterior as well as dorsal surface of the forearm, which can occur variably. A precise course of these venous vessels, which are grouped together, is therefore not definable. Depending on the anatomical condition and the current situation, they can be palpated in qualitatively different ways. One way to make them more visible is to apply proximal circular compression to the upper arm, which stagnates the blood and thus leads to swelling of the veins. Athletic exertion or grasping of the hands can also serve to temporarily enlarge the vessels.

For palpation, the client is positioned in a supine or seated position. The palpator first orientates visually on the forearm and looks for bluish vessels extending over the forearm on the palmar and dorsal sides. Often, the palmar or anterior lateral veins are easier to find. Then the elastic vessels can be felt with gentle pressure over the fingertips and moved in relation to surrounding tissue.

Implementation Note

Preparatory measures that stimulate blood circulation in the forearm area improve the location of the superficial veins on the forearm (Fig. 7.41).

7.2.3.7 Palpation of the Rete Venosum Dorsale Manus

The venous network on the dorsum of the hand is an individually developed system which conveys venous blood from the dorsal metacarpal veins into the cephalic vein on the radial side and into the basilic vein on the ulnar side. The

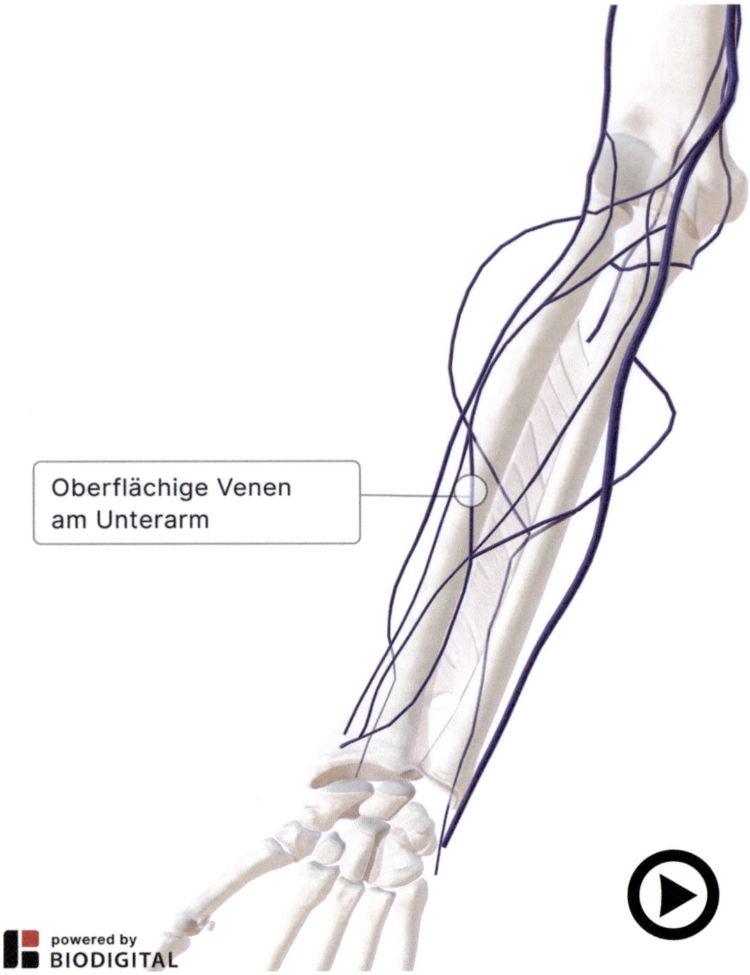

Fig. 7.41 Anatomy and palpation of the superficial veins of the forearm (▶ https://doi.org/10.1007/000-cyb)

rete venosum dorsale manus is epifascial, so that the individual vessels can usually already be found in the visual findings. Depending on the anatomical conditions and the current state of the vessels, they emerge. Due to their location and nature, the veins are often used for the placement of a venous catheter [15].

For palpation of the venous network on the back of the hand, the client is positioned in a supine or sitting position. If the veins are already visible, they can be grasped directly with the fingertips. The special characteristics such as the bluish colouring, the rounded and elastic shape as well as the displaceability under the skin as a prime example come to light. If the veins are not directly visible, a briefly applied circular compression on the forearm as well as a short but intensive activation of the hand or forearm musculature can serve for better visualisation.

Implementation Note

Preparatory measures that stimulate the blood circulation in the hand and forearm area improve the location of the rete venosum dorsale manus (Fig. 7.42).

7.2.4 Veins in the Area of the Head

Numerous veins drain deoxygenated blood from the head as well as the neck region into large collecting veins such as the V. jugularis externa, anterior and interna, the V. subclavia, the V. vertebralis and the V. cervicalis profunda. These flow via the V. brachiocephalica as well as the V. cava superior at the atrium dexter of the heart to carry the oxygen-depleted blood into the pulmonary circulation and then pump it oxygen-rich into the systemic circulation. Drainage requires numerous venous vessels on the skull that transport the blood. From this group, only those that are palpable are presented in the following chapters. These include the superficial temporal vein, the facial vein, the angular vein, the posterior auricular vein and the occipital vein. Their proximity to the arteries often assists the palpator in locating the roundish, elastic and bluish vessels. When presenting them, it should be noted that the veins run centripetally and thus allow blood to flow in the opposite direction to the arteries. Therefore, the order will be from the smaller to the larger vessels.

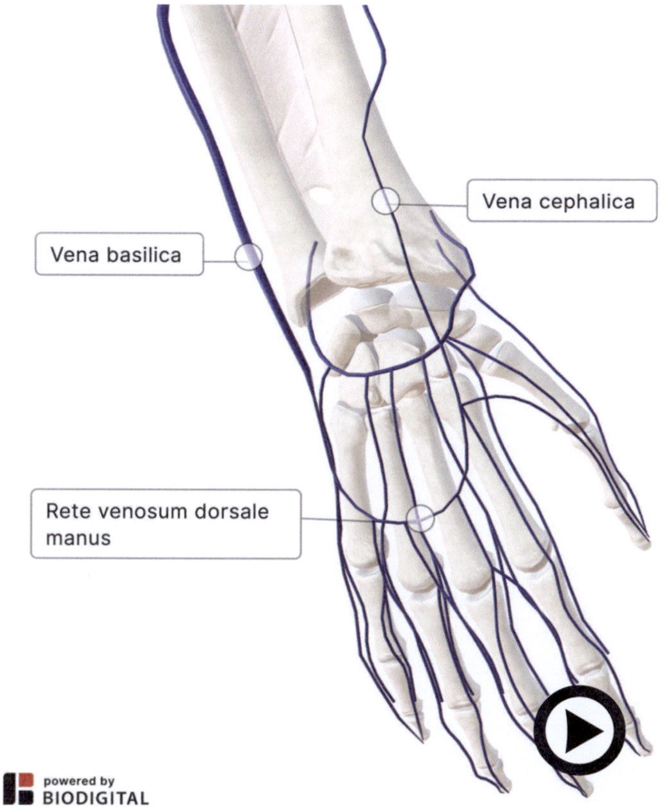

Fig. 7.42 Anatomy and palpation of the Rete venosum dorsale manus (▶ https://doi.org/10.1007/000-cyc)

After the presentation of the anatomical position, the palpation instructions for the respective veins in the area of the head follow. It is recommended to position the client in a relaxed position for the head. The supine position is suitable.

7.2.4.1 Palpation of the Superficial Temporal Vein

The superficial temporal vein, with its slightly occipital companion artery of the same name, runs directly in front of the ear from superior to inferior and receives venous blood from the lateral facial region and the top of the head and conveys it into the retromandibular vein.

The rather short venous vessel can be felt in front of the meatus acusticus externus. The client is positioned supine or in a sitting position while the therapist first feels the pulse of the superficial temporal artery (see Sect. 7.1.4.3) in this region with the finger berries placed flat. If the fingers move in an anterior direction, they directly encounter the round, elastic and easily movable superficial temporal vein, which also runs vertically. They can then follow the vessel across its course.

Implementation Note

The pressure should be moderate at first in order to be able to perceive the vein (Fig. 7.43).

7.2.4.2 Palpation of the Facial Vein

Under the levator anguli oris, the facial vein arises from the angular vein and runs steeply caudoposteriorly towards the posterior third of the mandible. In its course, it is covered by numerous structures such as the Bichat's fat plug, the risorius muscle or the platysma. In its course, it is accompanied by the artery of the same name. Directly in front of the masseter muscle, it passes over the lower edge of the mandible, takes in the retromandibular vein in the region of the mandibular angulus and passes through the trigonum caroticum into the internal jugular vein. Due to its numerous tributaries, it drains oxygen-depleted blood from the facial region.

For palpation, with the client in the supine or sitting position, the therapist stands sideways at the level of the head and contacts the masseter muscle (see Sect. 5.11.1) of the homolateral side with the fingertips. Directly anterior to the anterior edge of the muscle, they meet the facial artery, the pulse wave of which is easily palpable when pressure is applied against the lower jaw. To palpate the venous vessel of the same name, the fingertips must move slightly posteriorly again so that they meet the facial vein between the anterior edge of the muscle and the artery. The roundish and easily displaced vessel can be gently grasped transversely to the course of the index and middle fingertips.

Implementation Note

Precise anatomical knowledge is of great importance to be able to locate the facial vein. A gentle approach should be taken in order to be able to feel the delicate vessel (Fig. 7.44).

7.2.4.3 Palpation of the Angular Vein

Lateral to the os nasale, the V. angularis arises from the confluence of the V. supraorbitalis and the V. frontalis. It is accompanied in its course caudally at the edge of the nose by the artery of the same name and opens into the facial vein at about the level of the nostrils slightly laterally below the levator anguli oris muscle. In its course, it receives numerous venous branches from the area of the eye as well as the nose and thus drains deoxygenated blood from these regions. Furthermore, it anastomoses with the superior ophthalmic vein and thus forms a bridge between the facial vein and the cavernous sinus.

For palpation, the patient is positioned supine or seated while the therapist orients the fingertips on the lateral edge of the nose to the angular artery (see Sect. 7.1.4.6). Starting from the artery, the fingertips move a little further posteriorly and meet directly with the angular vein, on which, laid flat, they can exert a stimulus.

Implementation Note

Depending on the anatomical condition, the vein can be felt across its course (Fig. 7.45).

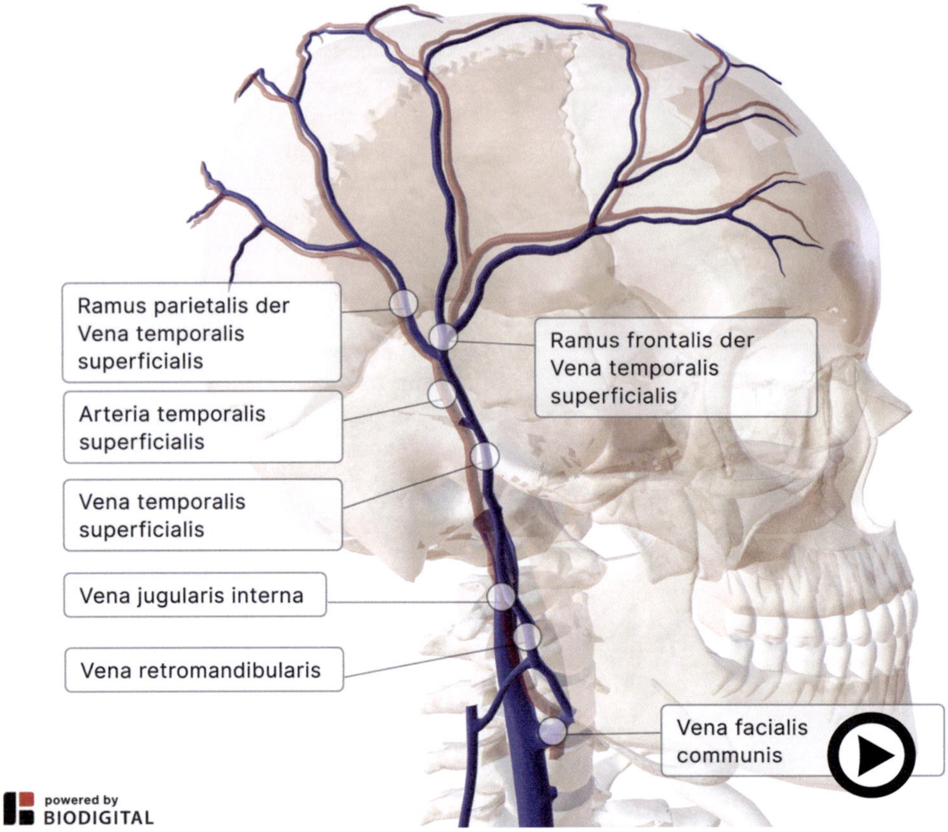

Fig. 7.43 Anatomy and palpation of the V. temporalis superficialis (▶ https://doi.org/10.1007/000-cyd)

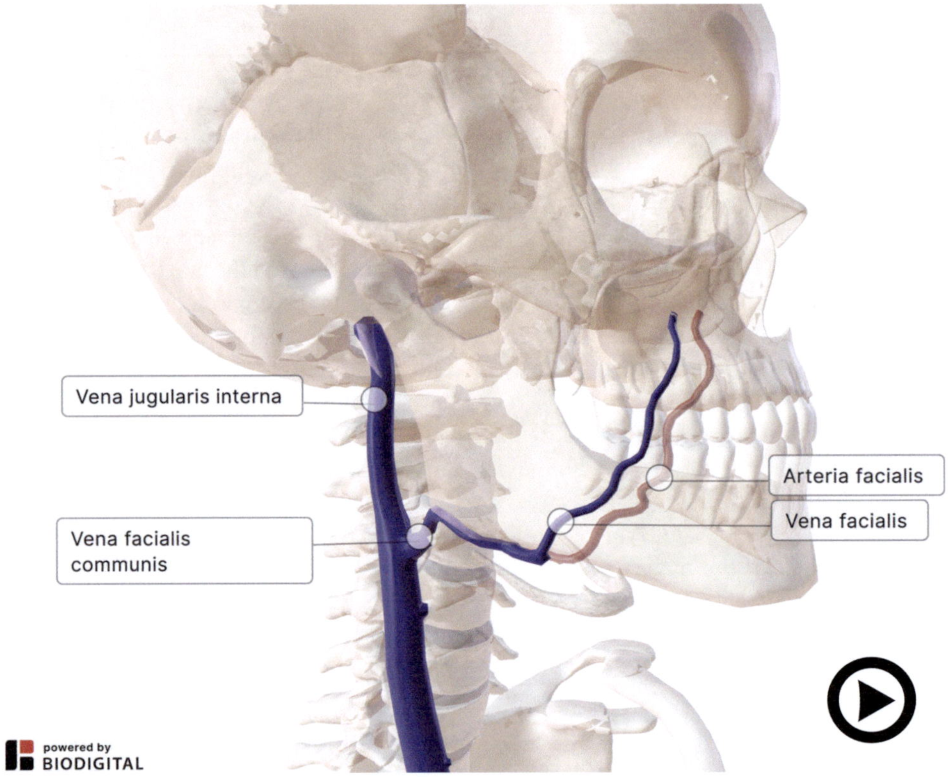

Fig. 7.44 Anatomy and palpation of the V. facialis (▶ https://doi.org/10.1007/000-cye)

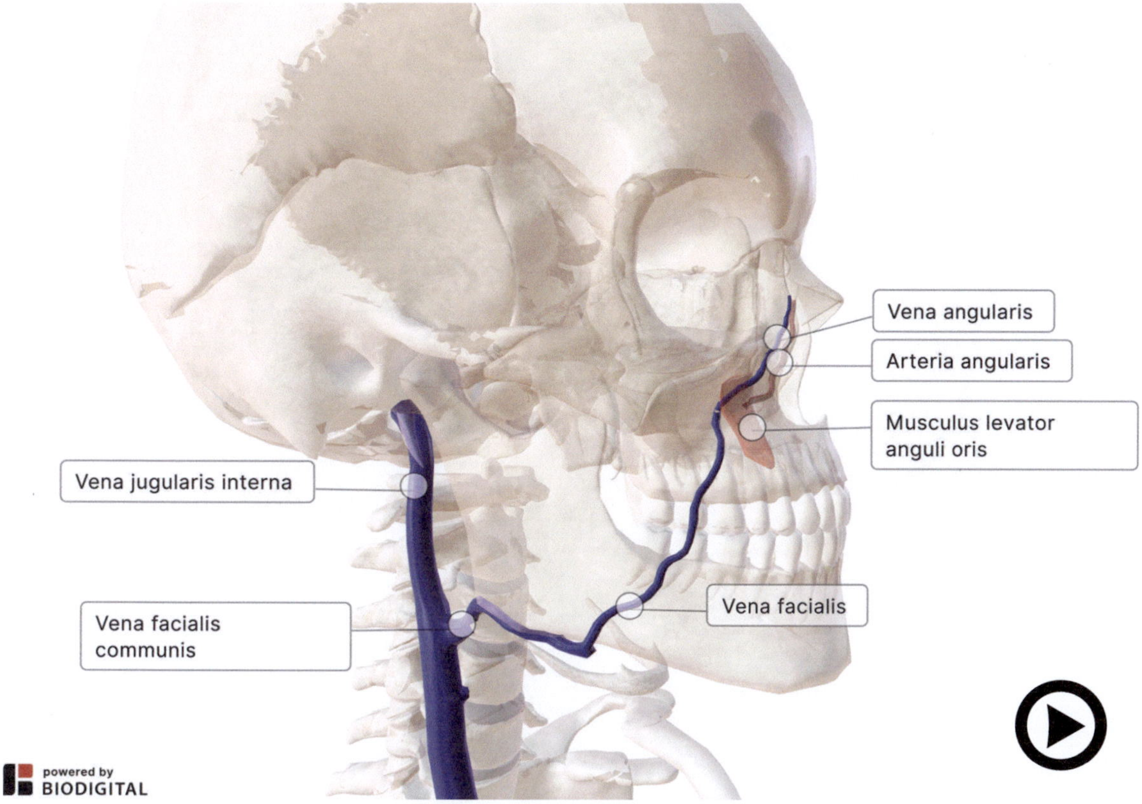

Fig. 7.45 Anatomy and palpation of the V. angularis (▶ https://doi.org/10.1007/000-cyf)

7.2.4.4 Palpation of the Posterior Auricular Vein

The areas behind the ear are drained by the posterior auricular vein, which is fed by the superficial temporal and occipital venous plexuses. Behind the auricle, it runs caudoanteriorly and is accompanied by the artery of the same name. After the venous vessel crosses the external carotid artery anterocaudally of the earlobe, it then joins the external carotid artery.

For palpation, the palpator orients to the posterior auricular artery (see Sect. 7.1.4.10) in the caudal region of the ear. In this region, the skin is very tender, which facilitates palpation. The client is in a supine or seated position, and the fingertips of the index and middle fingers first feel the pulse by placing them flat and gently. If they move caudally, they directly hit the small, roundish, elastic and easily movable venous vessel. However, this can easily be confused with the nerve branch of the posterior auricular nerve, which is directly connected caudally and can be felt more as a firm, round and movable structure.

Implementation Note

Palpation must be superficial and gentle; otherwise, the delicate vessels will be squeezed, making precise palpation impossible. Often, therefore, only stimulation is possible (Fig. 7.46).

7.2.4.5 Palpation of the Occipital Vein

The occipital region is drained by the occipital vein. It receives oxygen-poor blood from the venous plexuses of the occiput, especially the skin and the muscles, and directs it occipitally into the cervical vein and in the lateral area of the head into the vertebral vein and the external jugular vein. Its course is therefore from occipital to rostral. It is accompanied by the artery of the same name and the associated nerve.

The palpation is done from the sitting or prone position so that the back of the head is easily accessible. The therapist stands at the level of the skull and orients himself to the occipital artery in the area of the back of the head (see Sect. 7.1.4.11). If pressure is applied slightly superior to the artery, the occipital vein receives a stimulus via the finger berries that are placed flat. Due to the direct proximity, it is difficult to feel the vein separately. It can then be recorded in its course with the artery.

Implementation Note

During palpation, pressure is often exerted simultaneously on the occipital nerve, which can lead to unpleasant sensations (Fig. 7.47).

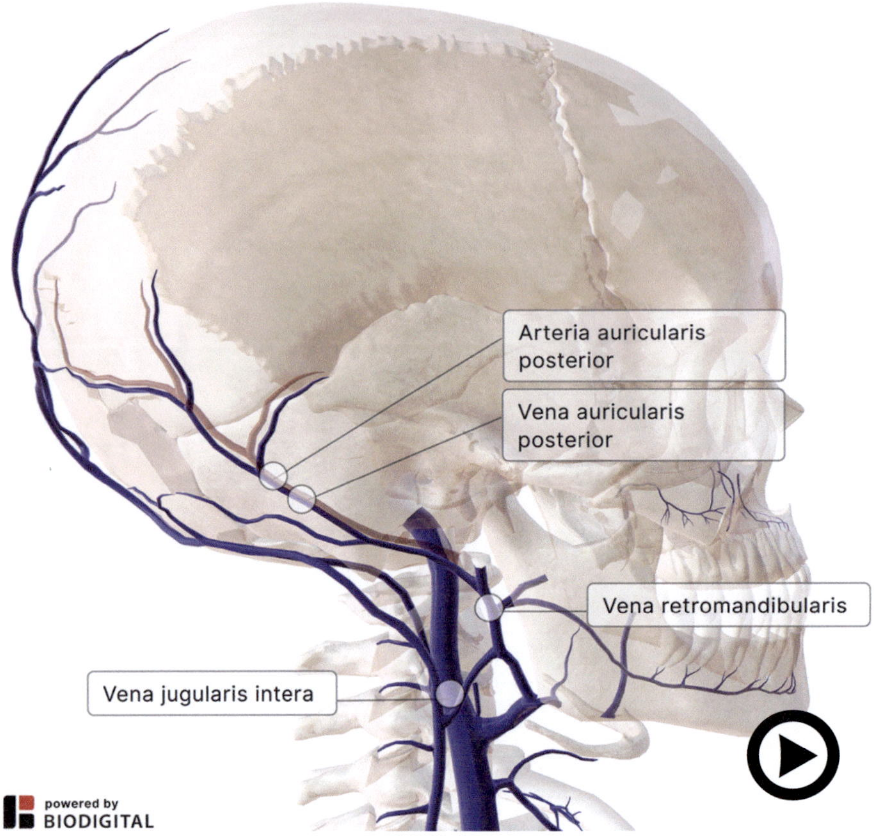

Fig. 7.46 Anatomy and palpation of the V. auricularis posterior (▶ https://doi.org/10.1007/000-cx3)

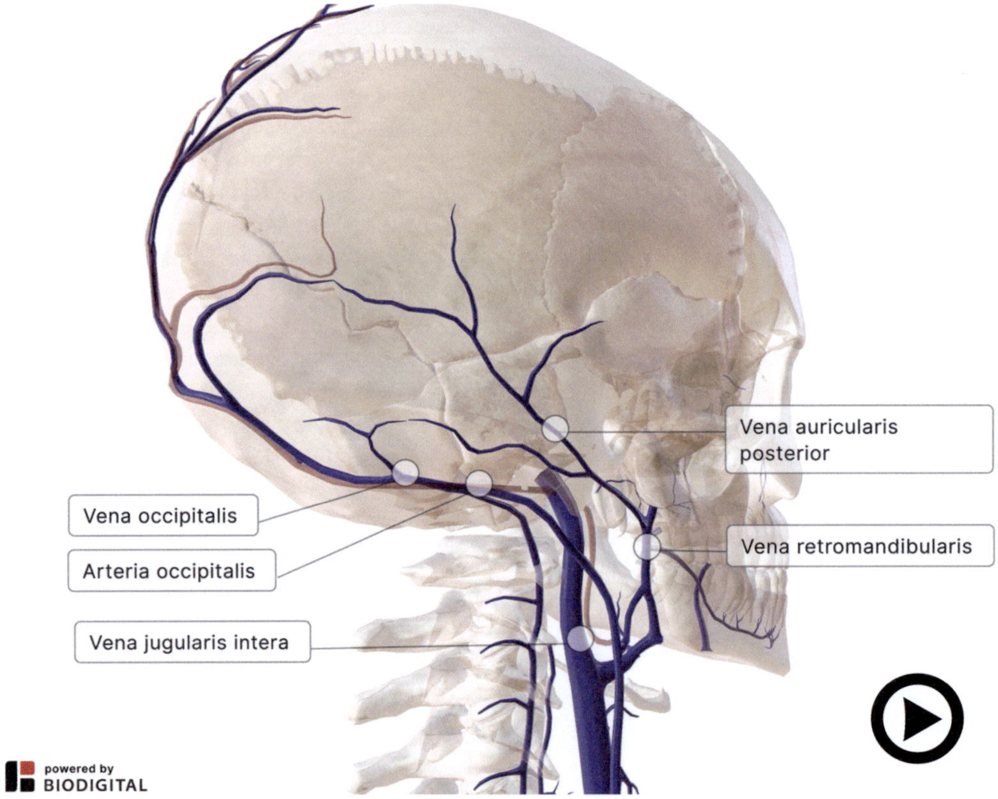

Fig. 7.47 Anatomy and palpation of the V. occipitalis (▶ https://doi.org/10.1007/000-cyh)

References

1. Sobinsky, K., Borozan, P., Gray, B., Schuler, J., & Flanigan, D. (1984). Is femoral pulse palpation accurate in assessing the hemodynamic significance of aortoiliac occlusive disease? *The American Journal of Surgery, 148*(2), 214–216. https://doi.org/10.1016/0002-9610(84)90223-X
2. Vorobeichik, L., & Abdallah, F. (2019). Femoral artery dissection after adductor canal block. *Anesthesiology, 130*(6), 1037–1038. https://doi.org/10.1097/ALN.0000000000002627
3. Smith, J., Hariri, N., Oriowo, B., & Lurie, F. (2020). Cystic adventitial disease of the popliteal artery presenting with features of entrapment syndrome. *Journal of Vascular Surgery Cases and Innovative Techniques, 6*(1), 75–79. https://doi.org/10.1016/j.jvscit.2019.10.009
4. Conte, S., & Vale, P. (2018). Peripheral arterial disease. *Heart, Lung and Circulation, 27*(4), 427–432. https://doi.org/10.1016/j.hlc.2017.10.014
5. Ntuli, S., Nalla, S., & Kiter, A. (2018). Anatomical variation of the dorsalis pedis artery in a South African population—A cadaveric study. *The Foot (Edinburgh, Scotland), 35*, 16–27. https://doi.org/10.1016/j.foot.2018.01.002
6. Sakalihasan, N., Limet, R., & Defawe, O. (2005). Abdominal aortic aneurysm. *The Lancet, 365*(9470), 1577–1589. https://doi.org/10.1016/S0140-6736(05)66459-8
7. Cevirme, D., Aksoy, E., Adademir, T., & Sunar, H. (2015). A perplexing presentation of entrapment of the brachial artery. *Case Reports in Vascular Medicine, 2015*, 236193. https://doi.org/10.1155/2015/236193
8. König, P., Hage, J., Bloem, J., & Prosé, L. (1994). Variations of the ulnar nerve and ulnar artery in Guyon's canal: A cadaveric study. *The Journal of Hand Surgery, 19*(4), 617–622. https://doi.org/10.1016/0363-5023(94)90270-4
9. Markert, B., Fraenzle, S., & Tieben, C. (2009). Information und Informationsverarbeitung. *Umweltwissenschaften und Schadstoff-Forschung, 21*, 483–486. https://doi.org/10.1007/s12302-009-0088-7
10. Younger, D. (2019). Giant cell arteritis. *Neurologic Clinics, 37*(2), 335–344. https://doi.org/10.1016/j.ncl.2019.01.008
11. Ercan, S., Çetin, C., Yavuz, T., Demir, H., & Atalay, Y. (2018). Effects of isokinetic calf muscle exercise program on muscle strength and venous function in patients with chronic venous insufficiency. *Phlebology, 33*(4), 261–266. https://doi.org/10.1177/0268355517695401
12. Portugal, I., Ribeiro, I., Sousa-Rodrigues, C., Monte-Bispo, R., & Rocha, A. (2014). Distribution of saphenous vein valves and its practical importance. *Brazilian Journal of Cardiovascular Surgery, 29*(4), 564–568. https://doi.org/10.5935/1678-9741.20140038
13. Millington, S., Lalu, M., Boivin, M., & Koenig, S. (2019). Better with ultrasound: Subclavian central venous catheter insertion. *Chest, 155*(5), 1041–1048. https://doi.org/10.1016/j.chest.2018.12.007
14. Harding, I., Mannakkar, N., Gonna, H., Domenichini, G., Leung, L., Zuberi, Z., & Gallagher, M. (2020). Exclusively cephalic venous access for cardiac resynchronisation: A prospective multicentre evaluation. *Pacing and Clinical Electrophysiology, 43*(12), 1515–1520. https://doi.org/10.1111/pace.14046
15. Takeshita, J., Nakayama, Y., Nakajima, Y., Sessler, D., Ogawa, S., Sawa, T., & Mizobe, T. (2015). Optimal site for ultrasound-guided venous catheterisation in paediatric patients: An observational study to investigate predictors for catheterisation success and a randomised controlled study to determine the most successful site. *Critical Care, 19*(1), 15. https://doi.org/10.1186/s13054-014-0733-4

Glossary

Australopithecus Extinct African ape species that lived 2–4 million years ago.

Clinical reasoning Clinically oriented logical thinking.

Entrapments Constriction through which structures such as nerves and vessels pass in their anatomical course.

Holism Wholeness theory, in relation to the holistic/integral view in therapy and findings.

Magic tissue Magical tissue, in this context the periosteum due to its multitude of receptors.

Mushy sign Indicates the accumulation of fluid, such as blood, in the muscle when palpated.

Periosteal-diaphyseal or chondral-apophyseal approaches Bony and cartilaginous transition regions for various attachment tissues such as musculature.

Range of motion Extent of movement of joints.

Referred pain Transmitted pain radiating from one region to another.

Tabatière Term for the radial foveola, which is bounded by the tendons of the abductor pollicis longus muscle and the tendon of the extensor pollicis longus and brevis muscles.

Tensegrity model Support system that is stable in itself but also dependent in itself. Therapeutic abnormalities and symptoms can occur due to tension-belt mechanisms away from the causative region.

Thixotropic Property of non-Newtonian fluids. Due to external influences such as movement, the viscosity of the fluid can decrease, which it regains after the movement has ended.

Viscoelastic material Adaptable, viscous property of tissues.

R. Bauer, S. Wolfram, *Atlas of Palpation*, https://doi.org/10.1007/978-3-662-69186-1

Index

R. Bauer, S. Wolfram, *Atlas of Palpation*, https://doi.org/10.1007/978-3-662-69186-1

MIX
Papier aus verantwortungsvollen Quellen
Paper from responsible sources
FSC® C105338

If you have any concerns about our products,
you can contact us on
ProductSafety@springernature.com

In case Publisher is established outside the EU,
the EU authorized representative is:
Springer Nature Customer Service Center GmbH
Europaplatz 3, 69115 Heidelberg, Germany

Printed by Libri Plureos GmbH
in Hamburg, Germany